D1179634

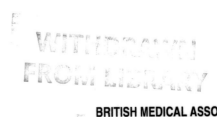

Recurrent
Pregnancy Loss

SERIES IN MATERNAL-FETAL MEDICINE

Published in association with the

Journal of Maternal-Fetal & Neonatal Medicine

Edited by

Gian Carlo Di Renzo and Dev Maulik

Howard Carp, *Recurrent Pregnancy Loss*, ISBN 9780415421300

Vincenzo Berghella, *Obstetric Evidence Based Guidelines*, ISBN 9780415701884

Vincenzo Berghella, *Maternal-Fetal Evidence Based Guidelines*, ISBN 9780415432818

Moshe Hod, Lois Jovanovic, Gian Carlo Di Renzo, Alberto de Leiva, Oded Langer, *Textbook of Diabetes and Pregnancy, Second Edition*, ISBN 9780415426206

Simcha Yagel, Norman H. Silverman, Ulrich Gembruch, *Fetal Cardiology, Second Edition*, ISBN 9780415432658

Fabio Facchinetti, Gustaaf A. Dekker, Dante Baronciani, George Saade, Stillbirth: *Understanding and Management*, ISBN 9780415473903

Vincenzo Berghella, *Maternal–Fetal Evidence Based Guidelines, Second Edition*, ISBN 9781841848228

Vincenzo Berghella, *Obstetric Evidence Based Guidelines, Second Edition*, ISBN 9781841848242

Howard Carp, *Recurrent Pregnancy Loss: Causes, Controversies, and Treatment, Second Edition*, ISBN 9781482216141

Recurrent Pregnancy Loss
Causes, Controversies, and Treatment
Second Edition

Edited by

Howard J. A. Carp, MB BS, FRCOG
Clinical Professor, Obstetrics and Gynecology,
Sheba Medical Center, Tel Hashomer, Israel and
Sackler School of Medicine,
Tel Aviv University, Israel

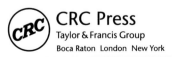

CRC Press
Taylor & Francis Group
Boca Raton London New York

CRC Press is an imprint of the
Taylor & Francis Group, an **informa** business

CRC Press
Taylor & Francis Group
6000 Broken Sound Parkway NW, Suite 300
Boca Raton, FL 33487-2742

© 2015 by Taylor & Francis Group, LLC
CRC Press is an imprint of Taylor & Francis Group, an Informa business

No claim to original U.S. Government works

Printed on acid-free paper
Version Date: 20141029

International Standard Book Number-13: 978-1-4822-1614-1 (Hardback)

This book contains information obtained from authentic and highly regarded sources. While all reasonable efforts have been made to publish reliable data and information, neither the author[s] nor the publisher can accept any legal responsibility or liability for any errors or omissions that may be made. The publishers wish to make clear that any views or opinions expressed in this book by individual editors, authors or contributors are personal to them and do not necessarily reflect the views/opinions of the publishers. The information or guidance contained in this book is intended for use by medical, scientific or health-care professionals and is provided strictly as a supplement to the medical or other professional's own judgement, their knowledge of the patient's medical history, relevant manufacturer's instructions and the appropriate best practice guidelines. Because of the rapid advances in medical science, any information or advice on dosages, procedures or diagnoses should be independently verified. The reader is strongly urged to consult the relevant national drug formulary and the drug companies' printed instructions, and their websites, before administering any of the drugs recommended in this book. This book does not indicate whether a particular treatment is appropriate or suitable for a particular individual. Ultimately it is the sole responsibility of the medical professional to make his or her own professional judgements, so as to advise and treat patients appropriately. The authors and publishers have also attempted to trace the copyright holders of all material reproduced in this publication and apologize to copyright holders if permission to publish in this form has not been obtained. If any copyright material has not been acknowledged please write and let us know so we may rectify in any future reprint.

Visit the Taylor & Francis Web site at
http://www.taylorandfrancis.com

and the CRC Press Web site at
http://www.crcpress.com

Contents

Foreword

Children are the anchors that hold a mother to life

Phaedra, **Sophocles**

In almost all traditions, the importance of procreation is inherent in man's very creation; both Old and New Testaments of the Bible refer to the tragic plight of barren women, eloquently describing the pain and agony of childlessness. However, records dated far earlier than the Bible confirm that fertility has been a constant fundamental priority and preoccupation, in all societies, throughout the ages of man. Fertility symbols are clearly identified in the relics of prehistoric times, of ancient civilizations in all parts of the world, a recognition of the concept that man's existence depends upon the renewal of fertility. The above quotation was written by Sophocles 2500 years ago. The ancient Canaanites and Greeks had gods of fertility—Ashtarte and Hermes. Today infertility is recognized as a disease by the World Health Organization, and numerous health care providers throughout the world. Recurrent pregnancy loss represents one aspect of disordered fertility. Recurrent pregnancy loss has been described as the "orphan" of infertility as this condition is often overlooked in the larger process of research and management of fertility. Recurrent pregnancy loss is a heterogeneous condition, with numerous causes, and numerous treatment options. It is multidisciplinary, involving gynecology, genetics, endocrinology, immunology, pediatrics and internal medicine. Whatever the cause and possible treatment, the psychological implications are enormous. Both partners may feel that they have failed in their parenting role. Couples have divorced with mutual recriminations, each blaming the other. Even when pregnancy does succeed, the pregnancy may be fraught with the fear of another loss. This anxiety is multiplied when the diagnosis remains unexplained.

The second edition of this book will be welcomed by many investigators and clinicians working in the field of recurrent pregnancy loss. As in the first edition, there are chapters governing basic scientific topics such as genetics, cytokines, mechanisms of action of antiphospholipid antibodies, and signaling between mother and fetus. The major advances in genetics, immunology, endocrinology, and thrombotic mechanisms have been described in depth. The methodology of clinical research and the application of evidence-based medicine to clinical practice have been explained comprehensively. The problems of mid-trimester loss and late obstetric complications are aired, including the problems associated with extreme prematurity and possible resulting handicaps. However, as is inevitable in clinical practice, there are many controversies, leaving the clinician in a quandary as to how to help the patient. The debates and opinion chapters have been thoroughly updated, but are still as debatable as they were in the first edition of this book. There is a new chapter on Chinese medicine (Chapter 41), and the underlying scientific evidence which is most thought-provoking and fascinating.

However, at the end of the line is a patient. Therefore the chapter on psychological mechanisms and the connection between psychological mechanisms, the immune and other systems is welcome. The story told by the patient in Chapter 42 is most touching, and reminds us of the real problem at hand.

It is hoped that this book will be read by specialists working in recurrent pregnancy loss clinics, and associated disciplines, who wish to keep up to date, and generalists who wish to gain a comprehensive view of developments in the field. It is to be hoped that the advances in scientific and clinical knowledge will continue as in the past, in order to improve the management of the patients and allow those still unable to have children, to fulfill this most basic of human desires.

Prof. Bruno Lunenfeld, MD PhD FRCOG FACOG (hon) POGS (hon)
Professor Emeritus at Faculty of Life Sciences Bar-Ilan University, President of the International Society for the Study of the Aging Male (ISSAM), General Secretary of the Asian-Pacific Initiative on Reproductive Endocrinology (ASPIRE), Member of the Israel government's National Council for Obstetrics, Genetics and Neonatology

Preface to the Second Edition

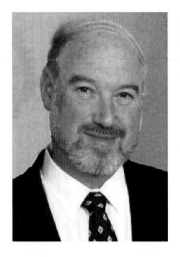

Although seven years have passed since the first edition of this book, recurrent pregnancy loss remains a distressing problem to couples, who understandably expect answers and solutions, and frustrating for the physician who often does not have these answers, particularly in the face of ever-changing and conflicting recommendations by guidelines from leading professional organizations. In the last seven years, there have been major advances in genetics, immunology, endocrinology, and other disciplines. However, recurrent pregnancy loss remains a vexing clinical problem as the cause often remains unexplained. Many treatment options remain controversial. In the first edition of the book, there were a number of debates on the place of various treatment options. It was hoped that by the time of the second edition, there would be no need for debates, and that the issues would have become clear by well-planned trials and that solid evidence would be available. Alas, this is not the case, and the debates remain as relevant as ever. This book tries to summarize the controversies, and discuss the scientific basis for various causes of pregnancy loss in depth, and to clarify the various treatment modalities which have been used in recent years, in the light of the major changes which have occurred over the last seven years

The book is planned for general gynecologists, and specialists working in the field. Each contributing author is an authority on a specific area of recurrent pregnancy loss. In the second edition, the chapters on genetics, the role of PGS, have been completely rewritten. There are new chapters on autoimmunity, third party reproduction, the use of immunostimulants such as CSF, and Chinese medicine. The chapter on second trimester loss has been modified to include the use of pessaries. All of the other chapters have undergone major revision to include the changes that have occurred over the last seven years.

I would like to thank each author for the time and effort taken in preparing the manuscripts to make publication of this book possible. I would also like to thank those responsible in a more indirect way for the publication of this book: my teachers over the years, and my collaborators. However, special recognition goes to the greatest teachers and collaborators of all, the patients.

Prof. Howard J. A. Carp, MB BS FRCOG
Clinical Professor, Obstetrics and Gynecology, Sheba Medical Center, Tel Hashomer, Israel and
Sackler School of Medicine, Tel Aviv University, Israel

Contributors

Nasser Al-Asmar
IVIOMICS USA Corp. Inc.
Miami, Florida

Gautam N. Allahbadia
Rotunda–The Center for Human
    Reproduction
Mumbai, Maharashtra, India

and

Rotunda IVF and Keyhole Surgery Center
Rotunda Blue Fertility Clinic and Keyhole
    Surgery Center
Rotunda Fertility Clinic and Keyhole Surgery
    Center
Sharjah, United Arab Emirates

Eytan R. Barnea
Society for the Investigation of Early
    Pregnancy
Cherry Hill, New Jersey

Peter Benn
Department of Genetics and Developmental
    Biology
University of Connecticut Health Center
Farmington, Connecticut

Harish M. Bhandari
Division of Reproductive Health
University of Warwick
and
Department of Obstetrics and
    Gynaecology
University Hospitals of Coventry and
    Warwickshire NHS Trust
Coventry, United Kingdom

Miri Blank
Zabludowicz Center for Autoimmune Diseases
    Sheba Medical Center
Sackler Faculty of Medicine
Tel-Aviv University
Tel-Aviv, Israel

Zvi Borochowitz
The Simon Winter Institute for Human
    Genetics
Bnai-Zion Medical Center
Technion-Rappaport Faculty of
    Medicine
Haifa, Israel

Benjamin Brenner
Department of Hematology and Bone Marrow
    Transplantation
Rambam Health Care Campus
and
Bruce Rappaport Faculty of Medicine
Israel Institute of Technology
Haifa, Israel

Paul R. Brezina
Fertility Associates of Memphis
Center for the Study of Recurrent
    Pregnancy Loss
Memphis, Tennessee

Richard Bronson
Department of Obstetrics and Gynecology
Stony Brook University Medical Center
Stony Brook, New York

Howard J. A. Carp
Department of Obstetrics and Gynecology
Sheba Medical Center
Tel Hashomer, Israel

and

Sackler School of Medicine
Tel Aviv University
Tel Aviv, Israel

Jerome H. Check
Cooper Medical School of Rowan
    University
Department of Obstetrics and Gynecology
Camden, New Jersey

Ole B. Christiansen
Fertility Clinic
Copenhagen, Denmark

and

Department of Obstetrics and
   Gynaecology
Aalborg University Hospital
Aalborg, Denmark

Carolyn B. Coulam
Reproductive Medicine Institute
Chicago, Illinois

Howard Cuckle
Department of Obstrics and Gynecology
Columbia University Medical Center
New York City, New York

Salim Daya
Newlife Fertility Centre
Mississauga, Ontario, Canada

P. Drakopoulos
Division of Obstetrics and Gynecology
University of Geneva
Geneva, Switzerland

A. R. Genazzani
Division of Obstetrics and Gynecology
University of Pisa
Pisa, Italy

Mariette Goddijn
Department of Obstetrics and
   Gynaecology
University of Amsterdam
Amsterdam, the Netherlands

Mordechai Goldenberg
Department of Obstetrics and Gynecology
Sheba Medical Center
Tel-Hashomer, Israel

and

The Sackler School of Medicine
Tel Aviv University
Tel Aviv, Israel

Mindy Gross
Raanana, Israel

Aisha Hameed
Department of Obstetrics and Gynaecology
Imperial College at St Mary's Hospital Campus
London, United Kingdom

Israel Hendler
Department of Obstetrics and Gynecology
Sheba Medical Center
Tel Hashomer, Israel

Aida Inbal
Beilinson Hospital
Rabin Medical Center
Sackler Faculty of Medicine
Tel Aviv University, Israel

Rotem Inbar
Zabludowicz Center for Autoimmune Diseases
and
Department of Obstetrics and Gynecology
Sheba Medical Center
Tel Hashomer, Israel

Raymond W. Ke
Fertility Associates of Memphis
Center for the Study of Recurrent
   Pregnancy Loss
Memphis, Tennessee

Pratap Kumar
Department of Obstetrics and Gynecology
Kasturba Medical College
Manipal University
Manipal, India

William H. Kutteh
Fertility Associates of Memphis
Center for the Study of Recurrent
   Pregnancy Loss
Memphis, Tennessee

Alana B. Levine
Hospital for Special Surgery
New York City, New York

Pelle G. Lindqvist
Malmö University Hospital
Malmö, Sweden

Michael D. Lockshin
Hospital for Special Surgery
New York City, New York

Andrea Lojacono
Department of Obstetrics and Gynaecology
Spedali Civili and University of Brescia
Brescia, Italy

S. Luisi
Division of Obstetrics and Gynecology
University of Pisa
Pisa, Italy

Shazia Malik
Consultant Subspecialist Reproductive
    Medicine
Imperial College at St Mary's Hospital
London, United Kingdom

Rubina Merchant
Rotunda–The Center for Human Reproduction
Mumbai, India

Aviv Messinger
Complementary Medicine Services
Department of Obstetrics and Gynecology
Sheba Medical Center
Tel Hashomer, Israel

Pere Mir
IVIOMICS India
New Delhi, India

Anna M. Musters
Department of Obstetrics and Gynaecology
University of Amsterdam
Amsterdam, the Netherlands

Thomas Philipp
Gynecology and Obstetrics
Danube Hospital
Vienna, Austria

N. Pluchino
Division of Obstetrics and Gynecology
University of Geneva
Geneva, Switzerland

Siobhan Quenby
Division of Reproductive Health
University of Warwick
and
Department of Obstetrics and Gynaecology
University Hospitals of Coventry and
    Warwickshire NHS Trust
Coventry, United Kingdom

Raj Rai
Department of Obstetrics and
    Gynaecology
Imperial College London
London, United Kingdom

Jane L. Reed
Laboratory for Reproductive Medicine and
    Immunology
San Jose, California

Lesley Regan
Head Department of Obstetrics and
    Gynaecology
Imperial College at St. Mary's Hospital
    Campus
London, United Kingdom

Lorena Rodrigo
Fundación Instituto Valenciano de Infertilidad
    (FIVI)
and
IVIOMICS S.L.
Parc Cientific of the University of
    Valencia
Paterna, Spain

Carmen Rubio
Fundación Instituto Valenciano de
    Infertilidad (FIVI)
and
IVIOMICS S.L.
Parc Cientific of the University of
    Valencia
Paterna, Spain

M. Russo
Division of Obstetrics and
    Gynecology
University of Pisa
Pisa, Italy

Shoshana Savion
Department of Cell and Developmental
    Biology
Sackler School of Medicine
Tel Aviv University
Tel Aviv, Israel

Marco Sbracia
Hungaria Center for Endocrinology and
    Reproductive Medicine (CERM)
Rome, Italy

Fabio Scarpellini
Hungaria Center for Endocrinology and
    Reproductive Medicine (CERM)
Rome, Italy

Daniel S. Seidman
Department of Obstetrics and Gynecology
The Chaim Sheba Medical Center
Tel-Hashomer, Israel

Keren Sela
The Institute for Fertility Research
Lis Maternity Center
Ichilov Hospital
Tel Aviv, Israel

Keren Shakhar
Department of Psychology
The College of Management Academic Studies
Rishon Lezion, Israel

Yehuda Shoenfeld
Zabludowicz Center for Autoimmune Diseases
Sheba Medical Center
Tel-Aviv University
Tel-Aviv, Israel

Carlos Simon
Fundación Instituto Valenciano de
    Infertilidad (FIVI)
and
IVIOMICS S.L.
Parc Cientific of the University of Valencia
Paterna, Spain

Joe Leigh Simpson
Department of Human and Molecular Genetics
Herbert Wertheim College of Medicine
Florida International University
Miami, Florida

and

Research and Global Programs
March of Dimes
White Plains, New York

Angela Tincani
Department of Rheumatology and
    Clinical Immunology
Spedali Civili
University of Brescia
Brescia, Italy

Vladimir Toder
Department of Cell and Developmental Biology
Sackler School of Medicine
Tel Aviv University
Tel Aviv, Israel

Arkady Torchinsky
Department of Cell and Developmental Biology
Sackler School of Medicine
Tel Aviv University
Tel Aviv, Israel

Marighoula Varla-Leftherioti
Head of the Immunobiology Department
"Helena Venizelou" Maternity Hospital
Athens, Greece

Akhila Vasudeva
Department of Obstetrics and Gynecology
Kasturba Medical College
Manipal University
Manipal, India

David Alan Viniker (Retired)
Whipps Cross University Hospital
London, United Kingdom

James Walker
Department of Obstetrics and Gynaecology
Clinical Science Building
St James University Hospital
Leeds, United Kingdom

J. M. Wenger
Division of Obstetrics and Gynecology
University of Geneva
Geneva, Switzerland

Edward E. Winger
Laboratory for Reproductive Medicine and
    Immunology
San Jose, California

Flora Y. Wong
Monash Newborn NHMRC
and
The Ritchie Centre
and
Department of Paediatrics
Monash University
Melbourne, Australia

Victor Y. H. Yu
Department of Paediatrics
Monash University
Melbourne, Australia

Sonia Zatti
Department of Obstetrics and Gynaecology
Spedali Civili
University of Brescia
Brescia, Italy

1

The Epidemiology of Recurrent Pregnancy Loss

Ole B. Christiansen

Introduction

Epidemiology can be defined as "the scientific study of disease frequency, determinants of disease, and the distribution of disease in a population." The determinants of disease considered in epidemiological studies are normally demographic parameters (age, sex, occupation, economic status) in addition to some clinical parameters relevant for the specific disease (e.g., tobacco and alcohol consumption, reproductive and family history)—all information that can be obtained through registers and questionnaires—whereas parameters requiring special interventions such as blood samples are normally not included in purely epidemiological studies.

Definition of Miscarriage and Recurrent Pregnancy Loss

The term miscarriage (or abortion) is used to describe a pregnancy that fails to progress, resulting in death and expulsion of the embryo or fetus. The generally accepted definition stipulates that the fetus or embryo should weigh 500 g or less, a stage that corresponds to a gestational age of up to 20 weeks (World Health Organization).[1] Unfortunately, this definition is not used consistently, and pregnancy losses at higher gestational ages are also, in some studies, classified as miscarriage instead of stillbirth or preterm neonatal death. Thus, from a definition perspective, it is important to characterize the population being studied so that comparisons across therapeutic trials can be made more appropriately and reliably.

Recurrent miscarriage should, according to the aforementioned definition of miscarriage, be defined as at least three consecutive miscarriages, whereas recurrent pregnancy loss (RPL) could also include pregnancy losses up to gestational week 28; however, unfortunately there is no consensus on the definition of recurrent miscarriage or RPL.[2] Pregnancy losses after week 20 are rare, so defining recurrent miscarriage and RPL as above will result in almost identical populations.

In some countries and according to some national guidelines only two miscarriages are required for diagnosis of RPL. More and more published studies of RPL therefore include women with only two previous miscarriages, which from an epidemiological point of view is very problematic. This issue will be discussed later.

Epidemiological Parameters Relevant for Recurrent Pregnancy Loss

Occurrence

Using the traditional definition, the incidence of RPL is the number of new women each year (or in another defined period) suffering their third consecutive pregnancy loss, and the prevalence of RPL is the number of women in a population who, at a specific time point, have had three or more consecutive pregnancy losses. The incidence/prevalence is often expressed as a rate of those individuals being at risk for the disorder. The number in the denominator could be all women in the population, women of fertile age or women who had attempted pregnancy at least two or three times. Indeed, the estimate of the incidence/prevalence of RPL is very uncertain since in most countries there is no nationwide registration of miscarriages or RPL, and many early miscarriages will not be treated in hospitals and are thus not registered. There is no valid estimate of the incidence of RPL whereas there are a few estimates of the prevalence rate of RPL. One of the most informative studies of the prevalence rate of RPL was performed by Alberman,[3] who asked female doctors to report retrospectively about the outcome of their previous pregnancies. Nine out of 742 + 355 women (0.8%) who had had three or four previous pregnancies reported three or more consecutive pregnancy losses. This study must still be considered the best estimate of the prevalence of RPL since the cohort was restricted to women who had attempted pregnancy at least three times, and because it consisted of doctors it is expected that misclassification of delayed menstruations, induced abortions, and ectopic pregnancies as miscarriages will be small. However, since the study is from before 1980 many early miscarriages may not have been registered due to lack of highly sensitive human chorionic gonadotropin tests and ultrasound examinations at that time. Furthermore, female doctors may not reflect the background population: on one side they may be healthier than other women, which may lower the miscarriage risk, but on the other side, due to their long education they are older than average when attempting pregnancy, which increases the miscarriage risk.

Other estimates of the population prevalence of RPL are roughly in accordance with that of Alberman. An RPL prevalence of 2.3% was found in 432 randomly identified women in a multicenter study.[4] In a group of 5901 Norwegian women with at least two pregnancies screened for toxoplasma antibodies, 1.4% had experienced RPL.[5] Data from a Danish questionnaire-based study[6] found, in a random sample of 493 women with at least two intrauterine pregnancies, that 0.6% had had at least three consecutive miscarriages, 0.8% at least three consecutive pregnancy losses during all trimesters, and 1.8% had had at least three, not necessarily consecutive, losses some time during pregnancy. Overall, these studies thus find the prevalence of RPL to be between 0.6% and 2.3%.

Number of Previous Miscarriages

Almost all prospective studies of RPL patients show remarkable consistency in finding an increasing risk of miscarriage as the number of previous miscarriages increases. The chance of subsequent live birth in untreated RPL patients with three, four, and five or more miscarriages has been found to be 42–86%, 41–72%, and 23–51%, respectively (Figure 1.1).[7–10] The significant variability in the estimate of the subsequent risk of miscarriage in RPL patients can probably be attributed to the time of ascertainment of the pregnancies (Figure 1.2) since the average age of the patients and the duration of follow-up in the various studies were not different. The information in Figure 1.2 is based on data directly given in the publications[8,10,11] or data that can unequivocally be deduced from the publications.

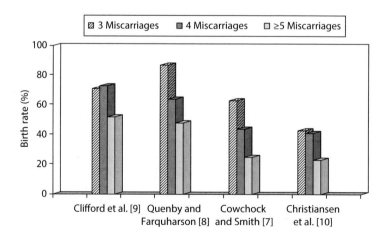

FIGURE 1.1 Subsequent birth rate according to the number of previous miscarriages in patients with recurrent pregnancy loss. Reported in four studies.

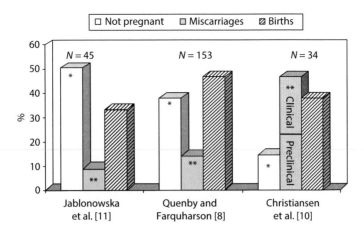

FIGURE 1.2 Incidence of subsequent live births and miscarriages. Frequency of women registered as not being pregnant, miscarrying or giving birth in three prospective cohorts of untreated patients with recurrent pregnancy loss. In Ref. 10 the proportion of miscarriages being preclinical and clinical is indicated. All miscarriages, except one in Ref. 11, and all in Ref. 8 were clinical. $*p = 0.001$; $**p < 0.0001$, χ^2 test.

In studies where the patients are urged to contact the department for inclusion in a treatment trial as soon as menstruation is 2–3 days overdue and the highly sensitive pregnancy test positive[10] almost all preclinical loss (including biochemical pregnancies) are identified and the patients will be registered as having a high fetal loss rate (47.1%) but a low nonpregnancy rate (14.7%) during the observation period. In studies where the patients are told to call the department in gestational week 6–7 and are included in treatment trials[11] or cohorts receiving standard care[8] only after ultrasonographic demonstration of fetal heart action most preclinical miscarriages are not ascertained and therefore significantly higher nonpregnancy rates (38.3–55.6%) and significantly lower miscarriage rates (11.1–14.4%) are registered compared with the former study (Figure 1.2). The subsequent probability of live birth in RPL can best be estimated using data from the placebo arm of studies in RPL (Refs. 10 and 11 in Figure 1.2) because in placebo-controlled trials the ascertainment of pregnancies is generally better than in nonrandomized studies since the patients are included according to a strict protocol and are more closely monitored in early pregnancy. More very early pregnancy losses are thus included in placebo-controlled trials and the live birth rate in the placebo-arm is expected to be lower than in nonrandomized studies. In accordance with this, Carp et al.[12] showed that the live birth rate among untreated patients in randomized studies was 15–20% lower than that of nonrandomized patients independently of the number of previous miscarriages.

The prognostical negative effect of the number of previous miscarriages could, in theory, be attributed to the fact that maternal age and the presence of age-related risk factors for miscarriages are positively correlated to gravidity. However, in multivariate analyses of clinical and paraclinical parameters of potentially prognostical impact in RPL, the number of previous miscarriages has without exception remained the strongest prognostical parameter also after adjustment for other risk factors.[7,13,14]

Instead of focusing on outcome of the first pregnancy after referral, a more reliable and clinically relevant way to estimate the prognosis after RPL may be to obtain information about the frequency of live birth per time unit after referral. From the Danish national birth register we obtained information about all subsequent live births happening in patients seen in our clinic. We found that five years after being referred to the clinic, 67% of the patients had got a living child.[15] The most important epidemiological determinants for live birth using this method were the number of previous miscarriages and maternal age.

Maternal Age

The age of women with RPL will influence the findings in studies of endocrinological and nongenetic immunological biomarkers. With progressing age the ovarian reserve will diminish and, both during

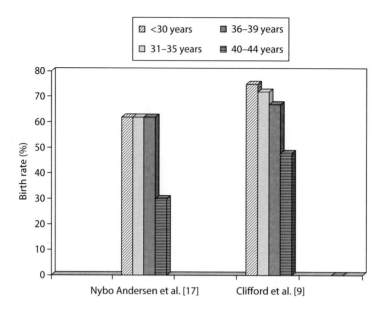

FIGURE 1.3 Subsequent birth rate according to maternal age in patients with recurrent pregnancy loss reported in two studies.

pregnancy and in the nonpregnant state, secretion of ovarian steroid hormones will be reduced. Immune parameters such as production of autoantibodies and T helper 2 cytokines are affected both directly by increased maternal age but also indirectly through diminished secretion of ovarian steroids.[16]

It is well-known that the risk of miscarriages increases with progressing maternal age in the general population.[15,17] However, in a register-based study of 634,272 Danish women achieving pregnancy between 1978 and 1992 who came into contact with a hospital during the pregnancy,[17] the miscarriage rates in women with RPL were almost identical in women of age 31–35 years and 36–39 years (38–40%) but increased to 70% in women of age 40–44 (Figure 1.3). It seems that the impact of age on miscarriage rate in RPL is quite modest until age 40, but beyond this age it is the strongest prognostical factor. In concordance with this several multivariate analyses[7,13,14] of prognostical variables for live birth in RPL patients (almost all of whom were younger than 40), found that maternal age was not a significant predictor of miscarriage after adjustment for other relevant independent variables. In the previously mentioned study of the long-term chance of live birth in RPL,[15] the live birth rate after five years ranged from 68% in women aged 30–34 years to 58% in women aged 35–39 years to 42% in women aged ≥40 years at the time of referral.

Subgroups of Recurrent Pregnancy Loss

The pregnancy history in women with RPL may include pregnancies that have ended in live birth. Thus, three different groups can be identified that should be assessed separately: (a) the primary RPL group consists of women with three or more consecutive pregnancy losses with no pregnancy progressing beyond 20 weeks' gestation; (b) the secondary RPL group consists of women who have had three or more pregnancy losses following a pregnancy that progressed beyond 20 weeks' gestation, which may have ended in live birth (most often), stillbirth or neonatal death; and (c) the tertiary RPL group, which is a group that has not been well characterized or studied and consists of women who have had several pregnancy losses before a pregnancy that progressed beyond 20 weeks' gestation followed by at least three more pregnancy losses.[12] In some studies, secondary RPL is defined as RPL after a live birth or a pregnancy that progressed beyond gestational week 28[12,18]; however, in this survey the definition in point (b) will be adopted.

Unfortunately, in many studies no separation of patients with primary and secondary RPL is made, which may indicate that the authors consider the two disorders as identical entities.

If primary and secondary RPL have different pathophysiological backgrounds we would expect different prognoses for the two conditions. Summarizing the placebo-treated patients included in our three placebo-controlled trials of immunotherapy[10,19] shows that the live birth rate in the first pregnancy was 17/35 = 48.6% in women with primary RPL compared with 11/34 = 32.4% in women with secondary RPL (not significantly different) with similar number of previous miscarriages and age. Other studies have reported success rates[8,9] in the two subsets that are not different, which must be considered the commonly accepted view, but more studies are needed.

Since patients with secondary RPL have carried a pregnancy to at least gestational week 20 they have been exposed to much higher quantities of fetal antigens derived from the placenta or from cells passing the placenta than patients with primary RPL. It has been estimated that in the third trimester several grams of syncytiotrophoblast debris are shed into the maternal circulation each day,[20] which often results in long lasting alloimmunization against paternal antigens.[21] The patients with secondary RPL have therefore been challenged to alloimmunization much more often than primary RPL patients and this is reflected in a higher frequency of alloantibodies (e.g., human leukocyte antigen (HLA) antibodies and antibodies against male-specific minor HY antigens) in the former.[22,23] Furthermore, fetal cells can survive for decades in the woman after a birth[24] and this feto–maternal microchimerism may play a role in inducing immunological tolerance to fetal antigens that may reduce immunological rejection of subsequent pregnancies.

In the secondary RPL group the sex of the firstborn seems to impact the prognosis which also emphasizes the belief that alloimmunization plays a role in the pathogenesis in this patient subset. In a study of a cohort of 305 patients with secondary RPL followed from 1986 to 2005,[25] the chance of giving birth to a child in the first pregnancy after a series of miscarriages was 23% lower in patients with a male compared with those with a female firstborn ($p < 0.001$). After adjustment for age, number of miscarriages and treatment the odds ratio (OR) for live birth in patients with a male firstborn was 0.37 (95% CI 0.2–0.7) compared with those with a female firstborn. The previous birth of a boy is therefore a strong prognostical negative factor in these patients, especially in patients carrying HLA class II alleles restricting immunity against male-specific minor HY antigens.[26]

RPL patients with second trimester losses also constitute a subset with particular characteristics. Drakeley et al.[27] found that 25% of their RPL patients had had at least one second trimester loss. Among 228 RPL patients admitted to our clinic from 2000 to 2004, 39 (17.1%) had experienced a mixture of first and second trimester miscarriages but only three had suffered exclusively second trimester losses. Since almost all patients with second trimester miscarriages had experienced at least one first trimester miscarriage, early and late RPL probably must have pathogenetic factors that are partially overlapping, but the observation that the overwhelming majority of patients only suffer first trimester miscarriages suggests that some pathogenetic factors are specific for those with early miscarriages. Several prospective studies indicate that a history of one or more second trimester pregnancy losses display a strong negative prognostical impact,[28,29] which also suggests that some pathogenetic factors are specific for patients with late losses.

Familial Aggregation

Quite a few studies have investigated the occurrence of RPL and sporadic miscarriage in families of women with RPL with normal parental karyotypes.[30–34] Results from relevant published studies are shown in Table 1.1. Alexander et al.[31] and Ho et al.[32] found significantly increased RPL rates in first-degree relatives of RPL women whereas Christiansen et al.[33] only found the RPL frequency significantly increased in sisters of RPL probands. Kolte et al.[34] in a questionnaire-based study where all stated miscarriages were confirmed from hospital records found a clinical miscarriage rate of 25.3% per pregnancy in siblings of RPL women, which is significantly higher ($p < 0.001$) than the rate of 13.1% in the background population.

Overall the risk of RPL in sisters of RPL women seems to be increased by a factor of seven and the risk of sporadic miscarriage by a factor of two compared with the background population. The relative frequency λ (the frequency of RPL in relatives divided by the frequency in the general population) is a measure of the degree of heritability of a disorder; the higher the value of λ, the higher is the genetic

TABLE 1.1

Studies of Occurrence of Recurrent Pregnancy Loss (RPL) in Relatives of Women with RPL

Reference and Kind of Relatives Studied	RPL Rate in Relatives (%)	RPL Rate in Controls (%)	*p*-value
Johnson et al.[30]			
Blood relatives	12.2	7.3	
Alexander et al.[31]			
Mothers and sisters	7.0	0.0	0.02
Ho et al.[32]			
First degree relatives	1.4	0.2	0.0001
Christiansen et al.[33]			
Sisters	10.6	1.8	0.00005
Brothers' wives	6.3	1.8	NS

NS: Not significant.

component.[35] λ for RPL is seven among sisters of RPL patients which points towards a moderate degree of heritability suggesting a substantial genetic contribution to the pathogenesis of RPL. However, a genetic linkage analysis was not able to find linkage to any major gene, suggesting that most RPL cases are probably caused by several genetic polymorphisms, each contributing only modestly to the total RPL risk (multifactorial inheritance).[34] This fits with the finding that several genetic polymorphisms, for example, HLA-DR3, the 14 base pair insertion in exon 8 of the HLA-G gene, genotypes associated with low plasma levels of mannose-binding lectin and heterozygocity for the factor II and factor V Leiden, have been reported to be associated with RPL with ORs between 1.3 and 2.7 compared with controls.[36]

Partner Specificity

In RPL research it has often been assumed that RPL is a partner-specific condition and a criterion that all pregnancies should be with the same partner has been included in the definition of RPL by some authors. The classic example of assumed partner-specificity is the theory of increased HLA sharing between spouses as a cause of RPL. It was suggested that due to a high HLA compatibility between spouses of RPL couples, the women failed to produce HLA antibodies and other so called blocking antibodies to the fetus that therefore became immunologically rejected.[37]

A prerequisite for this theory is that the woman will only experience RPL in a particular partnership but no epidemiological study has ever documented this. Indeed, in patients with secondary RPL, a logistic regression analysis of variables of importance for outcome in the first pregnancy after referral showed that a change of partner during the series of miscarriages was associated with an OR of 0.66 (95% confidence limits 0.3–1.3) for a succeeding live birth.[25] Although not statistically significant there was a tendency that a change of partner worsened rather than improved the prognosis for a live birth, which does not support the concept that RPL is partner-specific. The aforementioned HLA sharing theory was therefore without any epidemiological foundation and later studies of HLA sharing between spouses of RPL couples were not able to confirm the theory.[38,39] The observation that there is a clear familial predisposition to RPL at least in females (Table 1.1) also argues against RPL as being partner-specific.

Recurrent Pregnancy Loss and Associations with Obstetric and Perinatal Outcome

Numerous studies have reported that women with RPL exhibit an increased risk of obstetrical and perinatal complications in ongoing pregnancies both before and after having experienced a series of miscarriages and the women themselves also seem to have been born with a significantly reduced birthweight.[40] The association between RPL and obstetrical complications are fully described in Chapter 37. I think that the existence of these associations supports the theory that factors impairing placental growth play a role in both conditions.

Lifestyle Factors

Lifestyle factors rarely, if ever, are major causes of RPL; however, epidemiological studies have given evidence that a series of lifestyle factors can increase the risk of miscarriage. There is good evidence that obesity,[41,42] high daily caffeine intake,[43–45] alcohol consumption,[46] use of nonsteroidal anti-inflammatory drugs,[47,48] and too much high impact physical exercise[49] increase the risk of miscarriage significantly. Social class and occupation also impact the rate of miscarriage, with the greatest risk among women exposed to high physical or psychical stress during work.[50,51] Several studies now also indicate that a previous subfertility/infertility diagnosis or infertility treatment may increase the risk of miscarriage.[14,52]

Integration of the Epidemiological Knowledge in Research and Management of Recurrent Pregnancy Loss

Now that I have reviewed a series of epidemiological parameters that relate to the classification, appearance, and prognosis of RPL, I will discuss how knowledge about the influence of these parameters may help us in the understanding of the background of and assist in doing research in causes and treatments of RPL.

Occurrence

Estimating the prevalence rate of RPL in a valid and reproducible way has several applications: it can be used for comparing risks of RPL between different populations or in subgroups within the same population and it can be used for comparing changes in risk over time—a knowledge that is necessary for identifying, for example, environmental and lifestyle-related risk factors. Furthermore, the observation that the RPL prevalence in the population is >1% indicates that RPL in most cases is not a random event but rather a disorder affecting women who have an increased risk of pregnancy loss. In theory, a woman could get the diagnosis RPL because she by chance had experienced three consecutive pregnancy losses caused by the same factors causing "sporadic" miscarriages, especially fetal chromosome abnormalities. However, if all RPL cases were caused by a random accumulation of "sporadic" miscarriages, the prevalence of RPL would be $0.14^3 = 0.27\%$ (based on a frequency of sporadic miscarriage of 14% in the population) rather than 1%.[6] The observed prevalence thus indicates that at least three out of four RPL cases are caused by nonrandom factors: factors carried by the couples increasing the risk of miscarriage in each pregnancy.

Number of Previous Miscarriages

It is clear from the knowledge that the number of previous miscarriages is the most important prognostical factor in RPL that this parameter has to be taken into account when planning trials testing interventions and therapies, especially trials comparing different groups. The ideal randomized controlled trial should stratify for the number of previous miscarriages, with randomization undertaken between control and experimental treatments within each stratum. To date, such a study has not been undertaken. It is quite likely that by stratifying the sample by the number of previous miscarriages, the effect of the experimental intervention will become more easy to demonstrate in those women with higher numbers of previous miscarriages than in those with fewer previous miscarriages because the spontaneous success rate is so much lower in the former group.[12,53]

Unfortunately, in many RPL studies patients with only two previous miscarriages are included. Experiencing only two miscarriages may in many cases be a chance phenomenon caused by de novo fetal chromosomal abnormalities (in particular autosomal trisomies) rather than a recurrent maternal factor. Cytogenetic evaluations of specimens of sporadic abortions have revealed an overall incidence of chromosomal abnormalities of 43%.[54] Thus, in theory, in $0.43 \times 0.43 = 18.5\%$ of all women with two consecutive miscarriages, the cause is the occurrence of two chromosomally abnormal conceptions.

Including women with only two early miscarriages in a study will in most cases "dilute" the estimate of the risk factor (in case-control and cohort studies) or the treatment effect in randomized controlled trials. The proportion of RPL patients in whom the disorder can be explained by a random accumulation of "sporadic" miscarriages will be expected to decline and, conversely, the proportion of cases which can be explained by a factor increasing the risk of miscarriage of euploid embryos will be expected to increase with the number of previous miscarriages.[55] This is supported by findings that the frequency of many immunological risk factors increases,[56–58] the possible effect of immunotherapy increases,[12,53] and the frequency of chromosomally abnormal abortuses declines[59] with the number of previous pregnancy losses.

Maternal Age

Since many endocrine and nongenetic immunological and thrombophilic biomarkers change with increasing age, there should be tight age-matching of patients with RPL in both case-control studies and treatment trials. Because progressing maternal age increases the subsequent miscarriage rate, stratification for age should be undertaken in therapeutic trials. However, in RPL age seems only to display a significant impact on pregnancy outcome after age 40[15,17] (Figure 1.3) so it may be sufficient to undertake stratification or adjustment in multivariate analyses according to age below and above 40 years.

Subgroups of Recurrent Pregnancy Loss

The presence of specific thrombophilic and immunological biomarkers may predispose to specific reproductive histories, for example RPL with or without a previous birth, and on the other hand previous reproductive history, for example a previous birth, may display a long-term effect on immune biomarkers as previously discussed.

Secondary and primary RPL and RPL with first and second trimester losses may have different pathogenetic backgrounds, and therefore the frequency of recognized risk factors for RPL and the efficacy of treatments may differ between the groups. Indeed a series of studies have provided data suggesting that such differences exist (Table 1.2).

The factor V Leiden mutation is the commonest cause of activated protein C (APC) resistance, which is a risk factor for thrombosis and is probably also associated with RPL.[60] Wramsby et al.[61] found it significantly associated only with primary and not secondary RPL and others have also reported much higher prevalence of this polymorphism in primary than secondary RM.[62,63] Rai et al.[64] found that APC resistance was significantly associated with the absence of a previous live birth among patients with

TABLE 1.2

The Prevalence of Risk Factors or Effect of Treatments in Patients with Primary and Secondary Recurrent Pregnancy Loss (RPL) and RPL with Second Trimester Losses (Late RPL)

Factor to Evaluate	Prevalence/Effect in Secondary versus Primary RPL	Prevalence/Effect in Late versus Early Primary RPL
Parental chromosome abnormality	Equal	N/A
Antipaternal antibodies	Higher	Higher
Antiphospholipid antibodies	Lower or equal	Higher
Heriditary thrombophilia factors	Lower	Higher
NK cell activity	Lower	N/A
HLA-DR3	Higher	N/A
MBL deficiency	N/A	Higher
Allogeneic lymphocyte immunization	Lower	N/A
Treatment with i.v. immunoglobulin	Higher	N/A

N/A: Cannot be estimated.

RPL. In a study of three congenital thrombophilic factors (including the factor V Leiden mutation), 25.5% with primary RPL compared with 15.1% of those with secondary RPL were positive for at least one factor.[65] The literature thus points towards a lower prevalence of factor V Leiden/APC resistance and probably other thrombophilic factors in secondary compared to primary RPL patients. Most studies also point towards a higher prevalence of thrombophilic factors, especially the factor V Leiden mutation in patients with second trimester miscarriages compared with those with only early losses.[60,66]

It is unclear whether the occurrence of parental chromosome abnormalities (mainly balanced transloca-tions) is different between primary and secondary RPL. In a review[67] of 79 relevant studies a slightly higher incidence of aberrations (3.7%) was found in couples with RPL and one or more live births compared with primary aborters (2.9%). Franssen et al.[68] found that the frequency of parental chromo-some abnormalities was not different between couples with RPL including a live birth and RPL couples without a previous birth. The frequency of parental chromosome anomalies thus seems to be almost similar in primary and secondary RPL.

A series of immunological parameters have been described as being important for RPL and they are also expected to display a different distribution between the subgroups of RPL patients if the patho-genetic backgrounds are different. Research in immunological factors in RPL has concentrated on alloantibodies, autoantibodies, natural killer (NK) cells, complement regulating factors such as man-nose-binding lectin and HLA antigens.

As previously mentioned, there is much evidence that the maternal immune system recognizes and reacts to the trophoblast and fetus in an ongoing pregnancy: *alloantibodies* directed against paternal/ fetal HLA antigens are produced with increased gestation[69] due to traffic of fetal cells into the mother's circulation in the third trimester and at delivery. Anti-HLA and other alloantibodies often persist for years and can therefore be found more often in women with secondary compared with primary RPL.[22,23]

Most *autoantibodies* can be found with increased prevalence in patients with RPL and their presence is associated with a poor pregnancy prognosis[13]; however, few studies of autoantibodies in RPL have differentiated between primary and secondary RPL. In patients with primary RPL, the prevalence of positive anticardiolipin or antinuclear antibody concentrations has been reported to be higher than in those with secondary RPL.[13,70,71] None of the individual differences were statistically significant but the clear trend emphasizes the importance that future studies of autoantibodies in RPL distinguish between primary and secondary RPL. There is, however, consensus that antiphospholipid (aPL) antibodies dis-play a stronger association with late miscarriages than with early RPL,[66] a fact which is integrated in the definition of the antiphospholipid syndrome:[72] the aPL syndrome is considered to be present in an aPL positive patient with a history of one or more fetal deaths beyond 10 weeks.

NK cell cytotoxicity, an important factor in the innate immune defence, has been reported to be pre-dictive for a poor prognosis in patients with RPL.[73] Only one study has differentiated between primary and secondary RPL[18] finding that the NK cell activity in peripheral blood was significantly increased in women with primary but not secondary RPL compared with controls.

Deficiency of the plasma protein *mannose-binding lectin* is determined by genetic polymorphisms on chromosome no. 10. Several studies have reported that mannose-binding deficiency is found more often in RPL patients than controls[57] but the association with pregnancy losses in late pregnancy is much stronger. Genotypes associated with deficiency of mannose-binding lectin were found in 36.8% of women with recurrent late intrauterine fetal losses but only in 12.5% of control women ($p = 0.001$).[74]

Class II HLA alleles are associated with most immunological disorders. In the largest published case-control study of HLA-DR alleles in patients with RPL[58] the immunological high-responder allele HLA-DR3 was found significantly more often in the total patient group than in controls (OR 1.4, $p < 0.02$). However, among the 250 patients with secondary RM, the frequency of the HLA-DR3 phe-notype was 32.4% compared with 21.0% in controls ($p < 0.006$). In patients with primary RPL the fre-quency of the HLA-DR3 phenotype was 21.8%, which was clearly similar to that of controls. It is thus clear that HLA-DR3 is only associated with secondary RM but not with primary RM.

The finding that increased NK cytotoxicity is associated with primary RPL indicates that excessive innate immunity may be associated with primary RPL. However, the association between particular

HLA class II alleles and secondary RPL[26,58] and the evidence that immunization against male-specific HY-antigens plays a role in secondary RPL[23] point toward a role for adaptive immunity in secondary RPL since recognition of alloantigens by T lymphocytes restricted by specific HLA class II molecules and alloantibody production are characteristics of the adaptive immune system.

Familial Aggregation

As discussed previously, family studies (Table 1.1) found that the RPL prevalence in siblings of RPL probands was in accordance with a multifactorial model for inheritance of RPL. In internal medicine and other disciplines the development of many common diseases (e.g., arterial hypertension, diabetes mellitus, schizophrenia) are thought to be determined by a multifactorial threshold model. One risk factor is not sufficient to cause disease but when several intrinsic and extrinsic factors come together in the same individual (or couple) the risk exceeds a threshold level and disease develops. Research in recent years has identified a series of new factors of importance for RPL. So many risk factors have now been identified that it is very common to find several of them in the same patient. Thrombophilic risk factors seem to aggregate significantly more frequently than expected in RPL patients and the presence of several factors in the same patients affects the prognosis negatively.[75,76] Traditionally, the causes of RPL have been divided into single sufficient factors as slices of a pie: uterine malformations 10%, endocrine factors 10%, aPL 15%, and so on, which together with the unexplained group end up to be 100%. This model is probably not adequate due to aforementioned arguments. I therefore encourage scientists and clinicians working in the area of RPL to think in the threshold rather than the pie model.[77] The clinical implication is that in principle an RPL patient should be screened for all potential risk factors and the investigation should not, for economical or other reasons, stop as soon as the first risk factor has been identified. The recognition that RPL exhibits a high degree of heritability paves the way for the identification of susceptibility genes for RPL through the performance of genetic linkage analyses in families with several siblings experiencing miscarriage[34] or RPL but also genome-wide genetic screening of RPL patients and controls.[78]

Association with Obstetric and Perinatal Complications

Women with a history of RPL exhibit a significantly increased risk of late pregnancy complications. Hence all RPL patients should be offered increased surveillance in late pregnancy (e.g., repeated ultrasound examinations) to decrease perinatal mortality and morbidity. A series of factors associated with RPL—aPL, thrombophilia factors and mannose-binding lectin-deficiency—have also been associated with low birthweight[57,66] stressing the hypothesis that many cases of RPL are caused by maternal factors impairing trophoblast proliferation and growth. Since RPL per se seems to be associated with low birthweight, prospective studies of the effect of the mentioned factors on perinatal complications should be adjusted for the confounding effect of the number and type (mid-trimester losses) of previous miscarriages.

Lifestyle Factors

As mentioned above, a number of lifestyle factors—including obesity, occupation, alcohol and caffeine consumption, and subfertility—are important for the risk of miscarriage. RPL is a complex disorder where lifestyle factors are expected to modify the effect of nonlifestyle (intrinsic) factors previously discussed. The prevalence of the most important lifestyle factors among patients and controls should be given in publications in order to document that the groups studied for the occurrence of nonlifestyle risk factors or pregnancy outcome are comparable. Since it is likely that smoking aggravates the effect of thrombophilic risk factors on risk of pregnancy loss, details about smoking habits should therefore obviously be reported in all studies of RPL and thrombophilia reporting pregnancy outcomes. Another example illustrating the importance of adjusting for lifestyle factors is polycystic ovary syndrome (PCOS) and RPL. It is generally recognized that women with PCOS exhibit an increased rate of miscarriage and RPL. However, when adjustment for obesity is undertaken in multivariate analyses, the miscarriage rate in PCOS is not dependent on polycystic ovarian pathology or PCOS-associated endocrine abnormalities.[79]

Conclusions

In all medical science, epidemiological studies can provide knowledge that is indispensable when basic laboratory research, case-control studies or controlled treatment trials are planned and carried out. This is also true when we are dealing with RPL: however, it seems that epidemiological knowledge is integrated only to a very limited degree in the current clinical research and management of RPL. Knowledge of the epidemiology of RPL can be helpful in the understanding of causes of RPL and can be helpful when research studies on the topic are designed.

Implications for Understanding of Recurrent Pregnancy Loss

Studies of the epidemiology of RPL provide information that is indispensable for the generation of rational hypotheses of the pathogenesis of the syndrome. Knowledge about the prevalence of RPL and indicators for the prognosis makes us believe that the majority of RPL cases are not due to a random accumulation of "sporadic" aneuploid miscarriages but that many patients carry risk factors that increase the risk of miscarriage of euploid embryos.

The few studies addressing the question of partner-specificity in RPL have not documented that the condition in general is partner-specific and the contribution from the male genome to the condition is therefore probably minor. However, numerous studies have found a familial aggregation of miscarriage and RPL among first-degree relatives of RPL patients, especially sisters, which indicates a significant degree of heritability in the women's families. The pattern of inheritance is that of multifactorial inheritance which is in accordance with clinical evidence: several risk factors for RPL can very often be found in a single patient, and an aggregation of risk factors aggravates the pregnancy prognosis.

Numerous studies have unanimously reported that RPL is associated with a series of complications in late pregnancy: increased risk of preterm birth and intrauterine growth retardation. It remains to be clarified from multivariate analyses which clinical and paraclinical factors among RPL patients determine the risks in late pregnancy. However, the correlation between late pregnancy and perinatal complications suggests that factors impairing trophoblast growth in early and late pregnancy play an important role in RPL.

Implications for Research in Recurrent Pregnancy Loss

Most nongenetic immunological and thrombophilic biomarkers are known to be affected by demographic and other epidemiological parameters in RPL patients and controls. Several epidemiological parameters must therefore be matched or adjusted for in case-control and cohort studies involving measurement of these biomarkers.

The number of previous miscarriages is not only the strongest prognostical factor but with increased numbers of previous miscarriages fetal aneuploidy seems to play a decreasing role and maternal factors an increasing pathogenic role. Therefore stratification by the number of previous miscarriages is important both in association studies and treatment trials. Primary and secondary RPL, from an epidemiological point of view, also seem to be distinct entities and in many case-control and treatment studies these two subgroups have indeed been found to behave quite differently (Table 1.2). Therefore analyses in case-control studies should be made separately in the two subsets and in treatment trials outcome should be adjusted for primary and secondary RPL status.

Estimates of the future miscarriage risk in RPL patients vary significantly between studies, mainly due to different methods of ascertainment and monitoring—some studies have estimated the prognosis too optimistic because preclinical pregnancy losses have been classified as nonpregnancy. To overcome this potential source of error, in future prospective cohort studies or treatment trials the baby-take-home rate per time unit should substitute the miscarriage rate per first subsequently registered pregnancy.

Lifestyle factors are currently rarely mentioned or are only reported very superficially in clinical studies in RPL. Since lifestyle factors per se or through interactions with intrinsic factors can increase the risk of miscarriage, the most important should be reported in more detail in future studies and appropriate stratification be performed according to their presence or absence.

Finally, the recognition of the different natures and pathogenetic background of primary and secondary RPL and the different nature of RPL with few miscarriages as opposed to RPL with many miscarriages should help eliminate the practice of combining data from too heterogeneous studies for meta-analysis.

REFERENCES

1. World Health Organization. Recommended definitions; terminology and format for statistical tables related to the perinatal period. *Acta Obstet Gynecol Scand* 1977;56:247–53.
2. Farquharson R, Jauniaux E, Exalto N on behalf of the ESHRE Special Interest group for Early Pregnancy (SIGEP). Updated and revised nomenclature for the description of early pregnancy events. *Hum Reprod* 2005;20:3008–11.
3. Alberman E. The epidemiology of repeated abortion. In: Beard RW, Sharp F, eds. *Early Pregnancy Loss: Mechanisms and Treatment*. London: Springer Verlag; 1988. p. 9–17.
4. Warburton D, Strobino B. Recurrent spontaneous abortion. In: Bennet MJ, Edmonds DK, eds. *Spontaneous and Recurrent Abortion*. Oxford: Blackwell Scientific; 1987: p. 193–213.
5. Stray-Pedersen B, Lorentzen-Styr AM. The prevalence of toxoplasma antibodies among 11,736 pregnant women in Norway. *Scand J Infect Dis* 1979;11:159–65.
6. Fertility and Employment 1979. *The Danish Data Archives no. 0363*, Odense University.
7. Cowchock FS, Smith JB. Predictors for live birth after unexplained spontaneous abortions: Correlations between immunological test results, obstetric histories, and outcome of the next pregnancy without treatment. *Am J Obstet Gynecol* 1992;167:1208–12.
8. Quenby SM, Farquharson RG. Predicting recurring miscarriage: What is important? *Obstet Gynecol* 1993;82:132–8.
9. Clifford K, Rai R, Regan L. Future pregnancy outcome in unexplained recurrent first trimester miscarriage. *Hum Reprod* 1997;12:387–9.
10. Christiansen OB, Pedersen B, Rosgaard A, Husth M. A randomized, double-blind, placebo-controlled trial of intravenous immunoglobulin in the prevention of recurrent miscarriage: Evidence for a therapeutic effect in women with secondary recurrent miscarriage. *Hum Reprod* 2002;17:809–16.
11. Jablonowska B, Selbing A, Palfi M, Ernerudh J, Kjellberg S, Lindton B. Prevention of recurrent spontaneous abortion by intravenous immunoglobulin: A double-blind placebo-controlled study. *Hum Reprod* 1999;14:838–41.
12. Carp HJ, Toder V, Torchinsky A, Portuguese S, Lipitz S, Gazit E et al. Allogenic leukocyte immunization after five or more miscarriages. Recurrent Miscarriage Immunotherapy Trialists Group. *Hum Reprod* 1997;12:250–5.
13. Nielsen HS, Christiansen OB. Prognostic impact of anticardiolipin antibodies in women with recurrent miscarriages negative for the lupus anticoagulant. *Hum Reprod* 2005;20:1720–8.
14. Cauchi MN, Coulam CB, Cowchock S, Ho HN, Gatenby P, Johnson PM et al. Predictive factors in recurrent spontaneous abortion—A multicenter study. *Am J Reprod Immunol* 1995;33:165–70.
15. Lund M, Kamper-Jørgensen M, Nielsen HS, Lidegaard Ø, Andersen AM, Christiansen OB. Prognosis for live birth in women with recurrent miscarriage. What is the best measure of success? *Obstet Gynecol* 2012;119:37–43.
16. Raghupathy J, Al-Mutawa E, Al-Azemi M, Makhseed M, Azizieh H, Szekeres-Bartho J. Progesterone-induced blocking factor (PIBF) modulates cytokine production by lymphocytes from women with recurrent miscarriage or preterm birth. *J Reprod Immunol* 2009;80:91–9.
17. Nybo Andersen AM, Wohlfahrt J, Christens P, Olsen J, Melbye M. Maternal age and fetal loss: Population based register study. *BMJ* 2000;320:1708–12.

18. Shakhar K, Ben-Eliyahu S, Loewenthal R, Rosenne E, Carp H. Differences in number and activity of peripheral natural killer cells in primary versus secondary recurrent miscarriage. *Fertil Steril* 2003;80:368–75.

19. Christiansen OB, Mathiesen O, Husth M, Lauritsen JG, Grunnet N. Placebo-controlled trial of active immunization with third party leukocytes in recurrent miscarriage. *Acta Obstet Gynecol Scand* 1994;73:261–8.

20. Huppertz B, Kadyrov M, Kingdom JC. Apoptosis and its role in the trophoblast. *Am J Obstet Gynecol* 2006;195:29–39.

21. van Kampen CA, Versteeg-van der Voort Maarschalk MF, Langerak-Langerak J, Roelen DL, Claas FH. Pregnancy can induce long-persisting primed CTLs specific for inherited paternal HLA antigens. *Hum Immunol* 2001;62:201–7.

22. Nielsen HS, Witvliet MD, Steffensen R et al. The presence of HLA-antibodies in recurrent miscarriage patients is associated with a reduced chance of live birth. *J Reprod Immunol* 2010;87:67–73.

23. Nielsen HS, Wu F, Steffensen R, van Halteren AG, Spierings E et al. HY antibody titers are increased in unexplained secondary recurrent miscarriage and associated with low male:female ratio in subsequent live births. *Hum Reprod* 2010;25:2745–52.

24. Bianchi DW, Zickwolf GK, Weil GJ, Sylvester S, DeMaria MA. Male fetal progenitor cells persist in maternal blood for as long as 27 years postpartum. *Proc Natl Acad Sci U S A* 1996;93:705–8.

25. Nielsen HS, Andersen AM, Kolte AM, Christiansen OB. A firstborn boy is suggestive of a strong prognostic factor in secondary recurrent miscarriage: A confirmatory study. *Fertil Steril* 2008;89:907–11.

26. Nielsen HS, Steffensen R, Varming K, van Halteren AG, Spierings E, Ryder LP et al. Association of HY-restricting HLA class II alleles with pregnancy outcome in patients with recurrent miscarriage subsequent to a firstborn boy. *Hum Mol Genet* 2009;18:1684–91.

27. Drakeley AJ, Quenby S, Farquharson RG. Mid-trimester loss; appraisal of a screening protocol. *Hum Reprod* 1998;13:1471–9.

28. Cowchock FS, Smith JB, David S, Scher J, Batzer F, Carson S. Paternal mononuclear cell immunization therapy for repeated miscarriage: Predictive variables for pregnancy success. *Am J Reprod Immunol* 1990;22:12–7.

29. Goldenberg RL, Mayberry SK, Copper RL, Dubard MB, Hauth JC. Pregnancy outcome following a second-trimester loss. *Obstet Gynecol* 1993;81:444–6.

30. Johnson PM, Chia KV, Risk JM, Barnes RM, Woodrow JC. Immunological and immunogenetic investigation of recurrent spontaneous abortion. *Dis Markers* 1988;6:163–71.

31. Alexander SA, Latinne D, Debruyere M, Dupont E, Gottlieb W, Thomas K. Belgian experience with repeat immunization in recurrent spontaneous abortion. In: Beard RW, Sharp F, eds. *Early Pregnancy Loss: Mechanisms and Treatment.* London: Springer Verlag; 1988. p. 355–63.

32. Ho H, Gill TJ, Hsieh C, Yang YS, Le TY. The prevalence of recurrent spontaneous abortion, cancer, and congenital anomalies in the families of couples with recurrent spontaneous abortions or gestational trophoblastic tumors. *Am J Obstet Gynecol* 1991;165:461–6.

33. Christiansen OB, Mathiesen O, Lauritsen JG, Grunnet N. Idiopathic recurrent spontaneous abortion. Evidence of a familial predisposition. *Acta Obstet Gynecol Scand* 1990;69:597–601.

34. Kolte AM, Nielsen HS, Moltke I, Degn B, Pedersen B, Sunde L et al. A genome-wide scan in affected sibling pairs with idiopathic recurrent miscarriage suggests genetic linkage. *Mol Hum Reprod* 2011;17:279–85.

35. Emery AEH. *Methodology in Medical Genetics.* 2nd rev. ed. Edinburgh, London, Melbourne, New York: Churchill Livingstone; 1986.

36. Christiansen OB, Steffensen R, Nielsen HS, Varming K. Multifactorial etiology of recurrent miscarriage and its scientific and clinical implications. *Gynecol Obstet Invest* 2008;66:257–67.

37. Beer AE, Semprini AE, Zhu X, Quebbeman JF. Pregnancy outcome in human couples with recurrent spontaneous abortions: HLA antigen profiles, HLA sharing, female serum MLR blocking factors and paternal leukocyte immunization. *Exp Clin Immunogenet* 1985;2:137–53.

38. Christiansen OB, Riisom K, Lauritsen JG, Grunnet N. No increased histocompatibility antigen sharing in couples with idiopathic habitual abortions. *Hum Reprod* 1989;4:160–2.

39. Ober C, van der Ven K. HLA and fertility. In: Hunt JB, ed. *HLA and the Maternal-Fetal Relationship.* Austin: RG Landers; 1996. p. 133–56.

40. Christiansen OB, Mathiesen O, Lauritsen JG, Grunnet N. Study of the birthweight of parents experiencing unexplained recurrent miscarriages. *BJOG* 1992;99:408–11.

41. Fedorcsak P, Storeng R, Dale PO, Tanbo T, Abyholm T. Obesity is a risk factor for early pregnancy loss after IVF or ICSI. *Acta Obstet Gynecol Scand* 2000;79:43–8.

42. Andersen AM, Andersen PK, Olsen J, Grønbæk M, Strandberg-Larsen K. Moderate alcohol intake during pregnancy and risk of fetal death. *Int J Epidemiol* 2012;41:405–13.

43. Infante-Rivard C, Fernandez A, Gauthier R, David M, Rivard GE. Fetal loss associated with caffeine intake before and during pregnancy. *JAMA, J Am Med Assoc* 1993;270:2940–3.

44. Fenster L, Hubbard AE, Swan SH, Windham GC, Waller K, Hiatt RA et al. Caffeinated beverages, decaffeinated coffee, and spontaneous abortion. *Epidemiology* 1997;8:515–23.

45. Giannelli M, Doyle P, Roman E et al. The effect of caffeine consumption and nausea on the risk of miscarriage. *Paediatr Perinat Epidemiol* 2003;17:316–23.

46. Rasch V. Cigarette, alcohol, and caffeine consumption: Risk factors for spontaneous abortion. *Acta Obstet Gynecol Scand* 2003;82:182–8.

47. Nielsen GL, Sorensen HT, Larsen H, Pedersen L. Risk of adverse outcome and miscarriage in pregnant users of non-steroidal anti-inflammatory drugs: Population based observational study and case-control study. *BMJ* 2001;322:266–70.

48. Li DK, Liu L, Odouli R. Exposure to nonsteroidal anti-inflammatory drugs during pregnancy and risk of miscarriage: Population based cohort study. *BMJ* 2003;327:368–72.

49. Madsen M, Jørgensen T, Jensen ML, Juhl M, Olsen J, Andersen PK et al. Leisure time physical exercise during pregnancy and the risk of miscarriage: A study within the Danish National Birth Cohort. *BJOG* 2007;114:1419–26.

50. Brandt LP, Nielsen CV. Job stress and adverse outcome of pregnancy: A causal link or recall bias? *Am J Epidemiol* 1992;35:302–11.

51. Florack EI, Zielhuis GA, Pellegrino JE, Rolland R. Occupational physical activity and the occurrence of spontaneous abortion. *Int J Epidemiol* 1993;22:878–84.

52. Wang JX, Norman RJ, Wilcox AJ. Incidence of spontaneous abortion among pregnancies produced by assisted reproductive technology. *Hum Reprod* 2004;19:272–7.

53. Daya S, Gunby J and The Recurrent Miscarriage Trialists Group. The effectiveness of allogeneic leukocyte immunization in unexplained primary recurrent abortion. *Am J Reprod Immunol* 1994;32:294–302.

54. Creasy R. The cytogenetics of spontaneous abortion in humans. In: Beard RW, Sharp F, eds. *Early Pregnancy Loss: Mechanisms and Treatment*. London: Springer Verlag; 1988. p. 293–304.

55. Christiansen OB. A fresh look at the causes and treatment of recurrent miscarriage, especially its immunological aspects. *Hum Reprod Update* 1996;2:271–93.

56. Pfeiffer KA, Fimmers R, Engels G, van der ven H, van der ven K. The HLA-G genotype is potentially associated with idiopathic recurrent spontaneous abortion. *Mol Hum Reprod* 2001;7:373–8.

57. Kruse C, Rosgaard A, Steffensen R, Varming K, Jensenius JC, Christiansen OB. Low serum level of mannan-binding lectin is a determinant for pregnancy outcome in women with recurrent spontaneous abortion. *Am J Obstet Gynecol* 2002;187:1313–20.

58. Kruse C, Steffensen R, Varming K, Christiansen OB. A study of HLA-DR and –DQ alleles in 588 patients and 562 controls confirms that HLA-DRB1*03 is associated with recurrent miscarriage. *Hum Reprod* 2004;19:1215–21.

59. Ogasawara M, Aoki K, Okada S, Suzumori K. Embryonic karyotype of abortuses in relation to the number of previous miscarriages. *Fertil Steril* 2000;73:300–4.

60. Rey E, Kahn SR, David M, Shrier I. Thrombophilic disorders and fetal loss: A meta-analysis. *Lancet* 2003;361:901–8.

61. Wramsby ML, Sten-Linder M, Bremme K. Primary habitual abortions are associated with high frequency of factor V Leiden mutation. *Fertil Steril* 2000;74:987–91.

62. Alintas A, Pasa S, Akdeniz N, Cil T, Yurt M, Ayyildiz O et al. Factor V Leiden and G20210A prothrombin mutations in patients with recurrent pregnancy loss: Data from the southeast of Turkey. *Ann Hematol* 2007;86:727–31.

63. Hussein AS, Darwish H, Shelbayeh K. Association between factor V Leiden mutation and poor pregnancy outcomes among Palestinian women. *Thromb Res* 2010;126:e78–e82.

64. Rai R, Shlebak A, Cohen H, Backos M, Holmes Z, Marriott K et al. Factor V Leiden and acquired activated protein C resistance among 1000 women with recurrent miscarriage. *Hum Reprod* 2001;16:961–5.
65. Carp H, Salomon O, Seidman D, Dardik R, Rosenberg N, Inbal A. Prevalence of genetic markers for thrombophilia in recurrent pregnancy loss. *Hum Reprod* 2002;17:1633–7.
66. Roque H, Paidas MJ, Funai EF, Kuczynski E, Lockwood CJ. Maternal thrombophilias are not associated with early pregnancy loss. *Thromb Haemostasis* 2004;91:290–5.
67. Tharapel AT, Tharapel SA, Bannerman RM. Recurrent pregnancy losses and chromosome abnormalities: A review. *BJOG* 1985;92:899–914.
68. Franssen MTM, Korevaar JC, Leschot NJ, Bossuyt PM, Knegt AC, Gerssen-Schorl KB et al. Selective chromosome analysis in couples with two or more miscarriages: Case-control study. *BMJ* 2005;331:137–41.
69. Regan L. A prospective study of spontaneous abortion. In: Beard RW, Sharp F, eds. *Early Pregnancy Loss. Mechanisms and Treatment*. London: Springer-Verlag; 1988. p. 23–37.
70. Cowchock S, Bruce Smith J, Gocial B. Antibodies to phospholipids and nuclear antigens in patients with repeated abortions. *Am J Obstet Gynecol* 1986;155:1002–10.
71. Rai R, Regan L, Clifford K, Pickering W, Dave M, Mackie I et al. Antiphospholipid antibodies and beta2-glycoprotein-I in 500 women with recurrent miscarriage: Results of a comprehensive screening approach. *Hum Reprod* 1995;10:2001–5.
72. Myakis S, Lockshin MD, Atsumi T, Branch DW, Brey PL, Cervera R et al. International concensus statement on an update of the classification criteria for definite antiphsopholipid syndrome (APS). *J Thromb Haemostasis* 2006;4:295–306.
73. Aoki K, Kajiura S, Matsumoto Y, Ogasawara M, Okada S, Yagami Y et al. Preconceptional natural-killer activity as a predictor of miscarriage. *Lancet* 1995;345:1340–2.
74. Christiansen OB, Nielsen HS, Lund M, Steffensen R, Varming K. Mannose-binding lectin-2 genotypes and recurrent late pregnancy losses. *Hum Reprod* 2009;24:291–9.
75. Coulam CB, Jeyendran RS, Fishel LA, Roussev R. Multiple thromobophilic gene mutations rather than specific gene mutations are risk factors for recurrent miscarriage. *Am J Reprod Immunol* 2006;55:360–8.
76. Jivraj S, Rai R, Underwood J, Regan R et al. Genetic thrombophilic mutations among couples with recurrent miscarriage. *Hum Reprod* 2006;21:1161–5.
77. Christiansen OB, Nybo-Andersen AM, Bosch E et al. Evidence-based investigations and treatments of recurrent pregnancy loss. *Fertil Steril* 2005;83:821–39.
78. Nagirnaja L, Palta P, Kasak L, Rull K, Christianen OB, Nielsen HS et al. Structural genomic variation as a risk factor to idiopathic recurrent miscarriage. *Hum Mut* 2014;35:972–82.
79. Wang JX, Davies MJ, Norman RJ. Polycystic ovarian syndrome and the risk of spontaneous abortion following assisted reproductive technology treatment. *Hum Reprod* 2001;16:2606–9.

2

Signaling between Embryo and Mother in Early Pregnancy: Basis for Development of Tolerance

Eytan R. Barnea

The Hypothesis

Viviparity is the hallmark of mammalian gestation, where progeny remains within the mother's body throughout fetal development. Once recognized and accepted, the embryo receives nutrition and protection. Thus, immunological acceptance and tolerance are paramount to the successful interaction between the embryo graft and its maternal host. Initial immunological awareness must take place prior to implantation. The semipermeable zona pellucida forms rapidly postfertilization and protects the embryo until it reaches the endometrium. The zona is surrounded by maternal immune cells, and this unit transmits the message that fertilization has occurred. The main question is when and how the embryo–maternal communication initiates and creates maternal recognition of pregnancy. This is the main topic of this chapter. Further, we will focus on preimplantation factor (PIF), a peptide secreted by viable embryos which plays an essential role in pregnancy promoting embryo development, uterine priming, trophoblast invasion, and systemic immune regulation. This recognition starts prior to direct embryo–maternal contact in the uterus. Finally, data generated using nonpregnant models of autoimmune disorders and transplantation also provide important insight into PIF's possible role in pregnancy.

Early Observations: Embryo–Maternal Recognition Initiates Prior to Implantation

In 1973, Beer and Billingham,[1] while working on immunological recognition mechanisms in mammalian pregnancy, suggested that the maternal system is aware of the presence of the early embryo, and actively responds to it. This was surprising considering the differences in genetic makeup of the mother and fetus (semi- or total), and contrary to the prevailing opinion at that time, which considered that the trophoblast was hypoantigenic, protecting it from cellular immunity. The same authors also suggested that unique human leukocyte antigens (HLA) are presented to the maternal system, the responses to which play a role in establishing and maintaining pregnancy. A decade later, it was suggested[2] that local, cell-based immunosuppressive and immunoprotective activity in the placenta was mediated by suppressor and other unknown cells. They further suggested that HLA sharing by parents leads to lack of maternal recognition and is therefore the basis for rejection, that is, miscarriage.

Hansel and Hickey[3] examined various compounds that might be involved in the maternal recognition of pregnancy, with an emphasis on domestic animals. They found several proteins, including the embryo-derived platelet activating factor (PAF), a trophoblastic protein with an antiluteolytic effect. Further progress regarding embryo–maternal recognition was provided by Weitlauf[4] who reported that embryo-conditioned media have a specific effect on the rat uterus compared with control media, or that produced by deciduomata (a nonpregnant environment). This strongly implied the presence of communication between the embryo and the mother before implantation, but specific factors involved were not identified.

Later studies have recognized that there are multiple types of placenta in mammals. The hemochorial placenta (found in the human and the mouse) is associated with intimate interaction, while in other species there is less invasiveness (such as the pig placenta which communicates with the endometrium through the histiotroph). In addition, the secretory products of different types of placentae also differ, human chorionic gonadotropin (hCG) in humans, prolactin in rodents,[5] and so on.

Despite such diversity at implantation, there are features which are common to the development of all mammals before implantation: egg and sperm fusion, progressive development of the fertilized embryo up to the blastocyst stage. In a recent review Moffet and Loke[6] concluded that pregnancy is not a classical acceptance/rejection phenomenon, and the specific compounds derived from the conceptus and the receptors present on immune cells need to be identified to better understand the unique interaction in pregnancy.

Rescue of the Corpus Luteum

Following ovulation, the corpus luteum (CL) is formed and secretes progesterone, which has a trophic effect on the endometrium. A variety of signals can rescue the CL. These include hCG in humans, prolactin in rodents, and estrogen in pigs, indicating that the CL rescuing signals are species-specific. When cow and mare uteruses are removed, PGF2α is not released and the CL persists long-term; therefore, the presence of the conceptus actually prevents luteolysis.[7] But the presence of an embryo is not necessary, and hCG injections, for example, can prolong the lifespan of the CL only to a certain degree. This contrasts with the uterus, in which a viable embryo must be present in order for the endometrium to become receptive. Thus, recognition of pregnancy and successful implantation takes place before the stage when rescue of the CL occurs, strongly suggesting that there is no linkage between tolerance and the CL.

Genomic Elements in Maternal Recognition of Pregnancy

Recent data show that the embryo expresses its genome as early as the two-cell stage. Thus in the earliest stages of development the embryo becomes a partial or total "non-self" from the perspective of the mother. Thus, development of the zona pellucida as a protection against maternal adversity becomes necessary. It has recently been observed that there is a major downregulation of genes in the preimplantation embryo compared to the unfertilized egg.[8] This downregulation may protect the embryo by minimizing its vulnerability, and in a mostly anaerobic environment it may be advantageous to shut down nonessential functions which are not necessary for survival. Additionally, the few genes that are upregulated may have an important physiological role. Novel genes that are expressed very early may lead to early maternal recognition of pregnancy.[9]

How Does Embryo Tolerance Develop?

The released mature egg reaches the ampular region and survives for only 12–24 hours unless it is fertilized. There is a one-in-three chance for fertilization to occur. Once the sperm penetrates the egg at fertilization, it becomes "invisible" to the maternal immune system. As expected, following egg/sperm fusion there is no maternally induced immune rejection, for as long as the egg membrane does not change its characteristics (expressing foreign antigens). Once foreign antigens are expressed, the fertilized egg rapidly becomes surrounded by the zona pellucida, a hard and impenetrable shell that wards off maternal immune cells. Further immune protection is provided by maternal cumulus oophorus cells, which further prevent direct access of maternal immune cells to the embryo. However, the cumulus cells persist only for a few days after fertilization, as their primary role is to facilitate tubal transport of the embryo towards the uterus. The cumulus has immune cells that secrete cytokines, and may serve as a first relay system for propagating embryo-derived signaling.[10] Indeed, it has been shown that within eight hours after fertilization there is emargination of platelets from the peripheral blood in mice.[11]

Embryonic cell proliferation up to the eight-cell stage is rather orderly. The blastomeres are totipotential (i.e., each of them could develop into a complete embryo). This process lasts approximately three days while the embryo travels within the fallopian tube. The speed of development is a good index to evaluate embryonic health with respect to the likelihood of implantation.

Lessons Learned from Assisted Reproductive Technology

The success in achieving healthy pregnancy and live birth using donor embryos in mammals and cross-species embryo transfer efficacy are two procedures that support the view that the embryo is self-driven. Pregnancy success, then, is dependent on effective embryo-driven signaling followed by an appropriate maternal response. Upon fertilization, the embryo actively signals its presence to the host/mother. Pinpointing exactly when the signals initiate and understanding their specific mechanisms are currently under investigation.[12,13] Certainly, the signaling must occur prior to the activation of the embryo genome. While in natural conception the presence of the sperm and its immune-activated compounds is clearly apparent to the maternal organism, this is not relevant when assisted reproductive technology (ART) is used. Following embryo transfer, four to five days pass until implantation takes place, indicating a lag between embryo presence and maternal acceptance. The delay suggests that this time is required to establish tolerance and prime the endometrium, making it both receptive and accommodating for the incoming embryo. In non-ART reproduction there is a similar delay (five to seven days). In both cases, the premise is that an embryo-driven signal makes the maternal organism responsive to the presence of the embryo.

Moreover, experience with transfer of donor (genetically dissimilar) embryos has shown high implantation and pregnancy success rates, further implicating the role of the embryo in the recognition process. Implantation can occur in sites outside the uterus, including the fallopian tube, ovary, or even (rarely) in the abdominal cavity on the bowel. The occurrence of ectopic pregnancy strongly indicates that maternal recognition of pregnancy must be systemic, not only localized to the uterus. Therefore, they must be exclusively embryo driven. However, the role of the endometrium in successful reproduction is still relevant since most successful pregnancies are intrauterine.

Autocrine signaling within the embryo depends initially on the successful fusion of an egg and sperm that are both chromosomally healthy. In both ART and non-ART settings, it is actually the sperm that compels development. While maternally-derived compounds penetrate the zona pellucida, they have limited access to the embryo itself and consequently only mildly impact the zygote.[14] Thus, the embryo emits more signals than it receives and the zona facilitates self-development and differentiation of the embryoblast and trophoblast. The importance of embryo-derived autocrine signaling is demonstrated in various experimental models utilizing culture media free of growth factors, where the embryo can self-perpetuate to easily reach an advanced blastocyst stage. Several culture models have been used to assess the effect of various compounds on embryo development, identifying maternal factors that clearly play a role in embryo growth and differentiation. Identification of maternal or nonembryo specific trophic compounds is pursued. There are IGF receptors in the embryo and the ligands have trophic effects and are modulated by embryonic IGFBP-3.[15–21] The process of implantation is highly intricate, and when embryo/maternal contact is direct, a myriad of compounds function in a coordinated manner.

Compounds Involved in Endometrial Priming and Immune Tolerance Development

Regulatory T cells (T_{reg}, CD4+/CD25+) increase prior to implantation, suggesting early embryo signaling which is not dependent on the presence of semen since it is also present post *in vitro* fertilization (IVF). There is a protolerant embryo-driven (T_H2) cytokine balance in pregnancy: increased IL4, IL5, and IL10 is coupled with reduced T_H1-type cytokines, such as IL2, interferon-γ (IFN-γ), and tumor necrosis factor-α (TNF-α).[3,22] However, excess T_H1 cytokines are associated with reproductive failure.[23] Activated NFκB cells cause a T_H1-type response, whereas increased peripheral T lymphocytes express progesterone receptors, and protect by releasing IL10 and TGFβ.[24] Other nonpregnancy-specific compounds may also be involved: sex steroids, integrins, and IL1b that have no mRNA for receptors in the embryo. Leukemia inhibiting factor and colony-stimulating factor which stimulate matrix metalloproteinase are also involved and inhibition of MUC-1 expression on the endometrial surface facilitates implantation.[25,26] Natural killer (NK) cells may also inhibit excessive trophoblast invasiveness by recognizing unusual fetal trophoblast major histocompatibility complex (MHC) ligands.[23] However, none of the above compounds are pregnancy-specific and therefore cannot be the prime signal for tolerance.

Implantation failure is frequent, disrupting the delicate balance between the uterine epithelial lining which becomes the decidua and the embryo. Endometrial adaptability to the incoming embryo has been studied.[27–31] Determining whether the endometrium acts as a sensor to weed out abnormal embryos, or whether abnormal embryos fail to create the necessary signaling for effective implantation is of great importance. New evidence suggests that the latter scenario may be more accurate. Also, it has been suggested that when two embryos are transferred one may support the other which may be of lower quality. These data raise a dual view that both the endometrium and the embryo itself participate actively in the success of the implantation process.

The endometrium can be hostile due to immune disruptors, such as high peripheral levels of NK cells, altered hormonal priming, infection, and deficient integrin expression. The role of antiphospholipid antibodies, for example, in failed implantation is still being debated.[32] The embryo can also fail to implant due to deficient expression of adhesion molecules (MMPs) as well as the lack of secretory and cellular elements that aid in the immune maternal recognition of pregnancy.[33] In addition, some embryos may only partially or temporarily implant, later dislodging into the fallopian tube leading to chemical or ectopic pregnancy. Recent data show an imbalance toward stimulatory over inhibitory NK cell receptors: CD158a and CD158b inhibitory receptor expression by $CD56^{dim}/CD16^+$ and $CD56^{bright}/CD16^-$ NK cells, decreased, while CD161-activating receptor expression by $CD56^+/CD3^+$ NKT cells increased in patients with implantation failures.[34]

Unique Phenomena Require Unique Signals

In order for a semi- or totally foreign embryo (or even a cross-species transfer) to implant and lead to successful progeny, unique embryo-derived signals must be present. However, immune tolerance is *conditional*, since rejection by the mother may take place at any moment until delivery. In order to emit such a specific signal the embryo must be viable and the maternal system receptive. The signal has to be expressed early in embryo development, potent, and has to have specific sites of action both on the maternal immune system and the endometrium. The signal must also be universally mammalian, because the same early phenomenon takes place in all mammals (and any diversity only occurs at the implantation phase).

What properties would such a signal have? It would *modulate* the maternal immune system without suppressing it. This is essential because during pregnancy the mother is exposed to pathogens and her ability to maintain an effective immune system to combat disease is necessary for survival, both for her and the embryo. Therefore, the signal would allow maternal immunity to function unimpeded, allowing it to fight pathogens, while maintaining tolerance toward the embryo. Signal intensity should not be excessive, impairing the maternal ability to reject defective embryos or seriously infected fetuses. The signal would prime the endometrium making the uterine environment hospitable for the embryo. Finally, as embryo–maternal interaction becomes intimate the dynamics change; complex events take place leading to *maintenance* of tolerance rather than the initiation, which is the topic of this chapter.

Evidence that the embryo may have an active role in immune recognition was suggested by studies showing that embryo-conditioned media have immune-suppressive properties.[35,36] However, the compounds responsible for this have not been fully characterized.

The main diagnostic marker for human pregnancy is hCG, but it does not reflect pregnancy viability, is detected later in embryo culture media, and persists in the circulation long-term after pregnancy has ended, greatly limiting its clinical use. hCG has an important role in the maintenance of the corpus luteum and, following implantation, is involved in altering the biochemical indices and morphology of endometrial cells, by acting on a specific binding site (CG/LH-R). A local immunological role has also been ascribed to hCG.[37] However, hCG is not pregnancy-specific, is unique to humans and, significantly, is also found in various cancers. It appears that most hCG effects involve support of pregnancy at implantation and beyond.

Platelet Activating Factor

PAF is an acetylated phosphoglyceride expressed by the embryo in both humans and rodents. Its role is mostly local within the fallopian tube aiding in the transfer of the embryo into the uterus.[38] However, in other species other compounds play similar roles; for example, in horses, prostaglandin E is secreted by the morula. PAF also has a trophic effect on the embryo.[39] PAF is not pregnancy-specific and is present in platelets, leukocytes, and endothelial cells. Therefore, it is clear that PAF could not be a unique signal required for pregnancy tolerance.

Early Pregnancy Factor

Early pregnancy factor (EPF) has been identified as chaperonin 10, a 12 kDa protein. It can be detected prior to implantation in the maternal circulation.[40] EPF has been shown to influence immune effects mediating the suppressive effect by binding T cells, NK cells, and monocytes. The receptor for EPF is not a functional homologue of chaperonin 10.[40] EPF activity in the serum is determined by decreased rosette formation using a cumbersome bioassay. A similar activity in mare and cow serum is related to a 26 kDa protein which is different from the chaperonin molecule.[41] In addition, EPF is not pregnancy-specific; it is also present in several nonpregnant tissues, including the serum of patients with ovarian cancer.[42]

Human Leukocyte Antigens

The embryo and trophoblast express nonclassical forms HLA-G, which may protect them against NK-mediated lysis, and lead to apoptosis of allogeneic cytotoxic CD8[+] T cells by Fas ligands.[43] But HLA-G-negative embryos may implant and therefore, HLA-G is not essential for implantation.[44] Recent data have shown that NK cells, which are dominant in the decidua, express a receptor for KIR2DL2, which interacts with HLA-G; however, a multiparous woman who lacked the receptor still had normal pregnancies.[45] Also, HLA-G polymorphism has been investigated in recurrent spontaneous abortion, but no difference has been found between the fertile and abortion-prone populations.[46] HLA-G can be detected in human embryo culture media by specific immunoassays. However, pregnancy can also occur in its absence. When HLA-G is present, there is a higher pregnancy rate and therefore its testing has been used to determine which embryos should be transferred after IVF.[47] However, the soluble forms are not secreted by the trophoblast, but are cleaved from membrane-bound HLA-G1. Thus, HLA-G may be necessary but is certainly not sufficient for initiating maternal tolerance of pregnancy.

Preimplantation Factor

Earlier work had shown that viable human and rabbit human embryo culture media contains unidentified immune modulatory compounds.[35,36] We developed a novel bioassay and reported that viable human and mouse embryo-conditioned culture media, and human and porcine pregnancy serum, contain immune-modulatory compounds that increase rosette formation between donor lymphocytes and platelets in the presence of CD2MAb due to PIF, a low molecular weight peptide(s).[48–54] A bioassay, unlike an immune assay, is a reflection of a biological phenomenon, which led us to study whether the compounds present in embryo culture media are also present in the maternal circulation. Using the PIF bioassay combined with affinity chromatography, followed by two-step high-performance liquid chromatography and identification by mass spectrometry, we have isolated and characterized PIF a 9–15 aa peptide that shares the first nine amino acids. Since the peptide replicated the bioassay results it was subsequently made synthetically, which replicated the native biological activity. Subsequently, both polyclonal and mouse monoclonal antibodies were generated that enabled detailed examination of the diagnostic and therapeutic potential of the embryo-derived peptide. The Barnea research group reported that PIF is secreted only by viable embryos and it can be measured shortly postfertilization at the two-cell stage in embryo culture media.[55] With its multitargeted effects, PIF plays an essential role in conditioning the mother for successful implantation. Viewing the embryo as a self-driven entity that enables itself to control its own destiny, *PIF could play an important role in this process.*

Preimplantation Factor—A Biomarker for Embryo Tolerance

The possibility that PIF plays a role in determining the embryo's destiny has been examined and documented in mouse, cow and human embryos.[55,56] The detection of PIF in culture media is associated with viability and, following embryo transfer, it is associated with successful pregnancy outcome. A more recent study provided further evidence for dependence of successful pregnancy outcome on the presence of PIF in human embryo culture media. Data generated by following single and multiple embryo transfer documented that lack of detection of PIF in the culture media correlates 100% with the lack of pregnancy following transfer. This aspect of PIF's potential as a biomarker of viable pregnancy is being investigated in multicenter clinical trials (Clinicaltrials.gov).

The use of βhCG as a pregnancy biomarker is well established. It is secreted by the embryo upon genome expression and it is detected in the maternal circulation within a few days postimplantation. However, such detection *per force* does not indicate that the pregnancy is viable since chemical pregnancies where βhCG is detected are rather common.[50] PIF may turn out to be a useful biomarker with practical advantages over hCG. Patients at risk for repeat pregnancy loss have been followed up by serial PIF bioassays.[50] PIF was not detected in the maternal circulation two to three weeks prior to a fall in hCG levels and clinical symptoms of spontaneous abortion. Morever, hCG was detected in the maternal circulation of all of these patients. Chemical pregnancies were also positive for hCG but not PIF.[50] Similarly PIF detection in the maternal circulation four days after embryo transfer was associated with a 71% live birth rate compared with 3% when PIF was not detected. PIF can also be detected in the pregnant woman's circulation by specific ELISA (enzyme-linked immunosorbent assay), which shows an increase in the first trimester, plateau in the second trimester and a fall in the third trimester. The bovine model closely approximates human pregnancy. We have reported that 10 days after artificial insemination, PIF identification led to live births in 91%, and at day 20 reached 100%.[57] Thus PIF detection is associated with a good pregnancy outcome. Prior to implantation the source of PIF is the embryo, whereas postimplantation, it is the placenta and possibly the fetus, as confirmed by immunohistochemistry and anti-PIF antibody studies.[57,58]

Preimplantation Factor Promotes Embryo Development and Prevents Recurrent Pregnancy Loss Serum-Induced Embryo Demise

Embryo viability is dependent on PIF. In the presence of anti-PIF-monoclonal antibody, a high rate of embryo demise was noted; the effect being dose-dependent.[55] PIF is taken up by viable embryos (mouse, cow, equine) confirming the autotrophic effect.[55] Specificity was demonstrated by using a scrambled peptide as a control—which failed to bind. Using a hardy bovine IVF model, where few embryos become blastocysts when cultured alone, PIF addition accelerated their development overcoming the block that bovine embryos have unless cultured in large groups.[59]

PIF's protective role aiding embryo survival in a potentially hostile environment has also been examined. In RPL, the embryo is exposed to circulating toxins, antibodies and oxygen radicals, among others. Since PIF targets the embryo directly, it negates embryo demise when serum containing the above toxins is added in culture, and the effect is dose-dependent.[59] It is the small molecules, which belong to the fraction less than 3 kDa (oxygen radicals, toxins), which delayed development as opposed to the high molecular weight molecules (antibodies and other proteins) which increased embryo demise. PIF interacts with the embryo and targets specific sites to exert both growth-promoting and protective properties. Specific PIF targets have been identified by passing 10 day old mouse embryo extracts using PIF-based affinity chromatography followed by quantitative mass spectrometry. This method has identified a number of classes of proteins; principally those related to oxidative stress (protein disulfide isomerase/thioredoxin) and heat shock proteins involved in preventing protein misfolding and actins/tubulins cytoskeleton/vascular/neural backbone. At day 10 (eight to nine weeks in human pregnancy) embryos transition from a hypoxic to an oxygenated environment due to formation of the placenta. PIF appears to play a significant protective role on the placenta. Thioredoxin protects against altered development in a hyperglycemic environment,[60] and anti-HSP antibody was shown to negatively affect cultured embryos' development.[61]

Implantation is an Embryo-Driven, Maternal-Responsive Process

Successful implantation requires intimate contact between the trophoblast and the decidua. Failed endometrial priming is frequently seen in cases of RPL. PIF, secreted by the embryo, may improve uterine receptivity by acting in concert with downstream expressed molecules to create the favorable environment in the endometrium.

We have examined whether PIF can affect beta integrin—a prime protein that is upregulated during the implantation window. In epithelial cells, but not in stromal cells, added PIF upregulates beta integrin expression.[62] Interestingly, upregulation took place independent of progesterone exposure. Hence, embryo specific signaling seems to be essential to create a maternal response to the incoming embryo. Others have shown that there are changes in a large number of genes' expression once the embryo becomes attached to the endometrium.[63] However, the change in gene expression is site-specific since this change is not observed in areas away from the implantation site. Consequently, it seems that the embryo is capable of creating a receptive environment, and this priming has to take place prior to implantation.

We have tested the effect of PIF on implantation by using an estrogen and progesterone primed stromal cell (HESC) model using global gene and protein analysis.[62,64] Notably the peptide acted as a proinflammatory agent. This is of interest because the endometrium, when irritated, increases implantation rates following embryo transfer.[65] Further, PIF promotes adhesion molecules that would facilitate embryo attachment and regulates apoptosis which is critical for implantation. Stromal cell separation and detachment enables the trophoblast to invade effectively. PIF regulates local immunity to eliminate apoptotic cells that could create a hostile proinflammatory environment. PIF also exerts antipathogenic effects by modulating TLRs (TOLL like receptors), thereby preventing implantation failure.

Remarkably, PIF promotes neural-related proteins in HESC perhaps protecting the notochord, the first embryonic structure.[64] Consequently, PIF may prevent adverse maternal environment-induced damage to the embryo.

The endometrial environment can be hostile. Using the equine model in endometrial cultures, PIF improved bacterial lipopolysaccharide (LPS)-induced inflammation by reducing PGF2a secretion and correlated with circulating progesterone levels.[66] Thus PIF may prevent implantation failure, the most vulnerable period of reproduction.

Following successful implantation, the decidua is formed. Using cultured decidual cells in culture, PIF's effect was examined, which showed a promoting effect on genes involved in protecting against an adverse environment.[64] In RPL, most losses occur in early gestation. Provided that the embryo is normal, the decidua is the site where the trophoblast derives its support and PIF could help to minimize adverse effects on the embryo.

The last phase in embryo/maternal interaction, which actually decides the fate of pregnancy, is trophoblast adherence and invasion. It was found that PIF promotes transformed trophoblastic cells' invasion.[67] However, it was not known whether this is also the case in primary trophoblastic cells. In a recent study, it was demonstrated that PIF also promotes primary human trophoblast invasion and mechanistically demonstrated that the effect on invasion operates through the matrix metalloproteinase (MMP)/tissue inhibitor of metalloproteinase-1 (TIMP)/integrin ratio through highly specific pathways. Further data showed that PIF is expressed in the trophoblast shortly after implantation (week five and above), and is highly localized in the extravillous (invasive) trophoblast. Uterine NK cells control against excessive invasion of the trophoblast and may lead to maternal hostility. Sequential *ex vivo* analysis showed the PIF secreted by the trophoblast is incorporated in uNK cells as evaluated at 10, 12, and 14 days of murine gestation. However, by day 14 PIF+ particles were released from uNK cells. Thus uNK hostility may be contained during gestation. However, in preparation for delivery, PIF levels decrease enabling the needed "rejection" phenomena to come into play. The gestational age-dependent expression of PIF (low in the human term placenta, and absent in the placenta at premature delivery) supports such a hypothesis.

The Role of Preimplantation Factor in Global Immune Regulation

Immunity drives reproduction and not vice versa. Systemic immunity is altered shortly postfertilization. Since PIF is detected in the maternal circulation prior to implantation, we examined the peptide's immune regulatory properties.[58,68,69] The results indicate that PIF has an important role in regulating maternal tolerance while keeping maternal defenses intact. PIF targets specific systemic immune cells, affecting cytokines and gene expression. PIF binds to naïve CD14+cells monocytes/neutrophils and, once activated, to T and B cells promoting the required Th2/Th1 cytokine ratio and expression. PIF promotes HLA-type genes related to tolerance in both naïve and anti-CD3/CD28 antibody induced PBMCs. In naïve cells, PIF promotes antipathogenic gene expression related to macrophage and NK cell action. In adaptive immunity, PIF controls genes involved in oxidative stress, protein misfolding and platelet activation. Thus the embryo, being a small antigen, creates only a limited signal indicating its presence regulating maternal immunity in order to be accepted. However, in the case of maternal adversity, there has to be a dual protective effect in which PIF participates. Firstly, PIF supports embryo preservation, and secondly, PIF may support maternal immunity to fight pathogens and disease. Examination of PIF/protein interactions revealed multitargeted interaction aided by the highly flexible folding structure of the peptide. Such observations may explain the profound differences observed between PIF's effect on innate and adaptive immunity.

Does the Embryo—Through Preimplantation Factor Action—Help Itself and the Mother to Prevent Adversity?

In RPL, systemic immunity plays an important role, especially overactive NK cells. We found that PIF reduces NK cell toxicity significantly, irrespective of whether the number of NK cells in the circulation was elevated or within the normal range.

Both immunoglobulin and intralipid have been suggested for treating RPL. Low dose PIF showed a similar inhibitory effect when tested side-by-side with high doses of the two other agents.[69] The effect of PIF is indirect, affecting CD69+ NK cell expression, a prime marker of NK activation. Thus, the embryo may be protected both by blocking serum and NK cytotoxicity, subsequently preventing further pregnancy losses in RPL.[59]

In order to further validate PIF's possible role in controlling systemic immune response, PIF's binding and effect on cytokines in peripheral blood mononuclear cells (PBMCs) of patients having >10 miscarriages and no viable birth were examined. There were significant changes both in binding characteristics and the cytokine secretion ratio compared to healthy controls. Therefore, PIF may identify patients prone to having altered systemic immune response that may lead to RPL.

Lessons Learned from Preimplantation Factor Efficacy in Nonpregnant Immune Disorder Models

Since pregnancy is a complex model for documenting the effect of a single agent, nonpregnant models have been utilized to test PIF. The observation that several autoimmune diseases are ameliorated in pregnancy, (except when severe) was recently reviewed.[70,71] It was found that PIF is effective in ameliorating approximately 20 different nonpregnant autoimmune/transplantation models. As the immunoregulatory effects of PIF are systemic as well as local, it is not surprising that PIF may affect other autoimmune processes. In juvenile diabetes and neuroinflammation models, the protection of target organs—pancreas and spinal cord—were noted, as were effects on circulating cytokines and immune phenotypes. As in pregnancy, the central mechanisms of protection are reduction of oxidative stress, protein misfolding and macrophage control.

Development of tolerance to the embryo without causing harmful immune-suppression is essential in reproduction. The use of the graft versus host model allowed us to examine this premise *in vivo*.[72,73] Semiallogeneic mesenchymal stem cells were transferred to a mouse where its immune cells were totally destroyed by radiation. PIF treatment prevented or reversed damage to skin, liver, and colon long-term. Since most pregnancies are semi- or allogeneic, such a model supports the observation that PIF has an important role in tolerance development. PIF also protects against a totally allogeneic transplant by preventing Graft vs host disease (GVHD) development. The donor embryo is a genetic mismatch, therefore PIF has an important role in the development of maternal tolerance. PIF also promotes autotransplantation of mesenchymal stem cells thereby facilitating the engraftment. Thereby, PIF may have a similar role in facilitating embryo implantation. Overall, the nonpregnant models investigating PIF's actions have enabled documentation of this peptide's multifaceted potential role in ensuring pregnancy success.

Summary

Overall, an integrated view of embryo–maternal interactions enables us to put in context the role of the conceptus and its unique secretory product PIF in reproductive success. (1) The embryo, a semi/ foreign entity, must sustain itself in an adverse environment. The embryo has an innate self-destructive potential, as poor quality embryos mostly fail to develop. The embryo also has autotrophic properties. (2) Uterine priming creates a favorable and nonhostile environment for the embryo. (3) Promotion of trophoblast invasion assures effective embryo–maternal interaction. (4) Regulation of systemic immunity has a dual role: protects itself and aids the maternal organism to fend off disease. Insight into these fundamental processes will provide a solid basis for development of effective diagnostic and therapeutic tools to reduce RPL. Finally, viewing pregnancy as embryo-centric and not maternal-centric will improve both our insight and management of RPL and other pathological conditions in pregnancy.

REFERENCES

1. Beer AE, Billingham RE, Yang SL. Maternally induced transplantation immunity, tolerance, and runt disease in rats. *J Exp Med* 1973;135:808–826.
2. Billingham RE, Head JR. Recipient treatment to overcome the allograft reaction, with special reference to nature's own solution. *Prog Clin Biol Res* 1986;224:159–85.
3. Hansel W, Hickey GJ. Early pregnancy signals in domestic animals. *Ann N Y Acad Sci* 1988;541:472–84.
4. Weitlauf HM. Embryonic signaling at implantation in the mouse. *Prog Clin Biol Res* 1989;294:359–76.
5. Soares MJ. The prolactin and growth hormone families: Pregnancy-specific hormones/cytokines at the maternal-fetal interface. *Reprod Biol Endocrinol* 2004;2:51.
6. Moffett A, Loke YW. The immunological paradox of pregnancy: A reappraisal. *Placenta* 2004;25:1–8.
7. Wright JM, Kiracofe GH, Beeman KB. Factors associated with shortened estrous cycles after abortion in beef heifers. *J Anim Sci* 1988;66:3185–9.
8. Alizadeh Z, Kageyama S, Aoki F. Degradation of maternal mRNA in mouse embryos: Selective degradation of specific mRNAs after fertilization. *Mol Reprod Dev* 2005;72:281–90.
9. Sharma S, Murphy SP, Barnea ER. Genes regulating implantation and fetal development: A focus on mouse knockout models. *Front Biosci* 2006;11:2123–37.
10. Piccinni MP, Scaletti C, Mavilia C, Lazzeri E, Romagnani P, Natali I et al. Production of IL-4 and leukemia inhibitory factor by T cells of the cumulus oophorus: A favorable microenvironment for pre-implantation embryo development. *Eur J Immunol* 2001;31:2431–7.
11. O'Neill C. Partial characterization of the embryo-derived platelet-activating factor in mice. *J Reprod Fertil* 1985;75:375–80.
12. O'Neill C. Thrombocytopenia is an initial maternal response to fertilization in mice. *J Reprod Fertil* 1985;73:559–66.
13. Somerset DA, Zheng Y, Kilby MD, Sansom DM, Drayson MT. Normal human pregnancy is associated with an elevation in the immune suppressive CD25+ CD4+ regulatory T-cell subset. *Immunology* 2004;112:38–43.
14. Turner K, Horobin RW. Permeability of the mouse zona pellucida: A structure-staining-correlation model using coloured probes. *J Reprod Fertil* 1997;111:259–65.
15. Block J, Hansen PJ. Interaction between season and culture with insulin-like growth factor-1 on survival of *in vitro* produced embryos following transfer to lactating dairy cows. *Theriogenology* 2007;67:1518–29.
16. Diaz-Cueto L, Stein P, Jacobs A, Schultz RM, Gerton GL. Modulation of mouse preimplantation embryo development by acrogranin (epithelin/granulin precursor). *Dev Biol* 2000;217:406–18.
17. Jousan FD, Oliveira LJ, Hansen PJ. Short-Term culture of *in vitro* produced bovine preimplantation embryos with insulin-like growth factor-i prevents heat shock-induced apoptosis through activation of the Phosphatidylinositol 3-Kinase/Akt pathway. *Mol Reprod Dev* 2008;75:681–8.
18. Kawamura K, Fukuda J, Kumagai J, Shimizu Y, Kodama H, Nakamura A et al. Gonadotropin-releasing hormone I analog acts as an antiapoptotic factor in mouse blastocysts. *Endocrinology* 2005;146:4105–16.

19. Kawamura K, Kawamura N, Kumagai J, Fukuda J, Tanaka T. Tumor necrosis factor regulation of apoptosis in mouse preimplantation embryos and its antagonism by transforming growth factor alpha/phosphatidylionsitol 3-kinase signaling system. *Biol Reprod* 2007;76:611–8.

20. Wei Z, Park KW, Day BN, Prather RS. Effect of epidermal growth factor on preimplantation development and its receptor expression in porcine embryos. *Mol Reprod Dev* 2001;60:457–62.

21. XU JS, Lee YL, Lee KF, Kwok KL, Lee WM, Luk JM et al. Embryotrophic factor-3 from human oviductal cells enhances proliferation, suppresses apoptosis and stimulates the expression of the beta1 subunit of sodium-potassium ATPase in mouse embryos. *Hum Reprod* 2004;19:2919–26.

22. Choudhury SR, Knapp LA. Human reproductive failure I: Immunological factors. *Hum Reprod Update* 2001;7:113–34.

23. Raghupathy R. Th1-type immunity is incompatible with successful pregnancy. *Immunol Today* 1997;18:478–82.

24. Druckmann R, Druckmann MA. Progesterone and the immunology of pregnancy. *J Steroid Biochem Mol Biol* 2005;97:389–96.

25. Kralickova M, Sima P, Rokyta Z. Role of the leukemia-inhibitory factor gene mutations in infertile women: The embryo-endometrial cytokine cross talk during implantation—A delicate homeostatic equilibrium. *Folia Microbiol (Praha)* 2005;50:179–86.

26. Aplin JD, Kimber SJ. Trophoblast-uterine interactions at implantation. *Reprod Biol Endocrinol* 2004;2:48.

27. Sadek KH, Cagampang FR, Bruce KD, Shreeve N, Macklon N, Cheong Y. Variation in stability of housekeeping genes in endometrium of healthy and polycystic ovarian syndrome women. *Hum Reprod* 2012;27:251–6.

28. Borthwick JM, Charnock-Jones DS, Tom BD, Hull ML, Teirney R, Phillips SC et al. Determination of the transcript profile of human endometrium. *Mol Hum Reprod* 2003;9:19–33.

29. Quezada S, Avellaira C, Johnson MC, Gabler F, Fuentes A, Vega M. Evaluation of steroid receptors, coregulators, and molecules associated with uterine receptivity in secretory endometria from untreated women with polycystic ovary syndrome. *Fertil Steril* 2006;85:1017–26.

30. Horcajadas JA, Pellicer A, Simon C. Wide genomic analysis of human endometrial receptivity: New times, new opportunities. *Hum Reprod Update* 2007;13:77–86.

31. Milne SA, Perchick GB, Boddy SC, Jabbour HN. Expression, localization, and signaling of PGE$_2$ and EP2/EP4 receptors in human nonpregnant endometrium across the menstrual cycle. *J Clin Endocrinol Metab* 2001;86:4453–9.

32. Francis J, Rai R, Sebire NJ, El-Gaddal S, Fernandes MS, Jindal P et al. Impaired expression of endometrial differentiation markers and complement regulatory proteins in patients with recurrent pregnancy loss associated with antiphospholipid syndrome. *Mol Hum Reprod* 2006;12:435–42.

33. Buckingham KL, Stone PR, Smith JF, Chamley LW. Antiphospholipid antibodies in serum and follicular fluid—Is there a correlation with IVF implantation failure? *Hum Reprod* 2006;21:728–34.

34. Ntrivalas EI, Bowser CR, Kwak-Kim J, Beaman KD, Gilman-Sachs A. Expression of killer immunoglobulin-like receptors on peripheral blood NK cell subsets of women with recurrent spontaneous abortions or implantation failures. *Am J Reprod Immunol* 2005;53:215–21.

35. Pinkas H, Fisch B, Tadir Y, Ovadia J, Amit S, Shohat B. Immunosuppressive activity in culture media containing human oocytes fertilized in vitro. *Arch Androl* 1992;28:53–9.

36. Fortin M, Ouellette MJ, Lambert RD. TGF-β$_2$ and PGE$_2$ in rabbit blastocoelic fluid can modulate GM-CSF production by human lymphocytes. *Am J Reprod Immunol* 1997;38:129–39.

37. Cameo P, Srisuparp S, Strakova Z, Fazleabas AT. Chorionic gonadotropin and uterine dialogue in the primate. *Reprod Biol Endocrinol* 2004;2:50.

38. O'Neill C. The role of paf in embryo physiology. *Hum Reprod Update* 2005;11:215–28.

39. Roudebush WE, Wininger JD, Jones AE, Wright G, Toledo AA, Kort HI et al. Embryonic platelet-activating factor: An indicator of embryo viability. *Hum Reprod* 2002;17:1306–10.

40. Ohnuma K, Ito K, Takahashi J, Nambo Y, Miyake Y. Partial purification of mare early pregnancy factor. *Am J Reprod Immunol* 2004;51:95–101.

41. Athanasas-Platsis S, Somodevilla-Torres MJ, Morton H, Cavanagh AC. Investigation of the immunocompetent cells that bind early pregnancy factor and preliminary studies of the early pregnancy factor target molecule. *Immunol Cell Biol* 2004;82:361–9.

42. Akyol S, Gercel-Taylor C, Reynolds LC, Taylor DD. HSP-10 in ovarian cancer: Expression and suppression of T-cell signaling. *Gynecol Oncol* 2006;101:481–6.

43. Fuzzi B, Rizzo R, Criscuoli L, Noci I, Melchiorri L, Scarselli B et al. HLA-G expression in early embryos is a fundamental prerequisite for the obtainment of pregnancy. *Eur J Immunol* 2002;32:311–5.

44. Bainbridge D, Ellis S, Le Bouteiller P, Sargent I. HLA-G remains a mystery. *Trends Immunol* 2001;22:548–52.

45. Gomez-Lozano N, De Pablo R, Puente S, Vilches C. Recognition of HLA-G by the NK cell receptor KIR2DL4 is not essential for human reproduction. *Eur J Immunol* 2003;33:639–44.

46. Yan WH, Fan LA, Yang JQ, Xu LD, Ge Y, Yao FJ. HLA-G polymorphism in a Chinese Han population with recurrent spontaneous abortion. *Int J Immunogenet* 2006;33:55–8.

47. Criscuoli L, Rizzo R, Fuzzi B, Melchiorri L, Menicucci A, Cozzi C et al. Lack of Histocompatibility Leukocyte Antigen-G expression in early embryos is not related to germinal defects or impairment of interleukin-10 production by embryos. *Gynecol Endocrinol* 2005;20:264–9.

48. Barnea ER, Lahijani KI, Roussev R, Barnea JD, Coulam CB. Use of lymphocyte platelet binding assay for detecting a preimplantation factor: A quantitative assay. *Am J Reprod Immunol* 1994;32:133–8.

49. Rosario GX, Modi DN, Sachdeva G, Manjramkar DD, Puri CP. Morphological events in the primate endometrium in the presence of a preimplantation embryo, detected by the serum preimplantation factor bioassay. *Hum Reprod* 2005;20:61–71.

50. Coulam CB, Roussev RG, Thomason EJ, Barnea ER. Preimplantation factor (PIF) predicts subsequent pregnancy loss. *Am J Reprod Immunol* 1995;34:88–92.

51. Roussev RG, Coulam CB, Kaider BD, Yarkoni M, Leavis PC, Barnea ER. Embryonic origin of preimplantation factor (PIF): Biological activity and partial characterization. *Mol Hum Reprod* 1996;2:883–7.

52. Roussev RG, Barnea ER, Thomason EJ, Coulam CB. A novel bioassay for detection of preimplantation factor (PIF). *Am J Reprod Immunol* 1995;33:68–73.

53. Barnea ER, Simon J, Levine SP, Coulam CB, Taliadouros GS, Leavis PC. Progress in characterization of pre-implantation factor in embryo cultures and in vivo. *Am J Reprod Immunol* 1999;42:95–9.

54. Barnea ER. Insight into early pregnancy events: The emerging role of the embryo. *Am J Reprod Immunol* 2004;51:319–22.

55. Stamatkin CW, Roussev RG, Stout M, Absalon-Medina V, Ramu S, Goodman C et al. PreImplantation Factor (PIF) correlates with early mammalian embryo development-bovine and murine models. *Reprod Biol Endocrinol* 2011;9:63.

56. Keramitsoglou T, Mentorou C, Promponas E, Perros GPT, Daves S, Mastrominas M et al. Preimplantation Factor (PIF*) contributes significantly to the prediction of pregnancy after single embryo transfer. *Joint International Congress of Asri and Esri*, Hamburg, Germany, 2012.

57. Ramu S, Stamatkin C, Timms L, Ruble M, Roussev R, Barnea ER. PreImplantation Factor (PIF*) detection in maternal circulation in early pregnancy correlates with live birth (bovine model). *Reprod Biol Endocrinol* 2013;11:105.

58. Barnea ER. Applying embryo-derived immune tolerance to the treatment of immune disorders. *Ann N Y Acad Sci* 2007;1110:602–18.

59. Stamatkin CW, Roussev RG, Stout M, Coulam CB, Triche E, Godke RA et al. Preimplantation factor negates embryo toxicity and promotes embryo development in culture. *Reprod Biomed Online* 2011;23:517–24.

60. Yang P, Reece EA. Role of HIF-1α in maternal hyperglycemia-induced embryonic vasculopathy. *Am J Obstet Gynecol* 2011;204:332 e1–7.

61. Matwee C, Kamaruddin M, Betts DH, Basrur PK, King WA. The effects of antibodies to heat shock protein 70 in fertilization and embryo development. *Mol Hum Reprod* 2001;7:829–37.

62. Barnea ER, Kirk D, Paidas MJ. Preimplantation Factor (PIF*) promoting role in embryo implantation: Increases endometrial Integrin-$\alpha2\beta3$ and amphiregulin and epiregulin while reducing betacellulin expression via MAPK in decidua. *Reprod Biol Endocrinol* 2012;10:50.

63. Kashiwagi A, Digirolamo CM, Kanda Y, Niikura Y, Esmon CT, Hansen TR et al. The postimplantation embryo differentially regulates endometrial gene expression and decidualization. *Endocrinology* 2007;148:4173–84.

64. Paidas MJ, Krikun G, Huang SJ, Jones R, Romano M, Annunziato J et al. A genomic and proteomic investigation of the impact of preimplantation factor on human decidual cells. *Am J Obstet Gynecol* 2010;202, 459:e1–8.

65. Gnainsky Y, Granot I, Aldo PB, Barash A, OR Y, Schechtman E et al. Local injury of the endometrium induces an inflammatory response that promotes successful implantation. *Fertil Steril* 2010;94:2030–6.

66. Kember J, Nash D, Barnea ER. PreImplantation Factor (PIF*) displays developmental-related evolving immune anti-inflammatory response of equine endometrial explants *in vitro*. *British Equine Veterinary Association (Beva) Congress*. Birmingham, UK, 2012.

67. Duzyj CM, Barnea ER, Li M, Huang SJ, Krikun G, Paidas MJ. Preimplantation factor promotes first trimester trophoblast invasion. *Am J Obstet Gynecol* 2010;203–402:e1–4.

68. Barnea ER, Kirk D, Ramu S, Rivnay B, Roussev R, Paidas MJ. PreImplantation Factor (PIF) orchestrates systemic antiinflammatory response by immune cells: Effect on peripheral blood mononuclear cells. *Am J Obstet Gynecol* 2012;207–313:e1–11.

69. Roussev R, Dons'koi B, Stamatkin C, Ramu S, Chernyshov V, Coulam CB et al. Preimplantation Factor inhibits circulating natural killer cell cytotoxicity and reduces CD69 expression: Implications for recurrent pregnancy loss therapy. *Reprod Biomed Online* 2012;26:79–87.

70. Barnea ER, Rambaldi M, Paidas MJ, Mecacci F. Reproduction and autoimmune disease: Important translational implications from embryo-maternal interaction. *Immunotherapy* 2013;5:769–80.

71. Paidas MJ, Annunziato J, Romano M, Weiss L, Or R, Barnea ER. Pregnancy and Multiple Sclerosis (MS): A Beneficial Association. Possible therapeutic application of embryo-specific Pre-implantation Factor (PIF*). *Am J Reprod Immunol* 2012;68:456–64.

72. Azar Y, Shainer R, Almogi-Hazan O, Bringer R, Compton SR, Paidas MJ, Barnea ER, Or R. PreImplantation factor reduces graft-versus-host disease by regulating immune response and lowering oxidative stress (Murine Model). *Biol Blood Marrow Transplant* 2013;19:519–28.

73. Shainer R, Azar Y, Almogi-Hazan O, Bringer R, Compton SR, Paidas MJ et al. Immune regulation and oxidative stress reduction by preimplantation factor following syngeneic or allogeneic bone marrow transplantation. *Conference Papers in Medicine* 2013;2013:1–8.

3

Genetics of Spontaneous Abortions

Joe Leigh Simpson

Introduction

Genetic factors are the most common causes of spontaneous abortion. From 50% to 80% of first trimester abortions show numerical chromosomal abnormalities. Other potential genetic causes include single-gene mutations or polygenic factors, almost unexplored in etiology of spontaneous abortions. In this chapter, we shall restrict discussion to the frequency and most common genetic causes of sporadic and recurrent abortions. We will not consider the unequivocal underlying genetic basis of so-called "nongenetic" causes that include heritable and nonheritable thrombophilias.

Chromosomal Abnormalities in Preimplantation Embryos

The frequency of losses in human preimplantation embryos has long been known to be very high.[1] Of morphologically normal embryos about 50–80% show numerical chromosomal abnormalities (aneuploidy or polyploidy), depending upon maternal age, initially based on couples undergoing preimplantation genetic diagnosis (PGD)[2] whose embryos were studied by fluorescent *in situ* hybridization (FISH) with five to seven chromosome-specific probes. Using array comparative genome hybridization (CGH) or single nucleotide polymorphism (SNP)-based methods allowing aneuploidy to be assessed in all 24 chromosomes, rates of aneuploidy are as high as 85–100% in women age 43 years and above.[3] These data are consistent with 6% aneuploidy in sperm from ostensibly normal males[4] and 20% aneuploidy in oocytes[5] obtained at time of *in vitro* fertilization. Aneuploidy rates in embryos and oocytes increase as maternal age increases.

Not surprisingly, chromosomal abnormalities are even more frequent in morphologically abnormal embryos than morphologically normal embryos.[2] Using FISH with five to seven chromosome-specific probes, abnormality rates of 75% are observed in morphologically normal cleavage stage embryos.[2] Contemporary studies utilizing 24 chromosome array CGH have not been reported, to my knowledge, in a morphologically abnormal cohort of embryos.

Chromosomal Abnormalities—in Clinically Recognized Spontaneous Abortion

Frequency

That 50% of clinically recognized pregnancy losses show a chromosomal abnormality[6–8] was initially based on analysis of spontaneously expelled products. If chorionic villus sampling (CVS) is performed after ultrasound diagnosis of fetal demise, the frequency is 75–90%.[9,10] Contemporary studies now utilize comparative genomic hybridization (CGH; microarray analysis) and have the advantage of not requiring cultured cells and in revealing abnormalities in abortuses more subtle than evident by karyotype (5–7 Mb sensitivity). Schaeffer et al.[11] performed CGH using microarrays on 41 abortuses that had previously been analyzed by karyotype and diagnosed as normal. Array CGH revealed heretofore unrecognized abnormalities in 4 of 41 cases. Coupled with data on abortuses recognized as deceased at the time of CVS, the frequency of chromosomal abnormalities in women age 35 or above can confidently be stated to be 60–75%.

In the second trimester, chromosomal abnormalities are less frequent, and the frequency is less certain. Some abortuses recognized in the second trimester are actually missed abortions that were retained *in utero* after a first trimester demise. It has long been recognized that fetal demise may precede spontaneous expulsion of the products of conception by several weeks.[12] Chromosomal abnormalities detected in second trimester abortions are similar to those observed in liveborn infants: trisomies 13, 18, and 21; monosomy X; and sex chromosome polysomies. The frequency of these anomalies is estimated to be approximately 15%.

In third trimester losses (stillborn infants), the frequency of chromosomal abnormalities has traditionally been stated to be 5% based on karyotypes. However, using array CGH the rate is higher.[13] This "increase" reflects tissue from stillborns often not growing *in vitro*, a requisite for performing a karyotype but not for array CGH. A major problem in assessing the frequency of chromosomal abnormalities is that maceration ensues soon after fetal death. This is obviously days in advance of delivery. Hefler et al.[14] found that 63% of 139 third trimester losses were macerated, impeding accurate morphological assessment and ability to perform cytogenetic studies. Irrespective, the frequency of chromosomal abnormalities in stillborns is lower than the 0.6% incidence found in liveborns in the general population.

Spectrum of Chromosomal Abnormalities

Autosomal Trisomy

Autosomal trisomies comprise approximately 50% of cytogenetically abnormal spontaneous abortions. Trisomy for every chromosome has been observed. Table 3.1 shows frequencies in one older series, still relevant. Trisomies of most relevance are 16, 22, 21, 15, 13, and 14 in that descending order. Trisomy 16 is rarely, if ever, observed in liveborns in nonmosaic form, but is the most common aberration in the abortus. These six chromosomes in aggregate account for 70% of trisomies—an important consideration in PGD. When less common aneuploidies occur, they are often accompanied by one of the sentinel trisomies (double trisomy). Thus, studying only the sentinel liveborn trisomies plus X and Y (perhaps nine chromosomes) can actually detect 90% of aneuploidies in embryos at PGD. Whether this holds for clinically recognized spontaneous abortions is less clear.

Correlations between placental or embryonic morphological abnormalities and specific trisomies are usually imprecise. Complications include nonspecific villous changes following fetal demise *in utero*. Thus, low predictive value exists when placental histology is used to distinguish aneuploid from euploid abortuses. A few correlations are valid. Fetuses with trisomies incompatible with life grow more slowly than those with trisomies compatible with life (e.g., trisomies 13, 18, 21). In one series crown-rump length for the latter was 20.65 mm, compared with only 10.66 mm for the former.[15] Either fetuses with nonlethal trisomies live longer than those with lethal trisomies, or fetuses with lethal trisomies exhibit greater intrauterine growth retardation, or both.

Abortuses from nonlethal trisomies (13, 18, and 21) also tend to show anomalies consistent with those found in full-term liveborn trisomic infants.[15,16] Malformations observed may be more severe than those found in induced abortions detected after prenatal diagnosis.

Most trisomies show a maternal age effect, but the relative effect varies among chromosomes. Maternal age correlates positively with errors at meiosis I, the most common cytological explanation for trisomies. The proportion of trisomies that arise at meiosis I versus meiosis II has traditionally been considered to vary among aneuploidies. Virtually all trisomy 16 cases are maternal in origin, and arise in meiosis I.[17] In trisomies 13 and 21, 90% are maternal, usually arising at meiosis I. In trisomy 18, however, two-thirds of the 90% of maternal origin cases arise at meiosis II.[18,19] These data have, however, traditionally been based on methods that have now been superseded. In particular, PGD aneuploidy testing has shown that premature chromatid separation is commonly observed during polar body analysis for PGD. Sometimes correction even occurs in meiosis II. Using these newer data, meiosis I errors seem only marginally higher (41.7% versus 35.2) in oogenesis than meiosis II errors; errors in both meiosis I and II are not uncommon. The relative distribution of errors seems to differ from that observed in trisomies recovered later in pregnancy.

TABLE 3.1

Chromosomal Completion in Spontaneous Abortions; Recognized
Clinically in the First Trimester

Completion	Frequency	Percentage
Normal:46,XX or 46,XY		54.1
Triploidy		7.7
69,XXX	2.7	
69,XYX	0.2	
69,XXY	4.0	
Other	0.8	
Tetraploidy:		2.6
92,XXX	1.5	
92,XXYY	0.55	
Not stated	0.55	
Monosmy X		18.6
Structural abnormalities		1.5
Sex chromosomal polysomy:		0.2
47,XXX	0.05	
47,XXY	0.15	
Autosomal monosomy (G)		0.1
Autosomal trisomy for chromosomes:		22.3
1	0	
2	1.11	
3	0.25	
4	0.64	
5	0.04	
6	0.14	
7	0.89	
8	0.79	
9	0.72	
10	0.36	
11	0.04	
12	0.18	
13	1.07	
14	0.82	
15	1.68	
16	7.27	
17	0.18	
18	1.15	
19	0.01	
20	0.61	
21	2.11	
22	2.26	
Double trisomy		0.7
Mosaic trisomy		1.3
Other abnormalities or not specified		0.9
		100.0

Source: Pooled data from several series, as gathered by Simpson J, Bombard A.
In: Edmunds DK, ed. *Spontaneous Abortion*, Oxford: Blackwell; 1987.
p. 51–76.

Maternal meiosis errors correlate not only with advanced maternal age, but also with decreased or absent meiotic recombination, which depend on synapse involving homologous sequences.[18–21] Location of the recombinant event on a given chromosome and the exact nature of recombination are pivotal, as discussed elsewhere.[22] Maternal age related aneuploidy is usually explained on the basis oocytes ovulated earlier in life are believed to be more likely to have undergone genetic recombination and, hence, be less predisposed to nondisjunction.[23] More recently it has been appreciated that premature chromatid separation is frequent in oocytes.[21]

Errors in paternal meiosis account for 10% of acrocentric (13, 14, 15, 21, and 22) trisomies.[24] In nonacrocentric trisomies, parental meiotic errors are equally likely to arise at meiosis I or II.[25] Paternal meiotic errors account for 10% of trisomy 21 cases, and for some cases of trisomy 2 abortuses. A paternal contribution is uncommon in other abortus trisomies.

Double Trisomy

The frequency of double trisomy in abortuses is more common than expected by chance. Frequency varies more than for other chromosomal abnormalities, which may reflect vicissitudes of culture (failure) or differences in sample characteristics (maternal age; gestational age). Double trisomies have traditionally been said to be slightly less than 1% of all abortuses[26,27] although a recent report of 517 abortuses found double trisomies in 2.2% of 321 successful karyotyped abortuses.[27]

Double trisomies most often involve the X chromosome, but may involve the Y chromosome or autosomes 21, 18, 16, 22, 13, 2, and 15 in descending order (Table 3.2). Diego-Alvarez et al.[27] tabulated the exact combination of the 178 reported double trisomies. In liveborns, approximately 50 double trisomies have been reported.[28] Usually one of the additional chromosomes is an X and the other is 13, 18, or 21. Advanced maternal age is a striking feature.[26–28] In the data of Diego-Alvarez et al.,[27] the mean maternal age was 39.7 ± 3.4 years. Almost all analyzed cases originated in maternal meiosis.

Gestational age was 8.7 ± 2.2 weeks at abortion in double trisomies in the series of Reddy,[26] compared with 10.1 ± 2.9 weeks for a single trisomy. In the series of Diego-Alvarez et al.[27] the gestation age was 8.2 ± 1.7 for double trisomies. The sex ratio was approximately 1 in both series.

Morphological examination usually reveals an empty sac[26,27] and only occasionally an embryo of normal morphology. In one study, five of seven double trisomies showed no morphological details;[28] one was anembryonic and the other (48,XXX + 18) showed hydrops fetalis.

Triploidy

In polyploidy, more than two haploid chromosomal complements exist. Nonmosaic triploidy ($3n = 69$) is more common than tetraploidy ($4n = 92$). Of general interest is the association between diandric (paternally inherited) triploidy and hydatidiform mole. A "partial mole" exists if molar tissue and fetal parts coexist. Partial (triploid) moles must be distinguished from the more common "complete" hydatidiform moles. Complete moles are 46,XX, exclusively of androgenetic origin, and exclusively villous tissue.[29]

TABLE 3.2

Recurrent Aneuploidy: Relationship between Karyotypes of Successive Abortuses

Complement of First Abortus	Complement of Second Abortus					
	Normal	Trisomy	Monosomy	Triploidy	Tetraploidy	De novo Rearrangement
Normal	142	18	5	7	3	2
Trisomy	33	30	1	4	3	1
Monosomy X	7	5	3	3	0	0
Triploidy	7	4	1	4	0	0
Tetraploidy	3	1	0	2	0	0
De novo rearrangement	1	3	0	0	0	0

Source: Data of Warburton D. et al. *Am J Hum Genet* 1987;41(3):465–83.

Placental findings in diandric triploid placentas include a disproportionately large gestational sac, focal (partial) hydropic degeneration of placental villi, and trophoblast hyperplasia.[30] Placental hydropic changes are progressive and, hence, difficult to identify in early pregnancy. Irrespective of chromosomal status, placental villi also undergo nonspecific hydropic degeneration following fetal demise. This makes correlations between histological and cytogenetic findings difficult. Embryonic/fetal malformations associated with triploid abortuses include neural tube defects and omphaloceles, both anomalies occurring in triploid conceptuses surviving to term. Facial dysmorphia and limb abnormalities have also been reported.[31] There is no apparent correlation between embryonic morphology and parental origin (diandry or digyny).[31]

Triploid abortuses are usually 69,XXY or 69,XXX. The origin has long been presumed to be due to dispermy.[29,32,33] Triploidy may follow either fertilization by two haploid sperm or fertilization by single diploid sperm.[33,34]

Tetraploidy

Tetraploidy ($4n = 92$) is less common than triploidy and rarely progresses beyond two to three weeks of embryonic life. This chromosomal abnormality can be associated with persistent trophoblastic disease, and thus needs to be identified in order to provide appropriate clinical follow-up. Tetraploidy in embryonic tissue should be distinguished from the not uncommon, and clinically insignificant, tetraploid cells found in amniotic fluid. True fetal tetraploidy does exist[35] and probably arises from failure of cytokinesis.[36] Failure of cytokinesis has been deduced on the basis of chromosomal complement (92,XXXX or 92,XXYY), and more recently confirmed by molecular studies.[37]

Monosomy

Autosomal monosomy appears to be lethal prior to or just beyond implantation, and thus seems not to persist to clinical recognition. Monosomy X, however, accounts for 15–20% of chromosomally abnormal specimens. Early monosomy X abortuses usually consist of only an umbilical chord stump. If survival persists until later in gestation, anomalies characteristic of Turner syndrome may be seen. These include cystic hygromas, generalized edema, and cardiac defects. Unlike liveborn 45,X individuals, 45,X abortuses show germ cells; however, germ cells rarely develop beyond the primordial stage. The pathogenesis of 45,X germ cell failure thus seems to be increased attrition of germ cells, rather than failure of germ cell development. Yet existence of germ cells during embryogenesis explains the rare but well-documented pregnancies occurring in 45,X individuals. Mosaicism (45,XX/46,XX) need not necessarily be invoked as the mechanism explaining these pregnancies.

Approximately 80% of monosomy X occurs as a result of paternal sex chromosome loss.[38] Consequently, there is a lack of a maternal age effect in 45,X. An inverse age effect has been reported.

Sex Chromosomal Polysomy (X or Y)

The complements 47,XXY and 47,XYY each occur in about 1 per 800 liveborn male births; 47,XXX occurs in 1 per 800 female births. X or Y polysomies are slightly (10%) more common in abortuses than in liveborn.

Recurrent Aneuploidy and its Clinical Consequences

In first trimester abortions recurrent aneuploidy occurs more often than expected by chance. Chromosomal complements of recurrent abortuses in a given family are more likely to be either recurrently normal or recurrently abnormal (Table 3.3). That is, if the complement of the first abortus is abnormal, the likelihood is increased that the complement of the second abortus will also be abnormal. This was originally based on data from Hassold[7] collected in Hawaii. Recurrence usually involves trisomy, for which ramifications exist with respect to the therapeutic management (or lack thereof). Controversy exists as to what extent the principle applies that numerical chromosomal abnormalities (aneuploidy) explain recurrent pregnancy losses. In the view of this author, recurrent aneuploidy should clinically apply until the number of losses reaches or exceeds four.

TABLE 3.3

Risk of Aneuploidy by Number of Prior Miscarriages; Stratified by Maternal Age

No. of Prior Spontaneous Abortions	Maternal Age <35 years	
	Adjusted OR for Trisomy 13, 18, 21[a]	Adjusted OR for All Aneuploidies[a]
0	1.00	1.00
1	1.27 (0.74–2.08)	1.19 (0.78–1.84)
2	1.31 (0.80–2.13)	1.21 (0.94–1.58)
≥3	1.36 (0.46–2.73)	1.41 (0.56–3.19)
No. of Prior Spontaneous Abortions	Maternal Age >35 years	
	Adjusted OR for Trisomy 13, 18, 21[a]	Adjusted OR for All Aneuploidies[a]
0	1.00	1.00
1	1.23 (1.04–1.52)	1.23 (1.00–1.52)
2	1.34 (1.01–1.82)	1.30 (0.99–1.74)
≥3	1.56 (1.03–2.31)	1.68 (1.12–2.52)

Source: Data from Bianco K et al. *Obstet Gynecol* 2006;107(5):1098–102.

Note: Comparison is with women with no spontaneous abortions, controlling for parity and indications for prenatal diagnosis.

[a] OR, odds ratio, 95% confidence intervals.

Some of the nonrandom distributions naturally reflect merely increasing incidence of aneuploidy with increasing maternal age. Adjustments for maternal age thus account for some of the ostensibly nonrandom distribution and, initially in the opinion of Warburton et al.,[39] precluded a relationship. That report by Warburton et al. pooled cases collected in New York City samples with the previously collected cohort from Hawaii;[7] however, a major confounder is that the New York City cases extended to 28 weeks' gestation. Second trimester cases predictably had a lower overall aneuploidy rate than the almost exclusive first trimester cases. Later studies of recurrent aneuploidy convinced Warburton that the concept of recurrent aneuploidy is indeed valid.[40]

Further support is derived from prenatal diagnosis samples, comparing results to predicted pregnancy outcome. Bianco et al.[41] studied 46,939 women undergoing prenatal genetic diagnosis (CVS or amniocentesis). The prevalence of aneuploidy increased progressively as the number of prior spontaneous abortuses increased (Table 3.3): 1.39% with no prior abortuses, 1.67% after one, 1.84% after two, and 2.18% after three abortions. After adjustments for maternal age, ethnicity, and type of invasive procedure (a surrogate indicator of gestational age), the odds ratios were 1.21 (95% confidence interval (CI) 1.01–1.47), 1.26, and 1.51, respectively. These findings thus confirmed an earlier study by Drugan et al.[42]

More recent support for the concept of recurrent aneuploidy is the occurrence of repeated trisomic preimplantation embryos in successive ART cycles. Comparing aneuploidy in cleavage stage embryos in women having aneuploid versus euploid embryos in prior cycles, Munne et al.[43] found aneuploidy rates to be 37% versus 21% in women under age 35 years, and 34% versus 31.5% in women over 35 years. Rubio et al.[44] reported increased aneuploid embryos in women undergoing PGD for repeated abortions, compared to women undergoing PGD for Mendelian indications. Frequencies of chromosomal abnormalities were 71% versus 45%, in abortuses, respectively.

Given the phenomenon of recurrent aneuploidy, and given that 50% of all abortuses are abnormal cytogenetically, aneuploidy should be as likely to be detected in a recurrent abortus as in a sporadic abortus. This has indeed proved to be true in most series. Among 420 abortuses obtained from women with repeated losses, Stephenson et al.[45] found 46% with chromosomal abnormalities. Their comparison was unselected pooled data, which showed 48% of abortuses to be abnormal; 27% of the original sample was trisomic.

Although recurrent aneuploidy should be assumed to apply with two or three losses, this does not necessarily hold for higher-order losses. These seem more likely to be cytogenetically normal.[46] Maternal factors ("nongenetic") thus become more plausible explanations, especially when numbers of losses exceed four. Consecutive losses of high number also favor nonaneuploid explanations because one would not necessarily expect every single abortus to be aneuploid.

Consistent with the above, Carp et al.[47] found that among women having three or more abortuses, the likelihood that the abortus would have an abnormal karyotype was only 29%. After an aneuploid abortus, the likelihood of a subsequent live birth was 68% (13 of 19). Yet if the abortus was euploid, the subsequent live birth rate was 41% (16 of 39). The likely explanation for the difference between studies is differences in samples, specifically increased gestational age in the sample of Carp et al.[47] That only 29% of abortuses in the series of Carp et al.[47] were chromosomally abnormal is consistent with their inclusion criteria extending to 20 weeks' gestation. There is less reason to expect recurrent aneuploidy in the second trimester, given the low (15%) frequency of chromosomal abnormalities and other explanations in the second trimester. There were also a higher mean number of previous pregnancy losses (4.7) in the series of Carp et al.[47]

Clinical Management of Recurrent Aneuploidy

If no information exists on chromosomal status of prior abortuses, chromosomal microarrays may yield information from paraffin block specimens.[48] If no information can be obtained, it is less clear whether prenatal genetic diagnosis is appropriate. However, the risk of an aneuploid offspring is definitely increased over background maternal age, and indeed can be calculated as discussed above.[41] The small but finite risk of amniocentesis or CVS is especially troublesome to couples who have had difficulty maintaining a pregnancy. Noninvasive approaches may be the preferable initial option, and with cell-free fetal DNA sensitivity for detecting trisomy 21 is over 99%. However, more information is obtained from the karyotype or array CGH possible with an invasive procedure. PGD is another option, allowing selective transfer of euploid embryos and clearly decreasing clinical abortions in couples with repeated abortions.[49] This is most applicable as maternal age advances; the frequency of aneuploid embryos increases from a background of 25% in younger women to over 90% at age 45 years.[3] These daunting odds mean pregnancy resulting in a liveborn is clinically unlikely. If one transfers euploid embryos, studies consistently show abortion rates only around 13–15% irrespective of maternal age. This strategy is more feasible with trophectoderm biopsy 24 chromosome array CGH.

Liveborn Consequences of Recurrent Abortions

To what extent are couples predisposed to recurrent aneuploidy at increased risk not only for aneuploid abortuses but also for aneuploid liveborns? The trisomic autosome in a subsequent pregnancy might not always confer lethality, but might be compatible with life (e.g., trisomy 21). Counseling for liveborn trisomy 21 following an aneuploid abortus has long been considered to confer a risk of about 1%.[50] Based on first trimester trisomies, which may or may not survive, Snijders and Nicolaides[51] reported a recurrence rate of 0.7% following trisomy 21 and 0.7% following trisomy 18. Both are higher than age-related background. Bianco et al.[41] provided data on the quantitative consequences of prior abortion after unknown karyotype. If the abortions are recurrent but no information is available on the chromosomal status, odds ratios provided by Bianco et al.[41] provide patient specific risk (Table 3.3). For example, if the a priori Down syndrome risk is 1 in 300, a woman's calculated risk after 3 abortions would be $1/300 \times 1.68$ or 1 in 179 if she were older than 35 years.

Structural Chromosomal Rearrangements—Translocations

Structural chromosomal rearrangements account for only 1.5% of all abortuses but a much higher proportion of abortuses that are recurrent. The presence of a balanced rearrangement in one parent can result in an unbalanced translocation in offspring. Phenotypic consequences depend on the specific duplicated or deficient chromosomal segments. A balanced translocation is found in 3–5% of couples experiencing repeated losses.[52–55] These individuals are themselves phenotypically normal, but their offspring (abortuses or abnormal liveborns) may show chromosomal duplications or deficiencies as a result of normal meiotic segregation. The prevalence of balanced translocations is higher in females than males,[53] and higher still if there is a family history of a stillborn or abnormal liveborn.[53,54]

Detecting a translocation heterozygote does not correlate with maternal age,[55] nor does the likelihood of detecting a balanced translocation substantially differ after 1, 2, or 3 miscarriages. In the tabulation by Simpson et al.,[53] detection rates in females after 2, 3, 4, and 5 losses were 0.8%, 1.7%, 2.3%, and 2.9%, respectively. For males, the respective rates were 1.2%, 1.9%, 2.4%, and 0 (0/39). Goddijn et al.[56] found that the odds ratios for finding a balanced translocation after 2, 3, and 4 or more losses were 1.4 (95% CI 0.4–4.8), 2.2 (0.4–12.5), and 2.1 (0.3–15.4), respectively.

Likelihood of Abnormal Liveborns

There are two general types of translocations: Robertsonian and reciprocal. Robertsonian translocations involve centric fusion of an acrocentric (13, 14, 15, 21, 11) chromosome. The theoretical risk of a parent with t(14q;21q) having a liveborn child with Down syndrome is 33%, but empirical risks are considerably less given the lethality of certain complements. Risks at the time of amniocentesis are 2% if the father carries a translocation-involving chromosome 21 and 10% if the mother carries such a translocation.[57,58] Robertsonian (centric fusion) translocations involving chromosomes other than chromosome 21 show lower empirical risks, based on liveborns or prenatal diagnosis samples. In t(13q;14q), the risk for liveborn trisomy 13 is 1% or less. This lower risk presumably reflects the lethality of many segregant products (trisomies and monosomies).

Reciprocal translocations involve interchanges between two or more metacentric chromosomes. Empirical data for specific translocations are usually not available, and generalizations are typically made on the basis of pooled data derived from many different translocations. In Robertsonian translocations, the theoretical risks for abnormal offspring (unbalanced reciprocal translocations) are also much greater than the empirical risks. Recurrence risk based on sex differences are less apparent. Empirical risks are 12% for offspring of either female heterozygotes or male heterozygotes.[57,58]

Mode of ascertainment is important. The frequency of unbalanced fetuses is lower if a parental balanced translocation was ascertained through repetitive abortions (3%) than through anomalous liveborns (nearly 20%).[57] Presumably this reflects the increased likelihood of severely unbalanced products (e.g., 3:1 segregations), greater in the former. Detecting a chromosomal rearrangement in a parent obviously dictates that prenatal cytogenetic studies should be offered. Even if there is normal transmission of chromosomes involved in the translocation, a different chromosome could be aneuploid (interchromosomal effect), irrespective of maternal age.

Likelihood of Subsequent Abortions in Structural Translocation

Distinct from the likelihood of unbalanced segregants in liveborns is the likelihood of subsequent abortion. Actually the cumulative likelihood does not differ from the expected 65–70% live birth rate observed in the general population with recurrent pregnancy loss (RPL). Goddijn et al.[56] reported only 26% miscarriages among 43 pregnancies in 25 carrier couples. Almost half the patients in a series of Goddijn et al.[56] (55/115) had only two miscarriages. Stephenson and Sierra[59] studied 1893 couples, 40 of whom had a balanced translocation (28 reciprocal and 12 Robertsonian). This series included 7 patients (14%) with two previous losses.

Among 35 monitored pregnancies in the reciprocal translocation group, the live birth rate was 63% (22/35); in the Robertsonian translocation group 69% (9/13). These data are comparable to those in the general repeated miscarriage population. Among abortuses of translocation heterozygote couples, 13 of 36 (36%) were unbalanced, 11 of 36 (30%) aneuploid for another chromosome (interchromosomal effect), and only 12 of 36 (33%) normal. Among recurrent miscarriage couples not having a translocation, the rates were 2%, 44%, and 54%, respectively.

Less favorable prognosis was reported by Sugiura-Ogasawara et al.,[60] the loss rates being 61% (11/18) for couples in which the male partner had a translocation and 72.4% (21/29) if the female partner had the translocation. Of 1184 couples with two or more miscarriages that had normal karyotypes, the miscarriage rate, by contrast, was only 28.3% (335/1184).[60] Carp et al.[61] reported that 45.2% (33/73) pregnancies of couples with a translocation heterozygote resulted in a live birth, compared with 55.3% (325/588) without a translocation. The same group later found a similar percentage of normal and balanced karyotypes (74%) in embryos of translocations heterozygotes as well as embryos of couples without a translocation (77%).[62] Carp et al.[62] concluded that any decrease in the live birth rate was due to factors unrelated to the chromosomal imbalance. However, one explanation is increased aneuploidy not detected in abortuses.

Irrespective of the above, the increased frequency of pregnancy losses raises the option of PGD in certain couples. The strategy is to identify and transfer only the (few) balanced embryos. Indeed, this unequivocally decreases the likelihood of abortion.[63]

PGD aneuploidy testing is particularly applicable to couples having a translocation in which the mother is of advancing age. Although couples having a balanced translocation become pregnant in percentages equivalent to the general population (60–70%), meiotic segregation unavoidably results in a much larger proportion of their embryos being imbalanced—at least 40% in Robertsonian translocations and over 60% in reciprocal translocations. The clinical consequence is longer time to achieve pregnancy.[59,60] In older women this delay (mean 6 years) can preclude liveborns. For this reason American Society of Reproductive Medicine guidelines recommend PGD be offered to identify the (few) balanced or genetically normal embryos suitable for transfer.[64]

Occasionally a balanced translocation precludes a normal liveborn infant. This occurs when a translocation involves homologous acrocentric chromosomes (e.g., t(13q;13q) or t(21q;21q)). The only possibility of normalcy is if trisomic rescue occurs; that is, the "additional" chromosome is "expelled" from the nucleus to yield the normal amount of chromosomal material. If the father carries a homologous structural rearrangement, artificial insemination may be appropriate. If the mother carries the rearrangement, donor oocytes or donor embryos should be considered.

Inversions

In an inversion, the order of the genes is reversed. The clinical consequence is analogous to translocation in that individuals heterozygous for an inversion are normal but their genes are rearranged. Likewise, these individuals suffer untoward reproductive consequences as a result of normal meiotic phenomena. The cytologic mechanism is more complex, involving not simply meiotic segregation but crossing over involving the inverted segment. It is a consequence of the recombinant event that produces unbalanced gametes. Duplication will exist for some regions and deficiencies for others. There are two types of inversions. In *pericentric* inversions, breaks occur in both arms. In *paracentric* inversions, the two breaks occur on the same arm. The frequency of inversions in couples having repetitive abortions is low; perhaps less than 1%.

Females with a *pericentric* inversion have a 7% risk of abnormal liveborns; males carry about a 5% risk.[65] Pericentric inversions ascertained through phenotypically normal probands are less likely to result in abnormal live infants, presumably reflecting the lethality of unbalanced products. Pivotal is whether crossing over occurs within the inverted segment. If so, this lends to imbalance in gametes. The clinical outcome is paradoxical. Inversions involving only a small portion of the total chromosomal length are usually lethal because when recombination occurs they yield large duplications or deficiencies. By contrast, in larger inversions (30–60% of the total chromosomal length) embryos are more likely to survive because imbalance is less. On a molecular level inversions less than 100 Mb appear not to exert undue untoward outcomes.[66] There were no recombinants in one tabulation when inversion was less than 50 Mb (40% of chromosome) length, and only a few for inversions around 50 Mb (40–50% of length); a much higher number occurred when the inversion was greater than 100 Mb.[66]

Data are limited on recurrence risk involving *paracentric* inversions. Theoretically, there should be almost zero risk of unbalanced products of clinical consequence than with pericentric inversions because nearly all paracentric recombinants should be lethal. However, both abortions and abnormal liveborns have been observed within the same kindred. The risk for unbalanced viable offspring has been tabulated to be 4%.[67]

Future Directions in Identifying Genetic Explanations for Pregnancy Loss

We have emphasized that 50–80% of first trimester abortuses show chromosomal abnormalities. In addition, microdeletions and microduplications (<1 Mb) can be detected by array CGH given higher resolution than karyotypes used simply to exclude aneuploidy.[11]

Casual logic has led some to conclude that the 20–50% of pregnancy losses not showing overt chromosomal abnormalities must be of "nongenetic etiology". However, this deduction would be incorrect because Mendelian and polygenic/multifactorial disorders universally fail to show chromosomal abnormalities. Indeed, single gene and polygenic etiologies more commonly explain congenital anomalies in liveborns than do chromosomal abnormalities. Thus, it would be illogical to assume that Mendelian and polygenic/multifactorial factors do not play pivotal roles in embryonic mortality. The difficulty is that few of the doubtless many genes required for differentiation have been identified. A myriad of potential candidate genes exist and are shown by animal studies, but difficulties in performing studies in humans exist.

Embryos that abort because of Mendelian or polygenic factors may or may not show structural anomalies. Lack of cytogenetic data on dissected specimens has made it difficult to determine the exact role that noncytogenetic mechanisms play in early embryonic maldevelopment. However, a structural anomaly found in an abortus having a normal chromosomal complement is still consistent with genetic etiology. Philipp and Kalousek[68] correlated the cytogenetic status of missed abortions with morphological abnormalities as observed at embryoscopy. Embryos with chromosomal abnormalities usually showed one or more external anomalies, but some euploid embryos also showed anatomical anomalies.

As the cost of sequencing plummets, whole exome sequencing or even whole genome sequencing will be applied to analysis of abortuses, and causative genes found. Recall that of the 22,000 human genes, function is known for only 5000–7000. It can be confidently predicted that many of the "unknown" genes code for embryonic or fetal development.

REFERENCES

1. Plachot M, Junca AM, Mandelbaum J, de Grouchy J, Salat-Baroux J, Cohen J. Chromosome investigations in early life. II. Human preimplantation embryos. *Hum Reprod* 1987;2(1):29–35.
2. Munne S, Alikani M, Tomkin G, Grifo J, Cohen J. Embryo morphology, developmental rates, and maternal age are correlated with chromosome abnormalities. *Fertil Steril* 1995;64(2):382–91.
3. Rabinowitz M, Ryan A, Gemelos G, Hill M, Baner J, Cinnioglou C et al. Origins and rates of aneuploidy in human blastomeres. *Fertil Steril* 2012;97(2):395–401.
4. Martin R. Chromosomal analysis of human spermatozoa. In: Verlinsky Y, Kuliev A, eds. *Preimplantation Genetics*, New York: Plenum Press; 1991. p. 91–102.
5. Plachot M. Genetics in human oocytes. In: Boutaleb Y, ed. *New Concepts in Reproduction*, Lancaster, UK: Parthenon; 1992. p. 367.
6. Boue J, Bou A, Lazar P. Retrospective and prospective epidemiological studies of 1500 karyotyped spontaneous human abortions. *Teratology* 1975;12(1):11–26.
7. Hassold TJ. A cytogenetic study of repeated spontaneous abortions. *Am J Hum Genet* 1980;32(5): 723–730.
8. Simpson J, Bombard A. Chromosomal abnormalities in spontaneous abortion: Frequency, pathology and genetic counseling. In: Edmunds, KB, ed. *Spontaneous Abortion*, Oxford: Blackwell; 1987. p. 51–76.
9. Sorokin Y, Johnson MP, Uhlmann WR, Zaldor IE, Drugan A, Koppitch FC 3rd et al. Postmortem chorionic villus sampling: Correlation of cytogenetic and ultrasound findings. *Am J Med Genet* 1991;39(3):314–16.
10. Strom CM, Ginsberg N, Applebaum M, Bozorgi N, White M, Caffarelli M et al. Analyses of 95 first-trimester spontaneous abortions by chorionic villus sampling and karyotype. *J Assist Reprod Genet* 1992;9(5):458–61.
11. Schaeffer AJ, Chung J, Heretis K, Wong A, Ledbetter DH, Lese Martin C. Comparative genomic hybridization-array analysis enhances the detection of aneuploidies and submicroscopic imbalances in spontaneous miscarriages. *Am J Hum Gen* 2004;74(6):1168–174.
12. Simpson JL, Mills JL, Holmes LB, Ober CL, Aarons J, Jovanovic L et al. Low fetal loss rates after ultrasound-proved viability in early pregnancy. *JAMA: J Am Med Assoc* 1987;258(18):2555–57.

13. American College of Obstetricians and Gynecologists Committee on Genetics. Committee Opinion No. 581: The use of chromosomal microarray analysis in prenatal diagnosis. *Obstet Gynecol* 2013;122(6):1374–7.

14. Hefler LA, Hersh DR, Moore PJ, Gregg AR. Clinical value of postnatal autopsy and genetics consultation in fetal death. *Am J Med Genet* 2001;104(2):165–8.

15. Warbuton D, Byrne J, Canik N. *Chromosomal Anomalies and and Prenatal Development: An Atlas*, New York: Oxford Publishing; 1991.

16. Kalousek D. Pathology of Abortion: Chromosomal and genetic correlations. In: Kraus F, Damjanov I, eds. *Pathology of Reproductive Failure*, Baltimore: Williams and Wilkins; 1991. p. 228.

17. Hassold T, Merrill M, Adkins K, Freeman S, Sherman S. Recombination and maternal age-dependent nondisjunction: Molecular studies of trisomy 16. *Am J Hum Genet* 1995;57(4):867–74.

18. Fisher JM, Harvey JF, Morton NE, Jacobs PA. Trisomy 18: Studies of the parent and cell division of origin and the effect of aberrant recombination on nondisjunction. *Am J Hum Genet* 1995;56(3):669–75.

19. Bugge M, Collins A, Petersen MB, Fisher J, Brandt C, Hertz JM et al. Non-disjunction of chromosome 18. *Hum Mol Genet* 1998;7(4):661–9.

20. Hassold TJ. Nondisjunction in the human male. *Curr Top Dev Biol* 1998;37:383–406.

21. Kuliev A, Zlatopolsky Z, Kirillova I, Spivakova J, Cieslak Janzen J. Meiosis errors in over 20,000 oocytes studied in the practice of preimplantation aneuploidy testing. *Reprod BioMed Online* 2011;22(1):2–8.

22. Lamb NE, Yu K, Shaffer J, Feingold E, Sherman SL. Association between maternal age and meiotic recombination for trisomy 21. *Am J Hum Genet* 2005;76(1):91–9.

23. Henderson SA, Edwards RG. Chiasma frequency and maternal age in mammals. *Nature* 1968;218(5136):22–8.

24. Hassold T, Abruzzo M, Adkins K, Griffin D, Merrill M, Millie E et al. Human aneuploidy: Incidence, origin, and etiology. *Environ Mol Mutagen* 1996;28(3):167–75.

25. Savage AR, Petersen MB, Pettay D, Taft L, Allran K, Freeman SB et al. Elucidating the mechanisms of paternal non-disjunction of chromosome 21 in humans. *Hum Mol Genet* 1998;7(8):1221–7.

26. Reddy KS. Double trisomy in spontaneous abortions. *Hum Genet* 1997;101(3):339–45.

27. Diego-Alvarez D, Ramos-Corrales C, Garcia-Hoyos M, Bustamante-Aragones A, Cantalapiedra D, Diaz-Recasens J et al. Double trisomy in spontaneous miscarriages: Cytogenetic and molecular approach. *Hum Reprod* 2006;21(4):958–66.

28. Li S, Hassed S, Mulvihill JJ, Nair AK, Hopcus DJ. Double trisomy. *Am J Med Genet, Part A* 2004;124A(1):96–8.

29. Beatty RA. The origin of human triploidy: An integration of qualitative and quantitative evidence. *Ann Hum Genet* 1978;41(3):299–314.

30. Jauniaux E, Burton GJ. Pathophysiology of histological changes in early pregnancy loss. *Placenta* 2005;26(2–3):114–23.

31. McFadden DE, Langlois S. Parental and meiotic origin of triploidy in the embryonic and fetal periods. *Clin Genet* 2000;58(3):192–200.

32. Jacobs PA, Angell RR, Buchanan IM, Hassold TJ, Matsuyama AM, Manuel B. The origin of human triploids. *Ann Hum Genet* 1978;42(1):49–57.

33. Egozcue S, Blanco J, Vidal F, Egozcue J. Diploid sperm and the origin of triploidy. *Hum Reprod* 2002;17(1):5–7.

34. McFadden DE, Robinson WP. Phenotype of triploid embryos. *J Med Genet* 2006;43(7):609–12.

35. Schluth C, Doray B, Girard-Lemaire F, Favre R, Flori J, Gasser B et al. Prenatal diagnosis of a true fetal tetraploidy in direct and cultured chorionic villi. *Genet Couns* 2004;15(4):429–36.

36. Rosenbusch BE, Schneider M. Separation of a pronucleus by premature cytokinesis: A mechanism for immediate diploidization of tripronuclear oocytes? *Fertil Steril* 2009;92(1):394 e395–8.

37. Baumer A, Dres D, Basaran S, Isci H, Dehgan T, Schinzel A. Parental origin of the two additional haploid sets of chromosomes in an embryo with tetraploidy. *Cytogenet Genome Res* 2003;101(1):5–7.

38. Chandley AC. The origin of chromosomal aberrations in man and their potential for survival and reproduction in the adult human population. *Ann Genet* 1981;24(1):5–11.

39. Warburton D, Kline J, Stein Z, Hutzler M, Chin A, Hassold T. Does the karyotype of a spontaneous abortion predict the karyotype of a subsequent abortion? Evidence from 273 women with two karyotyped spontaneous abortions. *Am J Hum Genet* 1987;41(3):465–83.

40. Warburton D, Dallaire L, Thangavelu M, Ross L, Levin B, Klein J. Trisomy recurrence: A reconsideration based on North American data. *Am J Hum Genet* 2004;75(3):376–85.

41. Bianco K, Caughey AB, Shaffer BL, Davis R, Norton ME. History of miscarriage and increased incidence of fetal aneuploidy in subsequent pregnancy. *Obstet Gynecol* 2006;107(5):1098–102.

42. Drugan A, Koppitch FC, 3rd, Williams JC, 3rd, Johnson MP, Moghissi KS, Evans MI. Prenatal genetic diagnosis following recurrent early pregnancy loss. *Obstet Gynecol* 1990;75(3 Pt 1):381–4.

43. Munne S, Sandalinas M, Magli C, Gianaroli L, Cohen J, Warburton D. Increased rate of aneuploid embryos in young women with previous aneuploid conceptions. *Prenatal Diagn* 2004;24(8):638–43.

44. Rubio C, Simon C, Vidal F, Rodrigo L, Pehlivan T, Remohi J et al. Chromosomal abnormalities and embryo development in recurrent miscarriage couples. *Hum Reprod* 2003;18(1):182–8.

45. Stephenson MD, Awartani KA, Robinson WP. Cytogenetic analysis of miscarriages from couples with recurrent miscarriage: A case-control study. *Hum Reprod* 2002;17(2):446–51.

46. Ogasawara M, Aoki K, Okada S, Suzumori K. Embryonic karyotype of abortuses in relation to the number of previous miscarriages. *Fertil Steril* 2000;73(2):300–4.

47. Carp H, Toder V, Aviram A, Daniely M, Mashiach S, Barkai G. Karyotype of the abortus in recurrent miscarriage. *Fertil Steril* 2001;75(4):678–82.

48. Benkhalifa M, Kasakyan S, Clement P, Baldi M, Tachdjan G, Demirol A et al. Array comparative genomic hybridization profiling of first-trimester spontaneous abortions that fail to grow in vitro. *Prenatal Diagn* 2005;25(10):894–900.

49. Munne S, Fischer J, Warner A, Chen S, Zouves C, Cohen J et al. Preimplantation genetic diagnosis significantly reduces pregnancy loss in infertile couples: A multicenter study. *Fertil Steril* 2006;85(2):326–32.

50. Alberman ED. The abortus as a predictor of future trisomy 21. In: Cruz DI, Gerald PS, eds. *Trisomy 21 (Down Syndrome)*, Baltimore: Raven Press; 1981.

51. Snijders RJ, Nicolaides KH. *Ultrasound Markers for Fetal Chromosomal Defects*, New York: Parthenon; 1996.

52. Fortuny A, Carrio A, Soler A, Cararach J, Fuster J, Salami C. Detection of balanced chromosome rearrangements in 445 couples with repeated abortion and cytogenetic prenatal testing in carriers. *Fertil Steril* 1988;49(5):774–9.

53. Simpson JL, Meyers CM, Martin AO, Elias S, Ober C. Translocations are infrequent among couples having repeated spontaneous abortions but no other abnormal pregnancies. *Fertil Steril* 1989;51(5):811–4.

54. De Braekeleer M, Dao TN. Cytogenetic studies in couples experiencing repeated pregnancy losses. *Hum Reprod* 1990;5(5):519–28.

55. Simpson JL, Elias S, Martin AO. Parental chromosomal rearrangements associated with repetitive spontaneous abortions. *Fertil Steril* 1981;36(5):584–90.

56. Goddijn M, Joosten JH, Knegt AC, van derVeen F, Franssen MT, Bonsel GJ et al. Clinical relevance of diagnosing structural chromosome abnormalities in couples with repeated miscarriage. *Hum Reprod* 2004;19(4):1013–7.

57. Boué A, Gallano P. A collaborative study of the segregation of inherited chromosome structural rearrangements in 1356 prenatal diagnoses. *Prenatal Diagn* 1984;4(7):45–67.

58. Daniel A, Hook EB, Wulf G. Risks of unbalanced progeny at amniocentesis to carriers of chromosome rearrangements: Data from United States and Canadian laboratories. *Am J Med Genet* 1989;33(1):14–53.

59. Stephenson MD, Sierra S. Reproductive outcomes in recurrent pregnancy loss associated with a parental carrier of a structural chromosome rearrangement. *Hum Reprod* 2006;21(4):1076–82.

60. Sugiura-Ogasawara M, Ozaki Y, Sato T, Suzumori N, Suzumori K. Poor prognosis of recurrent aborters with either maternal or paternal reciprocal translocations. *Fertil Steril* 2004;81(2):367–73.

61. Carp H, Feldman B, Oelsner G, Schiff E. Parental karyotype and subsequent live births in recurrent miscarriage. *Fertil Steril* 2004;81(5):1296–301.

62. Carp H, Guetta E, Dorf H, Soriano D, Barkai G, Schiff E. Embryonic karyotype in recurrent miscarriage with parental karyotypic aberrations. *Fertil Steril* 2006;85(2):446–50.

63. Harton GL, Munne S, Surrey M, Grifo J, Kaplan B, McColloh DH et al. Diminished effect of maternal age on implantation after preimplantation genetic diagnosis with array comparative genomic hybridization. *Fertil Steril* 2013;100(6):1695–703.

64. Fritz MA. Perspectives on the efficacy and indications for preimplantation genetic screening: Where are we now? *Hum Reprod* 2008;23(12):2617–21.

65. Gardner RJ, Sutherland GR, Shaffer LG. *Chromosome Abnormalities and Genetic Counseling.* New York: Oxford; 2012.
66. Anton E, Vidal F, Egozcue J, Blanco J. Genetic reproductive risk in inversion carriers. *Fertil Steril* 2006;85(3):661–6.
67. Pettenati MJ, Rao PN, Phelan MC, Grass F, Rao KW, Cosper P et al. Paracentric inversions in humans: A review of 446 paracentric inversions with presentation of 120 new cases. *Am J Med Genet* 1995;55(2):171–87.
68. Philipp T, Kalousek DK. Generalized abnormal embryonic development in missed abortion: Embryoscopic and cytogenetic findings. *Am J Med Genet* 2002;111(1):43–7.

4

Debate: Should Fetal Karyotyping Be Performed in Recurrent Pregnancy Loss? Yes

Howard J. A. Carp

Investigation of the embryonic chromosomal status in RPL allows an accurate diagnosis to be reached, affects the patient's subsequent prognosis and influences the treatment. In clinical practice the patient usually represents in the interval in between pregnancies, and often no information is available about the chromosomal status of previous miscarriages. Lack of information regarding the karyotype leads to inaccurate diagnosis. Embryonic chromosomal aberrations account for between 25% and 60% of recurrent miscarriages.[1–5] Dhillon et al.[6] have shown in a metaanalysis that chromosomal microarrays can detect an additional 13% of genetic abnormalities in the abortus than can conventional karyotyping. Moreover, embryonic chromosomal aberrations have been found in the presence of other presumptive causes of pregnancy loss. In antiphospholipid syndrome, two series have reported incidences of 20%[7] and 40%.[2] Carp et al.[8] have reported four chromosomal aberrations in patients with hereditary thrombophilias. In a series by Carp et al.,[3] trisomies were the most common form of aberration, occuring in 66.7% of chromosomally aberrant embryos, with trisomies 21, 16, and 18 being the most common, followed by monosomy X and triploidies. However, since the publication of that series numerous other aberrations have been seen.

Until recently standard banding techniques were used to diagnose genetic aberrations. However, banding techniques can only assess structural and numerical chromosomal rearrangements, and are liable to fail due to contamination, culture failure or overgrowth of maternal cells, and so on. Multiplex fluorescence in situ hybridization (M-FISH)[9] has been used to try to overcome these problems. The technique may allow additional genetic diagnoses to be made, such as uniparental disomy or skewed X chromosome inactivation.[10] Recently it has been possible to assess the entire genome by comparative genomic hybridization (CGH), usually incorporated into a microarray. If the patient presents between pregnancies with no information as to the chromosomal status of previous miscarriages, it may be possible to retrieve this information. Although the karyotype of previous miscarriages may not have been investigated, histological slides, and paraffin blocks are usually available from previous miscarriages. These blocks and slides have been used to extract DNA which can then be analyzed by CGH-based microarrays, as previously described.[11–13] Array-CGH may also be useful in detecting submicroscopic chromosomal changes in the parents with unexplained RPL and the abortuses hitherto reported to have normal karyotypes.[14] Hence, it is not possible to reach an accurate diagnosis of the cause of recurrent miscarriage unless the chromosomal status of the fetus is determined.

Karyotyping of the abortus allows the patient to be given prognostic information regarding subsequent pregnancy outcomes. Warburton et al.[14] summarized 273 women who had abortuses karyotyped. They concluded that, after a previous trisomic miscarriage, the prognosis is favorable. Two subsequent studies[2,3] have examined the outcome of the subsequent pregnancy according to the karyotype of the miscarriage. In a series by Ogasawara et al.[2] (Figure 4.1), there was a statistically significant trend for a patient with an aneuploidic abortion to have a better prognosis. The same trend was apparent in a series by Carp et al.[3] In women with three miscarriages and an aneuploidic miscarriage, reassurance of a good prognosis may be sufficient, and save the patient more extensive investigations and treatment of dubious value. This may not be the case in euploid abortions. The better prognosis after an aneuploid abortion is entirely logical as fetal aneuploidy is due to a fetal cause. Hence there is a greater chance that in a subsequent pregnancy, with a new embryo,

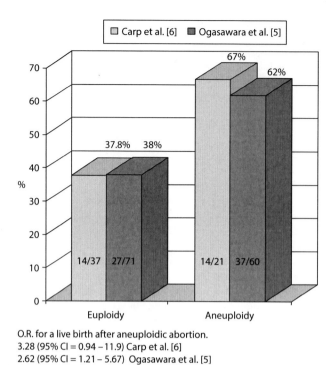

O.R. for a live birth after aneuploidic abortion.
3.28 (95% CI = 0.94 – 11.9) Carp et al. [6]
2.62 (95% CI = 1.21 – 5.67) Ogasawara et al. [5]

FIGURE 4.1   Outcome of subsequent pregnancy according to fetal karyotype.

the next fetus will be euploid. However, an euploid abortus indicates that the cause of miscarriage is more likely to be maternal, hence the same problem is liable to return in a subsequent pregnancy thus worsening the prognosis. Any prognosis is empirical if the karyotype of the abortus is unknown.

Fetal karyotyping has been assessed in a subsequent abortion in a study by Sullivan et al.[5] Of 30 patients with an aneuploid abortion, only three (10%) had a subsequent aneuploid abortion. In the author's series (unpublished) 43 abortuses were found to be aneuploid, and a subsequent abortion was karyotyped. Only eight of the 43 abortuses were aneuploid (19%). Hence, only approximately 15% of aneuploid abortions will be followed by a subsequent aneuploid abortion. Eighty-five percent of patients with an aneuploid abortion can be assured that the prognosis is good, and that the aneuploid abortion may be a chance occurrence. However, the other 15% may have a recurring cause of fetal aneuploidy, and can be offered pregestational diagnosis.

Fetal karyotyping also directs treatment. If the fetus is aneuploid, pregestational screening (PGS) can be used to give the mother a euploid embryo. However, if the fetus is normal, the maternal environment requires treatment. As all previous maternal treatment modalities have ignored the fetal karyotype, fetal aneuploidy has confounded the results of treatment directed to maternal factors. Hence, there are debates in this book as to whether hormone supplementation, thromboprophylaxis, immunopotentiation, and so on, should be used. Additionally, the place of surgery for uterine anomalies, and treatment of antiphospholipid syndrome are equally debatable. If these treatment modalities had only been used in patients miscarrying euploid embryos, the above mentioned therapies might be found to be efficacious, and their place might need no debate. The role of PGS is also controversial. When PGS is used on unselected patients with recurrent miscarriage, it has also been reported to be of little value.[15,16] It is our opinion that PGS has a place,[17,18] but that the place is limited to patients with repeat aneuploidies.

We have seen a 42-year-old patient with three consecutive aneuploid abortions. Her details are given in Figure 4.2. If fetal karyotyping had not been performed she would have been recommended paternal leucocyte immunization or immunoglobulin at that time. However, as the karyotype was available, immunotherapy would probably not have increased her chance of a live birth. In view of the advanced maternal age (increasing the likelihood of chromosomal aberrations), and the possibility that all the embryos may

Age 42, Obstetric history is as follows:

1st Pregnancy Artificial Abortion
2nd Pregnancy Normal Delivery, ♀ 3400 g
3rd Pregnancy Normal delivery ♂ 3500 g
4th Pregnancy Blighted ovum.
5th Pregnancy Left ectopic pregnancy, treated conservatively with Methotrexate
6th Pregnancy Blighted ovum
7th Pregnancy Terminated artificially at 20 weeks for 47 XXX, fetal karyotype
8th Pregnancy Biochemical pregnancy
9th Pregnancy Missed abortion 10 weeks, after treatment with aspirin & progesterone supplements. Fetal karyotyping showed a 48XX karyotype with both 14 and 15 trisomies
10th Pregnancy Missed abortion at 10 weeks. Fetal karyotyping showed 22 trisomy.

Previous investigations showed no maternal cause for miscarriage.
Parental karyotype 46XX/ 46XY

Treatment advised—ovum donation in view of; advanced maternal age, increasing chance of subsequent aneuploid abortion, impossibility for screening all 23 chromosomes at PGS. And low possibility of conceiving at IVF.

FIGURE 4.2   Patient with recurrent aneuploidy.

be aneuploid at PGS, she was advised ovum donation. These poor prognosis patients are outside the normal guidelines for treatment, and do not have the good prognosis of 70–75% as other patients. However, they still require appropriate management which rests on accurate diagnosis.

Chromosomal aberrations are often suspected to have a recurring basis due to either a structural anomaly, such as reciprocal or Robertsonian translocations, inversions, or mosaicism for numerical aberrations. Parental chromosomal aberrations have been found in 10.8% of recurrently aborting women in the author's series,[19] but the usually quoted prevalence is 3–5%.[20–22] If a parental chromosomal aberration is found, this is usually assumed to be the cause of recurrent miscarriage. However, parental karyotyping does not provide a diagnosis or prognosis, neither does it direct treatment. Carp et al.[23] have karyotyped 39 abortuses from recurrently miscarrying couples, with parental karyotypic aberrations. Seventeen of the 39 (26%) were euploid. Another 10 (26%) had the same balanced translocation as the parent. Hence 69% were chromosomally normal. Only five (13%) abortuses had unbalanced translocations, whereas seven (18%) of the abortuses had subsequent abortuses with numeric aberrations unrelated to the parental chromosomal disorder, (5 trisomies, 2 monosomy X).

Parental karyotyping does not provide a prognosis. Four papers,[19,24–26] have looked at the subsequent live birth rate in patients with recurrent miscarriage and parental chromosomal rearrangements. These are summarized in Table 4.1. Taken together, the live birth rate was 53.6% for patients with a mean of

TABLE 4.1

Subsequent Live Birth Rate with Parental Chromosomal Aberrations

	Carp et al.[19]	Goddijn et al.[25]	Stephenson and Sierra[26]	Sugiura-Ogasawara et al.[24]	Total
Pregnancies	75	42	58	47	222
Live births	33	30	41	15	119
Proportion live births	44%	70%	71%	32%	53.6%
Mean No. miscarriages	4.23	3.9	5.4	2.9	4.19

4.19 previous miscarriages. This live birth rate of 53.6% was somewhat higher than the expected rate for patients with 4.19 miscarriages, according to numerous series in the literature,[27,28] and may reflect the fact that patients losing aneuploid embryos have a better prognosis than patients losing euploid embryos.

Parental karyotyping, in addition to being nondiagnostic or prognostic, does not indicate treatment. Musters et al.[29] used parental structural chromosome aberrations as a basis for comparing pregestational diagnosis (PGD) to natural conception recurrent miscarriage. There were no randomized control trials for analysis. Seven studies were identified on the outcome after natural conception and five studies on the outcome after PGD. As expected, PGD lowered the incidence of miscarriage; however, due to the lower pregnancy rate after PGD, there were fewer live births. After natural conception, there were 42% live births in the first pregnancy (average miscarriage rate 28%). After PGD, there were 35% live births (average miscarriage rate 9%). Hence, parental karyotyping could not be used as the basis for recommending PGD to increase the live birth rates in couples with recurrent miscarriage and a structural chromosome abnormality.

Therefore, chromosomal analysis of the abortus seems the most important single investigation for the assessment of recurrent miscarriage, as recommended by the Royal College of Obstetricians and Gynaecologists in their 1998[30] guideline, revised in 2011.[31] We find this test invaluable, and its absence leads to an incomplete diagnosis, inaccurate prognosis, and possibly wrong advice as to management.

REFERENCES

1. Stern JJ, Dorfman AD, Gutierez-Najar MD et al. Frequency of abnormal karyotype among abortuses from women with and without a history of recurrent spontaneous abortion. *Fertil Steril* 1996;65:250–3.
2. Ogasawara M, Aoki K, Okada S et al. Embryonic karyotype of abortuses in relation to the number of previous miscarriages. *Fertil Steril* 2000;73:300–4.
3. Carp HJA, Toder V, Orgad S et al. Karyotype of the Abortus in Recurrent Miscarriage. *Fertil Steril* 2001;5:678–82.
4. Stephenson MD, Awartani KA, Robinson WP. Cytogenetic analysis of miscarriages from couples with recurrent miscarriage: A case-control study. *Hum Reprod* 2002;17:446–51.
5. Sullivan AE, Silver RM, LaCoursiere DY et al. Recurrent fetal aneuploidy and recurrent miscarriage. *Obstet Gynecol* 2004;104:784–8.
6. Dhillon R, Hillman S, Morris R, McMullan D, Williams D, Coomarasamy A et al. Additional information from chromosomal microarray analysis (CMA) over conventional karyotyping when diagnosing chromosomal abnormalities in miscarriage: A systematic review and meta-analysis. *BJOG* 2014;121:11–21.
7. Takakuwa K, Asano K, Arakawa M et al. Chromosome analysis of aborted conceptuses of recurrent aborters positive for anticardiolipin antibody. *Fertil Steril* 1997;68:54–8.
8. Carp HJA, Dolitzky M, Inbal A. Thromboprophylaxis improves the live birth rate in women with consecutive recurrent miscarriages and hereditary thrombophilia. *J Thromb Haemostasis* 2003;1:433–8.
9. Uhrig S, Schuffenhauer S, Fauth C et al. Multiplex-FISH for pre and postnatal diagnostic applications. *Am J Hum Genet* 1999;65:448–62.
10. Lanasa MC, Hogge WA, Kubik C et al. Highly skewed X chromosome inactivation is associated with idiopathic recurrent spontaneous abortion. *Am J Hum Genet* 1999;65:252–4.
11. Bell KA, Van Deerlin PG, Feinberg RF, du Manoir S, Haddad BR. Diagnosis of aneuploidy in archival, paraffin-embedded pregnancy-loss tissues by comparative genomic hybridization. *Fertil Steril* 2001;75:374–9.
12. de Jong D, Verbeke SLJ, Meijer D, Hogendoorn PC, Bovee JV, Szuhai K. Opening the archives for state of the art tumour genetic research: Sample processing for array-CGH using decalcified, formalin-fixed, paraffin-embedded tissue-derived DNA samples. *BMC Res Notes* 2011;4:1.
13. Fensterer H, Radlwimmer B, Sträter J, Buchholz M, Aust DE, Julié C et al. EORTC Gastrointestinal (GI) Group. Matrix-comparative genomic hybridization from multicenter formalin-fixed paraffin-embedded colorectal cancer tissue blocks. *BMC Cancer* 2007;7:58.
14. Warburton D, Kline J, Stein Z et al. Does the karyotype of a spontaneous abortion predict the karyotype of a subsequent abortion?—Evidence from 273 women with two karyotyped spontaneous abortions. *Am J Hum Genet* 1987;41:465–83.

15. Platteau P, Staessen C, Michiels A et al. Preimplantation genetic diagnosis for aneuploidy screening in patients with unexplained recurrent miscarriages. *Fertil Steril* 2005;83:393–7.
16. Go KJ, Patel JC, Cunningham DL. The role of assisted reproductive technology in the management of recurrent pregnancy loss. *Curr Opin Endocrinol Diabetes* 2009;16:459–63.
17. Carp HJA, Dirnfeld M, Dor J et al. ART in Recurrent Miscarriage: Pre-Implantation Genetic Diagnosis/ Screening or Surrogacy? *Hum Reprod* 2004; 19:1502–5.
18. Carp HJA. Commentary on 'Additional information from chromosomal microarray analysis (CMA) over conventional karyotyping when diagnosing chromosomal abnormalities in miscarriage: A systematic review and meta-analysis'. *BJOG* 2014;121:20–21.
19. Carp HJA, Feldman B, Oelsner G et al. Parental karyotype and subsequent live births in recurrent miscarriage *Fertil Steril* 2004;81:1296–301.
20. De Braekeleer M, Dao TN. Cytogenetic studies in couples experiencing repeated pregnancy losses. *Hum Reprod* 1990;5:519–28.
21. Portnoi MF, Joye N, van den Akker J et al. Karyotypes of 1142 couples with recurrent abortion. *Obstet Gynecol* 1988;72:31–4.
22. Fortuny A, Carrio A, Soler A et al. Detection of balanced chromosome rearrangements in 445 couples with repeated abortion and cytogenetic prenatal testing in carriers. *Fertil Steril* 1988;49:774–9.
23. Carp HJA, Guetta E, Dorf H et al. Embryonic karyotype in recurrent miscarriage with parental karyotypic aberrations *Fertil Steril* 2006;85:446–50.
24. Sugiura-Ogasawara M, Ozaki Y, Sato T et al. Poor prognosis of recurrent aborters with either maternal or paternal reciprocal translocations. *Fertil Steril* 2004;81:367–73.
25. Goddijn M, Joosten JH, Knegt AC et al. Clinical relevance of diagnosing structural chromosome abnormalities in couples with repeated miscarriage. *Hum Reprod* 2004;19:1013–7.
26. Stephenson MD, Sierra S. Reproductive outcomes in recurrent pregnancy loss associated with a parental carrier of a structural chromosome rearrangement. *Hum Reprod* 2006;21:1076–82.
27. Knudsen UB, Hansen V, Juul S et al. Prognosis of a new pregnancy following previous spontaneous abortions. *Eur J Obstet Gynecol Reprod Biol* 1991;39:31–6.
28. Carp HJA. Investigation and treatment for recurrent pregnancy loss. In: Rainsbury P, Vinniker D, eds. *A Practical Guide to Reproductive Medicine*. Carnforth, Lancs, UK: Parthenon and Co; 1997. p. 337–62.
29. Musters AM, Repping S, Korevaar JC, Mastenbroek S, Limpens J, van der Veen F, Goddijn M. Pregnancy outcome after preimplantation genetic screening or natural conception in couples with unexplained recurrent miscarriage: A systematic review of the best available evidence. *Fertil Steril* 2011;95:2153–7.
30. Royal College of Obstetricians and Gynaecologists, Guideline No. 17. *The Management of Recurrent Miscarriage*. London: RCOG; 1998.
31. Royal College of Obstetricians and Gynaecologists, Guideline No. 17. The *Management of Recurrent Miscarriage*. London: RCOG; 2011.

5

Debate: Should Fetal Karyotyping Be Performed in Recurrent Pregnancy Loss? No

Zvi Borochowitz

Introduction

The first report of a chromosomal abnormality in aborted material was of a triploidy in spontaneous abortion, four decades ago by Penrose and Delhanty.[1] It took several years before cytogenetic analysis of miscarriage became an option in laboratories, due to the difficulties of culturing fetal tissue. The development of techniques, which allowed chorionic villi to be used for "long-term cultures," and later "direct preparation of metaphases from villi," revolutionized the cytogenetic analysis of products of conception. Since then it is debatable whether it is either clinically justifiable or psychologically essential to determine the cause of pregnancy loss for counseling about further pregnancies. The crucial role of chromosomal imbalance in abnormal early human development is well established. It has been suggested that most chromosome abnormalities result in disordered development incompatible with prolonged intrauterine survival and live birth. The mechanism by which a chromosome abnormality could lead to regression of the conceptus is unclear. Approximately 50–60% of first trimester spontaneous abortions have karyotypic abnormalities, mainly numerical such as autosomal trisomy, monosomy X, and polyploidy. This conclusion is based on the results of cytogenetic studies conducted in laboratories throughout the world.[2] The majority (90%) of karyotypically abnormal pregnancies miscarry in the first trimester, and the majority (93%) of karyotypically normal pregnancies continue.[3] Most chromosomal abnormalities that result in spontaneous abortion are random events, and may be associated with recurrent spontaneous abortion. However, even in recurrent spontaneous miscarriage, parental carriership is found in 4–6%.[4–5]

Cytogenetic Abnormalities

Cytogenetic evaluation of sporadic spontaneous abortions has shown that 50–60% are chromosomally abnormal. This means that about 5–10.5% of all pregnancies result in sporadic abortions caused by chromosomal abnormalities. Pregnancy loss of chromosome origin is uncommon after 15 weeks gestation; therefore, this chapter concentrates on first trimester miscarriages. Fetal de novo chromosomal abnormalities are a major cause of sporadic first trimester spontaneous abortions, and some cases of recurrent miscarriage might be caused by repeat fetal chromosomal abnormalities. Although tissue sampling, culture technique, and direct preparation of chorionic villi have improved over time, the rate of chromosomal abnormality has remained similar with a detection rate of 49%. Numerical abnormalities are found in approximately 86% of these, with trisomies being the most frequent (52%) (trisomies 6, 13, 18, 21, and 22), followed by polyploidy (21%) and monosomy X (13%). Structural chromosome abnormalities can be classified as deletions, translocations, inversions, and duplications, but only translocations and inversions play a role in miscarriages. Structural chromosome abnormalities occur in less than 5% of chromosomally abnormal abortuses. In approximately 8% of cases, other chromosome abnormalities are found including double and triple trisomies (accounting for about 1.4% and 0.05%, respectively). These figures have remained constant over time, and independent of the culture method used or the success rate, which is now reported to be approximately 90%.[2,4,6] The recurrence risk of another miscarriage is not, or only slightly elevated (16%) when compared to the initial risk for all women (10–15%), and thus routine karyotyping of fetal material in miscarriages is thought not to be worthwhile and unnecessary.[4] Furthermore, it should be noted that karyotyping of abortuses has many pitfalls including the possibility of maternal tissue contamination, failure to seek other causes of RPL if cytogenetic assessment reveals an abnormal karyotype and the occurrence of non-cytogenetic embryonic abnormalities.[7] The recurrence risk of numerical abnormalities is low, so karyotyping of fetal material in case of a miscarriage does not seem to be worthwhile in daily practice. Half of the structural abnormalities may be inherited from a parent carrying a balanced chromosome translocation or inversion. This type of chromosomal abnormality would be found by parental karyotyping, however, based on the published literature, opinions are still divided regarding the incidence of carrier status, and if it is higher after three miscarriages rather than after two miscarriages. The Royal College of Obstetricians and Gynaecologists[8] recommends chromosome analysis after three miscarriages, whereas the American Society of Reproduction Medicine,[9] recommends chromosome analysis after two miscarriages. However, parental karyotyping is expensive and does not always give valuable information; therefore, its use could also be avoided in many couples.[10–11]

Prognosis

The presence of a cytogenetic abnormality in miscarriages explains the loss. However, in most couples with recurrent pregnancy loss, thorough evaluation, including parental karyotype testing will be negative. Therefore, the majority (approximately 50–75%) of couples with recurrent pregnancy loss have no definitive diagnosis. Live birth rates of between 35% and 85% are commonly reported in couples with unexplained recurrent pregnancy loss who undergo an untreated or placebo-treated subsequent pregnancy. Meta-analysis of randomized, prospective studies suggests that 60–70% of women with unexplained recurrent pregnancy loss will have a successful next pregnancy.[12] Recurrent pregnancy loss may be due to an abnormal embryo, which is incompatible with life. As the number of miscarriages increases, the prevalence of chromosomal abnormality decreases, and the chance of recurring maternal cause increases.[13–14]

Thus, many couples will view the prognosis as favorable.

Laboratory Technique

Conventional cytogenetic analysis of spontaneous abortion tissue is strongly dependent on tissue culturing and is associated with a significant culture failure rate, which varies from 5% to 42% in different laboratories. The banding technique for karyotyping can only assess structural and numeric rearrangements. It is laborious and liable to fail as a result of contamination, culture failure, or overgrowth of maternal cells. The mechanism of cell death *in vitro* has not been sufficiently investigated. Consequently, culture failure is common. Another possible disadvantage of the (semi-) direct preparation is the discrepancy that may occur between embryonic and chorionic villus cells. Such a discrepancy might be due to mosaicism only being found in placental tissue, that is, confined placental mosaicism. It is possible to assume that tissue culture failure is a marker of particular genomic imbalances incompatible with normal cell proliferation. If this hypothesis is true, then the standard cytogenetic analysis of spontaneous abortions may underestimate the frequency and diversity of chromosomal abnormalities. Thus, the fetal karyotype may not be represented correctly by the villous karyotype. The estimated percentage of mosaicism is 1–2% for (semi-) direct chromosome preparation in chorionic villous sampling. In view of these difficulties, it has been argued that other more sophisticated tests such as Comparative Chromosomal Microarray Analysis (CMA), aCHG may overcome these problems and allow additional genetic diagnoses to be made, such as uniparental disomy or skewed X chromosome inactivation. As CMA does not require dividing cells, it can be useful in fetal demise with culture failure.[15] In a recent study of samples from stillbirths, single nucleotide polymorfism (SNP) oligonucleotide microarray analysis has been found to be more likely to yield results than karyotype analysis (87.4% versus 70.5%, $p < 0.001$) and provided better detection of genetic abnormalities (aneuploidy or pathogenic copy number variants, 8.3% versus 5.8%; $p = 0.007$).[16] CMA may also be useful in the future as a diagnostic tool, *instead* of parental and/or abortus' karyotyping, when more data will be accessible and when the cost decreases. Further investigations of CNVs (Copy Number Variations are alteration of the DNA results in the cell having an abnormal or normal variation in the number of copies of one or more sections of the DNA), particularly those involving genes that are imprinted in the placenta, in women with RPL may be worthwhile. However, it should be noted that, at present, there are few data on the use of CMA in recurrent miscarriage. Current available guidelines for genetic evaluation and counseling of couples with recurrent miscarriage state that the use of specialized chromosomal studies such as comparative genome hybridization, subtelomeric studies, interphase studies on sperm and assays for skewed X-inactivation patterns are not warranted at this time, as their clinical utility has yet to be determined. Hence, current laboratory techniques prevent fetal karyotyping as a routine clinical test, and CMA techniques are still too expensive with little supportive evidence based data in RPL.

Below are some consensus remarks from various sources regarding fetal karyotyping.

Consensus Remarks

Gynecologists, obstetricians, and fertility specialists from 18 countries participated in a 3-day workshop held in Denmark in 2002–2005.[17]

Improved techniques in cytogenetics have permitted more accurate and reliable assessments of the products of conception. Given these improvements in our diagnostic ability, it is even more important that every effort be made to study the products of conception in every case of miscarriage *in therapeutic trials* so that a more valid evaluation can be made regarding the efficacy *of the experimental treatment*". They do not recommend karyotyping of abortus material.

National Society of Genetic Counselors—2005[10]

Parental karyotyping is expensive and does not always give valuable information; therefore, its use could be avoided in many couples.

Royal College of Obstetricians and Gynaecologists—2011[8]

"Cytogenetic analysis should be performed on products of conception of the third and subsequent consecutive miscarriage(s). Parental peripheral blood karyotyping of both partners should be performed in couples with recurrent miscarriage where testing of products of conception reports an unbalanced structural chromosomal abnormality."

(*This statement is under Category D* [based on non-analytical studies and expert opinion]). The college concluded—Cytogenetic testing is an expensive tool and may be reserved for patients who have undergone treatment in the index pregnancy or have been participating in a research trial.

American Society of Reproductive Medicine—2012[9]

"Testing of the products of conception may also be of psychological value to the couple, however, there are many pitfalls to this approach including the possibility of maternal contamination of the specimen, failure to seek other causes of RPL if the cytogenetic assessment reveals an abnormal karyotype and the occurrence of non-cytogenetic embryonic abnormalities."

Concluding Remarks

A. The recurrence risk of another miscarriage is not, or only slightly elevated (16%) when compared to the initial risk of all women (10–15%), and thus routine karyotyping of fetal material in miscarriages is thought not to be worthwhile or necessary in daily practice.

B. More than half of abortuses have normal chromosomes, while most of the abnormal chromosomes are numerical abnormalities (86%), in which trisomies of various chromosomes occur in more than 2/3 of these, giving rise to a randomly occurring effect.

C. Furthermore, with so many possible causes for recurrent miscarriage, it would be tempting to think that the prognosis for those women whose recurrent miscarriages are unexplained (more than half) is dire. But three quarters of these women will go on to have a successful pregnancy if offered nothing more, and nothing less, than tender love and care, and reassurance through ultrasound that nothing is abnormal.

D. The current technical tissue culturing in use of conventional cytogenetic analysis of the abortus is laborious and subject to problems such as external contamination, culture failure and selective growth of maternal cells, which varies from 5% to 42%. As current rates of chromosomal abnormalities have remained constant over time, and are independent of the culture method used in most laboratories, (even with the current success rate of 90%), there is no benefit to the use of such method.

E. CMA may be useful in the future as a diagnostic tool, *instead* of parental and/or karyotyping of the fetus, when more data are available, and when the cost decreases. However, CMA analysis is not warranted at this time.

F. The summaries of several major Consensus papers, quoted above, do not advise routine karyotyping of the embryo in recurrent pregnancy loss.

Consequently, one must conclude that there is no clinical justification, nor any psychological benefit for fetal karyotyping. This conclusion is well supported throughout this in-depth current literature survey, as well as in these consensus clinical guides of the leading professional societies.

REFERENCES

1. Penrose LS, Delhanty JD, Triploid cell cultures from a macerated foetus. *Lancet* 1961;10(1):1261–2.
2. Rubio C, Pehlivan T, Rodrigo L et al. Embryo aneuploidy screening for unexplained recurrent miscarriage: A minireview. *Am J Reprod Immunol* 2005;53:159–65.
3. Quenby S, Vince G, Farquharson R et al. Recurrent miscarriage: A defect in nature's quality control? *Hum Reprod* 2002;17(8):1959–63.
4. Goddijn M, Leschot NJ. Genetic aspects of miscarriage. *Bailliere's Best Pract Res Clin Obstet Gynaecol* 2000;14(5):855–65.
5. Griebel CP, Halvorsen J, Golemon TB et al. Management of spontaneous abortion. *Am Fam Physician* 2005;72(7):1243–50.
6. Yusuf RZ, Naeem R. Cytogenetic abnormalities in products of conception: A relationship revisited. *Am J Reprod Immunol* 2004;52(1):88–96.
7. Pfeifer S, Fritz M, Goldberg J et al. Evaluation and treatment of recurrent pregnancy loss: A committee opinion. *Fertil Steril* 2012;98(5):1103–11.
8. Royal College of Obstetricians and Gynaecologists. The investigation and treatment of couples with recurrent miscarriage. Guideline no.17, April 2011-www.rcog.org.uk.
9. Practice Committee of American Society for Reproductive Medicine. Definitions of infertility and recurrent pregnancy loss: A committee opinion. *Fertil Steril*. 2012; 98(5):1103–11.
10. Laurino MY, Bennett RL, Saraiya DS et al. Genetic evaluation and counseling of couples with recurrent miscarriage: Recommendations of the National Society of Genetic Counselors. *J Genet Counsel* 2005;14:165–181.
11. Alijotas-Reig J and Garrido-Gimenez C. Current concepts and new trends in the diagnosis and management of recurrent miscarriage. *Obstet Gynecol Surv* 2013;68(6): 445–466.
12. Jeng GT, Scott JR, Burmeister LF. A comparison of meta-analytic results using literature vs individual patient data. Paternal cell immunization for recurrent miscarriage. *JAMA, J Am Med Assoc* 1995;274(10):830–6.
13. Ogasawara M, Aoki K, Okada S et al. Embryonic karyotype of abortuses in relation to the number of previous miscarriages. *Fertil Steril* 2000;73(2):300–4.
14. Kwinecka-Dmitriew B, Zakrzewska M, Latos-Bielecska A et al. Frequency of chromosomal aberrations in material from abortions. *Ginekol Pol* 2010;81:896–901.

15. ACOG Committee Opinion No. 446: Array comparative genomic hybridization in prenatal diagnosis. *Obstet Gynecol* 2009;114:1161.

16. Reddy UM, Page GP, Saade GR et al. Karyotype versus microarray testing for genetic abnormalities after stillbirth. *N Engl J Med* 2012;367(23):2185.

17. Christiansen OB, Nybo Andersen AM, Bosch E et al. Evidence-based investigations and treatments of recurrent pregnancy loss. *Fertil Steril* 2005;83(4):821–39.

6

Debate: Should Preimplantation Genetic Screening Be Performed in Recurrent Pregnancy Loss? Yes

Pere Mir, Nasser Al-Asmar, Lorena Rodrigo, Carlos Simon, and Carmen Rubio

Spontaneous pregnancy loss can be due to several factors either maternal or fetal. Embryo/fetal chromosomal abnormalities are the most common factor involved in spontaneous miscarriages, accounting for about 50% of all pregnancy losses before the 15th week of gestation.[1] The term recurrent pregnancy loss (RPL) is widely accepted as the loss of two or more pregnancies from the same partners, and affects up to 5% of couples of reproductive age.[2] Common causes for RPL are immunological, endocrine, anatomic, or genetic factors, but about 50% of RPL cases still remain unexplained, or idiopathic. In this group of patients, fetal chromosomal abnormalities have been reported to be the most common cause of RPL, accounting for up to 55% of cases, thus leaving a remainder of 24.5% of truly unexplained RPLs.[3]

It has been proposed that couples suffering from idiopathic RPL who generate chromosomally abnormal embryos ending in miscarriage should undergo preimplantation genetic screening (PGS) in order to overcome this problem. PGS analyzes the chromosomal status of the embryo before embryo transfer, therefore only chromosomally normal embryos are placed into the maternal uterus. By transferring euploid embryos, free of chromosome abnormalities, PGS aims not only to increase pregnancy and implantation rates in infertile patients, but also to reduce the miscarriage rate in RPL patients, and to dramatically decrease the risk of having aneuploid offspring. Several years ago there was a significant debate about the usefulness of PGS because none of the randomized studies showed a clear benefit for the use of this technique (reviewed in Mastenbroek et al., 2011).[4] However, these negative results were due to the technical limitations of the fluorescence *in situ* hybridization (FISH) which was used at the time, and only allowed a limited number of chromosomes to be analyzed, and poorer embryo biopsy techniques and culture conditions than those available today.[5–8]

There is increasing evidence supporting the use of PGS in idiopathic RPL patients. In a study published by Bianco et al.,[9] in which prenatal diagnosis was performed in 46,939 women, an increased risk of karyotypic abnormalities was confirmed in the products of conception in idiopathic RPL patients. The first evidence demonstrating that RPL couples have an increased number of chromosomally abnormal embryos (ranging from 50% to 80%) was published by our group in 1998,[10] and these results were later confirmed by other studies.[11–17]

Using FISH for chromosomes 13, 15, 16, 18, 21, 22, X, and Y to select chromosomally normal embryos for transfer demonstrated that reproductive outcome is improved by PGS.[11] Our studies demonstrate that, after PGS, significantly higher implantation rates were obtained in couples who previously suffered aneuploid miscarriages. Secondly, similar embryo aneuploidy, pregnancy, and implantation rates were recorded in couples with RPL after fertility treatments as in those with previous spontaneous pregnancies. Thirdly, there were no miscarriages after PGS in couples in which the FISH assay first showed that the male partner's sperm was abnormal. Finally, lower implantation rates are observed in couples with ≥5 previous miscarriages, which is associated with a lower incidence of chromosomally abnormal embryos. We concluded that PGS should be recommended when RPL is associated with chromosomopathy in up to five previous miscarriages, and when there is a high incidence of chromosomal abnormalities in sperm.[11]

In fact, a systematic review of the evidence for the efficacy of PGS in patients with idiopathic RPL versus controls not undergoing PGS suggested that the miscarriage rate might be lower after undergoing PGS.[18] The technology has continued to evolve and it is now possible to assess all 24 human chromosomes using a new strategy known as comprehensive chromosomal screening (CCS) that overcomes the limitations of FISH. Several approaches towards 24-chromosome analysis have been developed, with array-comparative genomic hybridization (array-CGH) being the preferred diagnostic approach for aneuploidy screening.[19,20] In fact, IVF programs are moving towards PGS using array-CGH as the first option for CCS.[21–26]

Array-CGH analysis can be performed on the three cell types that can be biopsied: polar bodies, day-3 embryo blastomeres, or throphectoderm cells. In all three cases, DNA needs to be amplified and the quality of the process must be ensured (e.g., by gel electrophoresis). Following this, the amplified samples and control DNAs are labeled with Cy3 and Cy5 fluorophores following the manufacturer's instructions. Labeling mixes are combined and hybridized onto the arrays; each probe is specific for a different chromosomal region and occupies a discrete spot on the slide. Chromosomal loss or gain is revealed by the color adopted by each spot after hybridization. The technique involves the competitive hybridization of differentially labeled test and reference DNA samples, the fluorescence intensity is detected using a laser scanner, and specific software is used for data processing. The entire protocol can be completed in less than 24 hours. Therefore, embryo transfer and the vitrification of surplus euploid embryos can be scheduled on day-5 when day-3 biopsies are performed, or on day-6 for trophectoderm biopsies.

In a recently published retrospective case-control study which included CCS in cycles for RPL patients with a day-3 biopsy and an array-CGH, the implantation rate in the CCS group was clearly higher when compared to the control group (52.63% vs. 19.15%; $p = 0.001$), the clinical pregnancy rate was also higher (69.23% vs. 43.91%, $p = 0.0002$), the ongoing pregnancy rate almost doubled (61.54% vs. 32.49%, $p = 0.0001$), the multiple pregnancy rate decreased (8.33% vs. 34.38%, $p = 0.0082$) and the miscarriage rate showed a lower trend (11.11% vs. 26.01%, $p = 0.13$). The authors concluded that CCS on cleavage-stage embryos using the array-CGH approach was a feasible and safe option for aneuploidy screening in idiopathic RPL.[27]

In the last three years, we have performed 329 array-CGH cycles with day-3 biopsies on couples with two or more previous miscarriages. In RPL patients below 38 years of age, 62.6% of the embryos were identified as chromosomally abnormal; in 80.0% of the cycles we were able to select a euploid embryo for transfer, with a mean number of 1.6 (SD 1.0) embryos transferred. The clinical pregnancy rate per transfer was 60.0%, with an implantation rate of 47.0%, and a miscarriage rate of 11.7%. In RPL women ≥38 years of age, the number of aneuploid embryos was significantly increased to 83.7% ($p < 0.05$), with euploid embryos suitable for transfer remaining in 56.4% of the cycles, and a mean number of 1.3 (SD 1.0) embryos transferred. The clinical pregnancy rate per transfer for women with RPL and advanced maternal age was 52.2%, the implantation rate was 50.3%, and the miscarriage rate was 10.0%. These results showed a clear benefit of 24-chromosome screening in couples with RPL (data not published). Furthermore a retrospective study comparing PGS using FISH analysis for nine chromosomes versus PGS using array-CGH for 24 chromosomes in RPL patients, showed a significant increase in the pregnancy rates per transfer and pregnancy rates per initiated cycle in the array-CGH group versus FISH.[28]

In summary, accumulated evidence has demonstrated that chromosomal abnormalities are a major cause of RPL of unknown etiology, and clinical results have demonstrated a reduction in the miscarriage rate of RPL patients undergoing PGS, which is even greater when using a CCS technique. Regardless of the strategy used to prevent RPL, in the case of any miscarriage, both the routine tests used to evaluate women with RPL,[29] and a comprehensive chromosomal analysis of the products of conception should be carried out in order to identify which patients can benefit from PGS.

To properly demonstrate the clinical usefulness of CCS in RPL patients, a proper randomized controlled trial should be conducted; however, this may prove difficult because previous results from these patients have shown a reduced miscarriage rate, as presented in this chapter. Therefore, based on the data shown here, we conclude that PGS using a CCS approach reduces miscarriage rates when applied to RPL patients. Therefore we recommend that CCS should be used for all RPL patients.

REFERENCES

1. Warren JE, Silver RM. Genetics of pregnancy loss. *Clin Obstet Gynecol* 2008;51:84–95.
2. Stephenson MD, Awartani KA, Robinson WP. Cytogenetic analysis of miscarriages from couples with recurrent miscarriage: A case-control study. *Hum Reprod* 2002;17:446–51.
3. Sugiura-Ogasawara M, Ozaki Y, Katano K et al. Abnormal embryonic karyotype is the most frequent cause of recurrent miscarriage. *Hum Reprod* 2012;27:2297–303.
4. Mastenbroek S, Twisk M, van der Veen F et al. Preimplantation genetic screening: A systematic review and meta-analysis of RCTs. *Hum Reprod Update* 2011;17:454–66.
5. Cohen J, Wells D, Munne S. Removal of 2 cells from cleavage stage embryos is likely to reduce the efficacy of chromosomal tests that are used to enhance implantation rates. *Fertil Steril* 2007;87:496–503.
6. Simpson JL. What next for preimplantation genetic screening? Randomized clinical trial in assessing PGS: Necessary but not sufficient. *Hum Reprod* 2008;23:2179–81.
7. Rubio C, Gimenez C, Fernandez E et al. Spanish interest group in preimplantation genetics, Spanish society for the study of the biology of reproduction. The importance of good practice in preimplantation genetic screening: Critical viewpoints. *Hum Reprod* 2009;24:2045–7.
8. Mir P, Rodrigo L, Mateu E et al. Improving FISH diagnosis for preimplantation genetic aneuploidy screening. *Hum Reprod* 2010;25:1812–7.
9. Bianco K, Caughey AB, Shaffer BL et al. History of miscarriage and increased incidence of fetal aneuploidy in subsequent pregnancy. *Obstet Gynecol* 2006;107:1098–102.
10. Simón C, Rubio C, Vidal F et al. Increased chromosome abnormalities in human preimplantation embryos after in-vitro fertilization in patients with recurrent miscarriage. *Reprod Fertil Dev* 1998;10:87–92.
11. Rubio C, Buendía P, Rodrigo L et al. Prognostic factors for preimplantation genetic screening in repeated pregnancy loss. *Reprod BioMed Online* 2009;18:687–93.
12. Pellicer A, Rubio C, Vidal F et al. *In vitro* fertilization plus preimplantation genetic diagnosis in patients with recurrent miscarriage: An analysis of chromosome abnormalities in human preimplantation embryos. *Fertil Steril* 1999;71:1033–9.
13. Werlin L, Rodi I, De Cherney A et al. Preimplantation genetic diagnosis as both a therapeutic and diagnostic tool in assisted reproductive technology. *Fertil Steril* 2003;80: 467–8.
14. Wilding M, Forman R, Hogewind G et al. Preimplantation genetic diagnosis for the treatment of failed *in vitro* fertilization–embryo transfer and habitual abortion. *Fertil Steril* 2004;81:1302–7.
15. Platteau P, Staessen C, Michiels A et al. Preimplantation genetic diagnosis for aneuploidy screening in patients with unexplained recurrent miscarriages. *Fertil Steril* 2005;83:393–7.
16. Findikli N. Embryo aneuploidy screening for repeated implantation failure and unexplained recurrent miscarriage. *Reprod BioMed Online* 2006;13:38–46.
17. Garrisi JG, Colls P, Ferry KM et al. Effect of infertility, maternal age, and number of previous miscarriages on the outcome of preimplantation genetic diagnosis for idiopathic recurrent pregnancy loss. *Fertil Steril* 2009;92:288–95.
18. Musters AM, Repping S, Korevaar JC et al. Pregnancy outcome after preimplantation genetic screening or natural conception in couples with unexplained recurrent miscarriage: A systematic review of the best available evidence. *Fertil Steril* 2011;95:2153–7.
19. Handyside AH. 24 chromosome copy number analysis: A comparison of available technologies. *Fertil Steril* 2013;100:595–602.
20. Simpson JL. Preimplantation genetic diagnosis to improve pregnancy outcomes in subfertility. *Best Pract Res Clin Obstet Gynaecol* 2012;26:805–15.
21. Rubio C, Rodrigo L, Mir P et al. Use of array comparative genomic hybridization (array-CGH) for embryo assessment: Clinical results. *Fertil Steril* 2013;99:1044–8.
22. Schoolcraft WB, Fragouli E, Stevens J et al. Clinical application of comprehensive chromosomal screening at the blastocyst stage. *Fertil Steril* 2010;94:1700–6.

23. Forman EJ, Tao X, Ferry KM et al. Single embryo transfer with comprehensive chromosome screening results in improved ongoing pregnancy rates and decreased miscarriage rates. *Hum Reprod* 2012;27:1217–22.

24. Mir P, Rodrigo L, Mercader A et al. False positive rate of an arrayCGH platform for single-cell preimplantation genetic screening and subsequent clinical aplication on day-3. *J Assisted Reprod Genet* 2013;30:143–9.

25. Yang Z, Liu J, Collins GS et al. Selection of single blastocysts for fresh transfer via standard morphology assessment alone and with array CGH for good prognosis IVF patients: Results from a randomized pilot study. *Mol Cytogenet* 2012;5:24–9.

26. Hodes-Wertz B, Grifo J, Ghadir S et al. Idiopathic recurrent miscarriage is caused mostly by aneuploid embryos. *Fertil Steril* 2012;98:675–80.

27. Keltz MD, Vega M, Sirota I et al. Preimplantation genetic screening (PGS) with comparative genomic hybridization (CGH) following day 3 single cell blastomere biopsy markedly improves IVF outcomes while lowering multiple pregnancies and miscarriages. *J Assisted Reprod Genet* 2013;30(10):1333–9.

28. Rubio C, Rodrigo L, Mateu E et al. Array CGH vs. FISH in recurrent miscarriage couples. *Hum Reprod* 2013; Abstract Book ESHRE Annual meeting. p. 444.

29. Branch DW, Gibson M, Silver RM. Clinical practice: Recurrent miscarriage. *N Engl J Med* 2010;363:1740–7.

7

Debate: Should Preimplantation Genetic Screening or Preimplantation Genetic Diagnosis Be Performed in Recurrent Pregnancy Loss? No

Anna M. Musters and Mariette Goddijn

Introduction

The management of recurrent miscarriage (RM) is a clinical challenge considering that in the majority of the couples no evidence based treatment is available to increase live birth rates or decrease miscarriage rates. Unexplained pregnancy loss is a diagnosis of exclusion, and is used when no aetiological factor is found on routine investigation.[1] It is not a definitive diagnosis. Although there is no effective therapy for unexplained pregnancy loss, the condition is so distressing for the affected couple and frustrating for the clinician that nonevidence based diagnoses and treatment are often proposed rather than adhering to guidelines that state that treatment for these couples may not be indicated.[2]

Preimplantation genetic screening (PGS) has been proposed as a treatment for couples with unexplained RM as the aneuploidy of the embryo may be the cause of the miscarriages in a substantial number of patients. The prevalence of fetal chromosome abnormalities is 45% in couples with a single sporadic miscarriage.[3] This prevalence is based on 13 studies including 7012 miscarriage samples. The prevalence of fetal chromosome abnormalities in women experiencing a subsequent miscarriage after a preceding miscarriage is comparable: 39% (based on 6 studies, including 1359 samples).[3] Additionally, preimplantation genetic diagnosis (PGD) has been proposed as a treatment for couples suffering from recurrent miscarriage and diagnosed with parental structural chromosome abnormalities. Both PGS in unexplained recurrent miscarriage and PGD for parental structural chromosome abnormalities will be discussed in this chapter.

Women with RM are eager and willing to try any form of treatment.[4] In this debate we shall attempt to show that the use of PGS or PGD is unwarranted due to the requirement for invasive techniques (in vitro fertilization (IVF)/intra-cytoplasmic sperm injection (ICSI)), the fact that couples with RM already have a high live birth rate without intervention, and there is no improvement in live birth rates with PGS or PGD in these couples.

Preimplantation Genetic Screening

PGS is an intervention that has been proposed to increase pregnancy rates and also to lower miscarriage rates by preventing fetal aneuploidy. In PGS, embryos are selected for transfer based on the chromosomal status of a single blastomere biopsied from that embryo, polar body biopsies, or trophectoderm biopsies from day-5 blastocysts.[5–7] In 2007, a trial revealed that in women of advanced maternal age the application of PGS in fact decreased pregnancy rates.[8] The results showed a decreased ongoing pregnancy rate of 24% in the PGS group compared to 35% in the control group (rate ratio: 0.68; 95% CI: 0.50–0.92). These findings continued to be reconfirmed in a meta-analysis including nine randomized controlled trials (RCTs).[9]

Should Preimplantation Genetic Screening Be Performed in Documented Fetal Aneuploidy?

Opinions differ as to the usefulness of karyotyping in miscarriage samples for routine clinical practice. There is no clear relevance for clinical decision making, but a fetal genetic test result may provide information for the woman or couple in question.[3] It has been suggested that PGS should be offered only to couples with documented aneuploid miscarriages. However, three studies have shown that these patients even have a better prognosis than those with euploid miscarriages.[10–12] In these documented aneuploid cases, it is unlikely that PGS will increase the chance of a live birth, but this has not been substantiated. Results obtained from observational studies must always be analyzed with caution since most of these patients, especially young women, have a good chance of a subsequent live birth.

In cases of recurrent fetal aneuploidy, it should be kept in mind that fetal aneuploidy determined at seven to eight weeks gestational age after the occurrence of a miscarriage is not similar to the determination of aneuploidy tested in one single cell or two cells at the very early embryonal stage, and does not legitimize the use of PGS. Diploid aneuploid mosaicism is the most common chromosomal constitution in spare human preimplantation embryos after IVF. A reliable determination of the ploidy status of a cleavage-stage embryo based on the analysis of a single cell is therefore not feasible.[13] Whether aneuploidy is tested by a blastomere biopsied from that embryo, or polar body biopsies, or trophectoderm biopsies from day-5 blastocysts is irrelevant.[5–7] Chromosome techniques might differ in their aneuploidy detection rate, for example, whole genome analysis with array comparative genome hybridization (aCGH) can potentially detect larger numbers of aneuploidies compared to fluorescence in situ hybridization (FISH) analysis. Additionally, aCGH analysis may discover chromosomal variations of unknown significance (VOUS). At present VOUS embryos are not replaced, thus a certain number of normal embryos may be discarded, again compromising the subsequent live birth rate.

Should Preimplantation Genetic Screening Be Performed in Women with Unexplained Recurrent Miscarriage?

Couples with unexplained RM have been suggested as candidates for PGS. The rationale behind the use of PGS in cases of unexplained RM is that aneuploidy of the embryo, although not assessed, may be the cause of RM.[14–18] Since PGS is invasive and requires *in vitro* fertilization, the claim that PGS increases the live birth rate should be substantiated beyond reasonable doubt before PGS is introduced into daily clinical practice. However, PGS is currently performed in RM worldwide.[19] Data from the European Society of Human Reproduction and Embryology (ESHRE) PGD consortium shows an increase of PGS cycles for couples with RM from 285 in 2003 to 2100 in 2009.[19,20] The current guidelines from this consortium do not give a recommendation in favor or against PGS for RM couples.[19,21] The American Society of Reproductive Medicine (ASRM) guideline states that the available evidence does not support the use of PGS as currently performed to improve live birth rates in patients with recurrent pregnancy loss, because RCTs are not available.[22,23]

A recent review described four observational studies concerning unexplained RM and PGS.[24] The total number of included couples was 181 and varied from 10 to 58 per study. The mean previous miscarriage rate varied between 2.8 and 4.7 and the mean maternal age varied from 35.4 to 37.6 years. In all studies the embryos were biopsied at day three of development and one or two blastomeres were aspirated and analyzed. The FISH probes used for aneuploidy screening differed in each study (minimum of three and maximum of nine probes). Also the number of embryos transferred varied per study; from single embryo transfer to five embryos per transfer. There was an average of 1.3 cycles (ranging from 1.2 to 1.6 cycles) per couple in the four studies.[17,18,24–26] Live birth rates per couple in these four studies varied between 19% and 46% (mean 35%; median 40%) and miscarriage rate per couple ranged from 0% to 10% (mean 9%; median 9%). After the review was published, a recent study investigated PGS outcome per cycle in couples with RM—instead of per couple.[27] This study used aCGH, and reported a live birth rate per started cycle of 33% and a miscarriage rate per started cycle of 2%.

TABLE 7.1

Reasons to Advise against Preimplantation Genetic Screening/Preimplantation Genetic Diagnosis in Recurrent Miscarriage

a. Reasons to advise against *PGS* in women with unexplained RM
  No reported higher chances of live birth rate after PGS compared to natural conception
  Relatively good pregnancy outcomes after natural conception in women with unexplained recurrent miscarriage
  Requirement of invasive techniques (IVF/ICSI)
  IVF/ICSI procedures associated with complications and high costs

b. Reasons to advise against *PGD* in women with RM and parental chromosome abnormalities
  Viable chromosomally unbalanced offspring are hardly ever detected through a history of recurrent miscarriage.
  Parental karyotyping is no longer considered useful in RM without a family history of the birth of a congenitally handicapped child
  No reported higher chance of live birth rate after PGD compared to natural conception
  Relatively good cumulative pregnancy outcomes after natural conception
  Requirement of invasive techniques (IVF/ICSI)
  IVF/ICSI procedures associated with complications and high costs

A summary of the reasons to advise against PGS in women with unexplained RM is presented in Table 7.1. No RCTs or even nonrandomized comparative studies have been performed to directly compare the efficacy of PGS with natural conception for couples with unexplained RM. The need for RCTs on this topic is evident, considering the increasing numbers of PGS performed for this indication worldwide.[19,20]

Counseling Women with Unexplained Recurrent Miscarriage

Chapter 22 classifies patients with RM into good, medium and poor prognosis groups depending on the number of prior miscarriages, and so on. It should be borne in mind that the majority of couples fall into the "good prognosis" group and have a relatively good future live birth rate after natural conception. Providing patients with an individualized future spontaneous live birth rate[28] can be most helpful. Furthermore, the management of couples with recurrent miscarriage will improve if individualized support is applied to couples, taking account of their own preferences at the time of miscarriage and when pregnant again.[29,30]

It is our moral obligation as physicians to provide women with reliable data from the literature, preferably from well conducted clinical trials. The claim of reproductive medicine units' websites that PGS improves pregnancy outcomes is unjustified.

It should be borne in mind that PGS (with blastomere biopsy and FISH technique) performed in women at advanced maternal age even decreased pregnancy rates compared to women not undergoing PGS,[8,31] which reinforces our obligation to offer PGS with newer techniques like trophectoderm biopsies and aCGH only in the setting of well conducted trials. Currently, PGS using trophectoderm biopsies from day-5 blastocysts and aCGH is most often applied. Some recent trials have been published using these newer techniques but these trials have only included women with subfertility and a pre-existing indication for IVF.[32–34] For women with a history of recurrent miscarriage and natural conception, no clinical trials have been reported to date using these techniques.

With proper counseling, the offering of expensive, invasive, potentially harmful, and nonevidence-based treatments like PGS can be avoided.

Should Preimplantation Genetic Diagnosis Be Performed in Women with Recurrent Miscarriage and Parental Chromosomal Abnormalities?

PGD has been used as a means of preventing miscarriages in patients with a parental karyotype abnormality. The rationale was to prevent the balanced translocation being passed on to the embryo in an unbalanced form. Recurrent miscarriage is associated with carrier status of a parental chromosome abnormality in one of the partners, most frequently balanced chromosome translocations followed by chromosome inversions. However, even in the presence of parental chromosomal rearrangements, the products of conception can be of a normal karyotype, the same karyotype as the carrier parent, or an unbalanced karyotype. The latter can lead to miscarriage, stillbirth, or the birth of a child with major congenital impairments.

The risk of viable unbalanced offspring in carrier couples appears to be rather low (0.7%).[35,36] Carriers detected through a history of recurrent miscarriage seem to form a different subgroup and are facing other reproductive risks than carriers for example, detected through a previous birth of a child with an unbalanced karyotype or the birth of unbalanced offspring in the family. Viable unbalanced offspring are hardly ever detected through a history of recurrent miscarriage. The subgroup with recurrent miscarriage is mainly prone to miscarriages and counseling should therefore focus on this risk rather than on the risk of unbalanced offspring. It has been suggested that PGD should be offered to carrier couples. The aim of PGD would be to decrease the incidence of offspring with an unbalanced karyotype and reduce the risk of miscarriages. However, although the theory sounds plausible, review of the data does not concur. In a recently published systematic review,[37] no RCTs or nonrandomized comparative studies comparing the effects of PGD with natural conception were found.[38–40] Data could only be derived from observational studies and case reports. It was concluded that there are insufficient data indicating that PGD improves the live birth rate in women with carrier couples with RM compared with natural conception. A retrospective study was published after this review.[41] In this study, 192 carrier couples with RM undergoing PGD were described. PGD was performed with FISH analysis of polar bodies or blastomeres. Although favorable IVF–PGD results were shown, the study was prone to flaws.[42] It is therefore still important that the couples will be offered appropriate unbiased counseling.

PGD, with its expensive cost, therefore has no place in the treatment of carrier couples with recurrent miscarriage. In the case of concomitant subfertility leading to an IVF/ICSI treatment, the balance of outweighing benefits versus risks could be more in favor of a positive decision towards PGD. However, even in this situation, it should be kept in mind that existing data do not support the use of PGD because there is no convincing evidence that it improves live birth rates. A summary of the reasons to advise against PGD in women with RM and a parental chromosome abnormality is presented in Table 7.1.

In fact the evidence for parental chromosomal abnormalities causing viable unbalanced offspring in carrier couples points to a very low risk, such that parental karyotyping is no longer considered useful for couples with RM without a family history of the birth of a congenitally handicapped child.[35,36,43]

Counseling Women with Recurrent Miscarriage about Preimplantation Genetic Diagnosis

The majority of couples with RM and a parental chromosome abnormality have a relatively good future (cumulative) live birth rate after natural conception. Providing patients with an individualized future spontaneous live birth rate can be very helpful.[35] Also for these couples, the management and satisfaction may improve if a proper plan is planned for supportive care in a next spontaneously achieved pregnancy.[30] Currently, new knowledge calls for abandoning parental karyotyping in couples with RM without a family history of the birth of a congenitally handicapped child. Viable chromosomally unbalanced offspring are hardly ever detected through a history of recurrent miscarriage. Logically, there is no further place for PGD to prevent the negligible chance of unbalanced offspring in these couples.[35,36] The claim that PGD reduces miscarriage rates should be viewed in the context of an absence of clinical trials providing the evidence. With proper counseling the offering of expensive, invasive, potentially harmful, and nonevidence based treatments like PGD can be avoided.

Conclusions and Recommendations

Most women with RM have a good prognosis after natural conception and a high cumulative live birth rate.[28] By reviewing the literature on PGS and PGD in women with RM, there are insufficient data to indicate that PGS or PGD improves live birth rates compared to natural conception. There are insufficient arguments to introduce PGS, with its high costs and potential complications related to the IVF/ICSI procedures, into the daily clinical practice for couples with unexplained RM. The need for comparative studies of high quality is urgent. There is no further place for parental karyotyping in couples with RM without a family history of the birth of a congenitally handicapped child. As a result, there is no place for PGD to prevent the negligible chance of unbalanced offspring in these couples.

Acknowledgments

The authors wish to thank S. Mastenbroek, clinical embryologist, for carefully reading and commenting on the manuscript.

REFERENCES

1. Rai R, Regan L, Recurrent miscarriage. *Lancet* 2006;368:601–11.
2. Franssen MT, Korevaar JC, van der Veen F et al. Management of recurrent miscarriage: Evaluating the impact of a guideline. *Hum Reprod* 2007;5:1298–303.
3. van den Berg MM, van Maarle MC, van Wely M et al. Genetics of early miscarriage. *Biochim Biophys Acta* 2012;1822:1951–9.
4. van den Boogaard E, Hermens RP, Leschot NJ et al. Identification of barriers for good adherence to a guideline on recurrent miscarriage. *Acta Obstet Gynecol Scand* 2011;90:186–91.
5. Gianaroli L, Magli MC, Ferraretti AP et al. Preimplantation genetic diagnosis increases the implantation rate in human in vitro fertilization by avoiding the transfer of chromosomally abnormal embryos. *Fertil Steril* 1997;68:1128–31.
6. Munné S, Magli C, Cohen J et al. Positive outcome after preimplantation diagnosis of aneuploidy in human embryos. *Hum Reprod* 1999;14:2191–9.
7. McArthur SJ, Leigh D, Marshall JT et al. Pregnancies and live births after trophectoderm biopsy and preimplantation genetic testing of human blastocysts. *Fertil Steril* 2005;84:1628–36.
8. Mastenbroek S, Twisk M, van Echten-Arends J et al. *In vitro* fertilization with preimplantation genetic screening. *N Engl J Med* 2007;357:9–17.
9. Mastenbroek S, Twisk M, van der Veen F et al. Preimplantation genetic screening: A systematic review and meta-analysis of RCTs. *Hum Reprod Update* 2011;17:454–66.
10. Carp H, Toder V, Aviram A et al. Karyotype of the abortus in recurrent miscarriage. *Fertil Steril* 2001;75:678–82.
11. Sullivan AE, Silver RM, LaCoursiere Y et al. Recurrent fetal aneuploidy and recurrent miscarriage. *Obstet Gynecol* 2004;104:784–8.
12. Ogasawara M, Aoki K, Okada S et al. Embryonic karyotype of abortuses in relation to the number of previous miscarriages. *Fertil Steril* 2000;73:300–4.
13. van Echten-Arends J, Mastenbroek S, Sikkema-Raddatz B et al. Chromosomal mosaicism in human preimplantation embryos: A systematic review. *Hum Reprod Update* 2011;17:620–7.
14. Gianaroli L, Magli MC, Ferraretti AP et al. The role of preimplantation diagnosis for aneuploidies. *Reprod Biomed Online* 2002;4:31–6.
15. Werlin L, Rodi I, Decherney A et al. Preimplantation genetic diagnosis as both a therapeutic and diagnostic tool in assisted reproductive technology. *Fertil Steril* 2003;80:467–8.
16. Rubio C, Pehlivan T, Rodrigo L, Simón C et al. Embryo aneuploidy screening for unexplained recurrent miscarriage: A mini review. *Am J Reprod Immunol* 2005;53:159–65.
17. Munné S, Chen S, Fischer J et al. Preimplantation genetic diagnosis reduces pregnancy loss in women aged 35 years and older with a history of recurrent miscarriages. *Fertil Steril* 2005;84:331–5.
18. Mantzouratou A, Mania A, Fragouli E et al. Variable aneuploidy mechanisms in embryos from couples with poor reproductive histories undergoing preimplantation genetic screening. *Hum Reprod*, 2007;22:1844–53.
19. Harper JC, Boelaert K, Geraedts J et al. ESHRE PGD Consortium data collection V: Cycles from January to December 2002 with pregnancy follow-up to October 2003. *Hum Reprod* 2006;21:3–21.
20. Goossens V, Traeger-Synodinos J, Coonen E et al. ESHRE PGD Consortium data collection XI: Cycles from January to December 2008 with pregnancy follow-up to October 2009. *Hum Reprod* 2012;27:1887–911.

21. Harton GL, Harper JC, Coonen E et al. European Society for Human Reproduction and Embryology (ESHRE) PGD consortium. ESHRE PGD consortium best practice guidelines for fluorescence *in situ* hybridization-based PGD. *Hum Reprod* 2011;26:25–32.
22. ASRM The Practice Committee of the Society for Assisted Reproductive Technology and the Practice Committee of the American Society of Reproductive Medicine. Preimplantation genetic testing: A practice Committee opinion. *Fertil Steril* 2008;90:S136–46.
23. Practice Committee of the American Society for Reproductive Medicine (ARSM) Evaluation and treatment of recurrent pregnancy loss: A committee opinion. *Fertil Steril* 2012;98:1103–11.
24. Musters AM, Repping S, Korevaar JC et al. Pregnancy outcome after preimplantation genetic screening or natural conception in couples with unexplained recurrent miscarriage: A systematic review of the best available evidence. *Fertil Steril* 2011;95:2153–7.
25. Wilding M, Forman R, Hogewind G, Di ML, Zullo F, Cappiello F et al. Preimplantation genetic diagnosis for the treatment of failed *in vitro* fertilization-embryo transfer and habitual abortion. *Fertil Steril* 2004;81:1302–7.
26. Platteau P, Staessen C, Michiels A et al. Preimplantation genetic diagnosis for aneuploidy screening in patients with unexplained recurrent miscarriages. *Fertil Steril* 2005;83:393–7.
27. Hodes-Wertz B, Grifo J, Ghadir S et al. Idiopathic recurrent miscarriage is caused mostly by aneuploid embryos. *Fertil Steril* 2012;98:675–80.
28. Brigham SA, Conlon C, Farquharson RG. A longitudinal study of pregnancy outcome following idiopathic recurrent miscarriage. *Hum Reprod* 1999;14:2868–71.
29. Musters AM, Taminiau-Bloem EF, van den Boogaard E et al. Supportive care for women with unexplained recurrent miscarriage: Patients' perspectives. *Hum Reprod* 2011;26:873–7.
30. Musters AM, Koot YE, van den Boogaard NM et al. Supportive care for women with recurrent miscarriage: A survey to quantify women's preferences. *Hum Reprod* 2013;28:398–405.
31. Twisk M, Mastenbroek S, van Wely M et al. Preimplantation genetic screening for abnormal number of chromosomes (aneuploidies) in *in vitro* fertilisation or intracytoplasmic sperm injection. *Cochrane Database Syst Rev* 2006;(1):CD005291.
32. Yang Z, Liu J, Collins G et al. Selection of single blastocysts for fresh transfer via standard morphology assessment alone and with array CGH for good prognosis IVF patients: Results from a randomized pilot study. *Mol Cytogenet* 2012;5:24.
33. Forman E, Hong K, Ferry K et al. *In vitro* fertilization with single euploid blastocyst transfer: A randomized controlled trial. *Fertil Steril* 2013;100:100–7.
34. Scott R, Upham K, Forman E. Blastocyst biopsy with comprehensive screening and fresh embryo transfer significantly increases *in vitro* fertilization implantation and delivery rates: A randomized controlled trial. *Fertil Steril* 2013;100:697–703.
35. Franssen M, Korevaar J, van der Veen F et al. Reproductive outcome after chromosome analysis in couples with two or more miscarriages: Index-control study. *BMJ* 2006;29:759–63.
36. Barber JC, Cockwell AE, Grant E et al. Is karyotyping couples experiencing recurrent miscarriage worth the cost? *BJOG.* 2010;117:885–8.
37. Franssen MTM, Musters AM, van der Veen F et al. Reproductive outcome after preimplantation genetic diagnosis in couples with recurrent miscarriage carrying a structural chromosome abnormality: A systematic review. *Hum Reprod Update* 2011;17:467–75.
38. Sugiura-Ogasawara M, Aoki K, Fujii T et al. Subsequent pregnancy outcomes in recurrent miscarriage patients with a paternal or maternal carrier of a structural chromosome rearrangement. *J Hum Genet* 2008;53:622–8.
39. Carp HJA, Feldman B, Oelsner G et al. Parental karyotype and subsequent live births in recurrent miscarriage. *Fertil Steril* 2004;81:1296–301.
40. Stephenson M and Sierra S. Reproductive outcomes in recurrent pregnancy loss associated with a parental carrier of a structural chromosome rearrangement. *Hum Reprod* 2006;21:1076–82.
41. Fischer J, Colls P, Escudero T et al. Preimplantation genetic diagnosis (PGD) improves pregnancy outcome for translocation carriers with a history of recurrent losses. *Fertil Steril* 2010;94:283–9.
42. Stephenson M and Goddijn M, A critical look at the evidence does not support PGD for translocation carriers with a history of recurrent losses. *Fertil Steril* 2011;95:e1.
43. Royal College of Obstetricians and Gynaecologists (RCOG). The investigation and treatment of couples with recurrent miscarriage. *Green-Top Guideline 17*, 2011.

8

Debate: Screening for Chromosomal Aberrations in Recurrent Pregnancy Loss: Nonspecific Testing Is Sufficient

Howard Cuckle

Background

Women with recurrent miscarriages are at increased risk of fetal chromosomal abnormalities in subsequent pregnancies. However, apart from known carriers of balanced translocations, the risk is not high enough to automatically justify invasive prenatal diagnosis. In the past, I have argued that a policy of continual risk re-assessed using a sequential multiple marker antenatal screening protocol is sufficient.[1] In recent years, the potential of screening for common trisomies has been greatly improved by the use of so-called "noninvasive prenatal diagnosis" methods. I will argue here that this development far from undermining the basis for continuous screening with conventional markers, actually enhances such a policy.

Purpose of Routine Screening

Screening for chromosomal abnormalities has the simple aim of identifying pregnancies at sufficiently high risk of an affected birth to warrant the hazards and costs of invasive testing. On average, chorionic villus sampling (CVS) and amniocentesis leads to at least 0.5% fetal losses[2] although this may vary according to the skills and experience of the individual operator. In the USA, Medicare reimbursement for procedural and karyotyping costs are about $1500.[3]

Local policy and national convention on what counts as sufficiently high risk to warrant invasive testing has generally emerged from the push and pull of health care providers, reimbursement tariffs, and professional bodies. Chromosomal abnormalities are relatively rare at birth—about 0.6%, excluding mosaics, in 70,000 consecutive newborns karyotyped[4]—so from the earliest days universal unselective invasive testing was not considered an option; rather there was selection based on advanced maternal age and family history of chromosomal abnormality.

The maternal age-specific birth prevalence of Down syndrome increases to 0.11%, 0.26%, 0.98% and 3.5% by ages 30, 35, 40, and 45 respectively.[5] The estimated risk at term for all common autosomal trisomies—Down, Edwards or Patau syndrome—is 0.48% and 1.6% at age 35–39 and 40–44, and for all chromosomal abnormalities 0.81% and 2.4%, respectively.[6] A family history of chromosomal abnormality confers a much higher risk than this when a maternal balanced translocation is found,[7] whilst for paternal carriers and for noncarrier couples there is only a modest excess over their maternal age-specific risk. With a Down syndrome proband and noncarrier parents the excess at mid-trimester is 0.54% for the same disorder and 0.24% for other aneuploidies.[8]

Testing these two high risk groups can have little impact on birth prevalence as most chromosomal abnormalities occur in young women and they are sporadic. This consideration has led to the development of newer methods of selection for invasive testing.

Conventional Screening Modalities

Beginning in the mid 1980s a series of maternal serum markers of aneuploidy was discovered: human chorionic gonadotrophin (hCG), the free-β subunit of hCG, α-fetoprotein (AFP), unconjugated oestriol (uE$_3$), inhibin A, and pregnancy associated plasma protein (PAPP)-A. Meanwhile even more discriminatory ultrasound markers were found: nuchal translucency (NT), nasal bone (NB), tricuspid regurgitation (TR), and ductus venosus (DV).

Various marker combinations, determined concurrently, formed the basis for the first effective screening protocols. The efficacy of a given policy is generally measured by applying a statistical model to calculate the expected detection rate, proportion of affected pregnancies selected for invasive testing, and the false-positive rate, proportion of unaffected pregnancies selected. When applied to all women using a one in 250 term risk cutoff, the norm in the UK, the model-predicted Down syndrome detection rate and false-positive rate are 68% and 4.2% for the best early second trimester maternal serum combination (Quad test—AFP, free β-hCG, uE$_3$ and inhibin), compared with 82% and 2.4%, respectively, for the most widely used first trimester combination (Combined test—PAPP-A and free β-hCG at 10 weeks and NT at 11 weeks).[9] In the USA where a 1 in 270 mid-trimester risk cutoff is favored, equivalent to about one in 350 at term, the corresponding rates are 73%, 5.9%, 84%, and 3.2%, respectively.

The same markers can also detect a large proportion of Edwards syndrome cases; in the second trimester this requires a separate risk cutoff but in the first trimester most are detected because of increased Down syndrome risks. Many of the remaining severe but nonlethal chromosomal abnormalities are also detected incidentally because of high Down or Edwards syndrome risks.[10] Although even more are associated with extreme marker levels, particularly NT,[11] it is not routine practice to calculate risks for these other disorders.

Policies for High Risk Groups

Screening was not initially applied to all women but only those not already regarded as high risk based on age and history. It was argued, most forcefully in the USA, that women in the "traditional" high risk groups expect to be provided with a diagnostic testing and the offer of a less definitive screening alternative was unfair. Eventually it was recognized that this hybrid policy is inefficient since many women with potentially low risks were receiving invasive testing, and screening is uniformly offered.

Although women with recurrent miscarriages are at increased risk of a fetal chromosomal abnormality in subsequent pregnancies, this risk is not very great. A study of almost 47,000 women having invasive prenatal diagnosis found a steady increasing trend in aneuploidy risk according to the number of previous miscarriages.[12] After adjustment for age, parity, and the indication for testing, the odds ratio compared to no miscarriages was 1.21, 1.26, and 1.51 for 1, 2, and 3 or more miscarriages, respectively. For a woman aged 30 with recurrent miscarriages this would barely increase the risk to that of women aged 35 who are no longer considered automatic candidates for invasive testing.

An increased proportion of couples with recurrent miscarriages are carriers of structural chromosomal rearrangements and it is important to establish their carrier status. In carrier couples subsequent pregnancies are more likely to end in fetal loss[13,14] although unbalanced translocations neither account for the excess of miscarriages[15] nor do they contribute much to the overall chromosomal abnormality risk.[16]

Sequential Screening

Thus purely in terms of aneuploidy risk there is no compelling reason to offer invasive testing automatically to women with recurrent miscarriages, with the possible exception of couples known to have certain types of translocations. However, there may be an argument in favor of more intensive antenatal screening than currently provided routinely.

Sequential screening protocols have been developed which considerably increase the detection rate for Down syndrome and other common trisomies. Attendance for screening is required on two occasions which is easier to arrange for women with recurrent miscarriages who already receive continual surveillance. The simplest protocol starts with the first trimester Combined test described above but adopts an extremely high cutoff risk, selecting a small number for invasive testing. The remainder then have the second trimester Quad test described above except that all seven first and second trimester marker levels are incorporated into the calculation of risk. This is a "stepwise" sequential screen. The model-predicted Down syndrome detection rate and false-positive rate with a 1 in 250 term risk cutoff are 89% and 1.7%.[9] Incorporating the newer first trimester ultrasound markers—NB, TR, and DV—would substantially enhance detection both of the common trisomies and other chromosomal abnormalities. For example, based on the latest parameters[17] routinely adding NB to the risk calculation would improve the above rates to 95% and 1.1%.

Routine sequential screening is already offered in some programs, such as that provided by the State of California, but it is not widespread, although increasingly NB is being determined at the time of the NT scan. For women with recurrent miscarriages it could be argued that stepwise sequential screening is necessary to yield higher detection and provide greater reassurance. One could go even further by extending the sequence of tests to include further markers at different times in pregnancy. A continuous screening protocol is a form of risk re-assessment by turns reassuring many and focusing concerns on a few with extreme risks.

An extension of the protocol could also be envisaged by incorporating into the risk calculation additional second trimester ultrasound markers. One option is to determine three "facial profile" markers that can be measured in the same plane as the biparietal diameter: nuchal skin-fold (NF), nasal-bone length (NBL), and pre-nasal thickness (PT). Modelling predicts that combining these with the Quad test would yield a detection rate comparable with a standard first trimester Combined test.[18]

Furthermore, so-called "soft" markers determined by the late second trimester anomaly scan, or genetic sonogram, could be used to modify the risk. These are not very discriminatory markers of aneuploidy and it has been estimated that routine screening with them would have a Down syndrome detection rate of 69% for a false-positive rate of 5%.[19] However, some clinicians do use the scan ad hoc in women with "borderline" risks from first or second trimester screening tests. This is often done simplistically, whereby the presence of one or more marker is taken to be sufficient to tip the balance in favor of invasive testing, and the absence of any markers is sufficient to contra-indicate testing. This is no longer acceptable; instead the prior risk needs to be modified by a series of likelihood ratios derived from each soft marker.[20]

Screening is a public health activity and as such requires the definition of cutoff levels in order to predict use of resources. In practice though, there is often less than strict adherence to the cutoff, which is merely taken to be a guide to action. Given the high chance of pregnancy failure and the associated anxiety among women with recurrent miscarriages it might be particularly appropriate to have a loose interpretation.

Non-Invasive Prenatal Diagnosis

The determination of cell-free (cf)DNA in maternal plasma would appear to be ideal for women with recurrent pregnancy loss who would naturally want to avoid any iatrogenic losses due to invasive prenatal diagnosis. However, clinicians and patients both need to be aware of the limitations of the new technology.

It is misleading to consider cfDNA testing as prenatal diagnosis, rather it is a potentially highly effective screening test but not a test that could replace current invasive testing. Indeed when a cfDNA screening test is "positive" amniocentesis or CVS is required to confirm the result.[21]

Several studies have investigated the test in women about to undergo invasive testing because of high risk of aneuploidy. In one meta-analysis, the estimated detection rates were 99%, 97%, 79%, and 83% for Down, Edwards, Patau, and Turner syndromes with false-positive rates of 0.2%, 0.2%, 0.4%, and 0.2% respectively.[22] So when screening for the four common trisomies cfDNA the estimated accumulative false-positive rate is 1%, not dissimilar to some conventional screening protocols. Moreover, the method is targeted at the common aneuploidies and is unable to detect a range of chromosomal disorders, including triploidy.

These rates are average performance since the discriminatory power of the test differs between individual women, depending on the proportion of cfDNA that is fetal in origin. This "fetal fraction" is correlated with maternal weight, and to some extent with the PAPP-A and hCG levels, but there is no reason to believe that, on average, it is markedly different in those at high risk of aneuploidy. So far the detection and false-positive rates in cfDNA studies of women not selected because at high risk are consistent with the above rate, although these studies are either small or have incomplete follow-up. There have not been any cfDNA studies in women with recurrent miscarriages.

Some are already suggesting that the increased detection rate for Down syndrome at a lower false-positive rate means that universal cfDNA screening should replace conventional modalities. One of the limitations is the very high unit cost of a cfDNA test. From a public health perspective the most important financial consideration is the "marginal" cost of avoiding a Down syndrome birth where the pregnancy would have been missed by conventional screening. This has been estimated to be several times higher than the life-time costs associated with Down syndrome.[23]

Contingent Screening

Although routine use of cfDNA screening may be prohibitively expensive the test is likely to have a secondary role in conventional screening. The concept of contingent screening was initially developed in sequential testing for Down syndrome, as an alternative to stepwise screening where only about 15–20% of women with borderline risks from the Combined test have further Quad markers. This approach yields detection rates comparable to stepwise screening and requires much less testing.[24]

Contingent screening where the Quad markers are replaced by cfDNA is a cost effective use of the new technology.[23] It can be greatly enhanced by the use of additional markers at the time of the first trimester Combined test. Adding two markers, placental growth factor (PlGF) and AFP, has been estimated to yield a Down syndrome detection rate of 97–8% for a 0.4% false-positive rate with 15–20% requiring cfDNA.[25]

A sequential screening protocol designed to continuously reassure women with recurrent pregnancy about their aneuploidy risk will necessarily lead to a higher overall false-positive rate as the positive results accumulate. The value of secondary cfDNA testing prior to invasive testing would greatly ameliorate this downside.

Adverse Pregnancy Outcome

Nicolaides has proposed that when women attend for a Combined test they are also assessed for their risk of the common maternal–fetal conditions such as pre-eclampsia, growth restriction, preterm delivery, and fetal macrosomia.[26] This concept has been most fully developed for pre-eclampsia, where early prophylactic medication with low dose aspirin has been shown to reduce risk by about a half.[27]

As with aneuploidy screening, *a priori* risk is modified by the results of pregnancy related markers. At the time of the Combined test good results have been achieved using two biophysical markers, mean arterial pressure and Doppler uterine artery blood flow, together with two serum markers levels, PAPP-A and PlGF. The model-predicted detection rate for "early" pre-eclampsia, requiring delivery before 34 weeks, is 93% at a false-positive rate of 5%.[28]

By retaining the Combined test and adding PlGF, rather than replacing it with routine cfDNA screening, women with recurrent losses can benefit from these developments in the prevention of pre-eclampsia, and other adverse outcomes. Such outcomes are common in pregnancy; for example, the incidence of pre-eclampsia is 2–8% in different populations.[29]

Conclusion

Continuous sequential screening using conventional markers provides a rational policy for women with recurrent pregnancy loss. From a public health perspective their risk of a chromosomal abnormality is not sufficiently high to offer automatic invasive testing when this is not routinely available to other women. However, their poor past pregnancy experience and future expectations may justify greater surveillance. A continuous screening policy would maximize detection and offer reassurance throughout the first and second trimesters of pregnancy. Where possible, risk would be calculated and revised using all possible markers, not just those routinely available, including: (1) first trimester ultrasound NB, TR, DV, serum PlGF, AFP; (2) early second trimester NF, NBL, PT; (3) late second trimester soft markers. In addition to Down and Edwards syndromes, risks should be calculated and revised for all types of aneuploidy. A policy of universal cfDNA screening for the common trisomies is not currently recommended for financial and other reasons. There is no particular reason to recommend it for women with recurrent miscarriage. Instead cfDNA could be used for secondary screening in those found to be at high risk, in order to reduce the need for invasive testing. Retaining conventional marker testing in women with recurrent pregnancy loss provides the potential of assessing their chance of an adverse pregnancy outcome.

REFERENCES

1. Cuckle H. Should CVS or amniocentesis be performed in RPL without screening? In: Carp HJA, ed. *Recurrent Pregnancy Loss: Causes, Controversies and Treatment*, London: Informa Healthcare; 2007. p. 55–7.
2. Tabor A, Alfirevic Z. Update on procedure-related risks for prenatal diagnosis techniques. *Fetal Diagn Ther* 2010;27:1–7.
3. Garfield SS, Armstrong SO. Clinical and cost consequences of incorporating a novel non-invasive prenatal test into the diagnostic pathway for fetal trisomies. *J Managed Care Med* 2012;15:34–41.
4. Hook EB, Hammerton JL. The frequency of chromosome abnormalities detected in consecutive newborn studies; differences between studies; results by sex and severity of phenotypic involvement. In: Hook EB, Porter IH, eds. *Population Cytogenetics: Studies in Humans*, New York: Academic Press; 1977. p. 63–79.
5. Cuckle HS, Wald NJ, Thompson SC. Estimating a women's risk of having a pregnancy associated with Down syndrome using her age and serum alpha-fetoprotein level. *Br J Obstet Gynaecol* 1987;94:387–402.
6. Hook EBH. Chromosomal abnormalities: Prevalence, risks and recurrence. In: Brock DJH, Rodeck CH, Ferguson-Smith MA, eds. *Prenatal Diagnosis and Screening*, Edinburgh: Churchill Livingstone; 1992. p. 351–92.
7. Boué A, Gallano P. A collaborative study of the segregation of inherited chromosome arrangements in 1356 prenatal diagnoses. *Prenatal Diagn* 1984;4:45–67.
8. Arbuzova S, Cuckle H, Mueller R et al. Familial Down syndrome: Evidence supporting cytoplasmic inheritance. *Clin Genet* 2001;60:456–62.
9. Cuckle H, Benn P. Multianalyte maternal serum screening for chromosomal defects. In: Milunsky A, Milunsky JM, eds. *Genetic Disorders and the Fetus: Diagnosis, Prevention and Treatment*, 6th ed. Chichester: Wiley-Blackwell; 2010. p. 771–818.
10. Alamillo CML, Krantz D, Evans M et al. Nearly a third of abnormalities found after first-trimester screening are different than expected: 10-year experience from a single center. *Prenatal Diagn* 2013;33:251–6.
11. Kagan KO, Avgidou K, Molina FS et al. Relation between increased fetal nuchal translucency thickness and chromosomal defects. *Obstet Gynecol* 2006;107(1):6–10.
12. Bianco K, Caughey B, Shaffer BL et al. Spontaneous abortion and aneuploidy. *Obstet Gynecol* 2006;107:1098–102.
13. Carp H, Feldman B, Oelsner G et al. Parental karyotype and subsequent live births in recurrent miscarriage. *Fertil Steril* 2004;81:1296–301.
14. Sugiura-Ogasawara M, Ozaki Y, Sato T et al. Poor prognosis of recurrent aborters with either maternal or paternal reciprocal translocations. *Fertil Steril* 2004;81:367–73.
15. Carp H, Guetta E, Dorf H et al. Embryonic karyotype in recurrent miscarriage with parental karyotypic aberrations. *Fertil Steril* 2006;85:446–50.
16. Franssen MTM, Korevaar JC, van der Veen F et al. Reproductive outcome after chromosome analysis in couples with two or more miscarriages: Case-control study. *Br Med J* 2006;332:759–63.

17. Cicero S, Rembouskos G, Vandecruys H et al. Likelihood ratio for trisomy 21 in fetuses with absent nasal bone at the 11–14-week scan. *Ultrasound Obstet Gynecol* 2004;23:218–23.

18. Miguelez J, Maymon R, Cuckle H et al. Model predicted performance of second trimester Down syndrome screening with ultrasound prenasal thickness. *J Ultrasound Med* 2010;29(12):1741–7.

19. Aagaard-Tillery KM, Malone FD, Nyberg DA et al. Role of second-trimester genetic sonography after Down syndrome screening. *Obstet Gynecol* 2009;114:1189–96.

20. Agathokleous M, Chaveeva P, Poon LCY et al. Meta-analysis of second-trimester markers for trisomy 21. *Ultrasound Obstet Gynecol* 2013;41(3):247–61.

21. Benn P, Borell A, Chiu R et al. Position statement from the aneuploidy screening committee on behalf of the Board of the International Society for Prenatal Diagnosis. *Prenatal Diagn* 2013;33:622–9.

22. Benn P, Cuckle H, Pergament E. Non-invasive prenatal diagnosis for aneuploidy—Current status and future prospects. *Ultrasound Obstet Gynecol* 2013;42:15–33.

23. Cuckle H, Benn P, Pergament E. Maternal cfDNA screening for Down's syndrome—A cost sensitivity analysis. *Prenatal Diagn* 2013;33:1–7.

24. Cuckle HS, Malone FD, Wright D et al. Contingent screening for Down syndrome. *Prenatal Diagn* 2008;28:89–94.

25. Nicolaides KH, Wright D, Poon LC et al. First-trimester contingent screening for trisomy 21 by biomarkers and maternal blood cell-free DNA testing. *Ultrasound Obstet Gynecol* 2013;42:41–50.

26. Nicolaides KH. A model for a new pyramid of prenatal care based on the 11 to 13 weeks' assessment. *Prenatal Diagn* 2011;31:3–6.

27. Bujold E, Roberge S, Lacasse Y et al. Prevention of preeclampsia and intrauterine growth restriction with aspirin started in early pregnancy: A meta-analysis. *Obstet Gynecol* 2010;116(2 Pt 1):402–14.

28. Akolekar R, Syngelaki A, Poon L et al. Competing risks model in early screening for preeclampsia by biophysical and biochemical markers. *Fetal Diagn Ther* 2013;33:8–15.

29. Steegers EA, von Dadelszen P, Duvekot JJ et al. Pre-eclampsia. *Lancet* 2010;21:376(9741):631–44.

9

Debate: Screening for Chromosomal Aberrations in Recurrent Pregnancy Loss: Noninvasive Prenatal Testing, Cytogenetics, and Ultrasound Are Needed

Peter Benn

Introduction

In this debate I argue that combinations of specific cytogenetic and molecular cytogenetic testing on parents and spontaneous abortion tissues, noninvasive prenatal testing, minimal use of invasive prenatal diagnosis, and second trimester ultrasound for fetal abnormality are all needed for the optimal management of pregnancies in women with a history of RPL. Furthermore, I assert that currently available nonspecific screening (first trimester combined test, second trimester quadruple test, and various newer combinations)[1,2] are insufficient in the management of these pregnancies.

Fetal Chromosome Abnormalities

Classical cytogenetic studies based on karyotyping have shown that approximately a half of all recognizable spontaneous abortion tissues have a major chromosome abnormality.[3] Among those that are cytogenetically abnormal, the most common abnormalities are trisomy (58%), triploidy or other polyploidy (20%), monosomy X (16%), and structural abnormalities (mostly unbalanced translocations) (4%). Even for 47,XXY and 47,XXX that are associated with relatively mild phenotypes in infants, there is some evidence that a relatively large proportion of the affected fetuses do not survive.[4] The reason why so many conceptuses have cytogenetic abnormalities is unknown but it is clear that strong selective pressures operate against abnormality, particularly early in pregnancy.

The estimate that approximately 50% of miscarriages are chromosomally abnormal is probably an underestimate because it is based mostly on clinically recognized losses, typically identified after six weeks gestational age. It is likely that even more cytogenetic abnormalities are present in preclinical losses. Furthermore, recent studies with chromosome microarrays (CMA) indicate that additional cytogenetic abnormalities are present. CMA potentially allows a larger proportion of cases to be successfully analyzed, distinguishes between maternal and fetal genotypes, and identifies some additional smaller imbalances, some of which may be considered causal.[5]

Although, in practice, relatively few spontaneous abortion tissues are referred for chromosome analysis, there are considerable benefits in providing the testing, as shown by Borell and Stergioto,[6] and discussed in Chapter 4. Fetal chromosome analysis can help establish recurrence risks (discussed below) and provide an explanation for an often highly traumatizing experience. This can be particularly valuable for RPL couples where supportive management is of great importance.[7] See also Chapter 44. Testing is particularly appropriate when there is ultrasound evidence for fetal structural abnormalities that would be consistent with a chromosome abnormality.

Recurrence Risks

Couples with a history of RPL are at a higher than normal risk for a further recurrence.[8] Among those that have losses due to cytogenetic abnormalities, recurrence risk will be dependent on the specific abnormalities that were present in the prior pregnancies.

Chromosome Translocations and Inversions

Of particular importance are unbalanced chromosome rearrangements in the spontaneous abortion tissues. For these cases, cytogenetic analysis of the parents is indicated to determine whether one of them is a carrier of the balanced form of rearrangement. These studies require conventional karyotyping rather than CMA because the latter does not identify balanced translocations. Risk for a spontaneous loss in a future pregnancy, reduced infertility in the carrier parent, or risk for a liveborn with an unbalanced karyotype will depend on the specific rearrangement identified, and for some abnormalities, the gender of the carrier parent.[3,9] Consultation with a genetic counselor is useful to obtain an estimate of risk for any particular chromosome rearrangement.

Even when an unbalanced translocation has not been identified in fetal tissue, it is common practice to offer karyotyping to RPL couples. In couples with a history of one loss, 2.2% will have a translocation or inversion carrier parent, with two losses 4.8%, and with three losses 5.2%.[10] Policies as to which couples should receive chromosome analysis vary in different medical settings.[11–14] Despite these high rates, the policy of karyotyping parents has been challenged by Barber et al.,[15] and Carp et al.,[16] who suggested that karyotyping for couples with a history of RPL may not be cost effective since it only identifies a relatively small number of couples that subsequently have a prenatal diagnosis of a fetus with an unbalanced karyotype. However both analyses failed to consider the extent to which the identification of the rearrangement may have altered prospective family planning (i.e., deciding not to have additional children, utilization of preimplantation genetic diagnosis (PGD), or adoption). They also did not consider the potential secondary benefits to additional family members or the considerable value of the reassurance to parents with normal karyotypes. Van Leeuwen et al.,[17] suggest that offering amniocentesis for all ongoing pregnancies is the least expensive way of preventing handicapped offspring but their proposed strategy had the added problems of the low acceptability of invasive testing and late diagnosis of affected pregnancies.

I posit that optimal prospective family planning requires early identification of translocation carriers and therefore selective use of karyotyping in RPL couples is necessary.

Autosomal Trisomy

Relative to the general population, the risk of aneuploidy may be increased for women who had past pregnancies with one or more of the common autosomal trisomies. Many of the women classified as having RPL can be expected to be older than the general maternal age population since they had several past pregnancies. Moreover, most of the autosomal trisomies seen in spontaneous abortions are positively correlated with maternal age[18] and therefore the population of women with a history of a trisomic loss should include many older women. Even allowing for their higher age, women who had a previous liveborn child or pregnancy with trisomy 21 appear to have an excess risk for trisomy 21 or other aneuploidy in subsequent pregnancies.[19–21] This may well also be true for women experiencing a miscarriage of a trisomy 21 pregnancy. A previous pregnancy with some other trisomies may also be associated with increased risk for the same or a different, potentially viable, trisomy in a subsequent pregnancy.[20,22] Based on a retrospective review of amniocentesis and CVS results, Bianco et al.,[23] were able to show that there was an increased risk of an abnormal karyotype for women with a history of miscarriage. Furthermore, when women were grouped according to the number of past spontaneous abortions (0, 1, 2, ≥3), the risk for trisomy appeared to correlate with the number of past losses. Higher than expected numbers of chromosome abnormalities have also been detected in PGD tests when the indication was recurrent miscarriage or previous aneuploid pregnancy.[24–26]

However, some studies on RPL women actually show lower than expected numbers of aneuploid losses.[27–29] Furthermore, the rate of aneuploidy appears to decline when the number of past miscarriages was very high. This might be explained by an ascertainment bias. Although a past pregnancy with trisomy might increase the risk in a subsequent pregnancy, the increase in risk is modest and given enough attempts, women whose cause of loss has been aneuploidy will eventually have a successful normal pregnancy. These high gravida women are then no longer included in the RPL population. On the other hand, those women with euploid miscarriages may include many that are caused by factors that have a far stronger chance of causing a loss. Very high gravida RPL women may therefore indeed show lower proportions of aneuploid losses. Consistent with this, the chance of a successful outcome in high gravida RPL women has been shown to be lower when the past miscarriages showed a normal karyotype.[28,29]

Precise definition of the risk for RPL women is therefore problematic because it will likely be dependent on the number of past pregnancies, maternal age at the time of the past pregnancies, the specific trisomy under consideration and inclusion or exclusion of other factors that might have contributed to loss.[3,29] A crude and somewhat unsatisfactory approach used in nonspecific screening for Down syndrome is to assign an excess risk for all women who had a past affected pregnancy.[1] Another approach is to increase the risk for those women who had a prior viable, or potentially viable, trisomy by equating the risk to that seen in advanced maternal age women.[3] These approaches can be expected to increase both the detection rate and false-positive rate, relative to the use of an uncorrected a priori risk. However, there appear to be no prospective data available that evaluate how conventional, nonspecific, screening tests perform in women with a history of a prior pregnancy with a trisomy or RPL.

Sex Chromosome Abnormality

The presence of a prior pregnancy with a 45,X, 47,XXX or 47,XXY does not appear to materially increase the risk for trisomy in a subsequent pregnancy.[20] From the patient perspective, the relatively common finding of 45,X in abortus tissue can therefore be considered a good result in so far as it provides an explanation for the loss and does not increase the risk for future pregnancies.

Triploidy

Triploidy can be separated into those cases with an extra set of maternal (digynic) or paternal (diandric) chromosomes which can be recognized by phenotype[30] or from microarray tests that include single nucleotide polymorphisms (SNPs). Diandric cases show a partial molar placenta and for these cases risk for a (partial or complete) molar pregnancy in a subsequent pregnancy is about 1:60. This is about 20-fold background risk.[31] It is unknown whether risk is increased with digynic triploidy or higher ploidy levels.

Management of Patients with Recurrent Pregnancy Loss

Couples who experience RPL are often extremely concerned about their past history, may be aware that they are at increased risk for a recurrence, and are worried. Most abortus tissues will not have received cytogenetic testing and even when the karyotypes were known, recurrence risk may be very poorly defined. Moreover, many couples that have experienced losses are anxious to avoid any testing that could increase the risk of a further loss. The risks associated with invasive testing have been extensively debated and current estimates are generally considered to be 0.5–1.0% for both amniocentesis and CVS.[32] Importantly, the risk of invasive testing is uncertain for women with a history of RPL where a predisposition for loss might be present.[33]

Given the common problem of many anxious couples seeking reassurance that their pregnancy is normal and yet unwilling to undergo invasive testing, what is the optimal testing strategy? The following summarizes the proposed specific testing recommended for RPL. As previously noted, there are many couples that do not meet the formal definition of RPL or past reproductive history may be poorly documented. Individual case consideration by the physician is therefore often necessary.

   i. Conventional chromosome analysis (karyotyping) for parents with a history of two or more miscarriages of unknown etiology.

   ii. Whenever possible, CMA or karyotyping of spontaneous abortion tissues for women with miscarriage of unknown etiology. [The benefits of using CMA for abortus tissues need to be balanced against the significant difficulty of interpreting findings of unknown, uncertain, or unrelated medical significance and the fact that CMA will not identify balanced translocations. These issues have been discussed more fully by Carp.[34]] Identification of an unbalanced translocation would prompt karyotyping of the parents. Identification of trisomy or triploidy in the abortion tissue would prompt counseling about the risk for future pregnancies.

   iii. Invasive testing (amniocentesis or CVS) when a balanced chromosome abnormality has previously been identified in a carrier parent.

   iv. For other continuing pregnancies, after 10 weeks gestational age, noninvasive prenatal testing (NIPT) through the analysis of cell-free DNA in maternal plasma. For pregnancies with a positive NIPT result, confirmation by invasive testing is indicated.

   v. For continuing pregnancies, after 16 weeks gestational age, second trimester ultrasound examination to help exclude the presence of open neural tube defects (if not previously diagnosed), and other significant fetal anatomic abnormalities. Amniocentesis should be offered in those cases where major fetal anatomic abnormalities are identified.

This proposed testing differs from that offered to women without a history of losses in that nonspecific screening (first trimester combined test, second trimester quadruple test, and various combinations) are replaced by NIPT, offered at the earliest gestational age that the testing can be reliably performed.

Currently, NIPT is only recommended for women who are high risk on the basis of prior conventional screening tests, maternal age or family history of some specific chromosome abnormalities.[35–39] Relative to nonspecific screening, NIPT has higher sensitivity and a lower false positive rate for trisomies 21 and 18. It has also been shown to be efficacious for trisomy 13 and 45,X and will also identify a proportion of cases with other sex chromosome aneuploidies.[40] Use of NIPT will potentially result in fewer invasive tests and can provide earlier and higher levels of reassurance than can be achieved using the conventional screening modalities.

Conventional screening does identify many cases with nonchromosomal fetal anatomic abnormalities and pregnancy complications. Therefore these conventional tests do still have a role. But for women receiving NIPT, the use of the conventional screening will need to be justified based on the nonchromosomal conditions not otherwise identified in the protocol suggested above.

It is acknowledged that some of the proposed testing may not be available in all regions, may be inconsistent with local policy or guidelines or be in conflict with broader nonspecific prenatal screening policies designed to ensure universal availability of testing. I also acknowledge that offering NIPT to all RPL women would be associated with increased cost, relative to its use in only those women determined to be high risk by other screening. However, I suggest that this added cost is likely to be small and justifiable since there will be reduced conventional screening, fewer invasive tests, and fewer office visits as a result of the earlier reassurance.

Finally, it should be noted that in the future NIPT is likely to be applicable to the detection of additional chromosomal abnormalities than can be diagnosed today,[40] and may well become the standard of care for all women. Furthermore, developments in low-cost high-throughput sequencing may soon allow cytogenetic characterization of many more spontaneous abortion tissues.[41] The recommendations above reflect the current state-of-the-art.

Summary Comment

RPL couples constitute a special group for whom additional reassurance and physiological support is indicated.[7] Providing an explanation for losses through genetic analyses of fetal tissues, excluding translocation in the parents, providing the best possible risk estimates for future pregnancies, and providing early NIPT can optimize prospective family planning and considerably ease anxiety.

Currently available nonspecific conventional screening is insufficient because it fails to meet the full needs of these couples. It is based on tenuous assessments of a priori risk and combinations of assays that do not have the necessary high predictive values.

REFERENCES

1. Cuckle H, Benn P. Multianalyte maternal serum screening for chromosomal defects. In: Milunsky A, Milunsky JM, eds. *Genetic Disorders and the Fetus: Diagnosis, Prevention and Treatment.* 6th edn. Chichester, U.K.: Wiley-Blackwell, 2010:771–818.
2. Johnson J, Pastuck M, Metcalf A et al. First trimester Down syndrome screening using additional serum markers with and without nuchal translucency and cell free DNA. *Prenatal Diagn* 2013;33:1044–9.
3. Benn PA. Prenatal diagnosis of chromosome abnormalities through amniocentesis. In: Milunsky A, Milunsky JM, eds. *Genetic Disorders and the Fetus: Diagnosis, Prevention and Treatment.* 6th edn. Chichester, U.K.: Wiley-Blackwell, 2010:771–818.
4. Morris JK, Albeman E, Scott C et al. Is the prevalence of Klinefelter syndrome increasing? *Eur J Hum Genet* 2008;16:163–70.
5. Rajcan-Separovic E. Chromosome micro arrays in human reproduction. *Hum Reprod Update* 2012;18:555–67.
6. Borrell A, Stergiotou I. Miscarriage in contemporary maternal-fetal medicine: Targeting clinical dilemmas. *Ultrasound Obstet Gynecol* 2013;42:491–7.
7. Silver RM. Fetal Death. *Obstet Gynecol* 2007;109:153–67.
8. Roman E. Fetal loss rates and their relation to pregnancy order. *J Epidemiol Community Health* 1984;38:29–35.
9. Gardner RJM, Sutherland GR, Shaffer LG. Chromosome abnormalities and genetic counseling. 4th edn. New York: Oxford University Press, 2012.
10. De Braekeleer M, Dao TN. Cytogenetic studies in couples experiencing repeated pregnancy losses. *Hum Reprod* 1990;5:519–28.
11. ACOG Practice Bulletin. Management of recurrent pregnancy loss. Number 24, February 2001. American College of Obstetricians and Gynecologists. *Int J Gynecol Obstet* 2002;78:179–90.
12. Jauniaux E, Farquharson RG, Christiansen OB et al. Evidence-based guidelines for the investigation and medical treatment of recurrent miscarriage. *Hum Reprod* 2006;21:2216–22.
13. Dutch Society of Obstetrics and Gynaecology (NVOG). Guideline: Recurrent miscarriage. Utrecht, The Netherlands: NVOG; 2007.
14. Royal College of Obstetricians and Gynaecologists. The investigation and treatment for couples with recurrent miscarriage. Green top guideline 17. April 2011. http://www.rcog.org.uk/files/rcog-corp/GTG17recurrentmiscarriage.pdf.
15. Barber JC, Cockwell AE, Grant E et al. Is karyotyping couples experiencing recurrent miscarriage worth the cost? *BJOG* 2010;117:885–8.
16. Carp HJA, Feldman B, Oelsner G et al. Parental karyotype and subsequent live births in recurrent miscarriage. *Fertil Steril* 2004;81:1296–301.
17. van Leeuwen M, Vansenne F, Korevaar JC et al. Economic analysis of chromosome testing in couples with recurrent miscarriage to prevent handicapped offspring. *Hum Reprod* 2013;28:1737–42.
18. Hassold T, Chiu D. Maternal age specific rates of numerical chromosome abnormalities with special reference to trisomy. *Hum Genet* 1985;70:11–17.
19. Arbuzova S, Cuckle H, Mueller R et al. Familial Down syndrome: Evidence supporting cytoplasmic inheritance. *Clin Genet* 2001;60:456–62.

20. Warburton D, Dallaire L, Thangavelu M et al. Trisomy recurrence: A reconsideration based on North American Data. *Am J Hum Genet* 2004;75:376–85.
21. Morris JK, Mutton DE, Alberman E. Recurrences of free trisomy 21: Analysis of data from the National Down Syndrome Cytogenetic Register. *Prenatal Diagn* 2005;25:1120–8.
22. De Souza E, Halliday J, Chan A, Bower C, Morris JK. Recurrence risks for trisomies 13, 18, and 21. *Am J Med Genet, Part A* 2009;149A:2716–22.
23. Bianco K, Caughey AB, Shaffer BL et al. History of miscarriages and increased incidence of fetal aneuploidy in subsequent pregnancy. *Obstet Gynecol* 2006;107:1098–102.
24. Rubio C, Simon C, Vidal F et al. Chromosomal abnormalities and embryo development in recurrent miscarriage couples. *Hum Reprod* 2003;18:182–8.
25. Munné S, Sandalinas M, Magli C et al. Increased rate of aneuploid embryos in young women with previous aneuploid conceptions. *Prenatal Diagn* 2004;24:638–43.
26. Al-Asmar N, Peinado V, Vera M et al. Chromosomal abnormalities in embryos from couples with a previous aneuploid miscarriage. *Fertil Steril* 2012;98:145–50.
27. Sullivan AE, Silver RM, LaCoursiere DY et al. Recurrent fetal aneuploidy and recurrent miscarriage. *Obstet Gynecol* 2004;104:784–8.
28. Ogasawara M, Aoki K, Okada S et al. Embryonic karyotype of abortuses in relation to the number of previous miscarriages. *Fertil Steril* 2000;73:300–4.
29. Carp H, Toder V, Aviram A et al. Karyotype of the abortus in recurrent miscarriage. *Fertil Steril* 2001;75:678–82.
30. McFadden DE, Robinson WP. Phenotypes of triploid embryos. *J Med Genet* 2006;43:609–12.
31. Sebire NJ, Fisher RA, Foskett M et al. Risk of recurrent hydatidiform mole and subsequent pregnancy outcome following complete or partial hydatidiform molar pregnancy. *BJOG* 2003;110:22–6.
32. Tabor A, Alfirevic Z. Update on procedure-related risks for prenatal diagnosis techniques. *Fetal Diagn Ther* 2010;27:1–7.
33. Esrig SM, Leonardi DE. Spontaneous abortion after amniocentesis in women with a history of spontaneous abortion. *Prenatal Diagn* 1985;5:321–8.
34. Carp HJA. Commentary on 'Additional information from chromosomal microarray analysis (CMA) over conventional karyotyping when diagnosing chromosomal abnormalities in miscarriage: A systematic review and meta-analysis' *Br J Obstet Gynaecol* 2013;121:20–1.
35. ACOG Committee Opinion. 2012. Noninvasive prenatal testing for fetal aneuploidy. Committee Opinion No. 545. American College of Obstetricians and Gynecologists. *Obstet Gynecol* 2012;120:1532–4.
36. Gregg AR, Gross SJ, Best RG et al. ACMG statement on noninvasive prenatal screening for fetal aneuploidy. *Genet Med.* 2013;15:395–8
37. Langlois S, Brock J-A, Current Status in Non-Invasive Prenatal Detection of Down Syndrome, Trisomy 18, and Trisomy 13 Using Cell-Free DNA in Maternal Plasma. *J Obstet Gynaecol Can* 2013;35:177–81.
38. Wilson KL, Czerwinski JL, Hoskovec JM et al. NSGC practice guideline: Prenatal screening and diagnostic testing options for chromosome aneuploidy. *J Genet Couns* 2013;22:4–15.
39. Benn P, Borrell A, Chiu R et al. Position statement from the Aneuploidy Screening Committee on behalf of the board of the International Society for Prenatal Diagnosis. *Prenatal Diagn* 2013;33:622–9.
40. Benn P, Cuckle H, Pergament E. Non-invasive prenatal testing for aneuploidy–current status and future prospects. *Ultrasound Obstet Gynecol* 2013;42:15–33.
41. Xie W, Tan Y, Li X et al. Rapid detection of aneuploidies on a bench top sequencing platform. *Prenatal Diagn* 2013;33:232–7.

10

Does the Maternal Immune System Regulate the Embryo's Response to External Toxins?

Arkady Torchinsky, Vladimir Toder, Shoshana Savion, and Howard J. A. Carp

Introduction

The maternal immune system, in addition to regulating embryonic development, may determine the tolerance of the embryo to environmental teratogens[1] and other toxins. In the first edition of this book, we described some of the mechanisms determining the susceptibility of the embryo to teratogens, and the possible mechanisms whereby immune responses may affect the ability of the embryo to resist teratogenic insults. Chapters 11 and 12 describe the malformations affecting human fetuses which can present as miscarriage and possibly recurrent miscarriage. Chapter 11 shows examples of early embryos which cease development due to major malformations which are incompatible with life. Some of these early fetal demises can only be diagnosed by embryoscopy, and not by conventional techniques such as ultrasound. Philipp et al.[2] have reported that 30% of these malformed embryos are eukaryotypic. There are few explanations as to why these malformations may occur. In addition, Chapter 3 describes the genetic factors responsible for recurrent pregnancy loss. Today we know that there are compounds which affect genetic integrity such as ionizing radiation, and Bisphenol A (used to make certain plastics and epoxy resins). However, in the last five years, there have been few reports of the mechanisms whereby immune responses may affect the embryo's resistance or susceptibility to teratogens and other toxins. Therefore, further studies are necessary in order to determine whether the knowledge accumulated so far will have clinical applications allowing targeted therapies to be developed, which will increase the embryo's resistance to those agents.

Fetomaternal Immunoreactivity and Embryonic Development

As early as the mid-1960s immune responses were shown to have a regulatory role in embryonic development. The mean litter size and mean placental weight were found to be higher in allogeneic than in syngeneic pregnancies.[3,4] The survival of transplanted embryos was also shown to be significantly higher when there was a difference in MHC antigens between the parents.[5] Moreover, the litter size and placental weights are higher in mice preimmunized with allogeneic paternal strain lymphocytes.[6] However, in mice, immunization with syngeneic splenocytes prior to syngeneic mating results in perinatal and postnatal mortality and an increased number of malformations among the progeny.[7] The sera of habitually aborting women are toxic to rat embryos in culture.[8] However, immunization with paternal leucocytes improved blastocyst development in culture with the sera of habitually aborting women, and reversed the embryotoxic effect of sera from nonimmunized women with recurrent miscarriages.[9]

Finally, stimulation of the maternal immune response has been shown to improve the reproductive performance of mice with a high degree of spontaneous postimplantation embryonic loss. In the CBA/J × DBA/2J mouse mating combination which is prone to resorptions, alloimmunization of the female with leukocytes of paternal haplotype significantly decreased the proportion of resorbed pregnancies from approximately 40% to 10–15%.[10] The same effect has been achieved with nonspecific immunostimulation of mice with Complete Freund adjuvant (CFA).[11,12]

Fetomaternal Immunoreactivity and Teratological Susceptibility

The above studies demonstrated that embryo survival depends on immune responses in the embryonic microenvironment. Torchinskii et al.[13] compared the effect of two teratogens, cyclophosphamide (CP) and 2.3-quinoxalinedimethanol, 1,4-dioxide (CAS # 17311-31-8)[14] in syngeneically- and allogeneically-mated CBA/J and C57Bl/6 mice. Both strains showed higher sensitivity to both teratogens after syngeneic mating than allogeneic mating. However, genetic differences between inbred and F1 (CBA/J × C57Bl/6) embryos could have explained the different response to the teratogens. Further experiments were performed in C57Bl/6 females whose immune responses were either depressed by removing the para-aortic lymph nodes, or activated by intrauterine immunization with allogeneic paternal splenocytes.[15,16] Suppression of the maternal immune response significantly increased the sensitivity of F1 (C57Bl/6 × CBA/J) embryos to both teratogens[15] and virtually eliminated the different responses between allogeneically and syngenei-cally mated females. In mice undergoing extirpation of draining lymph nodes, CP produced a resorption rate of approximately 20%, and a malformation rate of 77%, whereas in sham-operated females these indices were 6% and 31%, respectively. In contrast, females primed with allogeneic paternal splenocytes before allogeneic mating showed enhanced tolerance to both teratogens.[16]

The response to the above teratogens has also been tested in the second pregnancy of C57Bl/6 mice.[16] The degree of embryotoxicity induced by both teratogens depended on the type of mating (allogeneic or syngeneic) in the first and second pregnancy, and that embryos of females mated twice allogeneically demonstrated a significantly higher resistance to both teratogens than embryos of allogeneically mated primigravid mice. Hence, the exposure of the maternal immune system to paternal antigens in the first pregnancy may modify the teratogenic response of embryos in repeated pregnancies.

Agents which activate macrophages have also been reported to increase tolerance to teratogens. ICR mice pretreated with Pyran copolymer or Bacillus Calmette–Guerin (BCG) vaccination exhibit increased tolerance to teratogens such as urethane, *N*-methyl-*N*-nitrosourea and ionizing radiation.[17] Additionally, injection of Pyran-activated macrophages to CL/Fr mice, which have a high incidence of cleft lip and palate, decreased the incidence of these anomalies. Many other immunostimulants also have similar effects. Nonspecific immune triggers such as xenogeneic rat splenocytes, increase the toler-ance of embryos to cyclophosphamide-induced teratogenic effects (Figure 10.1)[18]. Furthermore, it has

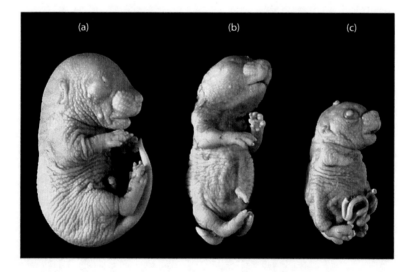

FIGURE 10.1   The teratogenic response of embryos of cyclophosphamide (CP)-treated intact and immunostimulated mice. Legend: CP induces a specter of gross structural anomalies such as open eyes, digit and limb reduction anoma-lies, exencephaly, gastroschisis and growth retardation in a dose-dependent fashion. Immunostimulation of females with xenogeneic rat splenocytes is followed by a decrease in the incidence and severity of these anomalies and an increase in fetal weight. (a) Fetus of an intact mouse; (b) fetus of immunostimulated CP-treated mouse; and (c) fetus of nonimmuno-stimulated CP-treated mouse.

been found that immunization if performed twice (21 day before mating and on day 1 of pregnancy) has a greater influence on the teratogenic response to CP than a single inoculation.[18]

The influence of the immune response on the susceptibility to teratogens has been investigated in insulin-dependent diabetes mellitus (IDDM) and heat shock. Meticulous metabolic control of diabetes has significantly decreased the risk of gross structural malformations in newborn infants. Nevertheless, the incidence of fetal malformations in women with IDDM (6–10%) is still three to five times higher than in nondiabetic women.[19] In laboratory animals, streptozocin (STZ) was used to induce diabetes in ICR mice treated with rat splenocytes 21 days before mating.[20] In STZ-induced diabetic ICR mice, approximately 9% of embryos show gross structural anomalies and the incidence of litters with malformed embryos reaches 63%.[21] Immunostimulation resulted in a decrease of both indices: only 18% of litters had malformed fetuses and the number of malformed embryos was, approximately, 2%. Moreover, immunostimulation was followed by an increase in the pregnancy rate: approximately 70% compared to 44% in nonimmunized diabetic females. Immunostimulation with CFA had a similar effect,[22] preventing cardiac developmental defects.

Heat shock-induced teratogenic effects in rodents are associated with the occurrence of anomalies in the brain and eye.[23] When ICR mice were immunized with rat splenocytes, a significantly decreased proportion of fetuses had exencephaly and open eyes.[24] The resorption rate in immunized mice was similar to that seen in intact ICR mice (approximately, 6–10%), whereas in nonimmunized mice exposed to heat shock it exceeded 20%.[24]

Holladay et al.,[25] showed that immune stimulation of pregnant mice with Pyran copolymer, BCG, or CFA increased the resistance of embryos to teratogens such as 2,3,7,8-tetrachlorodibenzo-*p*-dioxin [TCDD], urethane, methylnitrosourea and valproic acid. Additionally, immune stimulation with CFA, granulocyte-macrophage colony-stimulating factor (GM-CSF), or interferon-gamma (IFN-γ) protects murine embryos against diabetes-induced teratogenic effects.[26] In our studies,[27] maternal immunostimulation with GM-CSF increased the resistance of murine embryos to CP.

Neither ultrasound nor restraint stress were shown to have a teratogenic effect but induce postimplantation embryonic death.[28] Immunization of C3H/HeJ female mice with allogeneic paternal splenocytes of DBA/2J mice, seven days before mating, reduces the number of restraint stress-induced embryonic losses.[29] Immune stimulation of CBA/J female mice with paternal splenocytes of DBA/2J males, two weeks before mating, decreases the number of ultrasonic stress-induced resorptions. Finally, stimulation of female mice with the biostimulators PSK and OK432 decreased the susceptibility of embryos to the teratogen 5-azacytidine, whereas injection of interleukin-1 (IL-1) decreased the tolerance of embryos to this teratogen.[30]

The above studies provide evidence that immune responses occurring between mother and fetus may influence the susceptibility of embryos to both environmental teratogens and detrimental stimuli generated by the mother. The underlying mechanisms remain largely undefined. Some possible mechanisms are described below.

Possible Mechanisms of Interaction between Immune Responses and Developmental Toxicants

Molecules Regulating Apoptosis in the Embryo

Most teratogens act on the embryo itself. The mechanisms which determine the response of embryonic cells to teratogens seem to be mainly associated with mechanisms regulating apoptosis induced by teratogenic stress.[31] Apoptosis is known to play a crucial role in normal embryogenesis. Apoptosis is involved in eliminating abnormal, misplaced, nonfunctional, or harmful cells, sculpting structures, eliminating unwanted structures, and controlling cell numbers.[32] Many chemical and physical toxins which induce structural anomalies also induce excessive apoptosis in embryonic structures, which are subsequently malformed.[33,34] Toder et al.[35] investigated whether maternal immune stimulation affects the degree of teratogen-induced apoptosis, and reported that immune stimulation of females with xenogeneic rat splenocytes did indeed decrease the intensity of CP-induced excessive apoptosis in embryonic structures.

Apoptosis is a genetically regulated process, involving activation of death signaling cascades and prosurvival pathways. A number of molecules, reported to be crucial in mediating apoptosis have been implicated as powerful determinants of teratogenic susceptibility.[31] It may be that teratogen-induced alterations in the expression of these molecules may be neutralized or prevented by maternal immune potentiation. The tumor suppressor protein p53 is activated by various cellular stresses that induce DNA damage, and is thought to be a key regulator of apoptosis.[36] p53 targets several steps in the apoptotic pathway, ensuring that apoptosis proceeds according to a well-coordinated program.[36] p53 also seems to regulate the response of embryos to teratogens such as benzo[a]pyrene,[37] 2-chloro-2-deoxyadenosine,[38] ionizing radiation,[39,40] diabetes,[41] and CP.[42] A CP-induced teratogenic insult was followed by the accumulation of p53 protein in embryonic structures; maternal immune stimulation with xenogeneic rat splenocytes or GM-CSF increased the tolerance of murine embryos to CP and partially normalized the expression of p53.[27] Sharova et al.[43] have shown that mice exposed to ure-thane (which induces cleft palate in mice), had a lower incidence of malformed fetuses after injection of CFA or interferon-gamma. Moreover, CFA also normalized the urethane-induced alterations in the expression of the p53 gene and of the bcl-2 gene, which is thought to be one of the key anti-apoptotic proteins.[44]

Caspases are also considered to be executors of apoptosis and are classified as initiators and effectors. The activation of initiator caspases takes place after their binding to adapter molecules and mature initiator caspases activate effector caspases. The initiator caspase-9 (and possibly caspase-2) operate in the mitochondrial pro-apoptotic pathway, whereas the initiator caspases 8 and 10 act in the death-receptor pro-apoptotic pathway. Both pathways use effector caspases (caspases 3, 6, and 7).[45] It has been reported[31] that at least one of the main initiator caspases (8 or 9) and/or the main effector caspase-3 are involved in the response to teratogens such as diabetes, ionizing radiation, heat shock, CP, sodium arsenite and retinoic acid.[31] The possibility that maternal immune stimulation may modify teratological susceptibility by affecting the process of teratogen-induced activation of caspases has been supported by our recent study.[46] The level of active caspases 3, 8, and 9 was lower in the embryos of immunostimu-lated CP-treated mice than in embryos of mice exposed to the teratogen alone.[46]

The transcription factor NF-κB is also thought to be a key molecule preventing cell death via the activation of genes, the products of which function as anti-apoptotic proteins.[47] NF-κB is transcription-ally active in embryos during organogenesis. One subunit of NF-κB, p65, has been shown to be indis-pensable for the protection of the embryonic liver against the physiological apoptosis induced by Tumor Necrosis Factor α (TNFα).[48] NF-κB has been reported to regulate the response to teratogens such as thalidomide,[49] phenytoin,[50] and CP.[51] NF-κB may be a target for immune activity in the embryonic microenvironment.[46] Intrauterine immunostimulation with rat splenocytes attenuated CP-induced sup-pression of NF-κB DNA binding activity in mouse embryos.

The above data suggest some mechanisms by which maternal immune stimulation might alter tera-tological susceptibility. However, the pathways by which maternal immune stimulation affects these mechanisms remain elusive.

Cytokines and Growth Factors Operating at the Fetomaternal Interface

A balanced cytokine milieu is a necessary condition for maternal–fetal immune tolerance.[52–54] Cytokine imbalances which precede or accompany embryonic demise may also be involved in some of the mechanisms regulating the susceptibility of the embryo to detrimental stimuli.[55] CP-induced teratogenesis is accompanied by an increase in TNFα and a decrease in Transforming Growth Factor-beta 2 (TGFβ2), and colony stimulating factor-1 (CSF-1) expression at the fetomaternal inter-face.[56–58] Increased TNFα and decreased TGFβ2 expression have also been described in the uterus of diabetic mice.[59–61]

TNFα has been shown to activate both apoptotic and anti-apoptotic signaling cascades,[62] which sug-gests that TNFα may regulate the response of the embryo to various stresses. Indeed, our team[63] has found that the incidence and severity of CP-induced gross structural craniofacial and limb anomalies were higher in TNFα-knockout fetuses than in their TNFα-positive counterparts.[63] TNFα-knockout embryos have also been found to be sensitive to diabetes-induced teratogenic stimuli.[64]

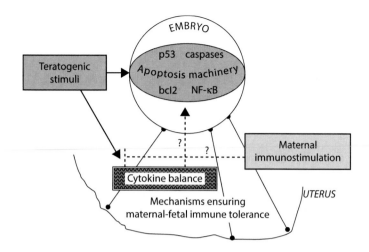

FIGURE 10.2 A simplified model depicting a possible pathway for maternal immunostimulation-induced modification of the teratological susceptibility. Legend: A teratogen affects the function of molecules regulating the teratogenic response (i.e., those regulating apoptosis) directly and, possibly, indirectly via inducing an imbalance of cytokines operating in the embryonic vicinity. Maternal immunostimulation influences the teratological susceptibility via modifying the expression pattern of these cytokines.

TGFβ, a multipotent growth factor, has been reported to be involved in regulating cell growth, differentiation, migration, and extracellular matrix deposition.[65] TGFβ family isoforms such as TGFβ1, TGFβ2 and TGFβ3 seem to be indispensable for normal embryogenesis. Indeed, TGFβ1-null embryos die before day 11 of pregnancy, whereas 25% of TGFβ2 knockout fetuses and 100% of TGFβ3 knockout fetuses exhibit cleft palate.[66] A number of studies have reported that TGFβ may be involved in mechanisms mediating teratogenesis. In experiments with the teratogenic dioxin TCDD, which induces cleft palate in mouse embryos, TGFβ3 was shown to counteract the effect of dioxin in blocking palatal fusion.[67] Additionally, TGFβ2-knockout embryos have been found to be more sensitive to retinoid-induced teratogenesis than their TGFβ2-positive counterparts.[68]

Hence, TNFα and TGFβ may determine the teratological susceptibility of embryos. Maternal immune stimulation, in addition to increasing the resistance of embryos to teratogenic stress, also tends to normalize the expression of these cytokines at the fetomaternal interface, implicating maternally-derived TNFα and TGFβ in pathways via which maternal immune stimulation modifies the responses of the embryo to teratogens. Although effective reciprocal signaling has been demonstrated between the uterus and preimplantation and peri-implantation embryos,[69,70] the effectiveness of reciprocal signaling during organogenesis (the period of greatest sensitivity to teratogens) remains undetermined. Nevertheless, the mechanisms thought to ensure maternal–fetal immune tolerance, cytokines and growth factors acting in the embryonic microenvironment, may primarily act as mediators, through which the maternal immune system regulates the response of the embryo to environmental teratogens. The above data suggest a model depicting a possible pathway by which maternal immunostimulation may modify teratological susceptibility (Figure 10.2). Within this model, modification of teratological susceptibility by maternal immunostimulation depends on both the type of teratogen and the type of immune stimulator.

Agents Affecting Genetic Integrity

The above paragraphs deal with resistance to teratogenic agents. However, a major cause of pregnancy loss is genetic aberrations. In human pregnancy, approximately 60% of miscarried pregnancies are accompanied by major chromosomal aberrations, such as 16 trisomy triploidy, and so on. Since the availability of whole genome analysis with molecular techniques, a further 15% of miscarried pregnancies are known to be genetically abnormal.[71] The cause of these aberrations is generally unknown. Copy number variants (CNV) are the basis of individual variations; however, at a certain stage, CNV become abnormal, leading to incompatibility with life. Numerous agents affect genetic integrity. Bisphenol A and ionizing radiation are two examples.

Bisphenol A

Bisphenol A (BPA) is used to manufacture certain plastics and epoxy resins; it has been in commercial use since 1957, for many consumer goods, (such as baby and water bottles, sports equipment, and CDs and DVDs) and for industrial purposes, like lining water pipes. BPA binds to an estrogen-related receptor γ (ERR-γ), which activates transcription, but not to the estrogen receptor itself.[72] ERR-γ is found in high concentration in the placenta, explaining BPA accumulation in the placenta.[73] BPA may be a teratogen as it has been reported to induce hypospadias and cryptorchidism[74] and be involved in the development of the female reproductive tract.[75] Additionally, down-regulation of mitotic cell-cycle genes has been observed in the ovaries of fetuses of BPA-exposed mice.[76] Finally, there has been one case-control study ($n = 45$) of recurrent miscarriage in relation to BPA, where higher serum BPA levels were found compared to controls.[77]

However, while exposure to BPA is widespread, the mechanisms whereby some embryos may be affected while others are not affected has hardly been investigated. Nevertheless, there is evidence to date that BPA acts via epigenetic mechanisms suppressing DNA methylation[78–80] and that dietary folic acid supplementation can reduce the effect of BPA on DNA methylation.[78] In parallel, data demonstrating that BPA can detrimentally affect T cell subsets, B cell functions, dendritic cell and macrophage functions,[81] and innate immunity,[82] suggesting that immune responses may be components of mechanisms underlying the effects of BPA on the genome.

Ionizing Radiation

Ionizing radiation causes atoms and molecules to become ionized or excited. These excitations and ionizations can produce free radicals, break chemical bonds, produce new chemical bonds and cross-link between macromolecules, and damage molecules that regulate vital cell processes (e.g., DNA, RNA, proteins). Although large doses are required for clinical effects in humans, small doses may affect cytokines and other parameters. Radiation is used clinically to prevent the multiplication of rapidly dividing cells in oncology. Ionizing radiation has been reported to affect the cerebral microcirculation associated with upregulation of proinflammatory cytokines and chemokines (including IL-6, IL-1α, and MCP-1), and increased apoptotic cell death.[83] Interferon gamma (IFN-γ) has been reported to be an essential cytokine required for the efficacy of immunotherapy in colon tumors in muridae.[84] As mentioned above, ICR mice pretreated with the Pyran copolymer or BCG vaccination exhibit increased tolerance to ionizing radiation.[17]

Implications for Clinical Practice

This review provides data that maternal immune responses may be involved in mechanisms determining the resistance of the embryo to teratogens and other environmental toxins. An important implication of this paradigm is that modulation of the maternal immune system may modify the embryo's sensitivity, not only to maternally-derived immune abortifacient stimuli, but also to environmental teratogens. These mechanisms may also be relevant in interpreting the mechanisms underlying "occult" pregnancy loss.[85] Modulation of the immune system has been used to prevent recurrent pregnancy loss in humans. The effects of immunotherapy are hotly debated in subsequent chapters of this book. Additionally, it is clear that the mother may miscarry structurally and genetically normal embryos, or aneuploid or malformed embryos. Until now it has been assumed that immunotherapy may affect the loss of normal embryos, and that the trials of immunotherapy are confounded by the loss of abnormal embryos. However, the opposite may be true. Immunotherapy may affect the loss of abnormal embryos. More data are necessary to determine the number of aneuploid embryos in trials of immunotherapy.

REFERENCES

1. Toder V, Torchinsky A. Immunoteratology: Where we are and where to go. *Am J Reprod Immunol* 1996;35:114–7.
2. Philipp T, Philipp K, Reiner A et al. Embryoscopic and cytogenetic analysis of 233 missed abortions: Factors involved in the pathogenesis of developmental defects of early failed pregnancies. *Hum Reprod* 2003;18:1724–32.
3. Billingham RE. Transplantation immunity and the maternal-fetal relation. *N Eng J Med* 1964; 270:667–72.
4. Billington WD. Influence of immunologic dissimilarity of mother and foetus on size placenta in mice. *Nature* 1964;202:317–8.
5. Kirby DKS. Transplantation and pregnancy. In: Rapoport FT, Dausser J, eds. *Human Transplantation.* New York: Grune and Stratton, 1968;565–8.
6. Beer AE, Scott JR, Billingham RE. Histocompatibility and maternal immune status as determinants of fetoplacental and litter weights in rodents. *J Exp Med* 1975;142:180–98.
7. Pechan PA. Syngeneic spleen immunization induces high mortality among progeny in mice. *Teratology* 1986;33:239–41.
8. Abir R, Ornoy A, Ben Hur H, Jaffe P, Pinus H. The effects of sera from women with spontaneous abortions on the *in vitro* development of early somite stage rat embryos. *Am J Reprod Immunol* 1994;32:73–81.
9. Zigril M, Fein A, Carp HJA et al. Immunopotentiation reverses the embryotoxic effect of serum from women with pregnancy loss. *Fertil Steril* 1991;56:653–69.
10. Chaouat G, Menu E, Bonneton C et al. Immunological manipulation in animal pregnancy and models of pregnancy failure. *Curr Opin Immunol* 1989;1:1153–6.
11. Toder V, Strassburger D, Irlin Y et al. Nonspecific immunopotentiators and pregnancy loss: Complete Freund adjuvant reverses high fetal resorption rate in CBA/J × DBA/2 mouse combination. *Am J Reprod Immunol* 1990;24:63–6.
12. Szekeres-Bartho J, Kinsky R, Kapovic M et al. Complete Freund adjuvant treatment of pregnant females influences resorption rates in CBA/J × DBA/2 matings via progesterone-mediated immuno-modulation. *Am J Reprod Immunol* 1991;26:82–3.
13. Torchinskii AM, Chirkova EM, Koppel MA et al. Dependence of the embryotoxic action of dioxidine and cyclophosphamide on the immunoreactivity of the maternal-fetal system in mice. *Farmakol Toksikol* 1985;48:69–73 (Russian).
14. Sweet DV. *Registry of Toxic Effects of Chemical Substances.* 1985–1986 ed. Washington: U.S. Government Printing Office; 1986;5:4305.
15. Torchinsky A, Fein A, Toder V. Immunoteratology: I. MHC involvement in the embryo response to teratogens in mice. *Am J Reprod Immunol* 1995;34:288–98.
16. Torchinsky A, Fein A, Carp H et al. MHC-associated immunopotentiation affects the embryo response to teratogen. *Clin Exp Immunol* 1994;98:513–9.
17. Nomura T, Hata S, Kusafuka T. Suppression of developmental anomalies by maternal macrophages in mice. *J Exp Med* 1990;172:1325–30.
18. Torchinsky A, Fein A, Toder V. Modulation of mouse sensitivity to cyclophosmamide-induced embryopathy by nonspecific intrauterine immunopotentiation. *Toxicol Methods* 1995;5:131–41.
19. Reece EA, Homko CJ, Wu YK. Multifactorial basis of the syndrome of diabetic embryopathy. *Teratology* 1996;54:171–83.
20. Torchinsky A, Toder V, Carp H et al. *In vivo* evidence for the existence of a threshold for hyperglycemia-induced major fetal malformations: Relevance to the etiology of diabetic teratogenesis. *Early Pregnancy* 1997;3:27–33.
21. Torchinsky A, Toder V, Savion S et al. Immunopotentiation increases the resistance of mouse embryos to diabetes- induced teratogenic effect. *Diabetologia* 1997;40:635–40.
22. Claudio Gutierrez J, Prater MR, Hrubec TC et al. Heart changes in 17-day-old fetuses of diabetic ICR (Institute of Cancer Research) mothers: Improvement with maternal immune stimulation. *Congenital Anomalies (Kyoto)* 2009;49:1–7.
23. Edwards MJ, Shiota K, Smith MRS et al. Hyperthermia and birth defects. *Reprod Toxicol* 1995; 9:411–25.

24. Yitzhakie D, Torchinsky A, Savion S et al. Maternal immunopotentiation affects the teratogenic response to hyperthermia. *J Reprod Immunol* 1999;45:49–66.
25. Holladay SD, Sharova L, Smith BJ et al. Nonspecific stimulation of the maternal immune system. I. Effects on teratogen induced fetal malformations. *Teratology* 2000;62:413–19.
26. Punareewattana K, Holladay SD. Immunostimulation by complete Freund's adjuvant, granulocyte macrophage colony-stimulating factor, or interferon-gamma reduces severity of diabetic embryopathy in ICR mice. *Birth Defects Res, Part A* 2004;70:20–7.
27. Savion S, Kamshitsky-Feldman A, Ivnitsky I et al. Potentiation of the maternal immune system may modify the apoptotic process in embryos exposed to developmental toxicants. *Am J Reprod Immunol* 2003;49:30–41.
28. Scialli AR. Is stress a developmental toxin? *Reprod Toxicol* 1988;1:163–72.
29. Clark DA, Banwatt D, Chaouat G. Stress-triggered abortion in mice is prevented by alloimmunization. *Am J Reprod Immunol* 1993;29:141–7.
30. Hatta A, Matsumoto A, Moriyama K et al. Opposite effects of the maternal immune system activated by interleukin-1beta vs. PSK and OK432 on 5-azacytidine-induced birth defects. *Congenital Anomalies (Kyoto)* 2003;43:46–56.
31. Torchinsky A, Fein A, Toder V. Teratogen-induced apoptotic cell death: Does the apoptotic machinery act as a protector of embryos exposed to teratogens? *Birth Defects Res, Part C* 2005;75:353–61.
32. Jacobson MD, Weil M, Raff MC. Programmed cell death in animal development. *Cell* 1997; 88:347–54.
33. Knudsen TV. Cell death. In: Kavlock RJ, Daston GP, eds. *Drug Toxicity in Embryonic Development I.* Berlin, Heidelberg: Springer-Verlag; 1997. p. 211–44.
34. Mirkes PE. 2001 Warkany lecture: To die or not to die, the role of apoptosis in normal and abnormal mammalian development. *Teratology* 2002;65:228–39.
35. Toder V, Savion S, Gorivodsky M et al. Teratogen-induced apoptosis may be affected by immunopotentiation. *J Reprod Immunol* 1996;30:173–85.
36. Fridman JS, Lowe SW. Control of apoptosis by p53. *Oncogene* 2003;22:9030–40.
37. Nicol CJ, Harrison ML, Laposa RR et al. A teratologic suppresser role for p53 in benzo[a]pyrene-treated transgenic p53-deficient mice. *Nat Genet* 1995;10:181–7.
38. Wubah JA, Ibrahim MM, Gao X et al. Teratogen-induced eye defects mediated by 53-dependent apoptosis. *Curr Biol* 1996;6:60–9.
39. Norimura T, Nomoto S, Katsuki M et al. p53-dependent apoptosis suppresses radiation-induced teratogenesis. *Nat Med* 1996;2:577–80.
40. Wang B, Ohyama H, Haginoya K et al. Prenatal radiation-induced limb defects mediated by Trp53-dependent apoptosis in mice. *Radiat Res* 2000;154:673–9.
41. Pani L, Horal M, Loeken MR. Rescue of neural tube defects in Pax-3-deficient embryos by p53 loss of function: Implications for Pax-3-dependent development and tumorigenesis. *Genes Dev* 2002;16:676–80.
42. Moallem SA, Hales BF. The role of p53 and cell death by apoptosis and necrosis in 4-hydroperoxycyclophosphamide-induced limb malformations. *Development* 1998;125:3225–34.
43. Sharova LV, Sura P, Smith BJ et al. Non-specific stimulation of the maternal immune system. I. Effects on fetal gene expression. *Teratology* 2000;62:420–8.
44. Tsujimoto Y, Shimizu S. Bcl-2 family: Life-or-death switch. *FEBS Lett* 2000;466:6–10.
45. Pommier Y, Antony S, Hayward RL et al. Apoptosis defects and chemotherapy resistance: Molecular interaction maps and networks. *Oncogene* 2004;23:2934–49.
46. Torchinsky A, Gongadze M, Zaslavsky Z et al. Maternal immunopotentiation affects caspase activation and NF-kappaB DNA-binding activity in embryos responding to an embryopathic stress. *Am J Reprod Immunol* 2006;55:36–44.
47. Karin M, Lin A. NF-κB at the crossroad of life and death. *Nat Immunol* 2002;3:221–7.
48. Beg AA, Sha WC, Bronson RT et al. Embryonic lethality and liver degeneration in mice lacking the RelA component of NF-kappa B. *Nature* 1995;376:167–70.
49. Hansen JM, Harris C. A novel hypothesis for thalidomide-induced limb teratogenesis: Redox misregulation of the NF-kappaB pathway. *Antioxid Redox Signaling* 2004;6:1–14.
50. Kennedy JC, Memet S, Wells PG. Antisense evidence for nuclear factor-kappaB-dependent embryopathies initiated by phenytoin-enhanced oxidative stress. *Mol Pharmacol* 2004;66:404–12.

51. Torchinsky A, Gongadze M, Savion S et al. Differential teratogenic response of TNFα$^{+/+}$ and TNFα$^{-/-}$ mice to cyclophosphamide: The possible role of NF-κB. *Birth Defects Res, Part A* 2006;76:437–44.

52. Raghupathy R. Pregnancy: Success and failure within the Th1/Th2/Th3 paradigm. *Semin Immunol* 2001;13:219–27.

53. Niederkorn JY. See no evil, hear no evil, do no evil: The lessons of immune privilege. *Nat Immunol* 2006;7:354–9.

54. Trowsdale J, Betz AG. Mother's little helpers: Mechanisms of maternal-fetal tolerance. *Nat Immunol* 2006;7:241–6.

55. Arck PC. Stress and pregnancy loss: Role of immune mediators, hormones and neurotransmitters. *Am J Reprod Immunol* 2001;46:117–23.

56. Gorivodsky M, Zemliak I, Orenstein H et al. Tumor necrosis factor alpha mRNA and protein expression in the uteroplacental unit of mice with pregnancy loss. *J Immunol* 1998;160:4280–8.

57. Gorivodsky M, Torchinsky A, Zemliak I et al. TGF beta 2 mRNA expression and pregnancy failure in mice. *Am J Reprod Immunol* 1999;42:124–33.

58. Gorivodsky M, Torchinsky A, Shepshelovich J et al. Colony-stimulating factor-1 (CSF-1) expression in the uteroplacental unit of mice with spontaneous and induced pregnancy loss. *Clin Exp Immunol* 1999;117:540–9.

59. Fein A, Kostina E, Savion S et al. Expression of tumor necrosis factor-α in the uteroplacental unit of diabetic mice: Effect of maternal immunopotentiation. *Am J Reprod Immunol* 2001;46:161–8.

60. Fein A, Magid N, Savion S et al. Diabetes teratogenicity in mice is accompanied with distorted expression of TGF-b2 in the uterus. *Teratog, Carcinog, Mutagen* 2002;22:59–71.

61. Pampfer S. Dysregulation of the cytokine network in the uterus of the diabetic rat. *Am J Reprod Immunol* 2001;45:375–81.

62. Baud V, Karin M. Signal transduction by tumor necrosis factor and its relatives. *Trends Cell Biol* 2001;11:372–7.

63. Torchinsky A, Shepshelovich J, Orenstein H et al. TNF-alpha protects embryos exposed to developmental toxicants. *Am J Reprod Immunol* 2003;49:159–68.

64. Torchinsky A, Gongadze M, Orenstein H et al. TNF-alpha acts to prevent occurrence of malformed fetuses in diabetic mice. *Diabetologia* 2004;47:132–9.

65. Massague J. How cells read TGF-beta signals. *Nat Rev Mol Cell Biol* 2000;1:169–78.

66. Nawshad A, LaGamba D, Hay ED. Transforming growth factor beta (TGFbeta) signalling in palatal growth, apoptosis and epithelial mesenchymal transformation (EMT). *Arch Oral Biol* 2004;49:675–89.

67. Thomae TL, Stevens EA, Bradfield CA. Transforming growth factor-beta3 restores fusion in palatal shelves exposed to 2,3,7,8-tetrachlorodibenzo-p-dioxin. *J Biol Chem* 2005;280:12742–6.

68. Nugent P, Pisano MM, Weinrich MC et al. Increased susceptibility to retinoid-induced teratogenesis in TGF-beta2 knockout mice. *Reprod Toxicol* 2002;16:741–7.

69. Dominguez F, Pellicer A, Simon C. Paracrine dialogue in implantation. *Mol Cell Endocrinol* 2002;186:175–81.

70. Stamatkin CW, Roussev RG, Stout M. et al. PreImplantation Factor (PIF) correlates with early mammalian embryo development-bovine and murine models. *Reprod Biol Endocrinol* 2011;9:63.

71. Dhillon R, Hillman S, Morris R et al. Additional information from chromosomal microarray analysis (CMA) over conventional karyotyping when diagnosing chromosomal abnormalities in miscarriage: A systematic review and meta-analysis. *BJOG* 2014;121:11–21.

72. Matsushima A, Kakuta Y, Teramoto T et al. Structural evidence for endocrine disruptor bisphenol A binding to human nuclear receptor ERR gamma. *J Biochem* 2007;142:517–24.

73. Takeda Y, Liu X, Sumiyoshi M et al. Placenta expressing the greatest quantity of bisphenol A receptor ERR{gamma} among the human reproductive tissues: Predominant expression of type-1 ERRgamma isoform. *J Biochem* 2009;146:113–22.

74. N'Tumba-Byn T, Moison D, Lacroix M et al. Differential effects of bisphenol A and diethylstilbestrol on human, rat and mouse fetal leydig cell function. *PLoS One* 2012;7:e51579 doi: 10.1371/journal.pone.0051579

75. Smith CC, Taylor HS. Xenoestrogen exposure imprints expression of genes (Hoxa10) required for normal uterine development. *FASEB J* 2007;21:239–46.

76. Lawson C, Gieske M, Murdoch B et al. Gene expression in the fetal mouse ovary is altered by exposure to low doses of bisphenol A. *Biol. Reprod.* 2011;84:79–86.

77. Sugiura-Ogasawara M, Ozaki Y, Sonta SI et al. Exposure to bisphenol A is associated with recurrent miscarriage. *Hum Reprod.* 2005;20:2325–9.

78. Bagchi D, Lau F, Bagch M. (Eds) *Genomics, Proteomics and Metabolomics in Nutraceuticals and Functional Foods.* Chapter 21, Wiley & Blackwell, Hoboken NJ, 2010. p. 319.

79. Susiarjo M, Sasson I, Mesaros C et al. Bisphenol A exposure disrupts genomic imprinting in the mouse. *PLoS Genet.* 2013;9(4):e1003401. doi: 10.1371/journal.pgen.1003401. Epub 2013 Apr 4.

80. Dolinoy DC, Huang D, Jirtle RL. Maternal nutrient supplementation counteracts bisphenol A-induced DNA hypomethylation in early development. *Proc Natl Acad Sci USA* 2007;104:13056–61.

81. Rogers JA, Metz L, Yong VW. Endocrine disrupting chemicals and immune responses: A focus on bisphenol-A and its potential mechanisms. *Mol Immunol* 2013;53:421–30.

82. Roy A, Bauer SM, Lawrence BP. Developmental exposure to bisphenol A modulates innate but not adaptive immune responses to influenza A virus infection. *PLoS One.* 2012;7(6):e38448. doi: 10.1371/journal.pone.0038448. Epub 2012 Jun 4.

83. Ungvari Z, Podlutsky A, Sosnowska D et al. Ionizing radiation promotes the acquisition of a senescence-associated secretory phenotype and impairs angiogenic capacity in cerebromicrovascular endothelial cells: Role of increased DNA damage and decreased DNA repair capacity in microvascular radiosensitivity. *J Gerontol, Ser A* 2013;68:1443–57.

84. Gerber SA, Sedlacek AL, Cron KR et al. IFN-γ mediates the antitumor effects of radiation therapy in a murine colon tumor. *Am J Pathol* 2013;182:2345–54.

85. Clark DA, Chaouat G, Gorczynski RM. Thinking outside the box: Mechanisms of environmental selective pressures on the outcome of the materno-fetal relationship. *Am J Reprod Immunol* 2002;47:275–82.

11

Fetal Structural Malformations—Embryoscopy

Thomas Philipp

Introduction

A failed pregnancy is often an emotional event and the parents demand answers about the probable cause and risk of recurrence in future pregnancies. To answer these questions, as well as to initiate appropriate treatment, particularly if the couple has experienced recurrent spontaneous abortion, an *accurate diagnosis* of the most likely cause has to be made.

All the protocols for the investigation of recurrent spontaneous abortion focus on maternal factors such as maternal thrombophilic disorders,[1-4] structural uterine anomalies,[5-6] endocrine abnormalities,[7] and parental chromosomal anomalies.[8,9] However, over 40% of couples with recurrent miscarriage are classified as having unexplained or idiopathic recurrent miscarriage.[10,11] Whether embryonic maldevelopment is a cause of recurrent early pregnancy loss is currently unknown. The demised embryo or early fetus is rarely subjected to a detailed morphologic and cytogenetic evaluation for several practical reasons. If the crown–rump length (CRL) is less than 30 mm when the embryo ceases development, the resolution of ultrasound is insufficient for precise visualization. Due to its minute size and fragility, the demised embryo cannot usually be subjected to detailed pathological examination. Dead embryos are extremely fragile, particularly if macerated, and mechanical trauma, either during spontaneous passage or instrumental evacuation of the uterus, frequently leads to destruction of the embryo and consecutive loss of the embryonic parts.[12]

Embryoscopy, however, allows visualization of the embryo *in utero*. With the transcervical approach, before curettage in cases of missed abortion, subtle morphologic details, undetectable by ultrasound, can accurately be assessed without any artificial damage (Figure 11.1).[13,14] In this chapter the diagnostic value of a detailed morphologic and cytogenetic evaluation of the demised embryo is discussed.

Technique of Transcervical Embryoscopy in Early Spontaneous or Missed Abortions

Transcervical embryoscopy requires an average of 10 minutes (range, 3–25 minutes). We perform the procedure under intravenous general anesthesia. Embryoscopy can be classified as five different steps:

Insertion of Hysteroscope and Exploration of the Uterine Cavity

With the patient in the lithotomy position, a speculum is inserted into the vagina. After disinfection with Betadine solution, the cervix is dilated. A rigid hysteroscope (12° angle of view, with both biopsy and irrigation working channels, Circon Ch 25–8 mm) is passed through the cervix under direct vision. If vision is lost, the hysteroscope is withdrawn slightly, and reinserted. A continuous normal saline flow is used throughout the procedure (pressure, 40–120 mm Hg) to help distend and clean the cervical canal and the endometrial cavity, thus providing a clear view. In failed first trimester pregnancies, the decidua capsularis and parietalis have not yet fused, so the uterine cavity can be assessed.

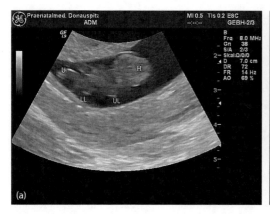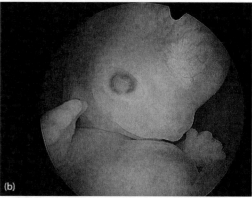

FIGURE 11.1   (a) Ultrasound prior to embryoscopy showed an embryo measuring 24 mm CRL without heartbeat. Head (H), umbilical cord (U), and upper (UL) and lower limbs (LL) can be seen. (b) Embryoscopic anteriolateral view of the upper portion revealed a well preserved embryo. Delicate structures like the nostrils are clearly discernible. Note the developing eyelids. Distinct fingers can be clearly seen.

Localization of the Gestational Sac and Incision of Chorion and Amnion

After inspection of the uterine cavity, the gestational sac is localized. The chorion is opened with microscissors (CH 7–2 mm), due to its opacity, and the embryo first viewed through the amnion. The small size of the embryo makes high demands on image resolution. At the end of the eighth week the CRL measures 30 mm but the embryo already possesses several thousand named structures. Therefore, the embryoscope should be advanced as close as possible to the embryo in order to document the minute developing structures such as the limbs (Figure 11.1). The amnion usually obscures vision by reflecting light. In failed pregnancies, there is no need to avoid rupturing the amnion with microscissors. The hysteroscope can then be inserted into the amniotic cavity. Documentation of the embryo's details can be better achieved from within the amniotic cavity.

Morphologic Evaluation of the Embryo

A complete examination of the conceptus includes visualization of the head, face, dorsal and ventral walls, limbs, and umbilical cord. The incidence of developmental defects is particularly high in early abortion specimens.[14,15] The development of the human embryo is a dynamic process with constantly changing anatomy and hence, appearance. Early diagnosis of developmental defects by embryoscopy requires basic knowledge of the anatomy of the developing human embryo. Therefore, the investigator must develop the ability to evaluate the developmental age of embryos accurately, as the diagnosis of an embryonic defect is dependent on precise aging.[16,17] The term gestational age, which is used in clinical and ultrasound terminology, should not be used for studying missed abortions, as most of these specimens are usually retained *in utero* after embryonic demise. The actual developmental age (DA) is derived from the CRL, measured by ultrasonography, and from the developmental stage assessed by embryoscopy.[16]

Tissue Sampling

In couples with recurrent miscarriage, and in cases of phenotypically abnormal embryos, accurate cytogenetic analysis of pregnancy tissue is essential.[18,19] The value of karyotyping early abortion specimens is limited by frequent false negative results, caused by maternal tissue contamination. The finding of a 46, XX karyotype in the curettage material is not always a reliable result.[20] Transcervical embryoscopy allows selective and reliable sampling of chorionic tissues with minimal potential for maternal contamination.[21] Direct chorion biopsies can be taken embryoscopically at the end of the morphologic

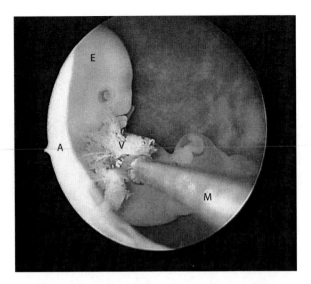

FIGURE 11.2 Direct chorionic villus sampling is performed under visual monitoring using a microforceps (M). Note the chorionic villi (V) at the tip of the microforceps. (A) Marks remnants of the amnion. A microcephalic 45,X0 embryo (E) with a CRL of 28 mm is visible in the background of the picture.

examination (Figure 11.2).[21,22] In our service, direct chorionic villus sampling is performed under direct vision, through the hysteroscope using microforceps (CH 7–2 mm).

In twin pregnancy, both chorionic sacs can be biopsied separately (Figure 11.3). At the end of the procedure chorionic villi are placed in normal saline and carefully dissected. The chorionic villi are then placed in culture medium and immediately forwarded to the cytogenetic laboratory for further processing. In our service, the tissue is subsequently cultured and analyzed cytogenetically, using standard G-banding cytogenetic techniques. Figure 11.4 shows the distribution of chromosome anomalies in our series of 359 specimens with an abnormal karyotype.

Instrumental Evacuation of the Uterus

At the end of the procedure instrumental evacuation of the uterus is performed.

Common Morphologic Defects in Early Abortion Specimens Diagnosed Embryoscopically

The following section is an overview of developmental defects that could be diagnosed with transcervical embryoscopy. Abnormal embryonic development can be local or general. General embryonic maldevelopment is known as:

Embryonic Growth Disorganization

There are four grades, which are based on the degree of abnormal embryonic development.[23] An empty or anembryonic sac is known as Grade 1 (GD 1). The amnion, if present, is usually closely applied to the chorion, (fusion of the amnion to the chorion is abnormal prior to 10 weeks of gestation). GD2 conceptuses show embryonic tissue of 3 to 5 mm in size, but with no recognizable external embryonic landmarks and no retinal pigment. It is not possible to differentiate caudal and cephalic poles (Figure 11.5). The embryo is often directly attached to the chorionic plate. GD 3 embryos are up to 10 mm long. They lack limb buds but retinal pigment is often present. A cephalic and caudal pole can be

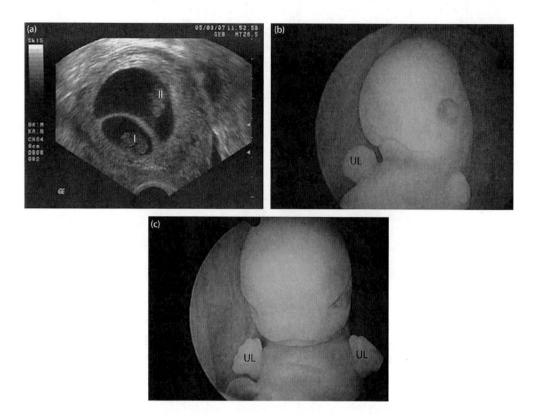

FIGURE 11.3   (a) Transvaginal ultrasonogram before embryoscopy examination of a patient's fourth consecutive pregnancy loss showed bichorionic twin pregnancy with two embryos (I + II), measuring 14 and 19 mm in CRL. No abnormalities were identified on sonography. (b) Embryoscopic examination from an anterolateral view of the upper part of twin I. External developmental defects are severe microcephaly and facial dysplasia. The hand plates are formed (UL) but finger ray development is missing indicating retarded upper limb development relative to the CRL. (c) Anterior view of the upper part of twin II. Distinct grooves are formed between the fingers of the microcephalic embryo, but the upper limbs are not bent at the elbows, indicating retarded development for an embryo of this size. The two chorionic sacs were biopsied separately. Chromosome analysis revealed trisomy 15 (47,XX, +15) (twin I) and trisomy 21 (47,XX, +21)(twin II).

differentiated. The GD 4 embryos have a CRL over 10 mm with a discernible head, trunk and limb buds. The limb buds show marked retardation in development and the development of the facial structures is highly abnormal.

In our experience growth disorganized embryos show a high frequency (92%) of autosomal trisomies, trisomy 16 being the most common, accounting for 46% of abnormal karyotypes.[13]

Localized Defects

Localized defects (Figures 11.3, 11.6 through 11.10) may be isolated or combined. Morphologically they are similar to developmental defects seen in fetuses. Malformations which have external manifestation and we were able to diagnose embryoscopically include the following.

Head Defects

Microcephaly, anencephaly, encephalocele, facial dysplasia, cleft lip, cleft palate, fusions of the face to the chest, absence of eyes, unfused eye globes, and proboscis are some of the defects which we have seen embryoscopically.

Microcephalic embryos may be seen on embryoscopy with a poorly developed cranium with loss of normal vascular markings. In particular the usual bulge of the frontal area, which is expected in

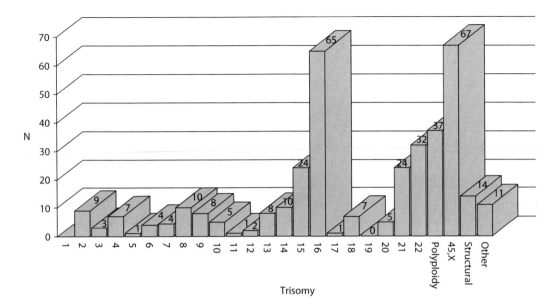

FIGURE 11.4 Frequency of trisomy for each chromosome, polyploidy, monosomy X, and structural chromosome anomalies among 359 specimens with an abnormal karyotype.

embryos of this size, is absent. Embryos with a dysplastic face show poorly developed branchial arches and midface structures on embryoscopic examination. Microcephaly and facial dysplasia are usually observed in combination. Chromosomal anomalies are the most common cause of these developmental defects. Encephaloceles present as a bulge in the cranium, often covered by adherent discoloured skin on embryoscopy. Embryoscopy has identified encephaloceles in the frontal and parietal regions of the embryonic head, unlike the situation in the fetus, where the defect usually occurs in the occipital area. The size of an encephalocele may range from small encephaloceles to large defects involving most of the cranium.[19,24]

In anencephalic embryos, the brain tissue may still be present and this condition is called exencephaly. The developing cerebral structures subsequently undergo varying degrees of destruction,

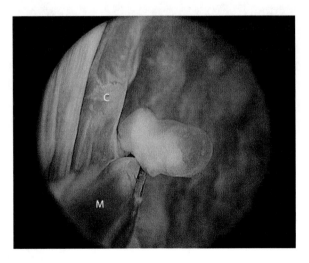

FIGURE 11.5 The microscissor (M) is pointing to a growth disorganized embryo (GD2) measuring 3 mm CRL. No recognizable external embryonic landmarks can be seen embryoscopically. An abnormal karyotype (47,XX, +4) was diagnosed cytogenetically. C shows the chorionic plate.

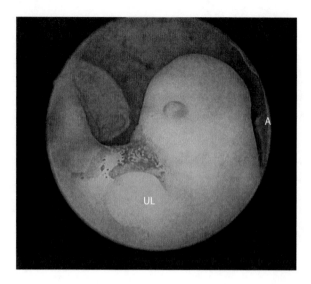

FIGURE 11.6   Close-up lateral view of the upper part of an embryo measuring 14 mm CRL after the amniotic membrane (A) had been opened. The microcephalic embryo showed a fusion face to the chest. Upper limbs (UL) showed hand plate formation, but not digital rays indicating retarded development of the limbs for an embryo of this size. Chromosome analysis revealed an abnormal karyotype (69,XXY).

leaving a mass of vascular structures and degenerated neural tissue. Neural tube defects (anencephaly, encepalocele, spina bifida) can be multifactorial in origin, caused by a lethal gene defect or nongenetic mechanisms such as amniotic bands. Chromosomal anomalies are the most common cause of embryonic neural tube defects.[19,24–27] The most common associations with chromosome abnormalities are triploidy and spina bifida,[28] 45,X0, and trisomies 9 and 14 with encephalocele.[29]

Lateral and median cleft lip can be distinguished embryoscopically. Lateral clefts may be unilateral or bilateral. Cleft lip occurs when the maxillary prominence and the united medial nasal prominences

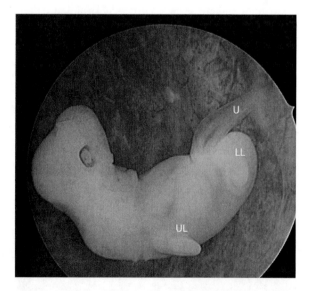

FIGURE 11.7   Embryoscopic lateral view of an embryo measuring 13 mm in length. External developmental defects of the embryo are severe microcephaly, facial dysplasia, profoundly retarded upper (UL) and lower (LL) limb development. (U) marks the umbilical cord. The missed abortion was the patient's third consecutive pregnancy loss and resulted from IVF. An apparently normal karyotype was diagnosed cytogenetically (46,XY).

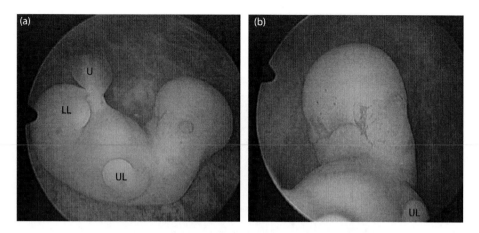

FIGURE 11.8   Lateral (a) and close up anterior view of the upper part (b) of an embryo measuring 12 mm CRL. External developmental defects of the embryo are severe microcephaly, facial dysplasia, profoundly retarded upper (UL) and lower (LL) limb development and an abnormal short cord (U). The dark brown areas in the facial region are due to maceration. The missed abortion was the patient's sixth consecutive pregnancy loss. An apparently normal karyotype was diagnosed cytogenetically (46,XY).

fail to fuse. The midline cleft lip represents a fusion defect of the median nasal swellings. In the embryo, cleft lip cannot be diagnosed until after seven weeks of development, since fusion does not occur until that time. Cleft lip may be part of a malformation syndrome. Irregular clefting may be caused by amniotic bands. In embryos clefting defects occur commonly with chromosomal aberrations, especially trisomy 13.

Cleft palate occurs if the primary anterior palate, lateral palatine processes, and nasal septum fail to unite. Cleft palate can only be diagnosed in the fetal period, since fusion is completed after the 10th week of development.

Trunk Defects

Trunk defects include spina bifida, omphalocele, and gastroschisis. The phenotype of spina bifida is different in the early developmental stages than the well-known appearance in the fetus or neonate.

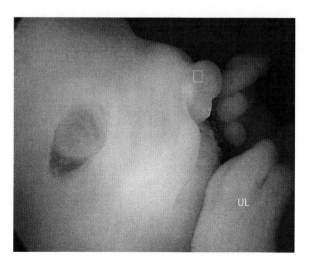

FIGURE 11.9   Close-up of the face of an embryo with a CRL of 27 mm. A median cleft lip (arrow) is present. (UL) marks the right upper limb. Trisomy 9 (47,XY, +9) was diagnosed.

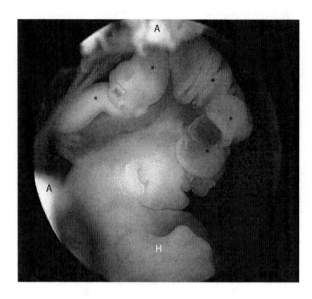

FIGURE 11.10 Embryoscopic lateral view of the upper portion of a well preserved embryo with anencephaly. The exposed brain tissue (*) is still intact (exencephaly). The digital rays of the hand (H) are notched. Parts of the external ear (E) are clearly discernable. Remnants of the amnion are labeled (A). A normal karyotype was diagnosed cytogenetically (46,XX).

In the embryo, spina bifida is frequently observed as a plaque-like protrusion of neural tissue over the caudal spine.[30] It is not clear whether the spina bifida seen in the embryo is due to a different mechanism to those seen in the fetus, or whether they are merely precursors to the lesions observed in the fetus. Myeloceles vary in size and location. The most common site in the embryo is the lumbar and sacral regions. Chromosomal aberrations are the most common cause of embryonic myeloceles.

The physiological midgut herniation is a macroscopically visible process which starts in the 6th week after fertilization. The midgut only fully returns to the abdominal cavity at the end of the 10th week of development. Herniation is still physiological at eight developmental weeks, hence omphalocele can only be diagnosed in the fetal period. Gastroschisis differs from the physiological herniation of the midgut as the umbilical cord is not involved and no sac is present. Gastroschisis is rarely observed in the embryo and occurs when the bowel protrudes from a defect that is generally located to the right side of the umbilicus. The pathogenesis of this defect is controversial, and a variety of different theories have been proposed.[31–33] The theory of abdominal wall disruption as a result of an *in utero* vascular accident has gained most acceptance. Therefore, gastroschisis is considered to be a sporadic event with a negligible risk of recurrence. Since the defect is usually not associated with chromosome aberrations it is rarely observed in early spontaneous abortions.

Limb Defects

Polydactyly, oligodactyly, syndactyly, split-hand/split-foot malformation, and transverse limb reduction defects are the most commonly observed malformations.

Polydactyly is one of the most common limb abnormalities found in the embryo. Polydactyly may be on the radial (preaxial) or ulnar (postaxial) side of the limb. Polydactyly may occur as isolated malformation or may be part of malformation syndromes. Postaxial polydactyly is common in trisomy 13.[34] In syndactyly two or more of the fingers or toes are joined together. At the end of the eighth developmental week, fingers become free and syndactyly can be diagnosed embryoscopically. Syndactyly may be part of a malformation syndrome. Syndactyly of digits III and IV is common in triploidy.[34,35]

The split-hand/split-foot malformation involves ectrodactyly. The hand is divided into two parts which are opposed like a lobster claw. In the second anatomical type the radial rays are absent with only the fifth digit remaining.[36] Split hand can be a part of numerous syndromes. In embryos with split hand malformation chromosome 15 trisomy can be found. In transverse limb reduction defect distal structures of the limb are absent with proximal parts being more or less normal. These limb defects are regarded as a disruption sequence which is presumed to be a result of peripheral ischemia.[37] The recurrence risk in future pregnancies is minimal.[34]

Umbilical Cord Defects

The following complications may affect the umbilical cord: knots, torsion, stricture, cysts, and abnormal thin and/or short cords. The mechanical lesions of the cord (knots, torsion, stricture) are rarely observed embryoscopically. Torsion of the umbilical cord can often be found in macerated specimens, but are usually postmortem artifacts. Umbilical cord cysts and abnormal thin and/or short cords are usually found in chromosomally abnormal embryos.

Duplication Anomalies

Chorangiopagus parasiticus (CAPP) or acardiac conjoined twins, and other conjoined twins have been observed embryoscopically.[38] The most severe defect in the acardiac conceptus is usually seen at the cranial pole. The parasitic twin is usually seen as a markedly edematous mass. The upper portion of the conceptus has missing or highly abnormal facial structures. There are usually only remnants of the upper extremities, but the lower limbs are often well developed. The "pump" twin is also usually developmentally abnormal.[39] The circulation is through the normal pump twin by a return reversed flow from artery directly to artery, or vein to vein, anastomoses of the cord or chorionic surface vessels. The observed anomalies of the parasitic twin are presumed to be caused by a combination of primary developmental defects and decreased oxygenation of the recipient twin with disruption of organogenesis.

Conjoined twinning is the result of late and incomplete twin formation at the latest possible moment when the embryonic axis is being laid down (between 13 and 15 days postconception). Most classifications are descriptive and based on the anatomical zones of coalescence. Fusion of the thorax (thoracopagus) is most commonly (70%) reported.

The importance of identifying these rare duplication anomalies cannot be overemphasized; parents can be reassured that the anomalies are accidental sequela of twinning, with no additional risk of recurrence in future pregnancies.[35]

Amnion Rupture Sequence

There are numerous theories concerning the pathogenesis of amniotic bands.[40] The theory of early amnion rupture, as proposed by Torpin,[41] has gained most acceptance. Amniotic rupture leads to subsequent amniotic band formation which interferes with normal embryonic development by causing malformations or disruptions. This sequence of events is known as the amnion rupture sequence (ARS).[42] Although this sequence is uncommon in live born infants, its frequency may be as high as one in 56 in previable fetuses. Bands that constrict the umbilical cord are recognized as the main cause of death in this sequence.[43] ARS may cause abnormalities that are detectable by embryoscopy, such as encephaloceles, cleft lip, and amputations. When aberrant sheet or bands of tissue are seen on embryoscopy, which are attached to the conceptus with characteristic deformities in a nonembryologic distribution, a diagnosis of amniotic band syndrome or ARS can be made.[44] Amniotic bands can occur as a result of abdominal trauma,[45] chorionic villus sampling,[46] and connective tissue abnormalities.[47] However, in most cases of ARS no such cause can be identified. Therefore, most authors consider ARS a sporadic event with a negligible risk of recurrence.

Aneuploidy/Polyploidy as the Main Cause for Abnormal Embryonic Development

The highest incidence of chromosome anomalies (86%) can be found in conceptuses with combined localized developmental defects. Among growth disorganized embryos, 70% are cytogentically abnormal. The lowest incidence of chromosomal abnormalities (41%) is found in phenotypically normal

TABLE 11.1

Specimen Morphology and Karyotype of 514 Missed Abortions

Morphology	Total Specimens		Total Specimens Successfully Karyotyped		Specimens with Abnormal Karyotype	
	No.	%[a]	No.	%[b]	No.	%[c]
Normal	58	11.3	56	96.2	23	41.1
Growth disorganization	237	46.1	225	95	156	69.3
Combined defects	198	38.5	193	97.3	166	86.0
Isolated defects	21	4.1	21	100	14	66.7
Total	514	100	495	96.3	359	72.5

[a] Percentage of total number of specimens with that morphology.
[b] Percentage of each morphologic category successfully karyotyped.
[c] Percentage of each morphologic category with an abnormal karyotype.

specimens (Table 11.1).[14] In summary, contrary to fetuses, aneuploidy/polyploidy is the major factor affecting normal embryonic development in early intrauterine deaths and may explain why spontaneous abortion is usually a sporadic event in a patient's reproductive history although the incidence of developmental defects is high. Most (95%) of the observed chromosomal mutations are not hereditary and carry no increased risk for future pregnancies. They originate de novo either in gametogenesis (trisomy and monosomy) or may result from polyspermic fertilization or failure of normal cleavage (triploidy and tetraploidy). Therefore all embryoscopic findings should be supplemented by the results of cytogenetic analysis to distinguish between nonchromosomal and chromosomal causes of anomalies. Cytogenetically diagnosed aneuploidy/polyploidy provides a causal explanation for these developmental defects in cases of a phenotypically abnormal embryo, and also indicates that the recurrence risk for the observed developmental defect and chromosomal abnormality in these couples is not increased.[48]

Clinical Significance of Detailed Morphologic and Cytogenetic Evaluation of Early Spontaneous Abortion

A cytogenetic examination of early intrauterine deaths is indicated if the pregnancy loss is a recurrent event[49] and/or occurred after IVF and/or after a prolonged period of infertility. If a chromosomal abnormality (autosomal trisomy, sex chromosome monosomy, and polyploidy) of the embryo is diagnosed, a causal explanation for the pregnancy loss is usually found, as most of the observed chromosomal abnormalities are incompatible with survival to the fetal period or to term.

However, karyotyping the products of conception following recurrent miscarriage is often not performed as cytogenetic evaluation of early intrauterine deaths has many drawbacks. The investigation is often hampered by tissue culture failure and by false negative results due to maternal contamination of the collected tissue.

Transcervical embryoscopy allows selective reliable sampling of chorionic tissues with minimal potential for maternal contamination.[21] In addition, abnormal embryonic development, as documented by embryoscopy in patients with apparently normal chromosomes, might add valuable information. This information would be completely lost if morphologic examination of the demised embryo had not been carried out and abnormal embryonic development would have remained undetected. Embryoscopy diagnoses subtle morphologic defects currently undetectable by ultrasound. A grossly abnormal embryo with a normal karyotype is a particularly valuable finding as it points to etiologic factors usually not considered to be etiologically related to early pregnancy loss (Figures 11.7 and 11.8).

If cytogenetic evaluation of the conceptus is performed, it is currently assumed that the absence of a genetic disorder of the conceptus indicates that women with recurrent miscarriage lose normal embryos, and these patients are given expensive treatment with potential side effects (e.g., steroids, heparin, i.v. immunoglobulin, paternal leukocyte immunization, etc.) to prevent miscarriage.

TABLE 11.2

Summary of Specimen Morphology and Karyotypic Outcome in 53 Patients with Recurrent Miscarriages (Three or More Consecutive Miscarriages)

	Total Specimens		Total Specimens Successfully Karyotyped		Specimens with Abnormal Karyotype	
Morphology	No.	%[a]	No.	%[b]	No.	%[c]
Normal	8	15.1	7	87.5	3	42.9
Growth disorganization	26	49.1	24	92.3	15	62.5
Combined defects	18	34	18	100	13	72.2
Isolated defects	1	1.9	1	100	1	100
Total	53	100	50	94.3	32	64

[a] Percentage of total number of specimens with that morphology.
[b] Percentage of each morphologic category successfully karyotyped.
[c] Percentage of each morphologic category with an abnormal karyotype.

Table 11.2 shows a summary of embryoscopic and cytogenetic findings in 53 patients with recurrent miscarriage (more than two consecutive early pregnancy losses). 50(94.3) were successfully karyotyped. 32 (64%) embryos had an abnormal karyotype. 14 (28%) embryos had a morphologic defect with an apparently normal karyotype and no morphologic and cytogenetic abnormality was seen in four (8%) specimens. Among specimens with an apparently normal karyotype, developmental defects, (embryonic growth disorganization, G1–G4) which are never observed in fetuses or the newborn, can be observed embryoscopically. Grossly abnormal development suggests a severe disturbance of growth and morphogenesis in early human development likely to be incompatible with survival into the second trimester.

Other embryos with an apparently normal karyotype often show developmental defects (craniofacial defects, limb defects, neural tube defects) comparable to those observed in fetuses and live born infants.

It is unlikely that maternal factors such as antiphospholipid antibodies, thrombophilic disorders, endocrine factors or uterine anomalies cause the developmental defects observed embryoscopically. After exclusion of a chromosomal disorder these developmental defects might be heterogeneous in their origin. In fetuses or live born infants, congenital malformations are commonly explained by Mendelian and multifactorial disorders, and there is no reason to believe that embryonic developmental defects have a different etiology. Recent studies, using molecular cytogenetic techniques, have shown that submicroscopic genetic imbalances containing genes required for embryonic growth and morphogenesis exist in karyotypically apparently normal spontaneous miscarriages,[50] malformed fetuses,[51] and embryos with developmental abnormalities documented by embryoscopy.[52] Consequently, we challenge the prevailing assumption that the absence of a genetic disorder of the conceptus on routine laboratory testing is a reason to look for nongenetic maternal causes for recurrent spontaneous abortion. A detailed morphologic and cytogenetic evaluation of early intrauterine deaths might have implications for future diagnosis and treatment of recurrent pregnancy loss.

In recurrent spontaneous abortion, current investigation protocols frequently do not permit a conclusive diagnosis because maternal factors are predominantly assessed. Currently used treatment protocols might not be effective if the losses are due to chromosomal aberrations or embryonic developmental defects. However, future studies might show that these therapy strategies might be highly effective, if they are restricted to the subgroup of patients recurrently miscarrying morphologically *and* cytogenetically normal pregnancies.

Acknowledgment

To a wonderful embryopathologist and teacher, who introduced me to embryopathology, Dr. DK Kalousek.

REFERENCES

1. Wilson WA, Gharavi AE, Koike T, Lockshin MD, Branch DW, Piette JC et al. International consensus statement on preliminary classification criteria for definite antiphospholipid syndrome: Report of an international workshop. *Arthritis Rheum* 1999;42:1309–11.

2. Rai RS, Regan L, Clifford K, Pickering W, Dave M, Mackie I et al. Antiphospholipid antibodies and beta 2-glycoprotein-I in 500 women with recurrent miscarriage: Results of a comprehensive screening approach. *Hum Reprod* 1995;10:2001–5.

3. Rai R, Backos M, Elgaddal S, Shlebak A, Regan L. Factor V. Leiden and recurrent miscarriage— Prospective outcome of untreated pregnancy. *Hum Reprod* 2002;17:442–5.

4. Kovalevsky G, Gracia CR, Berlin JA, Sammel MD, Barnhart KT. Evaluation of the association between hereditary thrombophilias and recurrent pregnancy loss: A meta-analysis. *Arch Intern Med* 2004;164:558–63.

5. Grimbizis GF, Camus M, Tarlatzis BC, Bontis JN, Devroey P. Clinical implications of uterine malformations and hysteroscopic treatment results. *Hum Reprod Update* 2001;7:161–74.

6. Salim R, Regan L, Woelfer B, Backos M, Jurkovic D. A comparative study of the morphology of congenital uterine anomalies in women with and without a history of recurrent first trimester miscarriage. *Hum Reprod* 2003;18:162–66.

7. Daya S. Efficacy of progesterone support for pregnancy in women with recurrent miscarriage. A meta-analysis of controlled trials. *Br J Obstet Gynaecol* 1989;96:275–80.

8. De Braekeleer M, Dao TN. Cytogenetic studies in couples experiencing repeated pregnancy losses. *Hum Reprod* 1990;5:519–28.

9. Franssen MTM, Korevaar JC, Leschot NJ, Bossuyt PMM, Knegt AC, Gerssen-Schoorl KBJ et al. Selective chromosome analysis in couples with two or more miscarriages: Case-control study. *BMJ* 2005;331:137–9.

10. Clifford K, Rai R, Watson H, Regan L. An informative protocol for the investigation of recurrent miscarriage: Preliminary experience of 500 consecutive cases. *Hum Reprod* 1994;9:1328–32.

11. Stephenson MD. Frequency of factors associated with habitual abortion in 197 couples. *Fertil Steril* 1996;66:24–9.

12. Kalousek DK. Anatomical and chromosomal abnormalities in specimens of early spontaneous abortions: Seven years experience. *Birth Defects* 1987;23:153–68.

13. Philipp T, Kalousek DK. Generalized abnormal embryonic development in missed abortion: Embryoscopic and cytogenetic findings. *Am J Med Genet 2002*;111:41–7.

14. Philipp T, Philipp K, Reiner A, Beer F, Kalousek DK. Embryoscopic and cytogenetic analysis of 233 missed abortions: Factors involved in the pathogenesis of developmental defects of early failed pregnancies. *Hum Reprod* 2003;18:1724–32.

15. Shiota K. Development and intrauterine fate of normal and abnormal human conceptuses. *Congenital Anomalies* 1991;31:67–80.

16. Moore KL. *The Developing Human—Clinically orientated Embryology*. 5th ed. Philadelphia, PA, USA: WB Saunders Co.; 1993.

17. Philipp T. *Atlas der Embryologie. Embryoskopische Aufnahmen der normalen und abnormen Embryonalentwicklung*. Wien: Facultas Verlag; 2004.

18. Wolf GC, Horger EO. Indication for examination of spontaneous abortion specimens: A reassessment. *Am J Obstet Gynecol* 1995;5:1364–7.

19. Philipp T, Kalousek DK. Neural tube defects in missed abortions—Embryoscopic and cytogenetic findings. *Am J Med Genet* 2002;107:52–7.

20. Bell KA, Van Deerlin PG, Haddad BR, et al. Cytogenetic diagnosis of "normal 46,XX" karyotypes in spontaneous abortions frequently may be misleading. *Fertil Steril* 1999;71:334–41.

21. Ferro J, Martinez MC, Lara C et al. Improved accuracy of hysteroembryoscopic biopsies for karyotyping early missed abortions. *Fertil Steril* 2003;80:1260–4.

22. Philipp T, Feichtinger W, Van Allen M et al. Abnormal embryonic development diagnosed embryoscopically in early intrauterine deaths after *in vitro* fertilization (IVF): A preliminary report of 23 cases. *Fertil Steril* 2004;82:1337–42.

23. Poland BJ, Miller JR, Harris M et al. Spontaneous abortion: A study of 1961 women and their conceptuses. *Acta Obstet Gynecol Scand* 1981;102(Suppl):5–32.

24. Mc Fadden DE, Kalousek DK. Survey of neural tube defects in spontaneously aborted embryos. *Am J Med Genet* 1989;32:356–8.
25. Bell JE, Gosden CM. Central nervous system abnormalities-contrasting patterns in early and late pregnancy. *Clin Genet* 1978;13:387–96.
26. Coerdt W, Miller K, Holzgreve W, Rauskolb R, Schwinger E, Rehder H. Neural tube defects in chromosomally normal and abnormal human embryos. *Ultrasound Obstet Gynecol* 1997;10:410–5.
27. Creasy MR, Alberman ED. Congenital malformations of the central nervous system in spontaneous abortions. *J Med Genet* 1976;13:9–16.
28. Philipp T, Grillenberger K, Separovic ER, Philipp K, Kalousek DK. Effects of triploidy on early human development. *Prenatal Diagn* 2004;242:276–81.
29. Canki N, Warburton D, Byrne J. Morphological characteristics of monosomy X in spontaneous abortions. *Ann Genet* 1988;31:4–13.
30. Patten BM. Overgrowth of the neural tube in young human embryos. *Anat Rec* 1952;113:381–93.
31. Shaw A. The myth of gastroschisis. *J Pediatr Surg* 1975;10:235–44.
32. De Vries PA. The pathogenesis of gastroschisis and omphalocele. *J Pediatr Surg* 1980;15:245–51.
33. Hoyme H, Higginbottom MC, Jones KL. The vascular pathogenesis of gastrochisis: Intrauterine interruption of the omphalomesenteric artery. *J Pediatr* 1981;98:228–31.
34. Ramsing M, Duda V, Mehrain Y et al. Hand malformations in the aborted embryo: An informative source of genetic information. *Birth Defects* 1996;30:79–94.
35. Dimmick JE, Kalousek DK. *Developmental Pathology of the Embryo & Fetus*. Philadelphia, PA, USA: JB Lippincott Co.; 1992.
36. Birch-Jensen A. *Congenital Deformities of Upper Extremities*. Copenhagen: Enjar Munksgaard; 1949.
37. Golden CM, Ryan LM, Holmes LB. Chorionic villus sampling: A distinctive teratogenic effect on fingers. *Birth Defects Res* 2003;67:557–62.
38. Philipp T, Separovic ER, Philipp K, et al. Transcervical fetoscopic diagnosis of structural defects in four first trimester monochorionic twin intrauterine deaths. *Prenatal Diagn* 2003;12:964–9.
39. Napolitani FD, Schreiber I. The acardiac monster. A review of the world literature and presentation of two cases. *Am J Obstet Gynecol* 1960;82:708–11.
40. Evans MI. Amniotic bands. *Ultrasound Obstet Gynecol* 1997;10:307–8.
41. Torpin R. Amniochorionic mesoblastic fibrous strings and amniotic bands. Associated constricting fetal anomalies or fetal death. *Am J Obstet Gynecol* 1965;91:65–75.
42. Kalousek DK. Bamforth S. Amnion rupture sequence in previable fetuses. *Am J Med Genet* 1988;3:63–73.
43. Hong CY, Simon MA. Amniotic bands knotted about umbilical cord. A rare cause of fetal death. *Obstet Gynecol* 1963;222:667–70.
44. Philipp T, Kalousek DK. Amnion rupture sequence in a first trimester missed abortion. *Prenatal Diagn* 2001;21:835–8.
45. Ossipoff V, Hall BD. Etiologic factors in the amniotic band syndrome. A study of 24 patients. *Birth Defects* 1977;13:117–32.
46. Firth HV, Boyd PA, Chamberlain P, Mackenzie IZ, Lindenbaum RH, Huson SM. Severe limb abnormalities after chorion villus sampling at 56–66 days gestation. *Lancet* 1991;337:762–3.
47. Young ID, Lindenbaum RH, Thompsen EM, Pemburg ME. Amniotic bands in connective tissue disorders. *Arch Dis Child* 1985;60:1061–3.
48. Warburton D, Kline J, Stein Z et al. Does the karyotype of a spontaneous abortion predict the karyotype of a subsequent abortion?—Evidence from 273 women with two karyotyped spontaneous abortions. *Am J Hum Genet* 1987;41:465–83.
49. Royal College of Obstetricians and Gynaecologists, Guideline No. 17. *The Management of Recurrent Miscarriage*. London: RCOG; 2003.
50. Schaeffer AJ, Chung J, Heretis K, Wong A, Ledbetter DH, Lese Martin C. Comparative genomic hybridization-array analysis enhances the detection of aneuploidies and submicroscopic imbalances in spontaneous miscarriages. *Am J Hum Genet* 2004;74:1168–74.
51. Le Caignec C, Boceno M, Saugier-Veber P, Jacquemont S, Joubert M, David A et al. Detection of genomic imbalances by array based comparative genomic hybridisation in fetuses with multiple malformations. *J Med Genet* 2005;42:121–8.
52. Rajcan-Separovic E, Qiao Y, Tyson C, Harvard C, Fawcett C, Kalousek D et al. Genomic changes detected by array CGH in human embryos with developmental defects. *Mol Hum Reprod* 2009;16(2):125–34.

12

Fetal Structural Malformations—Ultrasound

Akhila Vasudeva and Pratap Kumar

Introduction

The early pregnancy scan is an essential part of contemporary routine antenatal care. In patients with recurrent pregnancy loss (RPL), a normal early pregnancy scan can be highly reassuring. At the same time, abnormal sonological findings may herald a nonviable pregnancy, detect chromosomal or structural malformations which are more common among these women, or forecast higher risk of poor pregnancy outcome. The most commonly used transducers, are: linear array or sector transducer (3–5 MHz for abdominal examination), and the transvaginal probe (5–10 MHz). In first trimester ultrasound, transvaginal sonography (TVS) is necessary up to approximately 10 weeks, and thereafter a transabdominal probe is mostly used. However, a transvaginal probe is complementary to abdominal ultrasound in order to complete the anatomical evaluation.

With modern ultrasound machines, there is only a negligible rise in tissue temperature, usually less than 1°C. It is unlikely that there is any deleterious effect of ultrasound in the first trimester during embryogenesis with routine grey scale ultrasound.[1] Although the potential for embryonic effects from Doppler imaging exists, there is little evidence that it is teratogenic, as long as pulses are applied at low level with minimal usage of the Doppler.

Normal Sonological Findings in the First Trimester

Knowledge of the "normal" development of the embryo and fetus is essential when scanning in the first trimester. The primary goal of ultrasound examination in the first trimester is to determine whether the pregnancy is intrauterine, embryonic/fetal number, viability by ruling out missed abortion/molar pregnancy, gestational age assessment by gestational sac size or crown rump length (CRL), aneuploidy screening, and to rule out structural abnormalities. It is also important to rule out uterine anomalies, evaluate fibroids (if any), and to rule out adnexal pathology. In cases of multiple pregnancy, assessment of chorionicity is of paramount importance.

Four to Five Weeks

The gestational sac can first be imaged sonographically at about 4.4 to 4.6 weeks from the last menstrual period, when the sac is 2–4 mm in size. The intradecidual sign and the double decidual sac sign are specific for intrauterine pregnancy, and rule out the possibility of ectopic pregnancy.[1] The serum β hCG (human chorionic gonadotrophin) level at which an intrauterine gestational sac should be seen with a modern high resolution vaginal probe is called the discriminatory zone, usually between 1000 and 2000 IU/L. When β hCG is above the discriminatory zone, absence of an intrauterine sac significantly raises the possibility of ectopic pregnancy. When β hCG is below this level, one cannot be certain and the incremental rise of β hCG indicates the location/viability of pregnancy. In recurrent biochemical pregnancy losses, ultrasound is not very useful as there is no sonological evidence of pregnancy in presence of very low β hCG.

The yolk sac is a circular structure, located between the chorion and the amnion, and is first visualized at the fifth postmenstrual week. The size of the embryo ranges from 2 to 3 mm in size and appears as a linear structure attached to the yolk sac and close to the uterine wall. Although embryonic cardiac activity can be visualized at this time, rates of less than 100 beats per minute are not predictive of a poor outcome, and follow-up scanning is imperative.[2]

Week Six

Ultrasonographically, the embryo appears as an undifferentiated structure at this time, except for the heartbeat. An average heart rate of 130 beats per minute can be seen using M-mode scanning. If the embryo is less than 4 mm, the absence of cardiac activity is nondiagnostic. Once a fetal heartbeat is visualized, the risk of miscarriage decreases as most miscarriages are blighted ova. Towards the end of the sixth week, the embryo is seen separately from the yolk sac. After fetal cardiac activity, the next anatomical structure to become visible is the primitive neural tube. Sonographically, this appears as a hypoechoic longitudinal structure running the length of the embryo, visible in the form of two parallel lines.[2]

Weeks Seven to Nine

The head and trunk can be visualized separately. Within the head, an intracranial cystic structure is visualized corresponding to the fourth ventricle (rhombencephalon).[2] The cerebral hemispheres can be visualized in some embryos at this gestation. The initial sign of normal herniation of the gut can be seen as an echogenic area at the abdominal insertion of the cord.

Week eight (Figure 12.1): The choroid plexus becomes visible and grows correspondingly with the cerebral hemispheres, developing into a crescent shape traversing the roof of the fourth ventricle. The third ventricle (diencephalon) is wide. The stomach can first be visualized at this gestation as a small hypoechogenic area on the left side of the upper abdomen, and should be seen in all embryos by 11 weeks.[2] It is possible to identify the atrial and ventricular walls of the heart moving reciprocally at the end of week eight,[2] with the atrial component appearing larger than the ventricular component. Clear identification between the thoracic and abdominal contents is possible by the ninth week. The cerebral hemispheres should be visualized in all embryos by week nine. At nine weeks, the size of the lateral ventricles increase rapidly and the third ventricle narrows. The spine is still characterized by two

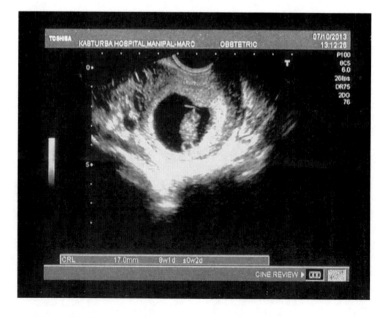

FIGURE 12.1   An eight-week TVS picture showing developing embryo and the yolk sac.

echogenic parallel lines. Normal mid-gut herniation can be seen as a large hyperechogenic mass. The long bones, hands and feet can be first imaged at this time.

Early Anomaly Scan at 10–14 Weeks

This scan needs a systematic approach to view the fetal anatomy, similar to that of a second trimester targeted scan. The aim is to obtain a transverse section of the head to demonstrate the ossified cranial bones, a midline echo, and the choroid plexuses should be seen in the ventricles (Figure 12.2);

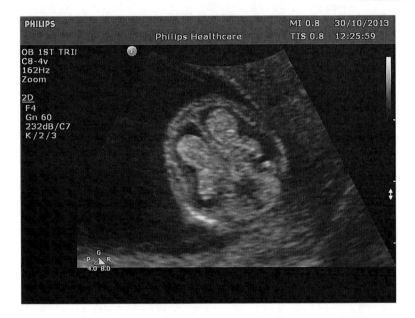

FIGURE 12.2 Developing choroid plexus in the 12th week fetus showing a typical "butterfly sign."

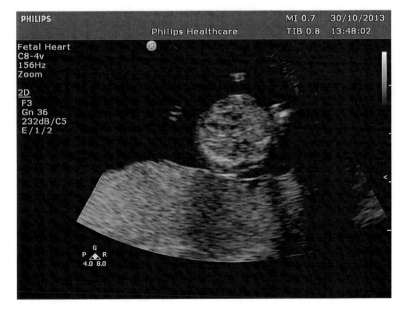

FIGURE 12.3 A four-chamber view demonstrated in a 12-week fetus.

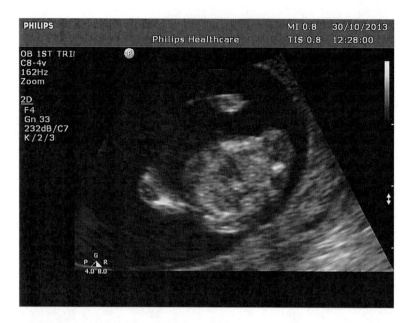

FIGURE 12.4   A three-vessel view demonstrated in a 12-week fetus.

a mid-sagittal view of the face should be obtained to demonstrate the nasal bone, orbits and a normal profile; sagittal section of the spine should be determined to view the presence of intact skin over the back, and transverse and longitudinal planes of the spine from neck to sacrum; a transverse section of the thorax should be sought to demonstrate the four-chamber view of the heart with a normal axis and also a three-vessel view (Figures 12.3 and 12.4); transverse and sagittal sections of the trunk and extremities should be obtained to demonstrate the stomach in the left upper quadrant, kidneys (Figure 12.5), the bladder (Figure 12.6), the abdominal insertion of the umbilical cord, and all the long bones, hands (Figure 12.7) and feet.

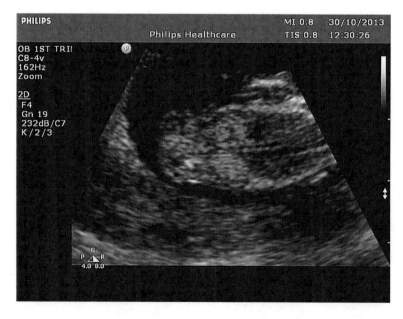

FIGURE 12.5   Kidneys visualized in an 11-week fetus.

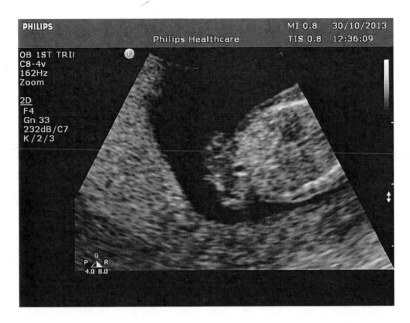

FIGURE 12.6 Bladder seen in an 11-week fetus.

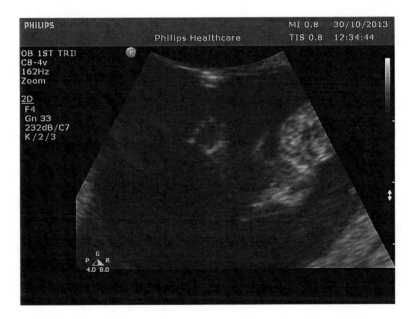

FIGURE 12.7 Open hand with five digits seen in an 11-week fetus.

Diagnosis of Miscarriage/Nonviable Pregnancy in Early Scans

The criteria for diagnosing a nonviable pregnancy or miscarriage by ultrasound have been under constant debate.[3] The RCOG in the UK has reviewed its guidance[4] to doctors and revised the ultrasound criteria used to define miscarriage to the following: (1) A mean gestation sac diameter of 25 mm (with no obvious yolk sac), or with a fetal pole with CRL 7 mm (the latter without evidence of fetal heart activity). (2) TVS should be performed in all cases for diagnosing nonviability. (3) Where there is any doubt about diagnosis and/or a woman requests a repeat scan, this should be performed at an interval of at least one week from the initial scan before medical or surgical measures are undertaken for uterine evacuation. No growth in gestation sac size or CRL is strongly suggestive of a nonviable pregnancy in the absence of embryonic structures on a repeat scan.

The routine use of TVS has led to improvements in the management of early pregnancy loss.[3,5,6] Once a certain diagnosis of miscarriage has been made, a proportion of women (up to 70%) will elect for expectant management.[5] Other women will choose medical or surgical management to deal with the miscarriage. However, expectant or medical management precludes genetic testing of the embryo in recurrent miscarriage. Whichever method is chosen, the diagnosis of a complete miscarriage is generally accepted as an endometrial thickness <15 mm with no evidence of retained products of conception. TVS is a sensitive tool for detecting residual trophoblastic tissue. Blood flow in the intervillous space in cases of first trimester miscarriage using color Doppler imaging predicts higher success of expectant management. The success of expectant management varies between 80 and 96% within two weeks in women with incomplete miscarriage and 59–62% in missed miscarriages and 52% in "anembryonic pregnancies".[5] It is generally accepted that evacuation of the retained products of conception should be offered after two weeks. Expectant management of miscarriage, using ultrasound parameters to determine eligibility, could significantly reduce the number of surgical evacuation procedures, unless accurate genetic testing is required. In the absence of a previous ultrasound scan documenting the presence of an intrauterine pregnancy, women with ultrasound features suggestive of a complete miscarriage should be managed as having a pregnancy of unknown location and have serum β hCG levels taken to check resolution of the pregnancy. This is needed so as not to miss a diagnosis of ectopic pregnancy.[3]

Threatened Miscarriage, Subchorionic Hematoma and Its Significance

Vaginal bleeding in very early pregnancy does not seem to be associated with any immediate or long-term consequences. Conversely, vaginal bleeding at 7–12 weeks, even in the presence of detectable fetal cardiac activity, is not only associated with a 5–10% miscarriage rate before 14 weeks of gestation but also with adverse pregnancy outcome.[5] The incidence of intrauterine hematoma in the first trimester in a general obstetric population is approximately 3.1%. The presence of a retroplacental hematoma (specially below the cord insertion) is significantly correlated with an increased risk for adverse pregnancy outcomes, such as miscarriage, pregnancy induced hypertension, placental abruption, preterm delivery, fetal growth restriction, fetal distress, meconium-stained amniotic fluid, operative delivery, neonatal intensive care unit admission, and also fetal demise/perinatal mortality.[7] The presence of a hematoma may be associated with a chronic inflammatory reaction in the decidua, resulting in persistent myometrial activity and expulsion of the pregnancy. The development of a hematoma may be the first sign of incomplete placentation and be associated with acute oxidative stress, which may impair subsequent placental and membrane development.

Predicting the Risk of Early Pregnancy Failure Based on Ultrasonographic Parameters

Gestational Sac

Once a gestational sac has been documented on ultrasound, subsequent loss of viability in the embryonic period remains around 11%. A smaller than expected gestational sac and a slower rate of growth (<1 mm/day), can predict poor pregnancy outcome, even in the presence of embryonic cardiac activity.[5] Small gestation sac size (before nine weeks) has been associated with chromosomal abnormalities, such as triploidy and trisomy 16.

Crown Rump Length

If an embryo has developed up to 5 mm in length, subsequent loss of viability occurs in 7.2% of cases. Loss rates drop to 3.3% for embryos of 6–10 mm and to 0.5% for embryos over 10 mm. A smaller than expected CRL has been associated with subsequent miscarriage, aneuploidy, fetal demise and poor pregnancy outcome including fetal growth restriction.[5,8,9]

Yolk Sac

The predictive value of SYS (secondary yolk sac) measurements in determining the outcome of an early pregnancy is limited. Most pregnancies which miscarry during the third month of pregnancy have normal SYS measurements at their initial scan before eight weeks of gestation. The yolk sac is found to persist inside the gestational sac after embryonic demise. Thus, variations in SYS size and sonographic appearance in most abnormal pregnancies are probably the consequence of poor embryonic development or embryonic death rather than being the primary cause of early pregnancy failure.[5]

Fetal Heart Activity

Fetal heart activity is the earliest proof of a viable pregnancy and it has been documented *in utero* by TVS as early as 36 days' menstrual age. From five to nine weeks of gestation there is a rapid increase in the mean heart rate from 110 to 175 beats per minute (bpm). The heart rate then gradually decreases to around 160–170 bpm. An abnormal developmental pattern of fetal heart rate (FHR) and/or bradycardia has been associated with subsequent miscarriage. In particular, a slow FHR at six to eight weeks appears to be associated with subsequent fetal demise. A single observation of an abnormally slow heart rate does not necessarily indicate subsequent embryonic death, but a continuous decline of embryonic heart activity is inevitably associated with miscarriage.[5]

Other Sonographic Markers

Abnormal shape of the gestational sac, increased echogenicity/thickness of the placenta, have all been proposed as sonographic markers associated with early spontaneous miscarriage.[5]

Aneuploidy Screening in 11–14 Weeks Scan

The most effective screening test for Down syndrome (and other aneuploidies) is the combined screening test performed between 11 and 14 weeks of gestation,[10] with the detection rates as high as 80–90%. This test involves the measurement of nuchal translucency and maternal serum estimation of free β hCG and pregnancy associated plasma protein-A (PAPP-A). Nuchal translucency has now evolved as the single most accurate ulrasonographic screening for Down syndrome. When the screening results are intermediate, there are other sonologic markers used to refine the risk of Down syndrome, for example nasal bone, ductus venosus Doppler, Tricuspid regurgitation, and so on. Wide application of this 11–14 week ultrasound for aneuploidy screening has improved our understanding of fetal anatomy and physiology.

Detection of Structural Abnormalities in the First Trimester Scan

In women with RPL, structural anomalies and aneuploidies are more common than in the general population. Many anomalies can be detected in the early scan, although not all are associated with RPL. Some anomalies are incompatible with intrauterine life. If fetal demise occurs in the first trimester, the patient will present with missed abortion. If demise occurs later, there may be mid-trimester fetal death. Other anomalies are compatible with intrauterine life, but not extrauterine life, presenting as stillbirth if there is no intervention prior to birth (e.g., anencephalus or renal agenesis). Others are compatible with life, but are associated with severe disability (e.g., open meningomyelocele). In such circumstances, the patient may elect to terminate the pregnancy. Therefore early detection should be the aim. The majority (80%) of common fetal malformations develop before 12 weeks of gestation. Advances in ultrasound technology and the improvement of high resolution transvaginal equipment

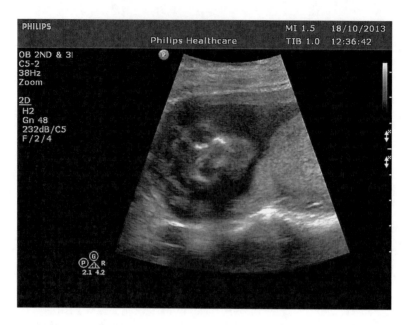

FIGURE 12.8   The "Mickey Mouse Sign" in an anencephalic fetus at 13th week of gestation.

have enabled detailed anatomical investigation of the fetus earlier than the classical mid-pregnancy scan.[11] However, the detection rate varies widely between studies, ranging from 26% to 70%.[11–15] There are several limitations to the detection of malformations in first trimester scanning. The resolution of ultrasound equipment is around 1 mm. consequently, the small size of fetal anatomical features is still a pivotal limiting factor before 12 weeks. Furthermore, many fetal anomalies develop at the end of organogenesis over a variable period of time and many anomalies may not be apparent before the end of the first trimester, such as agenesis of the corpus callosum. Some anomalies have sonographic features that are different from those usually seen during the routine mid-trimester anomaly scan (i.e., anencephalus). By contrast, normal fetal developmental features, such as midgut herniation, have the

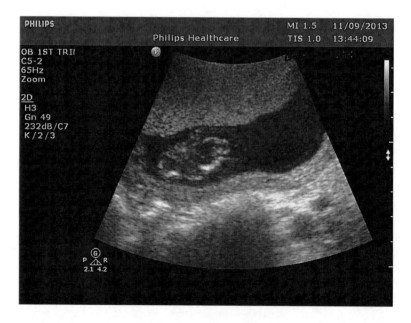

FIGURE 12.9   A hydropic fetus at nine weeks, also showing abnormal morphology for gestation.

same features as pathological exomphalos, hence confirmation of the exact gestational age is crucial for early diagnosis.

Some malformations will almost always be detected, such as anencephaly, and some will never be detected, such as microcephaly. There are also abnormalities that are potentially detectable depending on a number of factors: the objectives set for such a scan and consequently the time allocated for the fetal examination, the expertise of the sonographer and the quality of the equipment used; secondly, the presence of an easily detectable marker for an underlying abnormality; and thirdly, the evolution in the phenotypic expression of the abnormality with gestation.

It is outside of the scope of this chapter to summarize all the anomalies which can be diagnosed, and for a full review, the reader is directed elsewhere. However, multiple organ scanning is possible. First trimester scanning can detect defects of the cranium (e.g., anencephaly, Figure 12.8) and brain (e.g., holoprosencephaly[16]), spine,[17,18] face and palate, heart,[19,20] congenital diaphragmatic hernia, abdominal wall defects, bladder, kidneys, choledocal, hepatic and omental cysts, anorectal malformations, bowel atresia, skeletal dysplasias,[21] kyphoscoliosis, cystic hygroma, and fetal hydrops (Figure 12.9).

When an anomaly is discovered, it is often difficult for a patient to decide on which course of action to take. In the case of RPL, the problem is compounded, as the pregnancy with anomalies may be the first pregnancy to have survived until the early scan. It may also be the last pregnancy to survive.

Advances in Genetics

In the majority of cases with ultrasound abnormalities, the fetal karyotype is normal when banding techniques are used. However, advances in genetic testing have introduced high resolution testing which have enabled additional genetic anomalies to be diagnosed to explain the anomalous ultrasound findings. Array comparative genomic hybridization (CGH) can be applied to detect copy number variations (CNVs) down to a resolution as low as 1 Kb (see Chapter 3). By applying array CGH in prenatal diagnosis in conjunction with chromosomal analysis, approximately 3.6% additional clinically significant genomic imbalances can be detected when the karyotype is normal, regardless of the indication of the referral.[22–25] This detection rate increases to 5.2% when the pregnancy has a structural malformation on ultrasound. Array CGH is a useful tool for the detection of submicroscopic CNVs and for identifying candidate genes for euploid miscarriages.[26] Array CGH can be performed on the uncultured cells. Thus results are quicker, and it also overcomes the problem of culture failure, maternal contamination, and poor chromosome morphology associated with conventional karyotyping. The American College of Obstetrics and Gynecology and Society for Maternal and Fetal Medicine, in their recent committee opinion (Number 581, December 2013), have recommended array CGH as a preferred technique of prenatal diagnosis when there are fetal structural anomalies on the ultrasound. Specifically CGH is preferred in cases of fetal demise/stillbirth, as it is more likely to yield results with improved detection of causative abnormalities. However, committee opinion does not recommend CGH on first/second trimester pregnancy losses as of now, since limited data are currently available on the clinical utility in this setting.

Conclusion

This chapter summarizes the role of first trimester sonography in the diagnosis and prognosis of pregnancy. Visualization of normal fetal anatomy in the first trimester, along with a low risk of aneuploidy screening, affords patients reassurance and reduction in anxiety. Earlier detection of lethal or severe fetal structural abnormalities allows for earlier decision making for pregnancy termination or earlier referral to a tertiary center and coordination of care amongst the appropriate specialists.

REFERENCES

1. Callen PW. The obstetric ultrasound examination. In: Callen PW, ed. *Ultrasonography in Obstetrics and Gynecology*. Philadelphia: Saunders, Elsevier; 2008. p. 3–25.

2. Donnelly JC, Malone FD. Early fetal anatomical sonography. *Best Pract Res Clin Obstet Gynaecol* 2012;26:561–73.
3. Bourne T, Bottomley C. When is a pregnancy nonviable and what criteria should be used to define miscarriage? *Fertil Steril* 2012;98:1091–6.
4. Royal College of Obstetricians and Gynaecologists. The management of early pregnancy loss. Green-Top Guideline, No. 25, October 2006. Available at: Http://www.rcog.org.uk.
5. Jauniaux E, Johns J, Burton GJ. The role of ultrasound imaging in diagnosing and investigating early pregnancy failure. *Ultrasound Obstet Gynecol* 2005;25:613–24.
6. Luise C, Jermy K, May C et al. Outcome of expectant management of spontaneous first trimester miscarriage: Observational study. *BMJ* 2002;324:873–5.
7. Sándor N, Melissa B, Joanne S et al. Clinical significance of subchorionic and retroplacental hematomas detected in the first trimester of pregnancy. *Obstet Gynecol* 2003;102:94–100.
8. Pedersen NG, Sperling L, Wøjdemann KR et al. First trimester growth restriction and uterine artery blood flow in the second trimester as predictors of adverse pregnancy outcome. *Eur J Obstet Gynecol Reprod Biol* 2013;168:20–5.
9. Mukri F, Bourne T, Bottomley C et al. Evidence of early first-trimester growth restriction in pregnancies that subsequently end in miscarriage. *BJOG* 2008;115:1273–8.
10. Malone FD. First trimester screening for aneuploidy. In: Callen PW, ed. *Ultrasonography in Obstetrics and Gynecology.* Philadelphia: Saunders, Elsevier, 2008. p. 60–9.
11. Weisz B. Early detection of fetal structural abnormalities. *Reprod BioMed Online* 2005;10:541–53.
12. Novotná M, Hašlík L, Svabík K et al. Detection of fetal major structural anomalies at the 11–14 ultrasound scan in an unselected population. *Ceska Gynekol* 2012;77:330–5.
13. Pilalis A, Basagiannis C, Eleftheriades M et al. Evaluation of a two-step ultrasound examination protocol for the detection of major fetal structural defects. *J Matern Fetal Neonatal Med* 2012;25:1814–7.
14. Jakobsen TR, Søgaard K, Tabor A. Implications of a first trimester Down syndrome screening program on timing of malformation detection. *Acta Obstet Gynecol Scand* 2011;90:728–36.
15. Dane B, Dane C, Sivri D et al. Ultrasound screening for fetal major abnormalities at 11–14 weeks. *Acta Obstet Gynecol Scand* 2007;86:666–70.
16. Sepulveda W, Dezerega V, Be C. First-trimester sonographic diagnosis of holoprosencephaly: Value of the "butterfly" sign. *J Ultrasound Med* 2004;23:761–5.
17. Syngelaki A, Chelemen T, Dagklis T et al. Challenges in the diagnosis of fetal non-chromosomal abnormalities at 11–13 weeks. *Prenatal Diagn* 2011;31:90–102.
18. Peker N, Yeniel AO, Ergenoglu M et al. Combination of intracranial translucency and 3D sonography in the first trimester diagnosis of neural tube defects: Case report and review of literature. *Ginekol Pol* 2013;84:65–7.
19. Borrell A, Grande M, Bennasar M et al. First-trimester detection of major cardiac defects with the use of ductus venosus blood flow. *Ultrasound Obstet Gynecol* 2013;42:51–7.
20. Huggon IC, Ghi T, Cook AC et al. Fetal cardiac abnormalities identified prior to 14 weeks' gestation. *Ultrasound Obstet Gynecol* 2002;20:22–9.
21. Vimercati A, Panzarino M, Totaro I et al. Increased nuchal translucency and short femur length as possible early signs of osteogenesis imperfecta type III. *J Prenatal Med.* 2013;7:5–8.
22. Evangelidou P, Alexandrou A, Moutafi M et al. Implementation of high resolution whole genome array CGH in the prenatal clinical setting: Advantages, challenges, and review of the literature. *Biomed Res Int* 2013;2013:346762. doi: 10.1155/2013/346762. Epub March 4, 2013.
23. Fiorentino F, Caiazzo F, Napolitano S et al. Introducing array comparative genomic hybridization into routine prenatal diagnosis practice: A prospective study on over 1000 consecutive clinical cases. *Prenatal Diagn* 2011;31:1270–82.
24. Wapner RJ, Martin CL, Levy B et al. Chromosomal microarray versus karyotyping for prenatal diagnosis. *New Engl J Med* 2012;367:2175–84.
25. Hillman SC, Pretlove S, Coomarasamy A et al. Additional information from array comparative genomic hybridization technology over conventional karyotyping in prenatal diagnosis: A systematic review and meta-analysis. *Ultrasound Obstet Gynecol* 2011;37:6–14.
26. Viaggi CD, Cavani S, Malacarne M et al. First-trimester euploid miscarriages analysed by array-CGH. *J Appl Genet* 2013;54:353–9.

13

Endocrinology of Pregnancy Loss

N. Pluchino, P. Drakopoulos, J. M. Wenger, S. Luisi, M. Russo,
and A. R. Genazzani

Introduction

The maintenance of pregnancy is dependent on numerous endocrinological events that eventually lead to the successful growth and development of the fetus. Although the great majority of pregnant women have no preexisting endocrine abnormalities, a small number of women can have endocrine alterations that could potentially lead to recurrent pregnancy losses. It is estimated that approximately 8 to 12% of all pregnancy losses are the result of endocrine factors. Progesterone is essential for successful implantation and maintenance of pregnancy. Therefore, disorders related to inadequate progesterone secretion by the corpus luteum may affect the outcome of the pregnancy. Luteal phase deficiency, hyperprolactinemia, and polycystic ovarian syndrome are some examples of endocrine disorders affecting pregnancy. Several other endocrinological abnormalities such as thyroid disease, hypoparathyroidism, uncontrolled diabetes, and decreased ovarian reserve have been implicated as etiologic factors for recurrent pregnancy loss. Inhibins and activins are nonsteroidal glycoproteins thought to have important roles in reproductive physiology and are proposed as markers of fetal viability.

Luteal Phase Deficiency and Pregnancy Loss

Progesterone plays a paramount role in the maintenance of early pregnancy. It prepares the endometrium for blastocyst implantation and controls endometrial development. The preovulatory increase in the secretion of 17β-estradiol (E2) promotes the proliferation and differentiation of uterine epithelial cells. This is followed by the production of progesterone, which induces the proliferation and differentiation of stromal cells.[1] Progesterone acts on the endometrium via specific receptors, the expression of which is controlled by estrogens. By downregulating estrogen receptors, progesterone leads to a fall of both estrogen and progesterone receptors.[2] During the luteal phase of the menstrual cycle, the corpus luteum is the only source of progesterone. In early pregnancy the corpus luteum continues to produce progesterone until the luteal placental shift. Cyclic secretion of estrogens and progesterone triggers morphological and physiological changes of the endometrium and creates a suitable endometrial environment for embryo implantation during the implantation window (5–10 days after the luteinizing hormone (LH) surge) and subsequent maintenance of early pregnancy. These changes fail to develop if progesterone production is lower than normal. Luteal phase deficiency was originally thought to derive from inadequate production of progesterone by the corpus luteum and subsequent inadequate endometrial maturation to allow proper placentation. Luteal phase defect (LPD) may be due to poor follicular development, decreased progesterone production by the corpus luteum, and a dysfunctional endometrial response to normal progesterone levels. There are other causes for luteal phase deficiency, including stress, exercise, weight loss, hyperprolactinemia, and menstrual cycles at the onset of puberty or perimenopause.[3] Abnormalities of the luteal phase have been historically reported to occur in up to 35% of women with recurrent pregnancy losses (RPLs).[4] Today, the true role of LPD in RPL is controversial and endometrial biopsies are rarely indicated.

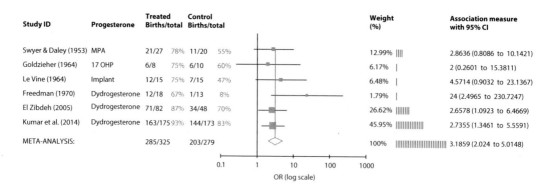

Study ID	Progesterone	Treated Births/total	Control Births/total		Weight (%)	Association measure with 95% CI
Swyer & Daley (1953)	MPA	21/27 78%	11/20 55%		12.99% ||||	2.8636 (0.8086 to 10.1421)
Goldzieher (1964)	17 OHP	6/8 75%	6/10 60%		6.17% |	2 (0.2601 to 15.3811)
Le Vine (1964)	Implant	12/15 75%	7/15 47%		6.48% |	4.5714 (0.9032 to 23.1367)
Freedman (1970)	Dydrogesterone	12/18 67%	1/13 8%		1.79% |	24 (2.4965 to 230.7247)
El Zibdeh (2005)	Dydrogesterone	71/82 87%	34/48 70%		26.62% ||||||||	2.6578 (1.0923 to 6.4669)
Kumar et al. (2014)	Dydrogesterone	163/175 93%	144/173 83%		45.95% |||||||||||||	2.7355 (1.3461 to 5.5591)
META-ANALYSIS:		285/325	203/279		100% ||||||||||||||||||||||	3.1859 (2.024 to 5.0148)

0.1   1   10   100   1000

OR (log scale)

FIGURE 13.1   Metaanalysis on progesterone support in recurrent miscarriage.

However, other mechanisms linked to physiopathology of the luteal phase could be associated with decreased progesterone production by the corpus luteum, decreased follicle stimulating hormone levels in the follicular phase and a decreased response to progesterone by the endometrium.[5,6] The methods used to diagnose luteal phase deficiency are not universally accepted. Serum progesterone levels greater than 10 ng/mL in the mid-luteal phase are rarely associated with an abnormal luteal phase when a targeted endometrial biopsy is performed.[7,8] The endometrium is considered to be out of phase when the histologic dating lags behind the menstrual dating by two days or more; as determined from the subsequent day of menses, the diagnosis requires endometrial biopsies in a minimum of two cycles. Endometrial biopsy, with evaluation of the morphological changes, was considered superior to serum progesterone determinations because of the pulsatile nature of progesterone secretion. Although serum progesterone levels below ≤12 ng/mL have been associated with increased risk of miscarriage,[9] serum progesterone levels can vary up to 10 times between blood drawn at a pulse peak or pulse nadir. More importantly, the morphological changes in the endometrium better represent the cumulative effect of cycle-specific patterns of corpus luteum function.[10] Despite the above-mentioned rationale, there is considerable interobserver and intraobserver variation in the interpretation of the endometrial biopsies. Hence endometrial biopsy is not often performed nowadays. Additionally, many women are unwilling to forego pregnancy for two cycles in order to undergo the biopsies.

The epidemiological studies of RPL appear to support the concept that luteal phase deficiency is in fact an etiologic factor. This is documented by studies demonstrating that hormone treatment to enhance progesterone production or supplementation is associated with an increased chance of a term pregnancy in women with RPL.[11] Figure 13.1 shows an updated meta-analysis of randomized and quasi randomized trials reported to date.

Progesterone supplementation after ovulation with or without the use of ovulation-induction agents can also be used two to three days after the basal body temperature increases (or after a positive urinary LH rest) and continued up to seven to 11 weeks of gestation.[12] Progesterone supplementation can be administered by intravaginal suppositories, intramuscular injection of progesterone in oil, as oral micronized progesterone, or as oral dydrogesterone. However, the subject of luteal phase deficiency and the association with RPL continues to be controversial. There have been no new trials. A Cochrane database systematic review by Oates-Whitehead[13] analyzed the same three papers used in Daya's[11] meta-analysis 10 years earlier. Recently a two center trial (PROMISE) is taking place. The results are eagerly awaited.

Hyperprolactinemia and Pregnancy Loss

Prolactin (PRL) is mainly synthesized and secreted by the lactotroph cells of the pituitary,[14] but also by other sites such as mammary gland, placenta, uterus, and T lymphocytes.[15] PRL, as well as placental lactogen (PL) and primate growth hormone (GH), binds the same PRL receptor (PRLR). Multiple isoforms of membrane-bound PRLR resulting from alternative splicing of the primary transcript have been identified in several species.[16] Many studies show that PRL play a role in reproductive function, being essential to female reproduction.[17] Past *in vitro* studies have shown that PRL plays a critical role in corpus luteum maintenance and progesterone production in rodents[18] and moreover, progesterone secretion by cultured granulosa cells obtained from human ovarian follicles is almost completely inhibited by high PRL concentrations (100 ng/mL) but not by lower concentrations (10 to 20 ng/mL).[19] These observations suggest the possibility that high PRL concentrations in the early phase of follicular growth may inhibit progesterone secretion, resulting in luteal phase defects. Instead, more recent researches on rodents have revealed that PRL receptors are involved not only in obtaining but also in maintaining pregnancy. PRLR−/− female mice showed an absence of pseudopregnancy and an arrest of egg development immediately after fertilization, with only a few reaching the stage of blastocysts.[20] The outcome is a complete sterility. Thus, whereas PRLR−/− females cannot implant blastocysts, the defect of the preimplantation egg development can be rescued by exogenous progesterone, indicating that one of the actions of PRL is to stimulate ovarian production of progesterone. However, although implantation occurs, full term pregnancy is not achieved,[21] most probably because of the absence of decidual PRLR. The precise cellular mechanism of PRL action in the human ovary remains to be elucidated; furthermore, a study of 64 hyperprolactinemic women with RPLs treated with bromocriptine was associated with a higher rate of successful pregnancy, and PRL levels were significantly higher in women that miscarried.[22]

In conclusion, normal PRL levels may play an important role in the growth and maintenance of early pregnancy but further studies are required clarify the role of PRL in the pathogenesis of recurrent miscarriages.

Thyroid Abnormalities and Pregnancy Loss

Hyperthyroidism

Hyperthyroidism occurs in approximately 0.1–0.4% of pregnancies.[23] It seems that excess production of thyroid hormone usually is not correlated with infertility or RPL. Women with subclinical or mild hyperthyroidism have evidence of ovulation when endometrial sampling is performed. Pregnant women with untreated overt hyperthyroidism are at increased risk for spontaneous miscarriage, congestive heart failure, thyroid storm, preterm birth, pre-eclampsia, fetal growth restriction, and increased perinatal morbidity and mortality.[24,25] Treatment of overt Graves' hyperthyroidism in pregnancy to achieve adequate metabolic control has been associated with improved pregnancy outcomes.[26] However, hyperthyroidism has not been reported commonly as an independent cause of RPL. Only a recent retrospective study has suggested that excess exogenous thyroid hormone is associated with an elevated rate of fetal loss.[27] A study by Nakayama et al.[28] study was performed in a unique population of patients with a genotype (Arg243-Gln mutation in the TH receptor β gene) showing resistance to thyroid hormone, and a high serum concentration of free thyroxine (FT_4) and tri-iodothyronine without suppressed thyrotropin. These women maintain a euthyroid state despite high thyroid hormone levels. Patients were analyzed in three different groups: affected mothers ($n = 9$), affected fathers ($n = 9$), and unaffected relatives ($n = 18$). The mean miscarriage rates were 22.9, 2.0, and 4.4%, respectively ($\chi^2 = 8.66$; $p = 0.01$). Affected mothers had an increased rate of miscarriage ($z = 3.10$; $p = 0.002$, by Wilcoxon rank-sum test).

Hypothyroidism

The most common cause of hypothyroidism in pregnant women, affecting approximately 0.5% of patients is chronic autoimmune thyroiditis (Hashimoto's thyroiditis).[29] Other causes of hypothyroidism include endemic iodine deficiency (ID), prior radioactive iodine therapy and thyroidectomy. There seems to be no doubt that hypothyroidism is associated with infertility. Untreated hypothyroidism in pregnancy has consistently been shown to be associated with an increased risk for adverse pregnancy complications, as well as detrimental effects on fetal neurocognitive development.[30] Specific adverse outcomes associated with maternal overt hypothyroidism include increased risks for premature birth, low birth weight, and miscarriage.[31]

Thyroid hormones have an impact on oocytes at the level of the granulosa and luteal cells that interfere with normal ovulation.[32] Low thyroxine levels have a positive feedback on thyroid-releasing hormone (TRH). Elevations in TRH have been associated with PRL elevation.[33] It is believed that elevated PRL alters the pulsatility of gonadotropin-releasing hormone (GnRH) and interferes with normal ovulation. Therefore, severe forms of hypothyroidism rarely complicate pregnancy because they are associated with anovulation and infertility. Even if an association exists between low thyroid function and pregnancy loss, direct evidence for a causal role is missing.[34] One postulated explanation for this relationship is that LPD has been linked to thyroid hypofunction. A study of thyroid function and pregnancy outcome in 2009 demonstrated a positive linear relationship between fetal loss and maternal thyroid-stimulating hormone (TSH) levels assayed in healthy women, without overt thyroid dysfunction.[35] Surprisingly, in this study any association was found between FT_4 levels and subsequent risk of child loss in these women.

We believe it is prudent to screen for thyroid disease and normalize thyroid function prior to conception when function is found to be abnormal. Even if there is no clear cause–effect relationship between hypothyroidism and RPL, there is some evidence that subclinical hypothyroidism is correlated with poor maternal outcome as well as prematurity and reduced intelligence quotient in the offspring.[36] There is disagreement as to the suitable upper limit of normal serum TSH in order to make the diagnosis of subclinical hypothyroidism. There is a trend with the new TSH assays to decrease the upper limit of normal TSH (range, 4.5 to 5.0 mU/L) to 2.5 mU/L. This upper limit is recommended by the National Academy of Clinical Biochemistry guideline, and based on the fact that 2.5 mU/L represents more than 2 standard deviations above meticulously screened euthyroid volunteers.[37] Clearly, this new upper limit will significantly increase the number of patients diagnosed with subclinical hypothyroidism, and its clinical benefit remains questionable.

Thyroid Autoimmunity and Pregnancy Loss

Autoimmune thyroid disease is the most common endocrine disorder in women of reproductive age with an overall prevalence in women of 10 to 15%[38] and among pregnant women, autoimmune thyroid disease has a prevalence of 5 to 20%.[39] In recent years many studies have found an association between thyroid autoimmunity (TA) and recurrent abortions; moreover it has been suggested that thyroid autoantibodies may be employed as a marker for at-risk pregnancies.[40,41] Many studies have linked TA with recurrent miscarriages, although the mechanism involved is unclear. Despite this, three mechanisms have been postulated to explain the possible association between TA and early pregnancy loss: (1) the presence of thyroid autoantibodies reflects a generalized activation of the immune system and a generally heightened autoimmune reactivity against the feto-placental unit;[42] (2) The presence of thyroid autoantibodies may act as an infertility factor and may delay conception. Thus, when women with thyroid autoantibodies do become pregnant, they are older and have a higher risk of miscarriage;[43,44] (3) The presence of thyroid autoantibodies in euthyroid women may be linked with a mild deficiency in thyroid hormone concentrations or a lower capacity of the thyroid gland to adapt to the demands of the pregnancy state. Indeed, the mean serum TSH values, while being within normal range, were significantly higher in thyroid autoantibody positive women compared to women with negative thyroid autoantibodies. This may reflect lower thyroidal reserve during pregnancy when a greater amount of thyroid hormones is demanded.[45] However, the various hypotheses mentioned above are not contradictory to each other, so it is possible that the mechanisms explained act in concert.

Thyroxine administration seems to be effective in reducing the number of miscarriages when given during the early stages of pregnancy, because miscarriages with maternal thyroid autoimmunity generally occur within the first trimester.[46] Poppe et al. have proposed that serum TSH, free FT_4 and thyroid autoantibodies should be measured in early gestation. When serum TSH is elevated or free FT_4 is below normal, levothyroxine (LT4) should be administered during pregnancy. In women with thyroid autoantibodies and serum TSH <2 mU/L, LT4 treatment is not warranted; however, serum TSH and free FT_4 should be measured later in gestation, preferably at the end of the second trimester. For women with thyroid autoantibodies and TSH between 2 and 4 mU/L in early gestation, treatment with LT4 should be considered. It is important to consider that serum TSH is downregulated during the first half of gestation by hCG.[47] However, further studies are required to understand if all women with positive thyroid autoantibodies should be started on LT4 therapy during their pregnancies to decrease miscarriage rate.

Diabetes Mellitus and Pregnancy Loss

Progestational diabetes including type 1, type 2 diabetes as well as other rare types of diabetes, complicates from 0.5% to 1% of all pregnancies.[48] Many studies showed that patients suffering from this clinical condition have significantly increased risk of spontaneous abortion, preterm labor, hypertensive disorders, and operative deliveries.[49–51] However, there are other known maternal risk factors that might increase this risk, like advanced maternal age, previous spontaneous abortion, alcohol consumption, cigarette smoking, excessive maternal weight, and maternal diseases other than diabetes, particularly hypothyroidism, which is observed in up to 30% of the patients with type 1 diabetes. Gutaj et al.,[52] in an observational, retrospective study, have analyzed some selected maternal parameters both in diabetic women in pregnancy with good perinatal outcome and in diabetic pregnant patients with a miscarriage. The results showed that women in the miscarriage group were older compared with those in the good outcome group and Hemoglobin A1c (HbA1c) was higher in the miscarriage group compared with the good outcome group. Moreover, it was found that maternal age and HbA1c were significant predictors of miscarriage. There was also a nonstatistically significant trend towards first trimester pregnancy loss in patients with hypertension, overweight/obesity, unplanned pregnancy, longer duration of diabetes, and diabetic vascular complications.[52] In conclusion, suboptimal metabolic control and increasing maternal age are the most significant risk factors for first trimester miscarriage in women with pregestational diabetes.

Polycystic Ovary Syndrome, Insulin Resistance, and Pregnancy Loss

It has been estimated that 40% of pregnancies in women with polycystic ovary syndrome (PCOS) will result in spontaneous loss.[53] PCOS is a complex disorder involving abnormalities in interactions between the pancreas, the hypothalamus/pituitary, the ovaries, the liver, and adipose tissues.[53] The underlying causes of RPL in PCOS patients may have several contributing and interrelated factors. These include obesity, hyperinsulinemia, hyperandrogenemia, insulin resistance (IR), poor endometrial receptivity, and elevated levels of LH.[54] It is thought that obesity acts on female reproductive function through hyperinsulinemia and consequently through its effect on androgen production. Some have argued that IR is a key factor to explain the association between obesity, PCOS and recurrent miscarriages.[55,56] Moreover, many studies have shown a possible association between IR and hyperhomocysteinemia.[57,58] Recent studies have highlighted the presence of hypofibronolysis associated with high levels of plasminogen activator inhibitor-1 (PAI-1) as a possible cause of RPL in women with PCOS.[59,60] The effects of elevated PAI-1 may also be increased by elevated homocysteine,[61] eventually leading to thrombosis. Moreover, plasma PAI-1 levels are associated with dyslipidemia, hyperinsulinemia and hypertension, which are three factors that contribute to the establishment of hyperhomocysteinemia.[62] Hence, PCOS involves several confounding factors that may contribute, individually or in combination, to thrombosis and eventually lead to RPL. The association of IR, hyperomocysteinemia and obesity in women with increased miscarriage rates is well-known. Chakraborty et al.[63] found that the incidence of hyperomocysteinemia and IR was significantly higher in RPL-affected PCOS patients when compared to the non-PCOS group. Moreover, the rates of abortion were significantly higher in hyperhomocysteinemic patients when compared to normohomocysteinemic women. Hyperinsulinemia and hyperandrogenemia are tightly associated, but the presence of an independent link between hyperandrogenemia and RPL remains contentious. Elevated androgens in the local microenvironment of the developing follicles impair follicular development and cause anovulation in PCOS patients. Elevated androgen levels and elevated insulin levels have detrimental effects on endometrial development. Elevated androgen levels decrease oocyte quality and embryo viability. Metformin enhances luteal phase uterine vascularity and blood flow and reduces the incidence of first trimester spontaneous abortions.[64,80] Metformin therapy throughout pregnancy in women with PCOS might reduce the otherwise high rate of first trimester spontaneous abortion,[65] but no properly designed placebo-controlled studies have been conducted.

Elevated Follicle-Stimulating Hormone and Pregnancy Loss

An increased level of basal follicle-stimulating hormone (FSH), a low level of antiMullerian hormone (AMH) and a low antral follicle count (AFC) have been shown to be linked to elevated miscarriage rates.[66] Also, a high incidence of decreased ovarian reserve has been observed among women with recurrent pregnancy loss.[67] The underlying challenge present in certain women with unexplained RPL may reside in the quality and quantity of their oocytes. In a retrospective comparative analysis, Trout and Seifer[68] measured FSH levels on day three of the cycle and estradiol (E2) in 36 patients with unexplained RPL and in 21 control RPL patients with a known etiology. These findings were reproduced subsequently in a similar analysis of 58 patients with RPL and unknown etiology.[67] Women with unexplained RPL were found to be more likely to have abnormal ovarian reserve. Among the 36 patients with unexplained RPL, 11 (31%) had elevated FSH, 14 (39%) had an elevated E2, and 21 (58%) had abnormal results for at least one or both tests. In the 20 patients of the control group, the findings were that one patient had elevated FSH (5%), three (14%) had an elevated E2, and four (19%) had abnormal results for at least one or both tests. In a different study, Hofman et al.[69] performed a clomiphene challenge test in 44 patients with RPL and found a similar incidence of diminished ovarian reserve when compared with 648 general infertility patients.

Women with abnormal ovarian reserve testing and unexplained RPL may have a higher incidence of embryonic chromosomal abnormalities. Thus, it may be prudent to incorporate ovarian reserve testing in the workup of patients with RPL. However, assessment of ovarian reserve is not a diagnostic test, but a screening tool. An abnormal test does not preclude the possibility of a live birth. Decreased ovarian reserve should not be presented to the patient as an absolute. Extensive counselling is recommended, given that no treatment, other than egg donation, is available.

Inhibins and Pregnancy Loss

Inhibins are nonsteroidal glycoproteins thought to have important roles in reproductive physiology. Inhibin A has a molecular weight of 34 kDa, and comprises an α-subunit linked by a disulfide bond to a highly homologous βA-subunit. Inhibin B is a similar dimeric glycoprotein with α and βB-subunits. Nonbioactive forms of the α-subunit include the amino-terminally extended product named inhibin pro-αC. Inhibin A is the major circulating bioactive inhibin found in early pregnancy. Inhibin B is not detectable in early pregnancy in the human.[70] Although their major function is in the negative feedback control of gonadotrophin secretion, the function in pregnancy may possibly be the promotion and modulation of placental secretory activity and placental immune modulation.

Circulating levels of inhibin A and pro-αC have been implicated in the process of implantation and early pregnancy development.[71] Inhibins have also been proposed as markers of fetal viability. In the nonpregnant female, inhibins are secreted and synthesized by both the developing Graafian follicle and corpus luteum.[72,73] Inhibins are also involved in the control of feto–maternal communication required to maintain pregnancy. Human placenta, decidua, and fetal membranes are the major sites of production and secretion of inhibin A and inhibin B in maternal serum, amniotic fluid, and cord blood.[74]

The corpus luteum has been shown to be the major site of inhibin A production. Production of inhibin A continues within the corpus luteum as pregnancy is established. During early pregnancy, mRNA for α, βA and βB have been demonstrated in the corpus luteum.[75] However, inhibins are also synthesized and secreted by the developing human placenta. Both α and βA-subunit mRNAs and proteins[76] have been localized in the human placenta, the major expression being from the syncytiotrophoblast.

The local actions during placental growth and differentiation are mirrored by changes in the circulating levels of dimeric inhibins and inhibin pro-αC as pregnancy progresses.[77] Circulatory concentrations of inhibin A increase progressively in early pregnancy.[78] There is a transient fall in the circulating concentration at approximately 12 weeks of gestation, followed by further increases in concentration from mid-gestation onwards.[71] Studies demonstrating lower levels of inhibin A in failing pregnancies have implicated inhibin A in the processes of successful implantation and early pregnancy development.[79]

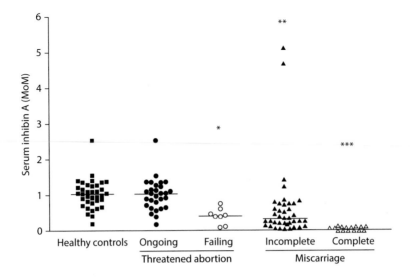

FIGURE 13.2 Maternal serum inhibin A levels in healthy pregnant women (control), patients with threatened abortion with ongoing and failing pregnancy, incomplete and complete miscarriage. Individual values are plotted (expressed as mean of mean) and horizontal bars represent the group medians. *p, 0.05, **p, 0.001, ***p, 0.001 versus healthy controls and threatened abortion with ongoing pregnancy.

Recently, inhibin A concentrations have been measured in the maternal circulation of healthy spontaneously pregnant women progressing to deliver a healthy term singleton baby, in patients with missed abortion [either fetal demise or anembryonic gestational sac] and with complete miscarriage,[74] in order to ascertain whether inhibin A measurement might provide a rapid and useful marker of early pregnancy viability, in comparison to hCG levels. Patients with complete miscarriage had the lowest hCG, and inhibin A levels, then missed abortion, and the highest levels were seen in ongoing pregnancies (Figure 13.2).

The potential value of inhibin A as a marker of early pregnancy complications should be examined in conjunction with other established biochemical markers such as serum β-hCG, progesterone, and glycodelin. Muttukrishna et al.[80] found a statistically significant correlation between serum concentrations of inhibin A and β-hCG (the degree of correlation varied according to the population group: normal controls $r = 0.55$, sporadic miscarriage $r = 0.79$, recurrent miscarriage $r = 0.66$). In the study, Muttukrishna et al.[80] confirm a statistically significant positive correlation between inhibin A and β-hCG in the women who had live births ($r = 0.46$, $p = 0.4$) but not in those that had a miscarriage. Given the small size of this and previous studies, it is not possible at this stage to establish whether serum inhibin A is a better marker than β-hCG, or whether combined inhibin A and β-hCG measurement is superior to β-hCG alone. Further studies are required to address these two questions.[81]

Endometriosis and Early Pregnancy Loss

Endometriosis is a clinical condition characterized by the presence of endometrium-like tissue outside of the uterine cavity. It is one of the most common causes of infertility and chronic pelvic pain affecting 1 in 10 women of reproductive age.[82] An association has also been reported between endometriosis and LPD and it is one of the putative determinants of infertility among endometriosis.[83,84] Furthermore, an increased prevalence of retarded endometrial development has been observed in women with endometriosis and infertility, compared with a fertile control population or a group of fertile women with tubal disease.[85] A high rate of pregnancy loss has also been reported,[86] which may involve LPD.

Loss of progesterone signaling in the endometrium may be a causal factor in the development of endometriosis, and progesterone resistance. Loss of progesterone signaling is often evident in women with this disease.[87–89] In endometriotic stromal cells, the number of progesterone receptors (PR), particularly the PR-B isoform, is significantly decreased, leading to a loss of paracrine signaling.[90,91] PR deficiency probably highlights the development of progesterone resistance in women with endometriosis who no longer respond to natural progesterone or progestin therapy.[92] Bulun et al. sought to clarify the molecular mechanisms leading to PR deficiency; in particular, it seems that changes in expression of estrogen receptor b (ERβ) and estrogen receptor a (ERα) may lead to PR loss and the progesterone resistance observed in endometriosis.[93]

However, further research is necessary in order to confirm that resistance to progesterone may be the mechanism involved in the development of recurrent miscarriage in women with endometriosis.

REFERENCES

1. Norwitz ER, Schust DJ, Fisher SJ. Implantation and the survival of early pregnancy. *N Engl J Med* 2001;345:1400–8.
2. Bergeron C. Morphological changes and protein secretion induced by progesterone in the endometrium during the luteal phase in preparation for nidation. *Hum Reprod* 2000;15:119–28.
3. Arredondo F, Noble LS. Endocrinology of recurrent pregnancy loss. *Semin Reprod Med* 2006;24:33–9.
4. Insler V. Corpus luteum defects. *Curr Opin Obstet Gynecol* 1992;4:203–11.
5. Tuckerman E, Laird SM, Stewart R et al. Markers of endometrial function in women with unexplained recurrent pregnancy loss. *Hum Reprod* 2004;19:196–205.
6. Jacobs MH, Balash J, Gonzalez-Merlo JM. Endometrial cytosolic and nuclear progesterone receptors in the luteal phase defect. *J Clin Endocrinol Metab* 1987;64:472–8.
7. Hensleigh PA, Fainstat T. Corpus luteum dysfunction: Serum progesterone levels in the diagnosis and assessment of therapy for recurrent and threatened abortion. *Fertil Steril* 1979;32:396–400.
8. Cumming DC, Honore LH, Scott JZ et al. The late luteal phase in infertile women: Comparison of simultaneous endometrial biopsy and progesterone levels. *Fertil Steril* 1985;43:715–9.
9. Arck PC, Rücke M, Rose M et al. Early risk factors for miscarriage: A prospective cohort study in pregnant women. *Reprod Biomed Online* 2008;17:101–13.
10. Coutifaris C, Myers ER, Guzick DS et al. Histological dating of rimed endometrial biopsy tissue is not related to fertility status. *Fertil Steril* 2004;82:1264–72.
11. Daya S. Efficacy of progesterone support for pregnancy in women with recurrent miscarriage: A meta-analysis of controlled trials. *Br J Obstet Gynaecol* 1989;96:275–80.
12. Karamardian LM, Grimes DA. Luteal phase deficiency effect of treatment on pregnancy rates. *Am J Obstet Gynecol* 1992;167:1391–8.
13. Oates-Whitehead RM, Haas DM, Carrier JA. Progestogen for preventing miscarriage. *Cochrane Database Syst Rev* 2003;4:CD003511.
14. Freeman ME, Kanyicska B, Lerant A et al. Prolactin: Structure, function, and regulation of secretion. *Physiol Rev* 2000;80:1523–631.
15. Ben-Jonathan N, Mershon JL, Allen DL et al. Extrapituitary prolactin: Distribution, regulation, functions, and clinical aspects. *Endocr Rev* 1996;17:639–69.
16. Bole-Feysot C, Goffin V, Edery M et al. Prolactin (PRL) and its receptor: Actions, signal transduction pathways and phenotypes observed in PRL receptor knockout mice. *Endocr Rev* 1998;19:225–68.
17. Horseman ND, Zhao W, Montecino-Rodriguez E et al. Defective mammopoiesis, but normal hematopoiesis, in mice with a targeted disruption of the prolactin gene. *EMBO J* 1997;16:6926–35.
18. Frasor J, Park K, Byers M et al. Differential roles for signal transducers and activators of transcription 5a and 5b in PRL stimulation of ER alpha and ER beta transcription. *Mol Endocrinol* 2001;15:2172–81.
19. McNatty KP, Sawers RS. Relationship between the endocrine environment within the graafian follicle and the subsequent secretion of progesterone by human granulosa cells in culture. *J Endocrinol* 1975;66:391–400.
20. Ormandy CJ, Camus A, Barra J et al. Null mutation of the prolactin receptor gene produces multiple reproductive defects in the mouse. *Genes Dev* 1997;11:167–78.
21. Binart N, Helloco C, Ormandy CJ et al. Rescue of preimplantatory egg development and embryo implantation in prolactin receptor-deficient mice after progesterone administration. *Endocrinology* 2000;14:2691–7.

22. Hirahara F, Andoh N, Sawai K et al. Hyperprolactinemic recurrent miscarriage and results of randomized bromocriptine treatment trials. *Fertil Steril* 1998;70:246–52.

23. Glinoer D. Thyroid hyperfunction during pregnancy. *Thyroid* 1998;8:859–64.

24. Millar LK, Wing DA, Leung AS et al. Low birth weight and preeclampsia in pregnancies complicated by hyperthyroidism. *Obstet Gynecol* 1994;84:946–9.

25. Kriplani A, Buckshee K, Bhargava VL et al. Maternal and perinatal outcome in thyrotoxicosis complicating pregnancy. *Eur J Obstet Gynecol Reprod Biol* 1994;54:159–63.

26. Momotani N, Noh J, Oyanagi H et al. Antithyroid drug therapy for Graves' disease during pregnancy. Optimal regimen for fetal thyroid status. *N Engl J Med* 1986;315:24–8.

27. Anselmo J, Cao D, Karrison T et al. Fetal loss associated with excess thyroid hormone exposure. *JAMA, J Am Med Assoc* 2004;292:691–5.

28. Nakayama T, Yamamoto T, Kanmatsuse K et al. Graves' disease associated with anticardiolipin antibody positivity and acquired protein S deficiency. *Rheumatol Int* 2003;23:198–200.

29. Allan WC, Haddow JE, Palomaki GE et al. Maternal thyroid deficiency and pregnancy complications: Implications for population screening. *J Med Screening* 2000;7:127–30.

30. Haddow JE, Palomaki GE, Allan WC et al. Maternal thyroid deficiency during pregnancy and subsequent neuropsychological development of the child. *N Engl J Med* 1999;341:549–55.

31. Abalovich M, Gutierrez S, Alcaraz G et al. Overt and subclinical hypothyroidism complicating pregnancy. *Thyroid* 2002;12:63–8.

32. Wakim AN, Polizotto SL, Buffo MJ et al. Thyroid hormones in human follicular fluid and thyroid hormone receptors in human granulosa cells. *Fertil Steril* 1993;59:1187–90.

33. Steinberger E, Nader S, Rodriguez-Rigau L et al. Prolactin response to thyrotropin-releasing hormone in normoprolactinemic patients with ovulatory dysfunction and its use for selection of candidates for bromocriptine therapy. *J Endocrinol Invest* 1990;13:637–42.

34. Clifford K, Rai R, Watson H et al. An informative protocol for the investigation of recurrent miscarriage: Preliminary experience of 500 consecutive cases. *Hum Reprod* 1994;9:1328–32.

35. Benhadi N, Wiersinga WM, Reitsma JB et al. Higher maternal TSH levels in pregnancy are associated with increased risk for miscarriage, fetal or neonatal death. *Eur J Endocrinol* 2009;160:985–91.

36. Casey BM, Dashe JS, Wells CE et al. Subclinical hypothyroidism and pregnancy outcomes. *Obstet Gynecol* 2005;105:239–45.

37. Baloch Z, Carayon P, Conte-Devolx et al. Guidelines Committee, National Academy of Clinical Biochemistry. Laboratory medicine practice guidelines. Laboratory support: For the diagnosis and monitoring of thyroid disease. *Thyroid* 2003;13:3–126.

38. Poppe K, Velkeniers B, Glinoer D. Thyroid disease and female reproduction. *Clin Endocrinol* 2007;66:309–21.

39. Glinoer D, Rovet J. Gestational hypothyroxinemia and the beneficial effects of early dietary iodine fortification. *Thyroid* 2009;19:431–4.

40. Singh A, Dantas ZN, Stone SC et al. Presence of thyroid antibodies in early reproductive failure: Biochemical versus clinical pregnancies. *Fertil Steril* 1995;63:277–81.

41. Marai I, Carp, HJA, Shai S et al. Autoantibody panel screening in recurrent miscarriages. *Am J Reprod Immunol* 2004;51:235–40.

42. Stagnaro-Green A, Roman SH, Cobin RH et al. Detection of at-risk pregnancy by means of highly sensitive assays for thyroid autoantibodies. *JAMA, J Am Med Assoc* 1990;264:1422–5.

43. Lejeune B, Grun JP, de Nayer P et al. Antithyroid antibodies underlying thyroid abnormalities and miscarriage or pregnancy induced hypertension. *Br J Obstet Gynaecol* 1993;100:669–72.

44. Menken J, Trussell J, Larsen U. Age and infertility. *Science* 1986;233:1389–94.

45. Lazarus JH, Kokandi A. Thyroid disease in relation to pregnancy: A decade of change. *Clin Endocrinol* 2000;53:265–78.

46. Negro R, Mangieri T, Coppola L et al. Levothyroxine treatment in thyroid peroxidase antibody-positive women undergoing assisted reproduction technologies: A prospective study. *Hum Reprod* 2005;20:1529–33.

47. Poppe K, Glinoer D, Tournaye H et al. Assisted reproduction and thyroid autoimmunity: An unfortunate combination? *J Clin Endocrinol Metab* 2003;88:4149–52.

48. Gabbe SG, Graves CR. Management of diabetes mellitus complicating pregnancy. *Obstet Gynecol* 2003;102:857–68.

49. Sibai BM. Risk factors, pregnancy complications, and prevention of hypertensive disorders in women with pregravid diabetes mellitus. *J Matern Fetal Med* 2000;9:62–5.

50. Melamed N, Hod M. Perinatal mortality in pregestational diabetes. *Int J Gynaecol Obstet* 2009; 104:S20–4.

51. Ramin N, Thieme R, Fischer S et al. Maternal diabetes impairs gastrulation and insulin and IGF-I receptor expression in rabbit blastocysts. *Endocrinology* 2010;151:4158–67.

52. Gutaj P, Zawiejska A, Wender-Ożegowska E et al. Maternal factors predictive of first–trimester pregnancy loss in women with pregestational diabetes. *Pol Arch Med Wewn* 2013;123:21–8.

53. Rai R, Backos M, Rushworth F et al. Polycystic ovaries and recurrent miscarriage—A reappraisal. *Hum Reprod* 2000;15:612–5.

54. Wang JX, Davies MJ, Norman RJ. Obesity increases the risk of spontaneous abortion during infertility treatment. *Obes Res* 2002;10:551–4.

55. Tian L, Shen H, Lu Q et al. Insulin resistance increases the risk of spontaneous abortion after assisted reproduction technology treatment. *Clin Endocrinol Metab* 2007;92:1430–3.

56. Maryam K, Bouzari Z, Basirat Z et al. The comparison of insulin resistance frequency in patients with recurrent early pregnancy loss to normal individuals. *BMC Res Notes* 2012;5:133.

57. Schachter M, Raziel A, Friedler S et al. Insulin resistance in patients with polycystic ovary syndrome is associated with elevated plasma homocysteine. *Hum Reprod* 2003;18:721–7.

58. Wijeyaratne CN, Nirantharakumar K, Balen AH et al. Plasma homocysteine in polycystic ovary syndrome: Does it correlate with insulin resistance and ethnicity? *Clin Endocrinol* 2004;60:560–7.

59. Sun L, Lv H, Wei W et al. Angiotensin-converting enzyme D/I and plasminogen activator inhibitor-1 4G/5G gene polymorphisms are associated with increased risk of spontaneous abortions in polycystic ovarian syndrome. *J Endocrinol Invest* 2010;33:77–82.

60. Gosman GG, Katcher HI, Legro RS. Obesity and the role of gut and adipose hormones in female reproduction. *Hum Reprod Update* 2006;12:585–601.

61. Atiomo WU, Bates SA, Condon JE et al. The plasminogen activator system in women with polycystic ovary syndrome. *Fertil Steril* 1998;69:236–41.

62. Bastard JP, Piéroni L, Hainque B. Relationship between plasma plasminogen activator inhibitor 1 and insulin resistance. *Diabetes Metab Res Rev* 2000;16:192–201.

63. Chakraborty P, Goswami SK, Rajani S et al. Recurrent pregnancy loss in polycystic ovary syndrome: Role of hyperhomocysteinemia and insulin resistance. *PLoS One* 2013;8:e64446.

64. Jakubowicz DJ, Iuorno MJ, Jakubowicz S et al. Effects of metformin on early pregnancy loss in the polycystic ovary syndrome. *Clin Endocrinol Metab* 2002;87:524–9.

65. Craig LB, Ke RW, Kutteh WH. Increased prevalence of insulin resistance in women with a history of recurrent pregnancy loss. *Fertil Steril* 2002;78:487–90.

66. Elter K, Kavak ZN, Gokaslan H et al. Antral follicle assessment after down-regulation may be a useful tool for predicting pregnancy loss in in vitro fertilization pregnancies. *Gynecol Endocrinol* 2005;21:33–7.

67. Gürbüz B, Yalti S, Ozden S et al. High basal estradiol level and FSH/LH ratio in unexplained recurrent pregnancy loss. *Arch Gynecol Obstet* 2004;270:37–9.

68. Trout SW, Seifer DB. Do women with unexplained recurrent pregnancy loss have higher day 3 serum FSH and estradiol values? *Fertil Steril* 2000;74:335–7.

69. Hofmann GE, Khoury J, Thie J. Recurrent pregnancy loss and diminished ovarian reserve. *Fertil Steril* 2000;74:1192–5.

70. Illingworth PJ, Groome NP, Duncan WC et al. Measurement of circulating inhibin forms during the establishment of pregnancy. *J Clin Endocrinol Metab* 1996;81:1471–5.

71. Muttukrishna S, George L, Fowler PA et al. Measurement of serum concentration of inhibin A (α-βA dimer) during human pregnancy. *Clin Endocrinol* 1995;42:391–7.

72. Groome NP, Illingworth PJ, O'Brien M et al. Detection of dimeric inhibin throughout the human menstrual cycle by two site enzyme immunoassay. *Clin Endocrinol* 1994;40:717–23.

73. Muttukrishna S, Fowler P, Groome NP et al. Serum concentrations of dimeric inhibin during the spontaneous human menstrual cycle and after treatment with exogenous gonadotrophin. *Hum Reprod* 1994;9:1634–42.

74. Luisi S, Florio P, Reis F et al. Inhibins in female and male reproductive physiology: Role in gametogenesis, conception, implantation and early pregnancy. *Hum Reprod Update* 2005;11:123–35.

75. Roberts VJ, Barth S, el-Roeiy A et al. Expression of inhibin/activin subunits and follistatin messenger ribonucleic acids and proteins in ovarian follicles and corpus luteum during the human menstrual cycle. *J Clin Endocrinol Metab* 1993;77:1402–10.

76. Petraglia F, Garuti C, Calza L et al. Inhibin subunits in human placenta: Localisation and messenger ribonucleic acids during pregnancy. *Am J Obstet Gynecol* 1991;165:750–8.

77. Ledger W. Measurement of Inhibin A and Activin A in pregnancy—Possible diagnostic applications. *Mol Cell Endocrinol* 2001;180:117–21.

78. Lahiri S, Anobile CJ, Stewart P et al. Changes in circulating concentrations of inhibins A and pro-α C during first trimester medical termination of pregnancy. *Hum Reprod* 2003;18:744–8.

79. Florio P, Lombardo M et al. Activin A, corticotrophin-releasing factor and prostaglandin F2 alpha increase immunoreactive oxytocin release from cultured human placental cells. *Placenta* 1995;17:307–11.

80. Muttukrishna S, Jauniaux E, Greenwold N et al. Circulating levels of inhibin A, activin A and follistatin in missed and recurrent miscarriages. *Hum Reprod* 2002;17:3072–8.

81. Prakash A, Laird S, Tuckerman S et al. Inhibin A and Activin A may be used to predict pregnancy outcome in women with recurrent miscarriage. *Fertil Steril* 2005;83:1758–63.

82. Giudice LC, Kao LC. Endometriosis. *Lancet* 2004;364:1789–99.

83. Moeloek FA, Moegny E. Endometriosis and luteal phase defect. *Asia–Oceania J Obstet Gynaecol* 1993;19:171–6.

84. Saracoglu OF, Aksel S, Yeoman RR et al. Endometrial estradiol and progesterone receptors in patients with luteal phase defects and endometriosis. *Fertil Steril* 1985;43:851–5.

85. Li TC, Warren MA, Dockery P et al. Human endometrial morphology around the time of implantation in natural and artificial cycles. *J Reprod Fertil* 1991;92:543–54.

86. Metzger DA, Olive DL, Stohs GF et al. Association of endometriosis and spontaneous abortion: Effect of control group selection. *Fertil Steril* 1986;45:18–22.

87. Kao LC, Germeyer A, Tulac S et al. Expression profiling of endometrium from women with endometriosis reveals candidate genes for disease-based implantation failure and infertility. *Endocrinology* 2003;144:2870–81.

88. Osteen KG, Bruner-Tran KL, Keller NR et al. Progesterone-mediated endometrial maturation limits matrix metalloproteinase (MMP) expression in an inflammatory-like environment: A regulatory system altered in endometriosis. *Ann N Y Acad Sci* 2002;955:37–47.

89. Zeitoun KM, Takayama K, Sasano H et al. Deficient 17beta-hydroxysteroid dehydrogenase type 2 expression in endometriosis: Failure to metabolize 17beta-estradiol. *J Clin Endocrinol Metab* 1998;83:4474–80.

90. Bulun SE, Cheng YH, Yin P et al. Progesterone resistance in endometriosis: Link to failure to metabolize estradiol. *Mol Cell Endocrinol* 2006;248:94–103.

91. Attia GR, Zeitoun K, Edwards D et al. Progesterone receptor isoform A but not B is expressed in endometriosis. *J Clin Endocrinol Metab* 2000;85:2897–902.

92. Vercellini P, Cortesi I, Crosignani PG. Progestins for symptomatic endometriosis: A critical analysis of the evidence. *Fertil Steril* 1997;68:393–401.

93. Bulun SE, Cheng YH, Pavone ME et al. Estrogen receptor-beta, estrogen receptor-alpha, and progesterone resistance in endometriosis. *Semin Reprod Med* 2010;28:36–43.

14

Debate: Should Progesterone Supplements Be Used? Yes

Jerome H. Check

In the first edition of *Recurrent Pregnancy Loss—Causes, Controversies and Treatment*, the "Role of Using Progesterone Supplementation" was presented as a debate: For—Jerome H. Check, Against—Shazia, Malik, and Lesley Regan.[1–3] There is no debate that completion of a pregnancy is not possible without progesterone (P). Surgical removal of the ovary with the corpus luteum of pregnancy prior to 8 weeks will lead to spontaneous miscarriage.[4] It is clear that a miscarriage will frequently ensue if the effect of progesterone is blocked by treating the woman with 600 mg of the progesterone receptor antagonist mifepristone at 600 mg for one day.[5]

Low levels of P during the first trimester have been found to be associated with a higher risk of miscarriage. Yeko et al. found that 17 of 18 women had a miscarriage with a serum P <15 pg/mL during the first trimester.[6] McCord et al. evaluated P levels in 3674 first trimester pregnancies and found a miscarriage rate of 85.5% with serum P <5 pg/mL, 65.8% with serum P 5 to <10 pg/mL, 31.3% with serum P 10 to 15 pg/mL, 9.8% with serum P levels 15 to <20 pg/mL and 7.7% with serum P 20 to <25 pg/mL.[7] The McCord et al. study did not show the extremely high miscarriage rate reported by Yeko et al. and had much more power but the principle was the same—low levels of P are associated with an increased miscarriage rate.

The association of increased chance of miscarriage with low serum P does not prove that the low P caused the miscarriage. Possibly the low serum P merely reflects a deteriorating placenta. One uncontrolled study aggressively treated women with serum P levels less than 15 pg/mL with P supplementation and produced a 70% live delivery rate.[8] Even women with serum P levels ≤8 pg/mL had a 60% viable rate following aggressive P therapy at the time of detection.[9] These salvage rates compare quite favorably to the high loss rate found by Yeko et al. in women with low serum P levels and even to the study by McCord et al. that did find an association of low serum P and miscarriage but not as high as found by Yeko et al.[6,7]

Evidence that placental deterioration may be the cause of the miscarriage in at least some women was provided by a study comparing serum estradiol (E2) in P supplemented women in those who miscarried versus those who were successful.[10] The serum E2 levels were significantly lower in those who miscarried versus those who were successful despite no difference in the serum P levels.[10] With the assumption that the majority of losses were from chromosomal defects, this study could be interpreted as supporting placental deterioration as a nonremedial cause of depletion of critical hormones during pregnancy. Progesterone supplementation would not be expected to prevent miscarriage if the cause is a failing fetal-placental unit.[10] On the other hand, one could argue that since the corpus luteum makes both P and E2, perhaps supplementing only P in some instances may be insufficient and thus these data could still be consistent with a failing corpus luteum not placental deterioration.[10]

Evidence that P Supplementation Decreases Miscarriage Rates in Women with Threatened Abortion

Women with low serum P frequently have bleeding and/or cramps which improve following P therapy. However, many women with threatened miscarriage deliver a live baby without P therapy. A Cochrane

Collaboration review entitled "Progestogen for treating threatened miscarriage" was published in 2011.[11] In this review the selection criteria included randomized or quasirandomized controlled trials that compared progestogen with placebo, no treatment, or other treatment given in an effort to treat threatened abortion.[11] Four studies met the inclusion criteria and provided the 421 participants for the meta-analysis.[12–15] There was evidence of a reduction in the rate of spontaneous miscarriage with the use of progestogens compared to placebo or no treatment (risk rate 0.53, 95% confidence interval 0.35 to 0.79). For two trials oral dydrogesterone 10 mg twice daily was given; one study only used 25 mg twice daily progesterone vaginal suppositories.[12–15] This Cochrane review also corroborated previous data suggesting no fetal risks by exposure to extra progesterone.[11,16] It is interesting that the benefit was greater for dydrogesterone than for micronized progesterone.

Thus these data suggest that progestogens can reduce the miscarriage rate when there is a threatened abortion. This, however, does not necessarily allow the conclusion that the use of progesterone can prevent miscarriage in women with a tendency for recurrent losses. The possibility exists that, fortuitously in some pregnancies, the corpus luteum of pregnancy may fail before the placenta is making adequate P. However, this may not occur on a repeated basis.

Luteal Phase Deficiency—Diagnosis

One way that recurrent miscarriage could be related to a progesterone insufficiency and be improved by progestogen therapy would be if there existed a recurrent problem of insufficient progesterone effect by the corpus luteum, that is, a luteal phase defect (LPD). An LPD could theoretically cause infertility or recurrent miscarriage. The concept is that if implantation does not occur in an endometrium that has been properly developed, the embryo may not implant at all or eventually result in a miscarriage.

It appears that only a small amount of P is needed to cause an adequate endometrial structure to allow implantation of the conceptus, at least as determined by endometrial biopsy and molecular markers.[17–25] No reliable marker has been identified that could detect a lack of progesterone leading to infertility.[19–25] It was suggested that merely a serum level of 5 pg/mL was needed not only to develop a normal secretory endometrium with normal classical histological changes but also to allow normal endometrial integrins and quantitative reverse transcription–polymerase chain reaction analysis for nine putative biochemical endometrial function markers.[25]

Presently being explored, but so far without any definitive conclusions in humans, is the relationship of the progesterone receptor initiating paracrine signaling within the uterine microenvironment during the preimplantation period.[26–29]

There is now a method for detection of the expression of a cluster of endometrial biomarker genes to assess endometrial receptivity.[30–33] One study failed to identify histological or biomarker abnormalities in women with suspected luteal phase defects but did find altered gene expression.[34]

Is Luteal Phase Deficiency Associated with Infertility or Recurrent Miscarriage?

A recent Practice Committee of the American Society of Reproductive Medicine published their opinion of the clinical relevance of LPD.[35] The committee was composed of 19 experts in the field of reproductive endocrinology. They stated that "No diagnostic test for luteal phase insufficiency has been proven in a clinical setting." They mention that "no treatment for luteal phase insufficiency has been shown to improve outcomes in natural unstimulated cycles."

The practice committee did not acknowledge a key publication that clearly demonstrated that the use of progesterone in the luteal phase could clearly improve pregnancy rates.[36] The study was a randomized drug comparison study comparing follicle maturing drugs in the follicular phase versus progesterone in the luteal phase in infertile women having an out-of-phase endometrial biopsy in the late luteal phase.[36] The first group compared were those who seemed to achieve a mature follicle (18 mm average diameter with serum E2 >200 pg/mL). For the 31 randomly assigned to P only, there were 24 pregnancies (77%) and only one of 24 (4.1%) miscarried compared to only three of 27 conceiving with clomiphene citrate or human menopausal gonadotropins (hMG) (11.1%) and two of three miscarried.[36] However, during the next six months 16 of 25 women conceived (64%) with P only who had failed with follicle maturing drugs with only one miscarriage (6.2%).[36]

Clinical experience suggests that women treated empirically with follicle maturing drugs achieve a six month pregnancy rate much higher than 11%. Indeed the 58 women with mature follicles were part of a prospective study of 100 consecutive infertile women with regular menses, patent fallopian tubes, and male partners with normal semen parameters. The other 42 women were randomly assigned to exclusive use of follicle maturing drugs (FMD) only or FMD with P luteal phase support versus P supplementation only.[36] For this group exclusive FMD resulted in a 70% clinical pregnancy rate (seven of 10) but with four miscarriages. In contrast for the 70% pregnancy rate with FMD and P (14 of 20) there was only one miscarriage. Progesterone alone resulted in a clinical pregnancy rate of only 25% (three of 12) with no miscarriages.[36] If one empirically placed all these women on follicle maturing drugs irrespective of follicular maturation 43.8% would have conceived with FMD versus 60.4% who would be treated exclusively with P.

The ASRM Practice Committee did not mention any study that refuted the benefits of treating infertility with P. If P deficiency can lead to an embryo that fails to implant causing infertility, it is not hard to envision that a slightly less severe problem could allow implantation but first trimester miscarriage. There actually has been a prospectively randomized placebo-controlled parallel group trial that did in fact find that P supplementation significantly reduced miscarriage rates in women with recurrent miscarriages.[37]

The Role of P in Reducing Immune Rejection of the Fetus

Progesterone enhances the expression by gamma/delta T cells of a unique 34 kDa protein known as the progesterone induced blocking factor (PIBF).[38] The PIBF protein has been found to allow the TH1/TH2 cytokine balance in favor of TH2 cytokines, which provides a more favorable immune environment for the fetus.[39] PIBF has been found to stabilize perforin granules in natural killer (NK) cells and thus inhibit release of perforin from these large storage granules which inhibits the main mechanism for NK cell cytotoxicity.[40]

Initially, both *in vitro* and *in vivo* studies suggested that the allogeneic stimulus of the fetal placental unit may be responsible for a hormone independent upregulation of P receptors by gamma/delta T cells.[41,42] Szekeres-Bartho et al. found significantly lower expression of PIBF in recurrent miscarriage patients compared with those with a healthy pregnancy.[43] Check et al. treated women in the first trimester aggressively with progesterone but found no difference in PIBF expression by lymphocytes.[44] This suggested that the main stimulus for PIBF may be P itself and perhaps whether some causes of miscarriage may be related to inadequate development of P receptors on gamma/delta T cells.[41,42,44,45] Indeed, it has been confirmed following the development of a more sensitive enzyme linked immunosorbent assay (ELISA) rather than the previously used less sensitive immunocytochemistry technique following the development of a monoclonal antibody, that P alone (even in males) is the main stimulus for PIBF expression once there has been adequate estrogen exposure to induce P receptors in the gamma/delta T cells, since there is a very high level of PIBF induced without exposure to a fetus.[46–48]

Progesterone may help to inhibit immune rejection of the fetus through other mechanisms than induction of PIBF and suppression of NK cell cytolysis. Progesterone can act rapidly by epigenetic (nongenomic) interaction with membrane receptors, for example, progesterone receptor membrane 1.[49] One study suggested that P interacting with P receptor 1 membrane may suppress, in an epigenetic manner, T cell rejection of the fetal semiallograft.[50]

Conclusions

One could debate whether there are "sufficient" evidence-based studies to warrant the treatment of women with recurrent miscarriage with progesterone, beginning in the luteal phase and continued throughout the first trimester. Since the good safety record of P has been well established, it makes no sense to withhold such therapy, advising the patient that the present opinion of the treating physician is that there is still an insufficient number of studies to convince that treating physician that the treatment is any better than careful vigilance and benign neglect.

Though the ASRM Practice Committee concluded that there is no evidence of LPD as a cause of miscarriage in lieu of documenting any structural endometrial defects, they failed to consider the effects of P on the immune system.[35] More support that LPD is a cause of infertility (and thus a logical cause of miscarriage with a slightly milder state of P deficiency) was a recent study using P therapy empirically in a group of women age ≤39.9 with over one year of unexplained infertility who were suspected of having LPD related to age (>30) or pelvic pain (suspicious of endometriosis with P resistance).[51,52] In six months 27 of 32 women (84.3%) had a serum beta-hCG (human chorionic gonadotropin) level >100 mIU/mL with luteal phase P as the sole treatment with a low rate of miscarriage.[51] In view of the aforementioned randomized comparison study finding better results with P than follicle maturing drugs when the follicle is mature but vice versa when there is release of the oocyte from an immature follicle, treatment of recurrent miscarriage from suspected LPD should include the use of mild follicular stimulation if there are inadequate mid-cycle estradiol levels attained or inadequate time of exposure to E2 during the follicular phase.[36,53] Estradiol is known to induce P receptors in the endometrium.[54,55] Studies of PIBF in males treated with P or E2 and P suggest that E2 induces P receptors in gamma/delta T cells also.[48]

The treating physician has the obligatory role of suggesting the most effective treatment paradigm with the least risk and least expense. How many erudite members of the ASRM Practice Committee on LPD would have suggested an alternative in lieu of empirical P usage for "unexplained" infertility. They may have suggested *in vitro* fertilization–embryo transfer (IVF-ET), which could be considered an extremely expensive, risky method of providing these women with P therapy from the early luteal phase, or recommended an even more expensive method of treating recurrent miscarriage—IVF-ET with comprehensive chromosome screening for recurrent miscarriage. The latter could be by far the most expensive way to administer P.

Present studies evaluating serum PIBF, now that a sensitive ELISA test has been created, will hopefully determine a discriminatory level below which there is an increased risk of nonconception or miscarriage. There is one caveat however. There is evidence that an intracytoplasmic occupation of PIBF may protect cancer cells from NK cell immune destruction.[56,57] The 90 kDa parent compound of PIBF is found in the cytoplasm of all highly proliferating cells.[58] It is possible that P is needed more for inhibiting the conversion of the intracytoplasmic 90 kDa PIBF form to intracytoplasmic split variants of 34–36 kDa products.[56,58] That, of course, would not allow easy detection of modification of P therapy during a pregnancy if that was the main operative mechanism.

REFERENCES

1. Carp HJA *Recurrent Pregnancy Loss: Causes, Controversies and Treatment*. Tel Aviv: Informa Healthcare; 2007.
2. Check JH. Debate: Should progesterone supplementation be used?—For. In: Carp HJA, ed. *Recurrent Pregnancy Loss: Causes, Controversies and Treatment*. London, UK: Informa Healthcare; 2007. ch. 6a. p. 89–92.
3. Malik S, Regan L. Debate: Should progesterone supplementation be used?—Against. In: Carp HJA, ed. *Recurrent Pregnancy Loss: Causes, Controversies and Treatment*. London, UK: Informa Healthcare; 2007. Ch. 6b. p. 93–6.
4. Csapo AI, Pulkkinen M. Indispensability of the human corpus luteum in the maintenance of early pregnancy: Lutectomy evidence. *Obstet Gynecol Surv* 1978;3:69–81.

5. Baulieu EE. Contragestion and other clinical applications of RU-486, an antiprogesterone at the receptor. *Science* 1989;245:1351–7.
6. Yeko TR, Gorrill MJ, Hughes LH, Rodi LA, Buster JE, Sauer MV. Timely diagnosis of early ectopic pregnancy using a single blood progesterone measurement. *Fertil Steril* 1987;48:1048–50.
7. McCord ML, Muram D, Buster JE et al. Single serum progesterone as a screen for ectopic pregnancy: Exchanging specificity and sensitivity to obtain optimal test performance. *Fertil Steril* 1996;66:513–6.
8. Check JH, Winkel CA, Check ML. Abortion rate in progesterone treated women presenting initially with low first trimester serum progesterone levels. *Am J Gynecol Health* 1990;IV(2):63/33–34/64.
9. Choe JK, Check JH, Nowroozi K et al. Serum progesterone and 17–hydroxyprogesterone in the diagnosis of ectopic pregnancies and the value of progesterone replacement in intrauterine pregnancies when serum progesterone levels are low. *Gynecol Obstet Invest* 1992;34:133–8.
10. Check JH, Lurie D, Davies E et al. Comparison of first trimester serum estradiol levels in aborters versus nonaborters during maintenance of normal progesterone levels. *Gynecol Obstet Invest* 1992;34:206–10.
11. Wahabi HA, Fayed AA, Esmaeil SA et al. Progestogen for treating threatened miscarriage. *Cochrane Database* 2011;CD005943.pub4.
12. El-Zibdeh MY, Yousef LT. Dydrogesterone support in threatened miscarriage. *Maturitas* 2009;65 Suppl 1:S43–6.
13. Gerhard I, Gwinner B, Eggert-Kruse W et al. Double-blind controlled trial of progesterone substitution in threatened abortion. *Biol Res Pregnancy Perinatol* 1987;8:26–34.
14. Palagiano A, Bulletti C, Pace MC et al. Effects of vaginal progesterone on pain and uterine contractility in patients with threatened abortion before twelve weeks of pregnancy. *Ann NY Acad Sci* 2004;1034:200–10.
15. Pandian RU. Dydrogesterone in threatened miscarriage: A Malaysian experience. *Maturitas* 2009;65 Suppl 1:S47–50.
16. Check JH, Rankin A, Teichman M. The risk of fetal anomalies as a result of progesterone therapy during pregnancy. *Fertil Steril* 1986;45:575–7.
17. Noyes RW, Hertig AI, Rock J. Dating the endometrial biopsy. *Fertil Steril* 1950;1:3–35.
18. Yashinaga K. Uterine receptivity for blastocyst implantation. *Ann N Y Acad Sci* 1988;541:424–31.
19. De Souza MM, Surveyor GA, Price RE et al. MUC1/episialin: A critical barrier in the female reproductive tract. *J Reprod Immunol* 1999;45:127–58.
20. Surveryor GA, Gendler SJ, Pemberton L et al. Expression and steroid hormonal control of Muc-1 in the mouse uterus. *Endocrinology* 1995;136:3639–47.
21. Creus M, Balasch J, Ordi J et al. Integrin expression in normal and out-of-phase endometria. *Hum Reprod* 1998;13:3460–8.
22. Margarit L, Gonzalez D, Lewis PD et al. L-selectin ligands in human endometrium: Comparison of fertile and infertile subjects. *Hum Reprod.* 2009;24:2767–77.
23. Wang B, Sheng JZ, He RH et al. High expression of L-selectin ligand in secretory endometrium is associated with better endometrial receptivity and facilitates embryo implantation in human being. *Am J Reprod Immunol* 2008;60:127–34.
24. Fukuda MN, Sato T, Nakayama J et al. Trophinin and tastin, a novel cell adhesion molecule complex with potential involvement in embryo implantation. *Genes Dev* 1995;9:1199–210.
25. Usadi RS, Groll JM, Lessey BA et al. Endometrial development and function in experimentally induced luteal phase deficiency. *J Clin Endocrinol Metab* 2008;93:4058–64.
26. Wetendorf M, DeMayo FJ. The progesterone receptor regulates implantation, decidualization, and glandular development via a complex paracrine signaling network. *Mol Cell Endocrinol* 2012;357:108–18.
27. Dominguez F, Garrido-Gomez T, Lopez JA et al. Proteomic analysis of the human receptive versus non-receptive endometrium using differential in-gel electrophoresis and MALDI-MS unveils stathmin 1 and annexin A2 as differentially regulated. *Hum Reprod* 2009;24:2607–17.
28. Parmar T, Gadkar-Sable S, Savardekar I et al. Protein profiling of human endometrial tissues in the midsecretory and proliferative phases of the menstrual cycle. *Fertil Steril* 2009;92:1091–3.

29. DeSouza L, Diehl G, Yang EC et al. Proteomic analysis of the proliferative and secretory phases of the human endometrium: Protein identification and differential protein expression. *Proteomics* 2005;5:270–81.

30. Garrido-Gomez T, Ruiz-Alonso M, Blesa D et al. Profiling the gene signature of endometrial receptivity: Clinical results. *Fertil Steril* 2013;99:1078–85.

31. Diaz-Gimeno P, Horcajadas JA, Martinez-Conejero JA et al. A genomic diagnostic tool for human endometrial receptivity based on the transcriptomic signature. *Fertil Steril* 2011;95:50–60.

32. Diaz-Gimeno P, Ruiz-Alanso M, Blesa D et al. The accuracy and reproducibility of the endometrial receptivity array is superior to histology as a diagnostic method for endometrial receptivity. *Fertil Steril* 2013;99:508–17.

33. Evans GE, Martinez-Conejero JA, Phillipson GTM et al. Gene and protein expression signature of endometrial glandular and stromal compartments during the window of implantation. *Fertil Steril* 2012;97:1365–73.

34. Young SL, Lessey BA, Balthazar U et al. Defining the relationship between progesterone dose, endometrial histology and gene expression using an *in vivo* luteal phase defect model. *Reprod Sci.* 2011;8:273A.

35. The Practice Committee of the American Society for Reproductive Medicine: The clinical relevance of luteal phase deficiency: A committee opinion. *Fertil Steril* 2012;98:1112–7.

36. Check JH, Nowroozi K, Wu CH et al. Ovulation–inducing drugs versus progesterone therapy for infertility in patients with luteal phase defects. *Int J Fertil* 1988;33(4):252–6.

37. El-Zibdeh MY. Dydrogesterone in the reduction of recurrent spontaneous abortion. *J Steroid Biochem Mol Biol.* 2005;97(5):431–4.

38. Szekeres-Bartho J, Kilar F, Falkay G et al. Progesterone-treated lymphocytes of healthy pregnant women release a factor inhibiting cytotoxicity and prostaglandin synthesis. *Am J Reprod Immunol Microbiol* 1985;9:15–8.

39. Szekeres-Bartho J, Wegmann TG. A progesterone-dependent immuno-modulatory protein alters the Th1/Th2 balance. *J Reprod Immunol* 1996;31:81–95.

40. Faust Z, Laskarin G, Rukavina D et al. Progesterone induced blocking factor inhibits degranulation of NK cells. *Am J Reprod Immunol* 1999;42:71–5.

41. Szekeres-Bartho J, Hadnagy J, Pacsa AS. The suppressive effect of progesterone on lymphocyte cytotoxicity: Unique progesterone sensitivity of pregnancy lymphocytes. *J Reprod Immunol* 1985;7:121–8.

42. Szekeres-Bartho J, Weill BJ, Mike G et al. Progesterone receptors in lymphocytes of liver-transplanted and transfused patients. *Immunol Lett* 1989;22:259–61.

43. Szekeres-Bartho J, Barakonyi A, Miko E et al. The role of γ/δ T cells in the feto-maternal relationship. *Semin Immunol* 2001;13:229–33.

44. Check JH, Ostrzenski A, Klimek R. Expression of an immunomodulatory protein known as progesterone induced blocking factor (PIBF) does not correlate with first trimester spontaneous abortions in progesterone supplemented women. *Am J Reprod Immunol* 1997;37:330–4.

45. Szekeres-Bartho J, Faust Zs, Varga P. The expression of a progesterone-induced immunomodulatory protein in pregnancy lymphocytes. *Am J Reprod Immunol* 1995;34:342–8.

46. Cohen R, Check JH, DiAntonio A et al. Progesterone induced blocking factor (PIBF), an immunosuppressive protein that inhibits natural killer (NK) cell cytolytic activity, detected 3 days after embryo transfer (ET). *Fertil Steril* 2012;98(3):Supplement:S28.

47. Check JH, Cohen R, Jaffe A et al. An allogeneic stimulus is not a prerequisite for the expression of the immunomodulatory protein the progesterone induced blocking factor (PIBF). *Am J Reprod Immunol*, ISIR 2013, Boston, MA.

48. Check JH, Cohen R, DiAntonio A et al. The demonstration that the immunomodulatory protein the progesterone induced blocking factor significantly rises in males with short term progesterone exposure provides new insights into the immunology of pregnancy. *Fertil Steril* 2013;99(3):S22–3.

49. Thomas P. Characteristics of membrane progestin receptor alpha (mPRα) and progesterone membrane receptor component 1 (PGMRC1) and their roles in mediating rapid progestin actions. *Front Neuroendocrinol* 2008;29:292–312.

50. Chien EJ, Liao CF, Chang CP et al. The non-genomic effects on NA(+)/H(+)-exchange 1 by progesterone and 20 alpha-hydroxyprogesterone in human T cells. *J Cell Physiol* 2007;211:544–50.

51. Check JH, Liss J, Check D. The beneficial effect of luteal phase support on pregnancy rates in women with unexplained infertility. *Fertil Steril* 2013;99(3) Suppl: S23, abstract #P-37.

52. Bulun SE, Cheng YH, Imir G et al. Progesterone resistance in endometriosis: Link to failure to metabolize estradiol. *Mol Cell Endocrinol* 2006;248:94–103.

53. Check JH, Liss JR, Shucoski K et al. Effect of short follicular phase with follicular maturity on conception outcome. *Clin Exp Obstet Gynecol* 2003;30:195–6.

54. Lessey BA, Killiam AP, Metzger DA et al. Immunohistochemical analysis of human estrogen and progesterone receptors throughout the menstrual cycle. *J Clin Endocrinol Metab* 1988;67:334–40.

55. Bergquist A, Ferno M. Oestrogen and progesterone receptors in endometriotic tissue and endometrium: Comparison of different cycle phases and ages. *Hum Reprod* 1993;8:2211–7.

56. Check JH, Cohen R. The role of progesterone and the progesterone receptor in human reproduction and cancer. *Exp Rev Endocrinol Metab* 2013;8:469–84.

57. Check JH, DiAntonio A, Check D et al. Clinical improvement of symptomatic advancing chronic lymphocytic leukemia following mifepristone therapy despite normal serum levels of the immunomodulatory protein the progesterone induced blocking factor (PIBF). American Association for Cancer Research Annual Meeting, Washington, DC, April 6–10, 2013.

58. Lachmann M, Gelbmann D, Kalman E et al. PIBF (progesterone induced blocking factor) is overexpressed in highly proliferating cells and associated with the centrosome. *Int J Cancer* 2004;112:51–60.

15

Debate: Should Progesterone Supplements Be Used? No

Aisha Hameed, Shazia Malik, and Lesley Regan

Introduction

The role of progesterone in the mammalian reproductive cycle is well described and undisputed. Its pharmaco-dynamics have been extensively studied and progesterone has been synthesized and commercially available since 1935. However, despite the putative role of progesterone in ameliorating unexplained recurrent pregnancy loss, the evidence base for its use in this setting is lacking, despite decades of clinical use. With this in mind, we argue that the use of progesterone supplementation for women, in whom no identifiable cause for three or more successive pregnancy losses before 20 weeks of gestation has been identified, is currently unjustified.

Scientific Basis

Luteal Phase Defect

Removal of the corpus luteum before the end of the seventh week of amenorrhoea leads to miscarriage. Rescue can be achieved with progesterone therapy but not with estrogen.[1] Corpus luteum deficiency, or luteal phase defect (LPD), has been cited as the underlying pathology in 35–40% of unexplained recurrent pregnancy losses manifesting in low serum progesterone levels and out-of-phase endometrial biopsies.[2,3] However, women with no history of recurrent miscarriage (RM) may exhibit endometrial histology suggestive of LPD in as many as 50% of single menstrual cycles and 25% of sequential cycles.[4] A prevalence study of out-of-phase endometrial biopsy specimens[5] failed to show any significant difference between fertile and infertile patients and recurrent pregnancy loss, which calls the role of this intervention into question. In a series of 74 women with RM before 10 weeks of gestation, there was no difference in pregnanediol excretion curves between those women who either miscarried, or went on to have a successful pregnancy.[6] In fact estriol was a better prognostic indicator, showing lower values in those destined to miscarry.

In a recent retrospective observational study of 132 women with unexplained RM, midluteal serum progesterone measurements were analyzed in a preconception cycle. Midluteal serum progesterone values were compared in women who went on to have a subsequent miscarriage and those who went on to have a live birth. The serum progesterone concentration in the live birth group ($n = 86$) and miscarriage group ($n = 46$) were 42.3 ± 2.4 nmol/L (mean ± SE) and 42.5 ± 3.2 nmol/L, respectively.[7] This study concluded that midluteal serum progesterone measurements do not predict the outcome of a subsequent pregnancy in women with unexplained RM. These results complement the findings of Peters et al.,[5] who proposed that LPD does not exist in the women with recurrent miscarriage group.

In 1993, Quenby and Farquharson[8] audited 203 consecutive couples attending their clinic and found that, compared to any other predictor, oligo-amenorrheic women were most likely to have further miscarriages, and further, that they exhibited low luteal phase estradiol levels but normal luteal progesterone and normal luteinising hormone (LH) profiles throughout the cycle. A more recent study found that a mid-luteal progesterone level of <10 ng/mL (as a marker of luteal phase deficiency), did not predict a future pregnancy loss in women with two successive unexplained first trimester miscarriages.[9]

Progesterone and Immuno-Modulation in Early Pregnancy

There is increasing evidence that progesterone is a key modulator in the immune response required to achieve a successful pregnancy outcome. The complexities of the adaptation between the maternal immune system and the semiallograft of the feto-placental unit are not clearly understood. The presence of progesterone and an upregulation of progesterone receptors on both decidual natural killer (NK) and placental lymphocytes appears to be required to defend the developing trophoblast from the maternal immune reaction.[10] These activated cells then synthesize progesterone-induced blocking factor (PIBF) mediating both the immuno-modulatory and antiabortive effects of progesterone.[11] In addition to the shift towards Th-2 cytokine production, NK cytolytic activity in human pregnancy is inversely related to the levels of PIBF-positive lymphocytes,[12] and neutralization in pregnant mice results in NK-mediated abortion.[11] The cellular T cell system, in particular the Th-1 cells, modulates this immune response releasing either Th-1 cytokines (such as TNF α) that induce cytotoxic and inflammatory reactions, or Th-2 cytokines (e.g., IL 10) associated with B cell production.[13] Serum cytokine profiles demonstrate a shift towards Th-2 in normal pregnancy whereas in RM sufferers the Th-1 response predominates.[14] A recent study reports that the administration of intramuscular progesterone injections to RM patients restored levels of soluble TNF receptors to values seen in women with no such history.[15] However, the treatment only commenced at eight weeks of gestation, included women up to 40 years of age and furthermore, it showed that in some of the cases no response in terms of receptor levels was seen in pregnancies which then went on to miscarry. PIBF appears to be the main modulator of the actions of progesterone, with significantly lower expression in RM patients compared to those with a healthy pregnancy.[16] Conversely, Check et al.[17] treated women in the first trimester aggressively with progesterone, but found no differences in PIBF expression by lymphocytes. However, Th cytokines were not measured in this study and could not be correlated either with PIBF levels or any given response to progesterone supplementation in specific patients. Murine experiments have shown a poor correlation between Th1/Th2 cytokines ratios and abortion rates implicating environmental selective pressures in eliminating "genetically weaker" embryos in early pregnancy.[18] Whilst some rodent data are enticing, PIBF data in human pregnancy are scanty and the mechanisms underlying immune-mediated pregnancy loss remain incompletely elucidated.[19]

Clinical Data

The uterine decidual and systemic levels of progesterone necessary to maintain an early pregnancy in humans are not understood[20] and hence clinical studies must by definition employ arbitrary doses/mode of delivery of supplementary drug. Furthermore, although the study criteria that should be fulfilled when designing a treatment trial for unexplained recurrent pregnancy loss have been proposed (see Table 15.1)[21] no published clinical trials that have systematically evaluated the role of progesterone treatment in recurrent pregnancy loss which fulfil these criteria are available.

Two meta-analyses published in the same journal reported conflicting results regarding the value of progesterone supplementation in miscarriage patients. Goldstein et al.[22] included trials of women with a "high risk" pregnancy, including a history of previous miscarriage, stillbirth or current preterm labour. In addition the authors used different preparations commenced at varying gestations and not surprisingly no benefit of treatment was identified. They subsequently recommended that randomized trials should be the only setting for the use of progestational agents in pregnancy. By contrast, Daya[23] presented a meta-analysis of controlled trials studying the efficacy of progesterone support for pregnancy in women with a history of RM. Although the odds ratio for pregnancies reaching at least 20 weeks of gestation was 3.09 (95% CI 1.28–7.42), even he concluded that RM patients with luteal phase deficiency should have the efficacy of progesterone assessed in prospective double-blind randomized controlled trials. Closer inspection of the data sets reveals why this conclusion was reached. Only three studies met the inclusion/exclusion criteria,

TABLE 15.1

Study Criteria for Recurrent Pregnancy Loss Treatments

---

1. Scientifically sound rationale
2. Power calculation ensuring sufficient numbers using reasonable assumption (e.g. 60% success without and 80% success with treatment)
3. Exclusion of patients with less than 3 unexplained clinical pregnancy losses
4. Exclusion of patients with presumed causes for prior pregnancy losses
5. Prospective study design
6. Pre-stratification of participants by age and number of prior losses (both independent risk factors for subsequent loss)
7. Effective randomisation after pre-stratification
8. Placebo controlled
9. Double-blind
10. No concomitant therapy
11. Karyotype of subsequent losses
12. Follow-up to ensure safety

Source: Hill JA. *J Soc Gynecol Invest* 1997;4:267–73.

and since the differences between the experimental groups were insignificant, they had to be pooled to achieve a statistically significant power calculation. None of these three studies demonstrated a significant progesterone deficiency; each employed a different progestogen, and each had different inclusion criteria but recruited patients only after they had reached at least eight weeks of gestation. In addition, only 50 treated and 45 control patients were identified in total. In the study by Levine,[24] patients were allocated to their treatment arm alternately as they presented, not randomly. Furthermore, the series published by Swyer and Daley[25] was similarly not "blinded"—treated patients were administered an implant whilst some controls were offered a placebo tablet. These data were again reviewed in the Cochrane meta-analysis published in 2003 which concluded that there was a statistically significant reduction in miscarriage which favored those women in the progestogen group, OR 0.37 (95% CI 0.17–0.91).[26]

In a subsequent small trial,[27] a significant reduction in the miscarriage rate was observed in women receiving dydrogesterone (10 mg orally) in early pregnancy compared to those who remained untreated ($p < 0.05$). In this trial women with an average of 3.3 previous unexplained recurrent abortions were randomized to receive either no treatment ($n = 30$), dydrogesterone ($n = 48$), or hCG (5000 IU IM every four days $n = 36$) from as soon as pregnancy was confirmed until the 12th week of gestation. This trial does not, however, conform to the gold standards cited in Table 15.1.

A further analysis of the available trials was published in 2011, drawing attention to the small participant numbers and the fact that they were of poor quality (the modified Jadad quality scores ranged from 0/5 to 2/5). These authors conceded that there was a trend towards progesterone supplementation being of benefit, with a 42–69% reduction in the rate of miscarriage, but emphasized the wide confidence intervals and the lack of statistically significant differences in all but one of the four studies. Furthermore, they highlighted that no data were available for other important and clinically relevant outcomes such as live birth.[28]

The most recent Cochrane meta-analysis of four trials involving 225 women with a history of three or more consecutive early miscarriages reported that progestogen treatment is associated with a statistically significant decrease in the miscarriage rate compared to placebo or no treatment (OR 0.39; 95% CI 0.21 to 0.72). However, once again the quality of the methodology was considered to be poor.[29]

Conclusions

The UK has licensed three progestogenic products for use in early pregnancy—intramuscular progesterone, vaginal progesterone and oral dydrogesterone, which have been available for between 10 and 20 years. However, the number of studies examining the efficacy of progesterone supplementation in early pregnancy are few and the total participants recruited remains small. In brief, they do not fulfil the criteria required to generate meaningful results. In addition, the diversity of biological and pharmacological variables does not allow extrapolation of the results across studies. Importantly, although no obvious adverse effects to mother or fetus have been reported, the relatively small population studied means that a low level of risk may as yet be unidentified.

The observed frequency of another miscarriage after three previous episodes is over 50% and the wish to prescribe an apparently safe and well-tolerated treatment is appealing, especially in light of the emerging scientific understanding of early pregnancy failure. As yet, however, the evidence for "tender loving care" shows a similar improvement in outcomes. The need "to do something" for a group of unfortunate patients often seems to override the use of an evidence-based approach to management. Whilst treatment does not appear to do harm, the evidence for the use of progesterone supplementation in recurrent pregnancy loss is contentious at best, dated and poor at worst.

In the UK, some 90% of physicians remain unconvinced of any beneficial effects and believe that evidence in the form of a large placebo-controlled randomized trial is required.[28] The results of such randomized controlled trials of progesterone supplementation for RM are eagerly awaited. The PROMISE (Progesterone in miscarriage) trial is a large multicentered study examining the effect of Cyclogest vaginal pessaries (micronized progesterone) versus placebo, funded by the Health Technology Assessment arm of the Medical Research Council (ISRCTN 92644181). It is hoped that the results of this study will provide clear evidence for the role of progesterone in the management of RM.

REFERENCES

1. Csapo AI, Pulkkinen MO, Ruttner B et al. The significance of the human corpus luteum in pregnancy maintenance. I. Preliminary studies. *Am J Obstet Gynecol* 1972;112:1061–7.
2. Jones GS. The luteal phase defect *Fertil Steril* 1976;27:351–6.
3. Daya S, Ward S. Diagnostic test properties of serum progesterone in the evaluation of luteal phase defects. *Fertil Steril* 1988;49:168–70.
4. Davis OK, Berkeley AS, Naus GJ et al. The incidence of luteal phase defect in normal, fertile women, determined by serial endometrial biopsies. *Fertil Steril* 1989;51:582–6.
5. Peters AJ, Lloyd RP, Coulam CB. Prevalence of out-of-phase endometrial biopsy specimens. *Am J Obstet Gynecol* 1992;166:1738–45; Discussion 1745–6.
6. Klopper A, Michie EA. The excretion of urinary pregnanediol after the administration of progesterone. *J Endocrinol* 1956;13:360–4.
7. Yan J, Liu F, Yuan X et al. Midluteal serum progesterone concentration does not predict the outcome of pregnancy in women with unexplained recurrent miscarriage. *Reprod Biomed Online* 2013;26:138–41.
8. Quenby SM, Farquharson RG. Predicting recurring miscarriage: What is important? *Obstet Gynecol* 1993;82:132–8.
9. Ogasawara M, Kajiura S, Katano K et al. Are serum progesterone levels predictive of recurrent miscarriage in future pregnancies? *Fertil Steril* 1997;68:806–9.
10. Roussev RG, Higgins NG, McIntyre JA. Phenotypic characterization of normal human placental mononuclear cells. *J Reprod Immunol* 1993;25:15–29.
11. Szekeres-Bartho J, Barakonyi A, Polgar B et al. The role of gamma/delta T cells in progesterone-mediated immunomodulation during pregnancy: A review. *Am J Reprod Immunol* 1999;42:44–8.
12. Szekeres-Bartho J, Faust Z, Varga P. The expression of a progesterone-induced immunomodulatory protein in pregnancy lymphocytes. *Am J Reprod Immunol* 1995;34:342–8.
13. Druckmann R, Druckmann MA. Progesterone and the immunology of pregnancy. *J Steroid Biochem Mol Biol* 2005;97:389–96.
14. Raghupathy R, Makhseed M, Azizieh F et al. Cytokine production by maternal lymphocytes during normal human pregnancy and in unexplained recurrent spontaneous abortion. *Hum Reprod* 2000;15:713–8.
15. Chernyshov VP, Vodyanik MA, Pisareva SP. Lack of soluble TNF-receptors in women with recurrent spontaneous abortion and possibility for its correction. *Am J Reprod Immunol* 2005;54:284–91.
16. Szekeres-Bartho J, Barakonyi A, Miko E et al. The role of gamma/delta T cells in the feto-maternal relationship. *Semin Immunol* 2001;13:229–33.

17. Check JH, Ostrzenski A, Klimek R. Expression of an immunomodulatory protein known as progesterone induced blocking factor (PIBF) does not correlate with first trimester spontaneous abortions in progesterone supplemented women. *Am J Reprod Immunol* 1997;330–4.
18. Clark DA, Chaouat G, Gorczynski RM. Thinking outside the box: Mechanisms of environmental selective pressures on the outcome of the materno-fetal relationship. *Am J Reprod Immunol* 2002;47:275–82.
19. Laird SM, Tuckerman EM, Cork BA et al. A review of immune cells and molecules in women with recurrent miscarriage. *Hum Reprod Update* 2003;9:163–74.
20. Azuma K, Calderon I, Besanko M et al. Is the luteo-placental shift a myth? Analysis of low progesterone levels in successful art pregnancies. *J Clin Endocrinol Metab* 1993;77:195–8.
21. Hill JA. Immunotherapy for recurrent pregnancy loss: "Standard of care or buyer beware". *J Soc Gynecol Invest* 1997;4:267–73.
22. Goldstein P, Berrier J, Rosen S et al. A meta-analysis of randomized control trials of progestational agents in pregnancy. *Br J Obstet Gynaecol* 1989;96:265–74.
23. Daya S. Efficacy of progesterone support for pregnancy in women with recurrent miscarriage. A meta-analysis of controlled trials. *Br J Obstet Gynaecol* 1989;96:275–80.
24. Levine L. Habitual Abortion. A controlled study of progestational therapy. *West J Surg, Obstet Gynecol* 1964;72:30–6.
25. Swyer GI, Daley D. Progesterone implantation in habitual abortion. *Br Med J* 1953;1:1073–7.
26. Oates-Whitehead RM, Haas DM, Carrier JA. Progestogen for preventing miscarriage. *Cochrane Database Syst Rev* 2003;(4):CD003511.
27. El-Zibdeh MY. Dydrogesterone in the reduction of recurrent spontaneous abortion. *J Steroid Biochem Mol Biol* 2005; 97:431–4.
28. Coomarasamy A, Truchanowicz EG, Rai R. Does first trimester progesterone prophylaxis increase the live birth rate in women with unexplained recurrent miscarriages? *Br Med J* 2011; 342.d1914
29. Haas DM, Ramsey PS. Progestogen for preventing miscarriage. *Cochrane Database Syst Rev* 2013;10:CD003511.

16

Opinion: Progestogens in Recurrent Miscarriage

Howard J. A. Carp

Chapters 14 and 15 have debated whether progesterone supplementation should be used in RPL. The theoretical basis, diagnosis of luteal deficiency and immunological actions of progesterone have been discussed. However, there are numerous progestogens available, and the reader may be in a quandary over which progestogen to prescribe, if at all. This chapter will try to assess the different types of progesterone and the evidence (or lack) of effect. Progestogen supplementation is used as a treatment for a presumed maternal cause of pregnancy loss, that is, luteal deficiency. Chapters 3, 11, and 12 have described the embryonic causes of RPL. 40% of recurrent miscarriages are due to chromosomal aberrations which are incompatible with life. It is against this background that the effect of progesterone has to be assessed. The relative merits of the different progestogens should be based on efficacy data and possible maternal and fetal side effects.

Assessment of Luteal Deficiency

Serum progesterone levels have been used to make prognoses about the continued development of pregnancy and even to diagnose pregnancy loss. The lowest progesterone level to be associated with a viable pregnancy was 5.1 ng/mL in the series by Stovall et al.[1] A single progesterone level ≥25 ng/mL was associated with a 97% likelihood of viable pregnancy. Al-Sebai et al.[2] summarized 358 threatened abortions <18 weeks; a single progesterone level ≤45 nmol/L (14 ng/mL) was reported to differentiate between aborting and ongoing pregnancies, (sensitivity 87.6%, specificity 87.5%). Arck et al.[3] have reported that low serum progesterone (≤12 ng/mL) is associated with an increased risk of miscarriage. However, serum progesterone levels are notoriously unreliable. Progesterone secretion pulsatile blood may be drawn at a pulse peak or nadir. These may vary ten-fold.[4] Hormone levels may be normal, but histology abnormal due to deficiency of progesterone receptors. Abnormal embryos produce low hCG levels. Low hCG levels lead to low progesterone levels. Consequently, low progesterone may be the mechanism rather than the cause of abortion. In these circumstances, diagnosis and treatment should probably be empirical rather than based on progesterone levels.

Before a trial of progesterone can be said to be conclusive, other predictive factors should be taken into account. These have been described in Chapter 1 and include the following. (1) The most important predictive factor is the number of previous miscarriages. The higher the number of previous miscarriages, the lower the live birth rate. As the number of previous losses increases, the chance of a live birth decreases.[5] Each subsequent miscarriage lowers the live birth rate by 23%[6] and (2) maternal age.

Evidence of Efficacy

Daya[7] reported a meta-analysis of controlled trials studying the efficacy of progesterone in RPL. The odds ratio for pregnancies to pass 20 weeks was 3.09 (95% CI 1.28–7.42). However, none of the three reports in Daya's[7] meta-analysis had sufficient power to show statistical significance. Each used a

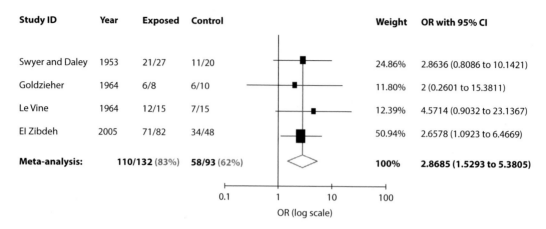

FIGURE 16.1   Meta-analysis on progestogen support in recurrent miscarriage.

different progesterone regimen. No trial matched for predictive factors, or chromosomal aberrations. Additionally, these trials came from the 1950s and 1960s. At that time there was no early ultrasound available. There was no matching for the presence of a fetal heart. Hence, some patients with missed abortions might have been treated after fetal demise. There was no matching for the start of treatment. Therefore some patients may have had treatment after fetal viability was assured. Oates-Whitehead et al.[8] reassessed the results of progesterone supplementation in RPL for the Cochrane Database. He was only able to find the same three papers for his meta-analysis as in Daya's[7] previous meta-analysis, and the results were similar. Oates-Whitehead et al. concluded, "There was evidence that women who have suffered three or more miscarriages may benefit from progestogen during pregnancy but more trials are needed." There have been two further trials.[9,10] Both assessed dydrogesterone. Both reported a statistically significant decrease in the number of subsequent miscarriages.

An updated meta-analysis is shown in Figure 16.1. This meta-analysis shows a statistically significant OR of 3.18 for a live birth (CI 2.02–5.10). There has been an additional attempt to carry out a randomized trial on dydrogesterone[11] which was abandoned due to lack of recruitment. A large multicenter study (PROMISE) is currently investigating micronized progesterone supplementation in women with unexplained RPL. However, as the PROMISE trial does not account for the confounding effect of embryonic chromosomal aberrations, it is likely to show a negative result. The results may then need to be added to the meta-analysis in Figure 16.1 to draw conclusions.

Which Progestogen

The term "natural progesterone" is often used. However, all progestogens including micronized progesterone are produced from plant steroids, found in *Dioscorea mexicana*, a plant of the yam family native to Mexico. *Dioscorea* contains a sterol called diosgenin. Diosgenin is converted to progesterone. Hence the source is always natural. However, progesterone is ineffective. In order to be used therapeutically, it can be micronized, converted with UV light to dydrogesterone, or compounded to 17-OHP. Hence, each progestogen is artificially manipulated. The next section deals with the progestogens in use in pregnancy.

Micronized Progesterone

Micronized progesterone can be administered orally or vaginally. The oral route is easiest, but progesterone is degraded in the liver. There is extreme variability in plasma concentrations.[12] Side effects include nausea, headache, and sleepiness. Vaginal administration avoids hepatic metabolism, there is rapid absorption, high bioavailability, and local endometrial effects.[13] It is not painful, and there are few side effects. However, there are problems with patient compliance. Vaginal administration is unacceptable in some societies. Vaginal progesterone is uncomfortable if there is bleeding or discharge and may be washed out if bleeding is severe.

In order to draw up Figure 16.1 a thorough literature search was carried out for all papers in EMBASE and Ovid MEDLINE® using search terms, progesterone, progestagens, micronised progesterone, 17-OH Progesterone, Duphaston or dydrogesterone. No reports were found on micronised progesterone for recurrent miscarriage.

Intramuscular Progesterone

Progesterone can be compounded for intramuscular injection, either as 17-hydroxy progesterone acetate, or as caproate in a depot form. The drug is suspended in oil for injection. Intramuscular progesterone achieves optimal blood levels. However, the side effects are many, including extreme pain, swelling, itching and other local reactions at injection site, abscess formation, hypersensitivity reactions, cough, dyspnea, tiredness, dizziness, genital itching, and increased risk of gestational diabetes, mood swings, headaches, bloating, abdominal pain, perineal pain, constipation, diarrhea, nausea, vomiting, joint pain, depression, decreased sex drive, nervousness, sleepiness, breast enlargement, breast pain, dysuria, polyuria, urinary tract infection (UTI), vaginal discharge, fever, flu-like symptoms, back pain, leg pain, sleep disorder, upper respiratory infection, asthma, acne, and pruritus.[14]

There are concerns regarding the vehicle, castor oil, which may induce labor by stimulating the release of prostaglandins.[15,16] Three clinical studies in singleton pregnancies have all shown an increased risk of miscarriage compared to placebo.[17–19] Hence, the U.S. Food and Drug Administration (FDA) has expressed concern about miscarriage at the 2006 advisory committee, and has stated that further study is required to evaluate the potential association of 17OHP-C with an increased risk of second trimester miscarriage and stillbirth.[14] Meantime, the only trial of 17-hydroxy progesterone acetate in RPL[20] found a small but statistically insignificant benefit in a small trial of 18 patients.

Dydrogesterone

Dydrogesterone is manufactured by treating progesterone with ultra-violet light, leading to a change in the spatial structure. Dydrogesterone is structurally and pharmacologically similar to progesterone, and acts through the progesterone receptor. In fact, dydrogesterone seems to bind the receptor approximately 50% more than progesterone itself.[21] Dydrogesterone has good oral bioavailability. Although metabolized in the liver, the metabolite 20-dihydrodydrogesterone is biologically active, unlike the metabolites of progesterone (pregnanediol, pregnanetriol and pregnanolone) which are inactive. As dydrogesterone binds the receptor directly, there is no change in serum progesterone levels, and consequently, no inhibition of progesterone formation in placenta.[22] There are minimal side effects,[23] In fact, it has been estimated that between 1977 and 2005 approx. 38 million women were treated with dydrogesterone, and more than 10 million fetuses exposed.[23] The drug is not washed out by bleeding or discharge. In the six papers quoted in Figure 13.1, only dydrogesterone had a statistically significant beneficial effect. The reports on each of the other three progestogens were underpowered to show any statistically significant benefit. They only included 95 patients. Whereas Kumar et al.'s[10] report on dydrogesterone in recurrent miscarriage includes 348 patients.

Congenital Malformations

The question of congenital malformations is essential regarding progestogens. Most reports of malformations have concentrated on the androgenic and antiandrogenic effects. Derivatives of 19-nortestosterone have been reported to cause virilization of the female embryo in rats. Virilization has never been reported in humans. However, the work in rats has led to progestogens derived from 19-nortestosterone not being used in pregnancy. Progesterone itself has antiandrogenic effects. There have been reports of progesterone being associated with an increased incidence of hypospadias. 17-Hydroxyprogesterone acetate has been associated with an increased chance of abortion.[14] Dydrogesterone has no effect on the androgen receptor. As stated above, Queisser Luft[23] has stated that 10 million fetuses have been exposed. There have been no increased risks of malformations with dydrogesterone.

Conclusions

Progesterone has numerous functions in pregnancy, and is essential for pregnancy to develop. Although there is a statistically significant 25% improvement in the live birth rate with progesterone supplementation, the figures, as for any treatment for maternal treatment of RPL, are confounded by fetal factors. As some of the papers in the meta-analysis in Figure 16.1 rely on papers published in the 1950s and 1960s it was questionable whether the previous metaanalyses were biologically or medically significant. However, the newer trials indicate that dydrogesterone has a significant effect. The results of the trial on micronized progesterone are eagerly awaited.

REFERENCES

1. Stovall TG, Ling FW, Carson SA et al. Serum progesterone and uterine curettage in differential diagnosis of ectopic pregnancy. *Fertil Steril* 1992;57:456–7.
2. Al-Sebai MA, Kingsland CR, Diver M et al. The role of a single progesterone measurement in the diagnosis of early pregnancy failure and the prognosis of fetal viability. *Br J Obstet Gynaecol* 1995;102:364–9.
3. Arck PC, Rücke M, Rose M et al. Early risk factors for miscarriage: A prospective cohort study in pregnant women. *Reprod Biomed Online* 2008;17:101–13.
4. Abraham GE, Maroulis GB, Marshall JR. Evaluation of ovulation and corpus luteum function using measurements of plasma progesterone. *Obstet Gynecol* 1974;44:522–5.
5. Daya S, Gunby J. The effectiveness of allogeneic leucocyte immunization in unexplained primary recurrent spontaneous abortion. *Am J Reprod Immunol* 1994;32:294–302.
6. Recurrent Miscarriage Immunotherapy Trialists Group. Worldwide collaborative observational study and metaanalysis on allogenic leucocyte immunotherapy for recurrent spontaneous abortion. *Am J Reprod Immunol* 1994;32:55–72.
7. Daya S. Efficacy of progesterone support for pregnancy in women with recurrent miscarriage. A meta-analysis of controlled trials. *Br J Obstet Gynaecol* 1989;96:275–80.
8. Oates-Whitehead RM, Haas DM, Carrier JA. Progestogen for preventing miscarriage. *Cochrane Database Syst Rev* 2003;CD003511.
9. El-Zibdeh MY. Dydrogesterone in the reduction of recurrent spontaneous abortion. *J Steroid Biochem Mol Biol* 2005;97:431–4.
10. Kumar A, Begum N, Prasad S, Aggarwal S, Sharma S. Oral dydrogesterone treatment during early pregnancy to prevent recurrent pregnancy loss and its role in modulation of cytokine production: A double-blind, randomized, parallel, placebo-controlled trial. Fertil Steril 2014;pii: S0015-0282(14)02022-6. doi: 10.1016/j.fertnstert.2014.07.1251. [Epub ahead of print]
11. Walch K, Hefler L, Nagele F. Oral dydrogesterone treatment during the first trimester of pregnancy: The prevention of miscarriage study (PROMIS). Adouble-blind, prospectively randomized, place bo-controlled, parallel group trial. *J Matern–Fetal Neonat Med.* 2005;18:265–9.
12. Di Renzo GC, Mattei A, Gojnic M et al. Progesterone and pregnancy. *Curr Opin Obstet Gynecol* 2005;17:598–600.
13. von Eye Corleta H, Capp E, Ferreira MB. Pharmacokinetics of natural progesterone vaginal suppository. *Gynecol Obstet Invest.* 2004;58:105–8.
14. FDA Reproductive Health Drugs Advisory Committee. August 29, 2006 Meeting to discuss NDA21-945.

15. Brancazio LR, Murtha AP, Phillps Heine R. Prevention of recurrent preterm delivery by 17 alpha-hydroxyprogesterone caproate. *N Engl J Med* 2003;349:1087–1088.

16. O'Sullivan MD, Hehir MP, O'Brien YM et al. 17 alpha-hydroxyprogesterone caproate vehicle, castor oil, enhances the contractile effect of oxytocin in human myometrium in pregnancy. *Am J Obstet Gynecol* 2010;202:453.

17. Yemini M, Borenstein R, Dreazen E et al. Prevention of premature labor by 17 alpha-hydroxyprogesterone caproate. *Am J Obstet Gynecol.* 1985;151:574–7.

18. Meis PJ et al. Prevention of recurrent preterm delivery by 17 alpha-hydroxyprogesterone caproate. *New Engl J Med* 2003;348:2379–85.

19. Keirse MJNC, Progestogen administration in pregnancy may prevent preterm delivery. *Br J Obstet Gynecol* 1990;97:149.

20. Goldzieher JW. Double-blind trial of a progestin in habitual abortion. *JAMA, J Am Med Assoc* 1964;188:651–4.

21. King RJ, Whitehead MI. Assessment of the potency of orally administered progestins in women. *Fertil Steril* 1986;46:1062–6.

22. Schindler AE, Campagnoli C, Druckmann R et al. Classification and pharmacology of progestins. *Maturitas* 2003;10:46Suppl 1:S7–S16.

23. Queisser-Luft A. Dydrogesterone use during pregnancy: Overview of birth defects reported since 1977. *Early Hum Dev* 2009;85:375–7.

17

Debate: Should Human Chorionic Gonadotropin Supplementation Be Used? Yes

James Walker

Introduction

In the late 1920s, Allen and Corner carried out experimental work demonstrating that preparations made from corpus luteum extracts could successfully support pregnancies in animals where the ovaries had been ablated.[1] Further work demonstrated that these preparations contained progesterone. However, initial work on the use of progesterone in maintaining early pregnancy in castrated rabbits failed and it was not until the study published in 1939 that a successful trial was achieved.[2] The difference in this study was that the castration was carried out after the 11th day following mating, when implantation of the embryos had occurred. Other work suggested an estrogen was more important in supporting the early pregnancy.[3] However, unlike in small animals, which almost inevitably abort after ovariectomy, the results in pregnancies in larger animals and humans were mixed with many cases cited in which abortion was seen to follow removal of the corpus luteum, while in others pregnancy appeared to continue successfully after ovariectomy in mid-pregnancy without hormonal support. It became clear that the effect was gestation dependent.[4] In human pregnancy, exogenous progesterone support was required only until around eight weeks gestation after which the pregnancy continued independently. The explanation of this became obvious with the realization that the corpus luteum is critical in early pregnancy, after which time the trophoblast takes over the hormonal support. This "hand over" time appeared to be between seven and eight weeks' gestation.

Because progesterone was thought to be important for the maintenance of normal pregnancy, the concept that a deficiency in progesterone might lead to miscarriage was a natural follow-on. By the late 1940s, it had been shown that functional reproductive deficits sufficient to cause infertility or recurrent abortion were present in women who appeared to be having regular menstrual cycles.[5] These abnormalities were due to a deficit in progesterone secretion during the luteal phase of the cycle (luteal phase deficiency). This disorder was characterized by inadequate endometrial maturation and was reported in up to 60% of women with recurrent miscarriage. However, these early studies are open to question since there was no reliable method of dating the cycle. Since many of these studies presumed that the patient's menstrual pattern is a normal 28-day cycle, these endometrial abnormalities could be related to prolonged cycles. However, more recent studies on the hormonal cycle have confirmed abnormalities of corpus luteal function with deficiency in progesterone levels in the luteal phase and early pregnancy of those with a history of miscarriage but in a lower percentage.[6] In one of the few prospective studies evaluating women with three or more consecutive miscarriages, luteal phase defect (LPD) was believed to be the cause in 17%.[7] Those found to have LPD are more likely to have early losses (prior to the detection of fetal heart activity) than later loss.[8]

The Evidence

Intervention—Estrogen

If hormonal lack is associated with miscarriage, hormonal support might be a possible therapy. The problem with steroid hormones is that they cannot be taken by mouth and synthetic substitutes are required. Because of the early work showing the benefit of an estrogen,[3] the first therapeutic trials were with diethylstilbestrol, a nonsteroidal estrogenic substance. This was given in large doses. None of these studies showed benefit and by the 1970s there was evidence of the effect of this medication on the female offspring.[9-11] Therefore, not only did estrogenic support not appear to be beneficial, it had major side effects in the female offspring. These included abnormalities of the cervix, recurrent pregnancy loss and, in extreme cases, clear cell carcinoma of the vagina. These studies had a significant influence on studies of hormonal support in pregnancy with the fear that hormones could have a detrimental effect on the unborn child.

Intervention—Progesterone

With previous studies suggesting that progesterone is the main supportive hormone in early pregnancy, there has been, in recent years, an interest in its use in *in vitro* fertilization. This support is given early, after embryo transfer, to support the luteal phase and the trials demonstrate an increase in successful pregnancies.[12] Interestingly, synthetic progesterone appeared to be superior to micronized progesterone. Because of the risk of ovarian hyperstimulation syndrome (OHSS), the use of human chorionic gonadotrophin (hCG) was not recommended.

A Cochrane systematic review of the studies on the use of progesterone to prevent spontaneous miscarriage show no benefit irrespective of the route of administration or type of progesterone used.[13] However, in the subgroup of patients with a history of recurrent miscarriage, there was significant increase in live birth rate. In all studies, there appear to be no obvious side effects. Therefore, there does appear to be some possible benefit of the use of progesterone in women with recurrent miscarriage to improve live birth rate and a large multicenter trial (PROMISE) is currently underway to assess the role of progesterone.[14]

Intervention—Human Chorionic Gonadotrophin

Human chorionic gonadotrophin is the hormone, produced by the placenta, responsible for the corpus luteal support in early pregnancy. If placentation is failing, levels of hCG may well be low resulting in low progesterone and leading to miscarriage.[15] Rather than giving exogenous progesterone, hCG treatment would stimulate the natural progesterone production and reduce the risks of abnormal effects on the fetus of progestogenic drugs. In recurrent miscarriage, two early small studies were supportive of benefit[16,17] which led to larger trials, some which were not confirmatory[18] and others supportive.[19] A meta-analysis of these four trials suggested treatment with hCG reduced the risk of miscarriage in women with a history of recurrent miscarriage (odds ratio 0.26, 95% confidence interval (CI) 0.14 to 0.52).[20] However, the authors cautioned the readers as they felt that there was some weakness in the older trials. Subanalysis in one of the trials suggested a particular benefit in women with oligomenorrhea.[19] Carp[21] has criticized both the methods of the underlying trials and called for larger better-structured design to answer the question. A more recent meta-analysis[22] in the Cochrane database included a fifth trial[23] which had included hCG as one arm of a randomized trial. With the inclusion of this trial, the meta-analysis suggested a statistically significant benefit in using hCG (risk ratio (RR) 0.51, 95% CI 0.32 to 0.81; five studies, 302 women). If an early trial[24] and a later large observation study,[21] are included in an updated meta-analysis, the results improve to a relative risk of 0.44 for preventing subsequent miscarriage, 95% CI 0.31 to 0.63; seven studies, 671 women (Figure 17.1).

These studies vary in their selection, randomization and blindness and, in most published meta-analyses, studies are removed if the methodology is thought to be of a lower standard and this always removes the statistical significance. The authors of the latest Cochrane systematic review[22] state that the evidence supporting hCG supplementation to prevent RM remains equivocal and that a well-designed randomized controlled trial of adequate power and methodological quality is required to determine whether hCG is beneficial in RM. However, it is important to notice that all the published studies show benefit. So the loss of significance is more related to the removal of numbers than the removal of bias papers. The subanalysis of studies yield interesting questions that highlight some of the problems of studies into recurrent miscarriage. Quenby and Farquharson[19] suggested benefit for those with a

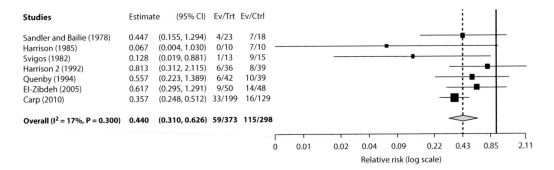

Studies	Estimate	(95% CI)	Ev/Trt	Ev/Ctrl
Sandler and Bailie (1978)	0.447	(0.155, 1.294)	4/23	7/18
Harrison (1985)	0.067	(0.004, 1.030)	0/10	7/10
Svigos (1982)	0.128	(0.019, 0.881)	1/13	9/15
Harrison 2 (1992)	0.813	(0.312, 2.115)	6/36	8/39
Quenby (1994)	0.557	(0.223, 1.389)	6/42	10/39
El-Zibdeh (2005)	0.617	(0.295, 1.291)	9/50	14/48
Carp (2010)	0.357	(0.248, 0.512)	33/199	16/129
Overall (I² = 17%, P = 0.300)	**0.440**	**(0.310, 0.626)**	**59/373**	**115/298**

Relative risk (log scale)

FIGURE 17.1 A Forrest plot of the cumulative studies into the use of hCG in recurrent miscarriage.

diagnosis of oligomenorrhea, and Carp[21] showed greater benefit for those with "poor prognosis", usually meaning those with a larger number of losses.

Problems of Interpretation

In all the published studies, the success rate of the treatment arm is 84% (range 82–100) and 61% (range 30–80) in the control arm. This suggests that the likelihood of a statistical difference is more to do with the poor outcome in the control group, which would reflect the background prognosis of those selected.[21]

Timing of Therapy

In many studies, treatment is commenced after viability has been confirmed by ultrasound. Since over 75% of recurrent miscarriages occur before this and only 25% after ultrasonic detection of a fetal heartbeat, if ultrasound detection of a fetal heart is required, the majority of miscarriages have already occurred. The early studies suggest that the benefit of hormonal therapy is early in the pregnancy and may not be beneficial after eight weeks' gestation. In the El-Zibdeh study,[23] early recruitment was used and demonstrated a significant benefit from both an oral progesten and, less so, hCG, in recurrent miscarriage.

Chromosomal Abnormality

HCG cannot be expected to influence karyotypic aberrations, only to affect the outcome of pregnancies with chromosomally normal embryos. In these studies, the results were not corrected for karyotypic aberrations in the embryo. In the Carp series[21] seven miscarriages in the hCG group were due to trisomies (2,15,16,16,21,22,22). Two of these patients had subsequent live births on hCG treatment. If these patients were excluded from the results, the benefit from hCG would be even higher.

Poor Prognosis

Although recurrent miscarriage is traditionally defined as three successive miscarriages, some trials use women after two miscarriages to allow for an increase in numbers. In his recent review of the problems of these trials, Carp states that those with a higher degree of loss (five or more) have a greater benefit from treatment, partly due to the greater likelihood of repeated failure leading to a higher loss rate in the control group.[25] This does not mean that those with a lower degree of loss do not benefit but, since their background success is better, the benefit provided by hCG is less and more difficult to prove.

Timing of Loss

It is likely that, if hCG is beneficial, it will be in women with a likelihood of hormonal deficiency in early pregnancy. One obvious group is those with oligomenorrhea[19] but also those with recurrent early (less than eight week) losses. It is at this time of pregnancy that the science would suggest that hormonal support is most beneficial.

Conclusions

HCG therapy is not a panacea for all cases of recurrent miscarriage, but it appears to be beneficial in a particular targeted group. The problem is selecting that target group. Certainly, those with a proven cause, such as antiphospholipid syndrome and chromosome abnormalities are unlikely to benefit. Those with repeated early loss (prior to a positive fetal heart) and those with an irregular cycle would appear to be more likely to benefit. By using these criteria, around 30% of cases of recurrent miscarriage could be offered hormonal support with a success rate of around 85%.[23] Whether to use a progestogen or hCG is a more difficult argument. However, with the concerns over the potential *in utero* effects of exogenous hormones, hCG has the advantage of being more "natural" with evidence of, at least, similar benefits.

I therefore support the use of hCG in the treatment of recurrent miscarriage in an appropriately assessed population.

REFERENCES

1. Allen WM, Corner, GW. Physiology of the corpus luteum: III. normal growth and implantation of embryos after very early ablation of the ovaries, under the influence of extracts of the corpus luteum. *Am J Physiol* 1929;88:340–6.
2. Allen WM, Heckel, GP. Maintenance of pregnancy by progesterone in rabbits castrated on the 11th day. *Am J Physiol* 1939;125:31–5.
3. Heckel GP, Allen, WM. Maintenance of the corpus luteum and inhibition of parturition in the rabbit by injection of estrogenic hormone. *Endocrinology* 1939;24:137–9.
4. Russ W. The maintenance of pregnancy in the human after removal of both ovaries—Case report. *Ann Surg* 1940;111(5):871–3.
5. Jones GES. Some newer aspects of the management of infertility. *JAMA, J Am Med Assoc.* 1949;141:1123–9.
6. Miller H, Durant, JA, Ross, DM, O'Connell, FJ. Corpus luteum deficiency as a cause of early recurrent abortion: A case history. *Fertil Steril* 1969;20(3):433–8.
7. Tulppala M, Bjorses UM, Stenman UH et al. Luteal phase defect in habitual abortion: Progesterone in saliva. *Fertil Steril* 1991;56(1):41–4.
8. Li TC, Iqbal T, Anstie, B. et al. An analysis of the pattern of pregnancy loss in women with recurrent miscarriage. *Fertil Steril* 2002;78(5):1100–6.
9. Lanier AP, Noller KL, Decker DG et al. Cancer and stilbestrol. A follow-up of 1,719 persons exposed to estrogens in utero and born 1943–1959. *Mayo Clin Proc* 1973;48(11):793–9.
10. Vessey MP, Fairweather DV, Norman-Smith B, Buckley J. A randomized double-blind controlled trial of the value of stilboestrol therapy in pregnancy: Long-term follow-up of mothers and their offspring. *Br J Obstet Gynaecol* 1983;90(11):1007–17.
11. Bamigboye AA, Morris, J. Oestrogen supplementation, mainly diethylstilbestrol, for preventing miscarriages and other adverse pregnancy outcomes. *Cochrane Database Syst Rev* 2003;(3):CD004271.
12. van der Linden M, Buckingham K, Farquhar C et al. Luteal phase support for assisted reproduction cycles. *Cochrane Database Syst Rev* 2011;(10):CD009154.
13. Haas DM, Ramsey PS. Progestogen for preventing miscarriage. *Cochrane Database Syst Rev* 2013;(10):CD003511.
14. PROMISE trial. http://www.controlled-trials.com/ISRCTN92644181.
15. Tong S, Wallace EM, Rombauts L. Association between low day 16 hCG and miscarriage after proven cardiac activity. *Obstet Gynecol* 2006;107(2 Pt 1):300–4.
16. Svigos J. Preliminary experience with the use of human chorionic gonadotrophin therapy in women with repeated abortion. *Clin Reprod fertil* 1982;1(2):131–5.
17. Harrison RF. Treatment of habitual abortion with human chorionic gonadotropin: Results of open and placebo-controlled studies. *Eur J Obstet Gynecol Reprod Biol* 1985;20(3):159–68.

18. Harrison RF. Human chorionic gonadotrophin (hCG) in the management of recurrent abortion; results of a multi-centre placebo-controlled study. *Eur J Obstet Gynecol Reprod Biol* 1992;47(3):175–9.
19. Quenby S, Farquharson RG. Human chorionic gonadotropin supplementation in recurring pregnancy loss: A controlled trial. *Fertil Steril* 1994;62(4):708–10.
20. Scott JR, Pattison N. Human chorionic gonadotrophin for recurrent miscarriage. *Cochrane Database Syst Rev* 1996(1):CD000101.
21. Carp HJ. Recurrent miscarriage and hCG supplementation: A review and metaanalysis. *Gynecol Endocrinol* 2010;26(10):712–6.
22. Morley LC, Simpson N, Tang T. Human chorionic gonadotrophin (hCG) for preventing miscarriage. *Cochrane Database Syst Rev* 2013;(1):CD008611.
23. El-Zibdeh MY. Dydrogesterone in the reduction of recurrent spontaneous abortion. *J Steroid Biochem Mol Biol* 2005;97(5):431–4.
24. Sandler SW, Baillie P. The use of human chorionic gonadotropin in recurrent abortion. *South Afr Med J* 1979;55(21):832–5.
25. Carp HJ. hCG supplementation in recurrent miscarriage: Pros and cons. In: *Gonadal and Nongonadal Actions of Gonadotropins.* Kumar ARC, Chaturvedi PK, Halder A, Rahman N eds. New Delhi: Narosa Publishing House; 2010.

18

Debate: Should Human Chorionic Gonadotropin Supplementation Be Used? No

Harish M. Bhandari and Siobhan Quenby

Introduction

Despite best efforts to identify the underlying causes of recurrent miscarriage (RM), it remains "unexplained" in the majority of cases. These couples request, and at times demand, treatment to achieve a successful reproductive outcome in a future pregnancy. As a result, many therapeutic interventions to supplement pregnancy hormones and/or to modify immune environment have evolved over the years. Most of the interventions have been used on an empirical basis with no strong evidence from well-designed studies. Here we argue that although human chorionic gonadotropin (hCG) supplementation has biological plausibility, it may have a detrimental effect on maternal decidualization, a crucial part of early pregnancy maintenance. A systematic review of the clinical evidence[1] does not support the use of hCG.

hCG is essential for the development of early pregnancy because it maintains the production of steroid hormone secretions from the corpus luteum. In addition, hCG has been found to have varied gonadal and extragonadal actions. hCG is a glycoprotein and is structurally similar to the other hormones in the glycoprotein hormone family, which includes luteinizing hormone (LH), follicle stimulating hormone (FSH), and thyroid stimulating hormone (TSH). These hormones have an identical α-subunit, but unique β-subunits that confer biological specificity. hCG is not a single molecule, but there are five different variants identified so far which share a common α-subunit and β-subunit amino acid sequence, but are found to have dissimilar functions.[2] The three important forms of hCG in early pregnancy are—(a) standard hCG produced by the syncytiotrophoblast, (b) sulfated hCG formed by the pituitary gonadotrophs[3] and (c) hyperglycosylated hCG (hCG-H) secreted exclusively by extravillous cytotrophoblasts.[4,5] The other two forms, hCGβ and hyperglycosylated hCGβ, are produced by most advanced cancers and may promote their invasion (except for choriocarcinoma and germ-cell tumors).[6,7]

Different isoforms of hCG have differing and multiple biological functions—standard hCG is responsible for promoting secretion of progesterone, involved in angiogenesis, differentiation of trophoblast cells and endometrial preparation for an implanting embryo. It is essential for preventing immune rejection of the invading feto-placental tissues, responsible for myometrial quiescence and also important for the development of fetal organs. Sulfated hCG, which has a higher circulating half-life than LH, supplements the action of LH in promoting ovulation, androstenedione production by theca cells and progesterone production by corpus luteal cells. The hCG-H enhances implantation by promoting the growth and invasion of cytotrophoblast cells. It has also been implicated in the evolution of choriocarcinoma and germ-cell cancers.[2]

hCG is detectable in the serum from the time of implantation and increases to a peak at 10 weeks of gestation, following which the levels remain stable throughout pregnancy. The principle function of hCG is to temporarily rescue the corpus luteum and to maintain the production of progesterone from the luteal cells. Progesterone production is taken over by the placenta at approximately seven weeks of pregnancy (luteo-placental shift).[8] Evidence from human studies suggests that the increasing amounts of hCG during the first few weeks of pregnancy are necessary for continued progesterone synthesis from the corpus luteum. In the absence of pregnancy, the administration of exogenous hCG is associated with prolonged corpus luteum function, provided that hCG was administered before the onset of luteal regression which occurs in the late luteal phase. In pregnant women with threatened miscarriage, hCG treatment is associated with a significant increase in hCG and progesterone levels.[9] In a series of clinical trials, Csapo and colleagues demonstrated that lutectomy prior to the seventh week of pregnancy caused a decrease in progesterone levels and subsequent miscarriage and that progesterone supplementation prevented the effect of lutectomy. However, when the corpus luteum was excised after the luteoplacental shift pregnancy was maintained, suggesting that the corpus luteum was no longer important for the production of progesterone.[8,10,11]

Spontaneous cyclical decidualization of the endometrial stromal compartment is an essential transformation that enables the endometrium to function as a biosensor and become receptive to, by responding to individual embryonic signals. Standard markers of decidualization are the induction of prokineticin-1 (PROK-1), a vital cytokine that regulates endometrial receptivity, prolactin (PRL) and insulin-like growth factor binding protein-1 (IGFBP-1). hCG strongly inhibits the expression of PROK-1, PRL[12] and IGFBP-1[13] in human decidualizing endometrial stromal cells from women with normal reproductive histories. Thus the trophoblast must be able to modulate the maternal decidual response. However, when this experiment was repeated with stromal cells from women with RM a different response, augmentation of PROK-1 and PRL expression occurred.[12] This very different response to hCG in stromal cells from women with RM suggests that hCG may not have a clinically beneficial effect on pregnancy outcome.

Suboptimal hCG levels reflect a failing early pregnancy and a number of observational clinical studies have found an association between the two. Ho et al.[14] found that early abnormal pregnancies were associated with insufficient hCG production, as reflected by lower hCG levels and an abnormal rate of increase. Additionally, the hCG was less biologically active than the hCG produced in normal pregnancies. However, Kato et al.[15] reported, in another observational study, that hCG levels and function in RM women suggested that the hCG levels were significantly lower compared to controls, but their biological activity was not different from that of normal women. This decreased production and possible altered function of the hCG may be due to the demise of trophoblast cells that precedes a miscarriage.

To summarize, it is apparent from these studies that hCG is critical to early pregnancy, ensuring active maintenance of steroid production from the corpus luteum and for endometrial preparation to facilitate implantation. The deficiency of this glycoprotein in early pregnancy is linked to adverse pregnancy outcomes such as miscarriage and RM. However hCG had, potentially, directly detrimental effects on decidualization *in vitro*.

Use of Human Chorionic Gonadotrophin Supplementation during Early Pregnancy

Threatened Miscarriage

Recent evidence is available from a Cochrane systematic review on hCG for threatened miscarriage.[16] The review included three studies, out of which two were prospective, double-blind, placebo-controlled trials (good-quality), involving a total of 312 women. The meta-analysis that compared hCG to placebo failed to demonstrate any benefit of hCG on the effect of miscarriage (RR 0.66; 95% CI 0.42–1.05). There was no significant difference in the outcome when only the two good-quality studies were analyzed separately (RR 0.83; 95% CI 0.46–1.46).

A recent Cochrane systematic review looking at "human chorionic gonadotrophin (hCG) for preventing miscarriage"[1] analyzed two studies (total 118 women) that were not in the previous review by Devaseelan et al.[16] No significant benefit was seen with hCG in minimizing the risk of threatened miscarriage (RR 0.52, CI 0.15–1.82).

It is important to note that, although the luteo-placental shift occurs at seven weeks of pregnancy and is complete by 12 weeks, suggesting that the physiological purpose of the corpus luteum is over by this time, the studies in this review had used hCG beyond this period.

Recurrent Miscarriage

There are many studies that have investigated the role of hCG supplementation for women with RM to improve subsequent pregnancy outcomes, and different results have been reported. A recently published Cochrane intervention review on hCG for preventing miscarriage[1] identified 12 studies, but included only five studies (Table 18.1)[17–21] that assessed the efficacy of prophylactic hCG in women with unexplained RM (302 women). The meta-analysis of these studies suggested that the use of hCG conferred an advantage over the placebo or no treatment by preventing miscarriage (RR 0.51, 95% CI 0.32–0.81). The mean number needed to treat (NNT) in order to achieve this benefit was seven.

Meta-analysis is a methodological tool used to pool the results of relevant trials on a specific topic in order to obtain a quantified synthesis, but "statistical heterogeneity" can be a problem for interpreting the results if excessive unexpected variation in the treatment effect occurs in one or some of the included studies. This meta-analysis was associated with heterogeneity and was mainly influenced by two studies,[17,18] which both intensely favored the use of hCG (Table 18.1). Additionally the various trials were not matched for known predictive factors such as maternal age, or number of miscarriages. Therefore, the random effects model would be more appropriate. When the random effects model was used to analyze these studies in order to minimize the heterogeneity, the authors found no significant difference in the treatment, placebo or no treatment arms. (RR 0.55, CI 0.28–1.09), but the heterogeneity still remained the same ($I^2 = 39\%$).

When the authors excluded the oldest two studies that had severe methodological weaknesses,[17,18] there was no significant benefit in using the hCG over the placebo or no treatment (RR 0.74, CI 0.44–1.23) (Table 18.2) and there was a greater homogeneity between the results ($I^2 = 0\%$). The authors finally concluded that there was not enough evidence to support the use of hCG in RM women and they reported that any improvement that could have occurred in the hCG group happened by chance.

A recent nonrandomized study, which involved 328 patients with three or more consecutive miscarriages, suggested that prophylactically administered hCG in early pregnancy statistically improved the

TABLE 18.1

hCG versus Placebo for Recurrent Miscarriage[a]

Study	Miscarriages per Treated Pregnancy		Risk Ratio (95% CI)
	Treatment	Control	
Svigos[17]	1/13	9/15	0.13 (0.02–0.51)
Harrison[18]	0/10	7/10	0.07 (0.00–1.03)
Harrison[19]	6/36	8/39	0.81 (0.31–2.11)
Quenby and Farquharson[20]	6/42	6/39	0.93 (0.33–2.64)
El-Zibdeh[21]	9/50	14/48	0.62 (0.30–1.29)
Total	22/151	44/151	0.51 (0.32–0.81)

Heterogeneity: $Chi^2 = 6.54$, df = 4 ($p = 0.16$); $I^2 = 39\%$.

[a] Figures quoted are the original figures of the papers in the Cochrane database.

TABLE 18.2

hCG versus Placebo for Recurrent Miscarriage Excluding Two Studies[a]

Study	Miscarriages per Treated Pregnancy		Risk Ratio (95% CI)
	Treatment	Control	
Harrison[19]	6/36	8/39	0.81 (0.31–2.11)
Quenby and Farquharson[20]	6/42	6/39	0.93 (0.33–2.64)
El-Zibdeh[21]	9/50	14/48	0.62 (0.30–1.29)
Total	21/128	28/126	0.74 (0.44–1.23)

Heterogeneity: $Chi^2 = 0.45$, df = 2 ($p = 0.80$); $I^2 = 0\%$.

[a] Figures quoted are the original figures of the papers in the Cochrane database.

TABLE 18.3

Results of a Randomized Controlled Trial of hCG in Women with Regular
Menstrual Cycles and Oligomenorrhea

Outcome	Oligomenorrhea		Regular Cycles	
	Placebo	hCG	Placebo	hCG
Miscarriages	6	2	4	4
Live births	4	11	25	25
Success rate (%)	40	85	86	86
p-value		<0.05		

live births by 15% (OR 1.88, 95% CI, 1.16–3.04).[22] The benefit was much higher (absolute benefit of 34%) in the group of women with five or more miscarriages (OR 4.33, 95% CI 1.7–11.3). Caution should be exercised in extrapolating the study results to the general population as the study is associated with selection bias and the groups are unlikely to be comparable.

There were no side effects of hCG reported in any of the studies and it appears that hCG remains safe for the mother. The risk of congenital defects was similar in both the groups suggesting that hCG did not increase the risk of congenital defects and was safe for the baby. The data were insufficient to comment on the effects of hCG on low birth weight, prematurity, neonatal death and cost.

Oligomenorrhea and Pregnancy Loss

Oligomenorrheic women may have associated endocrinological abnormalities which may put them at an increased risk of having an adverse pregnancy outcome. The incidence of oligomenorrhea in women with sporadic miscarriages is considerably higher (21%)[23] as compared to 0.9% in the general female population.[24] Hasegawa et al.[23] demonstrated that, in a population of 119 women with spontaneous first trimester miscarriage less than 11 completed weeks, more (34%) women who had a spontaneous miscarriage of an euploid pregnancy were oligomenorrheic when compared to women (12.5%) who had a pregnancy loss with an abnormal karyotype ($p < 0.01$). Further interesting observations from this study revealed that 57% of oligomenorrheic women miscarried a blighted ovum which was karyotypically normal. The findings are highly suggestive that oligomenorrhea and associated delayed ovulation are associated with miscarriage of euploid rather than aneuploid pregnancies. A prospective cohort study examined the role of using the medical history and investigation components of women to predict pregnancy outcome following RM.[25] Oligomenorrheic women were more likely to have a subsequent miscarriage whereas menstrual regularity predicted a successful pregnancy outcome. This group of oligomenorrheic women were found to have a difference in hormonal profile with low levels of oestradiol, but a normal progesterone profile in the luteal phase and a normal LH profile throughout the menstrual cycle when compared to women with regular cycles.

Quenby and Farquharson[20] performed a double-blind, placebo-controlled study investigating the role of hCG supplementation in women with idiopathic miscarriage (included in the Cochrane review of Morley et al.).[1] A subgroup analysis showed that, in women with RM and oligomenorrhea, administration of hCG in early pregnancy conferred a significant ($p = 0.039$) favorable outcome of a live birth (85%) when compared to placebo and supportive therapy (40%). There was no difference in the pregnancy outcome in women with regular cycles (Table 18.3). However subgroup analyses are prone to bias and the numbers were very small.

Conclusions

At present, the available evidence is insufficient to fully evaluate the effects of hCG supplementation during early pregnancy for women with unexplained RM. There are biological and clinical arguments both for and against its use as a treatment. At present, hCG support should be offered to women only within a research trial, and advocating empirical hCG treatment during the early stages of pregnancy, which can be very stressful, should be discouraged. There is an urgent need for an adequately powered, well-designed, prospective, randomized controlled trial comparing hCG supplementation to placebo, which may create an evidence-based role for using hCG to improve pregnancy outcome in women with RM. The design of any such trial should stringently follow standardized nomenclature and be restricted to women who miscarry chromosomally normal embryos. This type of trial is logistically possible, but would need to be multicentered because of the large number of women required to participate. There are therefore numerous financial implications to completing such a trial. A subgroup analysis should be carried out to accurately assess the efficacy of hCG in different subgroups, taking into consideration increased maternal age, number of prior miscarriages, obesity and menstrual irregularity. Recombinant hCG is pure compared to urinary hCG and a trial should also compare the safety and efficacy of these two forms of hCG.

REFERENCES

1. Morley LC, Simpson N, Tang T. Human chorionic gonadotrophin (hCG) for preventing miscarriage. *Cochrane Database Syst Rev* 2013;31;1:CD008611.
2. Cole LA. hCG, five independent molecules. *Clin Chim Acta* 2012;413:48–65.
3. Birken S, Maydelman Y, Gawinowicz MA et al. Isolation and characterization of human pituitary chorionic gonadotropin. *Endocrinology* 1996;137:1402–11.
4. Kovalevskaya G, Genbacev O, Fisher SJ et al. Trophoblast origin of hCG isoforms: Cytotrophoblasts are the primary source of chorio- carcinoma hCG. *Mol Cell Endocrinol* 2002;194:147–55.
5. Cole LA, Dai D, Butler SA et al. Gestational trophoblastic diseases: Pathophysiology of hyperglycosylated hCG-regulated neoplasia. *Gynecol Oncol* 2006;102:144–9.
6. Acevedo HF, Hartstock RJ. Metastatic phenotype correlates with high expression of membrane-associated complete ß-human chorionic gonadotropin in vivo. *Cancer* 1996;78:2388–99.
7. Regelson W. Have we found the "definitive cancer biomarker"? The diagnostic and therapeutic implications of human chorionic gonadotropin-beta statement as a key to malignancy. *Cancer* 1995;76:1299–301.
8. Csapo AI, Pulkkinen MO, Wiest WG. Effects of luteectomy and progesterone replacement therapy in early pregnant patients. *Am J Obstet Gynecol* 1973;115:759–65.
9. Qureshi NS, Edi-Osagie EC, Ogbo V et al. First trimester threatened miscarriage treatment with human chorionic gonadotrophins: A randomised controlled trial. *BJOG* 2005;112:1536–41.
10. Csapo AI, Pulkkinen MO, Ruttner B et al. The significance of the human corpus luteum in pregnancy maintenance. I. Preliminary studies. *Am J Obstet Gynecol* 1972;112:1061–7.
11. Csapo AI, Pulkkinen M. Indispensability of the human corpus luteum in the maintenance of early pregnancy. Luteectomy evidence. *Obstet Gynecol Surv* 1978;33:69–81.
12. Salker M, Teklenburg G, Molokhia M et al. Natural selection of human embryos: Impaired decidualization of endometrium disables embryo-maternal interactions and causes recurrent pregnancy loss. *PLoS One* 2010;5:e10287.
13. Licht P, Russu V, Lehmeyer S et al. Intrauterine microdialysis reveals cycle-dependent regulation of endometrial insulin-like growth factor binding protein-1 secretion by human chorionic gonadotropin. *Fertil Steril* 2002;78:252–8.
14. Ho HH, O'Connor JF, Nakajima ST et al. Characterization of human chorionic gonadotropin in normal and abnormal pregnancies. *Early Pregnancy* 1997;3:213–24.
15. Kato K, Mostafa MH, Mann K et al. Human chorionic gonadotropin exhibits normal biological activity in patients with recurrent pregnancy loss. *Gynecol Endocrinol* 2002;16:179–86.
16. Devaseelan P, Fogarty PP, Regan L. Human chorionic gonadotrophin for threatened miscarriage. *Cochrane Database Syst Rev* 2010;12:CD007422.
17. Svigos J. Preliminary experience with the use of human chorionic gonadotrophin therapy in women with repeated abortion. *Clin Reprod Fertil* 1982;1:131–5.
18. Harrison RF. Treatment of habitual abortion with human chorionic gonadotropin: Results of open and placebo-controlled studies. *Eur J Obstet Gynecol Reprod Biol* 1985;20:159–68.

19. Harrison RF. Human chorionic gonadotrophin (hCG) in the management of recurrent abortion; results of a multi-centre placebo-controlled study. *Eur J Obstet Gynecol Reprod Biol* 1992;47:175–9.
20. Quenby S, Farquharson RG. Human chorionic gonadotropin supplementation in recurring pregnancy loss: A controlled trial. *Fertil Steril* 1994;62:708–10.
21. El-Zibdeh MY. Dydrogesterone in the reduction of recurrent spontaneous abortion. *J Steroid Biochem Mol Biol* 2005;97:431–4.
22. Carp HJA. Recurrent miscarriage and hCG supplementation: A review and metaanalysis. *Gynecol Endocrinol* 2010;26:712–6
23. Hasegawa I, Takakuwa K, Tanaka K. The roles of oligomenorrhoea and fetal chromosomal abnormalities in spontaneous abortions. *Hum Reprod* 1996;11:2304–5.
24. Münster K, Schmidt L, Helm P. Length and variation in the menstrual cycle—A cross-sectional study from a Danish county. *Br J Obstet Gynaecol* 1992;5:422–9.
25. Quenby SM, Farquharson RG. Predicting recurring miscarriage: What is important? *Obstet Gynecol* 1993;82:132–8.

19

Antiphospholipid Syndrome—Pathophysiology

Rotem Inbar, Miri Blank, and Yehuda Shoenfeld

Introduction

The antiphospholipid syndrome (APS) was first defined as a syndrome in 1983,[1] consisting of recurrent thrombotic events and/or pregnancy loss, associated with the persistent presence of antiphospholipid antibodies (aPL). Several aPL subtypes are known, with the three formal diagnostic assays anticardiolipin (ACL), anti β-2 glycoprotein 1 (β_2GP1), and lupus anticoagulant (LAC).[2] Over the past few decades since initially defined, this syndrome has become known to be systemic, potentially affecting almost every organ system in the body. There is no single specific cause for APS but rather, as in other autoimmune diseases, a combination of environmental, hormonal, and genetic factors has been proposed.[3–5] Specifically within this definition, obstetric APS refers to pregnancy morbidity occurring in patients with persisting antiphospholipid antibodies.[6] Criteria used to define obstetric APS are one fetal loss after 10 weeks gestation; three or more early miscarriages with no other apparent explanation; preeclampsia or placental insufficiency, associated with a premature birth before 34 weeks of gestation.[7–9] It is recognized today that the presence of aPL represents the most frequent acquired risk factor for a treatable cause of recurrent pregnancy loss and associated obstetric complications.[2] The aPL are not only a diagnostic tool of APS, but rather participate in its pathophysiology with an active pivotal role, mediating several different manifestations of the syndrome.

Thrombosis of the placental vasculature was initially believed to be in the center of all adverse pregnancy outcomes related to this syndrome.[9] In more recent years, however, a heterogeneous group of clinical, experimental, and histopathological evidence has accumulated, showing how intraplacental thrombosis is far from being the sole mechanism involved.[10] Other mechanisms for placental and obstetric pathology have emerged, which will be discussed below. However, the basic immunology is summarized in Chapter 27.

The pathophysiology of APS involves all arms of the coagulation system, as well as other mechanisms not related to hypercoagulability. In fact antiphospholipid antibodies have been shown to be directly toxic to the developing fetus, as these antibodies can be passively transferred from humans to naive mice and will induce pregnancy loss in those mice.[11] Active immunization with human pathogenic monoclonal anticardiolipin antibody induces the clinical manifestations of antiphospholipid syndrome in BALB/c mice (Figure 19.1).[12] Additionally, the serum from women with APS is highly teratogenic to rat embryos in culture and also affects embryonic growth.[13] Moreover, purification of the IgG fraction of the sera of women with APS directly affects the embryo and yolk sac, reducing their growth.[14] This chapter discusses the etiology and pathophysiology of APS with a special emphasis on the obstetrical view and pregnancy loss.

Etiology of the Antiphospholipid Syndrome

Phospholipids (PL) are the basic components of all cell membranes where they are present in two layers. Each PL consists of a glycerol moiety attached to two esterified fatty acid chains (one saturated and one unsaturated) as well as a phosphodiester-linked alcohol side chain. In normal situations, the inner leaflet of the phospholipid bilayers is composed of negatively charged or anionic alcohol groups facing the cytoplasm, whereas the outer layer is composed of neutral or zwitterionic alcohol groups facing the

(a)

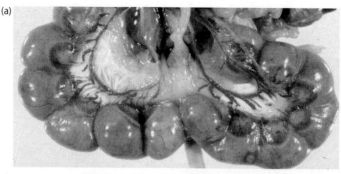

(b)

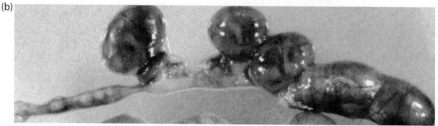

FIGURE 19.1   Healthy pregnant mouse versus APS pregnancy. (a) Healthy pregnancy and (b) mouse placental resorption equivalent to fetal loss in human.

extracellular fluid or blood stream.[15] Some conditions can break down the tolerance for "self" phospholipids and stimulate the formation of aPL. In the situation of ischemia, cell injury or abnormal immunoregulation (autoimmunity), negatively charged PLs can be exteriorized to the outer leaflet, while in the presence of excess calcium or low pH, cone-shaped, hexagonal phase phospholipid configurations can be formed. These changes may either provide an antigenic stimulus for the production of aPL or permit a number of serum proteins with procoagulant activity (β_2-glycoprotein I (β_2-GPI), prothrombin, protein C, protein S, and annexin V) to bind PL epitopes and to be presented to the immune system in unique "neoantigenic" conformations, which are recognized and give rise to aPL.[16] In the latter case, aPL may recognize either only the PL region of the complex or an epitope consisting of the portion of the PL and neighboring amino acids on the protein carrier or they clearly act with the protein alone.

Pregnancy itself appears to be a triggering event that allows protein cofactors to bind PL and become antigenic for aPL production. Placental tissues continuously change, and this major tissue remodeling results in externalization of inner surface PLs, which when appearing on the outer membrane may either be a direct stimulus for aPL production or permit plasma proteins to bind them so that neoantigens give rise to aPL. This has been documented for phosphatidylderine (PS). Despite the presence of an active membrane-associated adenosine triphosphate (ATP)-dependent aminophospholipid translocase that normally relocates PS from the outer to the inner monolayer, PS is exteriorized during trophoblast differentiation.[17] When exposed to the blood, PS allows $\beta2$-GPI to be immobilized and become antigenic for pathogenic aPL production.

Antiphospholipid antibodies have long been known to require a cofactor in order to exert their effects. This cofactor (apolipoprotein H or β_2-glycoprotein-1—β_2GP1), a negatively charged phospholipid binding protein, is the membrane antigen to which aPL bind. Binding of aPL to the β_2GP1 forms divalent IgG-β_2GP1complexes that have increased affinity for membrane phospholipid.[18] The physiological function of β_2GP1 is unknown. β_2GP1 deficiency is not associated with disease; homozygous β_2GP1 null mice also appear to suffer no pathological effects.[19] $\beta2$GP1-dependent aPL are thought to recognize their antigen on placental tissue, inhibit the growth and differentiation of trophoblasts, cause inflammation, defective angiogenesis and thrombosis, eventually leading to impaired placentation and subsequent placental function.

Similar to the majority of autoimmune diseases, it appears that APS too has a multifactorial etiology, in which genetic susceptibility is made apparent by environmental factors.

One such environmental factor that has been intensively investigated is infections. The infectious etiology of APS has been reported extensively. The infectious agents most commonly associated with APS are parvovirus B19, cytomegalovirus (CMV), toxoplasma, rubella, varicella, HIV, streptococcal and staphylococcal infections, gram-negative bacteria and mycoplasma pneumonia.[20,21] In a series of 100 APS patients, various infections have been shown to precede the development of APS, including skin infections (18%), HIV (17%), pneumonia (14%), hepatitis C virus (13%), and urinary tract infection (10%).[22] *Helicobacter pylori*, a common bacterial pathogen that colonizes the gastric mucosa and induces chronic gastric inflammation, has been associated with APS. In pregnant women, *H. pylori* infection can cause intrauterine fetal growth retardation, and increases the risk of reproductive disorders.[23,24]

As in other autoimmune disorders, molecular mimicry between (β_2GP1) and bacterial and viral epitopes is the principal mechanism by which infectious agents induce APS in genetically prone individuals. A molecular resemblance between β_2GP1 epitopes and infectious pathogens such as *Haemophilus influenzae*, *Neisseria gonorrhoeae*, *Helicobacter pylori*, CMV, and tetanus toxoid have been found.[25–28] Nevertheless, there are additional mechanisms by which infectious antigens induce autoimmunity and antibody production. Proteins sourced from infectious agents can cause polyclonal activation of a subset of T lymphocytes, or polyclonal B cell activation. Superantigens may also induce a nonspecific immune response. In the wide activation of the immune system, self- recognizing antibodies can be produced. Various infectious agents can modulate the release of cytokines and chemokines which are involved in growth, differentiation, and chemotaxis of the Th cell population and regulate MHC class 1 and 2 molecule expression.[27,30,31]

The β_2GP1 molecule seems to be the most significant antigen in APS. It has been widely investigated and found to be immunogenic *in vivo*. Passive transfer of anti-β_2GP1 antibodies induced experimental APS in naive mice.[11,32,33] Immunization of BALB/c, PL/J mice or New Zealand white rabbits with β_2GP1 resulted in the generation of anti-β_2GP1 antibodies. The high titers of mouse anti-β_2GP1 antibodies have been associated with an increased proportion of fetal resorption (the equivalent of fetal loss in humans), thrombocytopenia, and prolonged activated partial thromboplastin time (aPTT), indicating that lupus anticoagulant may also be active in experimental APS.[32] Oral administration of β_2GP1 to APS mice resulted in induction of tolerance to experimental APS.[34]

Direct experimental evidence for molecular mimicry of infectious pathogens has emerged from the effect of immunization with certain microbial pathogens that share epitope homology with the β_2GP1 molecule. Pathogenic anti-β_2GP1 autoantibodies directed against the TLRVYK epitope were formed in mice that were immunized with *H. influenzae* or *N. gonorrhoeae* that exhibit the TLRVYK sequence, or with tetanus toxoid that does not present linearly the sequence TLRVYK, but can still serve as a mimotope. The formed anti-β_2GP1 autoantibodies have been shown to be pathogenic and capable of inducing the clinical picture of experimental APS, manifested by a high proportion of fetal loss, thrombocytopenia, and a prolonged aPTT 27.[24] Induction of APS in two different nonautoimmune mice strains, the BALB/c and C57BL/6, was achieved by tetanus toxoid hyperimmunization using different adjuvants.[35,36] APS manifested differently in the two mice strains: fetal resorption or lowered fecundity. These observations demonstrate that environmental factors exert their effect based on the individual's genetic background. In a different study, the pathogenic effect of monoclonal antibodies to β_2GP1 was inhibited by the addition of synthetic peptides including the TLRVYK sequence. The latter prevented the development of APS in mice injected with monoclonal antibodies to β_2GP1, or decreased the degree of endothelial cell activation, monocyte adhesion and the expression of adhesion molecules *in vitro*.[37] Additionally, therapeutic alternatives for obstetric APS have been investigated. A CMV-derived synthetic peptide (TIFI) with specific affinity for the β_2GP1 phospholipid binding site has been shown to inhibit the adhesion of the aPL molecule to the trophoblast cell membrane *in vitro* in a dose-dependent manner.[38] These findings correlated with the protective effect of TIFI observed in *in vivo* animal models, in which injection of aPL at pregnancy day zero caused increased fetal loss rate and growth restriction, both significantly reduced by TIFI.[38]

It is important to note that while some infections, using the mechanisms listed above, may be the initiators of the cascade leading to APS development, others such as syphilis and Lyme disease cause the appearance of aPL antibodies that recognize phospholipids directly, without involving the phospholipid binding protein β_2GP1, thus not causing the antiphospholipid syndrome.

Another subset of environmental factors involved in immune mediated diseases including APS can be collectively termed "adjuvants". The role of adjuvants has become increasingly recognized in recent years. A novel syndrome has been introduced, ASIA (autoimmine syndrome induced by adjuvants), including vaccines, infectious agents, silicone, pristine, and aluminum salts under a common denominator.[39]

Over the past several decades it has become clear that infectious agents and vaccines have many similarities in their ability to facilitate antibody production, immune reactions and a wide spectrum of autoimmune phenomena.[30,31,40] The induction of autoimmunity is not surprising, as the essence of a vaccine is a live-attenuated or recombinant pathogenic antigen.[4,41,42] Apart from infectious antigen, vaccines contain additional substances which may harbor the ability to trigger an immune response. These are preservatives, adjuvants, and other manufacturing residues. The formal role of the adjuvant is augmentation of the immune response to the antigen. However, in recent years, many adjuvants have been found to trigger autoimmunity by themselves.[30,43-46] The ASIA syndrome incorporates previously distinguished medical conditions, and merges the diverse autoimmune and inflammatory conditions caused by different pharmaceutical, industrial or environmental compounds with the immune-mediating capabilities of causing the "adjuvant effect". Included in this category are not merely traditional vaccine-utilized adjuvants, but any substance having this immune triggering capacity. Some of the syndromes and phenomena included within ASIA are the Gulf War syndrome, chronic fatigue syndrome, macrophagic myofasciitis, and postvaccination phenomena, which appear to have surprising similarities and can be traced back to a common denominator—the adjuvant effect.[39] There are several lines of evidence by which APS can be related to the ASIA syndrome. In the literature, several vaccines have been correlated to the onset of APS, the common ones being tetanus toxoid vaccine, hepatitis B, and influenza.[47] In addition, induction of experimental APS, by immunization with tetanus toxoid added to different adjuvants, has led to different results regarding fertility in C57BL/6 mice.[48] Furthermore, immunization with complete Freund's adjuvant (CVA) or incomplete Freund's adjuvant (IFA—without *M. tuberculosis*) induced specific pathogenic β_2GP1 dependent autoantibodies in genetically hypercoagulation prone mice (heterozygous factor V Leiden mice). The central and intriguing finding in this study was the induction of high levels of aPL following adjuvant immunization alone.[49]

Mechanisms of Reproductive Failure in Antiphospholipid Syndrome

Thrombosis

Systemic thromboembolism is the principal manifestation of APS. Evidence for thrombi in the placental circulation and the beneficial effect of anti-thrombotic therapy in APS suggest that thrombosis has a central role in reproductive failure. The underlying basis for the hypercoagulable state in APS is complex, and involves altered activity of all three major components that govern hemostasis: platelets, fibrinolysis, and the coagulation cascade. The coagulation system in APS has been shown to be altered at different levels. aPL inhibit both protein C activation and the function of activated protein C (APC), thereby preventing the inactivation of activated factor V and VIII.[50] This inhibition is conditional upon the presence of β_2GP1 which is a prerequisite for the binding of aPL to protein C. In addition, autoantibodies directed against protein C, protein S, and thrombomodulin have been detected in some APS patients.[51]

Tissue factor, an initiator of the extrinsic coagulation cascade, which is not normally expressed by intravascular cells, has been shown to be altered in APS patients. It has been shown that tissue factor-related procoagulant activity and tissue factor mRNA levels in monocytes are increased in primary APS patients with thrombosis when compared to those without thrombosis.[52] Injection of purified IgG aCL from APS patients with previous thrombotic episodes induced a significant increase in both monocyte procoagulant activity and tissue factor expression, as compared with purified IgG or IgM aCL from two systemic lupus erythematosus (SLE) patients without thrombosis.[53] In addition, functional anti-tissue factor pathway inhibitor activity has been detected in the sera of a subset of APS patients, showing a correlation between the degree of inhibition and associated occurrence of arterial thrombosis and stroke.[54]

Endothelial cells are affected by aPL autoantibodies. Potentiation of human umbilical vein endothelial cells' (HUVEC) procoagulant activity by aPL contained in sera from SLE patients is strongly decreased after depleting IgG from the sera.[55] Human anti-β_2GP1 IgM monoclonal antibodies and polyclonal anti-β_2GP1 antibodies have been shown to induce tissue factor at both protein and mRNA level in HUVEC monolayers *in vitro*.[56] aPL can further upregulate adhesion molecules' (E-selectin, ICAM-1 and VCAM-1) expression and secretion of the proinflammatory cytokines IL-1b and IL-6.[57] Increased plasma levels of soluble VCAM-1 have been found in primary APS patients with recurrent thrombotic events, and elevated levels of tissue plasminogen activator and von Willebrand factor (as endothelial perturbation markers) have been associated with aPL in SLE.

Decreased endothelial cell prostacyclin 2 (PGI$_2$), the principal inhibitor of platelet aggregation, and increased thromboxane A2 (TXA$_2$) production by platelets have both been implicated as mechanisms predisposing to thrombosis in patients with APS. aPL enhance platelet TXA$_2$ production, and allow platelet activation to occur without a compensatory increment in the vascular biosynthesis of PGI$_2$.[58]

Hypofibrinolysis can further aggravate the prothrombotic state in APS. Endothelial cell dysfunction can increase plasma levels of type-1 plasminogen activator inhibitor and tissue-type plasminogen activator antigens.[59] In addition the hypofibrinolytic state can be further aggravated by the presence of autoantibodies against components of the fibrinolytic system such as anti-plasmin/plasminogen[60] and anti-tissue tPA (plasminogen activator).[61]

Platelets play a central role in primary hemostasis and are involved in the prothrombotic state of APS patients. Monoclonal aCL obtained from patients with APS increased platelet interaction with the subendothelium. It has been proposed that a minor degree of platelet activation can lead to exposure of phospholipids which can potentially be amplified to a much larger degree in the serum of APS patients than in controls.[53] β_2GP1 initially bind to these phospholipids, then bind aPL to form β_2GP1-phospholipid complexes. The latter can further activate platelet aggregation by allowing the interaction between the Fc portion and the platelet surface FcγRII receptors (the only FcγR molecules present on platelets).[53,62] In addition to activation of the FcγRII receptors, the β2GP1-phospholipid complexes can also exert their action through complement activation as complement generated in the presence of aPL binds to negatively charged phospholipids and activate platelets.[63]

In addition to the systemic prothrombotic effects, aPL may alter the placental circulation by attacking certain placental epitopes. Annexin A5, a potent anticoagulant protein that has a thrombomodulatory role in the placental circulation is such a target.[64] Annexin V is found on the apical surface of placental syncytiotrophoblast and forms clusters on exposed phospholipids, thereby forming a protective shield on the phospholipid surface. Annexin V blocks phospholipids from becoming available for coagulation reactions. The annexin V protective shield could be damaged by either binding to anti-annexin V or preventing its binding to the PL membrane, or by blocking autoantibodies against annexin V/PL.[65] Anti-annexin V autoantibodies have been detected in patients with SLE and APS associated with pregnancy loss, while reduced levels of annexin V have been observed on the placental villi of women having aPL and recurrent pregnancy loss and a thrombogenic background.[66]

Thrombosis in the placental vasculature was initially thought to be the main cause of adverse pregnancy outcome in women with APS. More recent data, however, and the heterogeneity of histological lesions seen in APS placentas, suggest that placental thrombosis is far from being the only accountable mechanism.

Arachidonic Acid and Prostacyclin

Antiphospholipid antibodies inhibit arachidonic acid release.[67] Arachidonic acid is an essential prerequisite for prostacyclin production. (Prostacyclin is a physiological inhibitor of thrombocyte aggregation, and a potent vasodilatator). aPL have been shown to increase the concentration of TXA$_2$ thus altering the thromboxane/prostacyclin balance.[68] The alteration in the PGI$_2$/TXA$_2$ balance has two effects, vasoconstriction which impedes the blood supply to the fetus, and platelet activation with the procoagulant effects as described above.

In a mouse model of experimental APS, Shoenfeld and Blank[69] infused ACL to pregnant mice in order to induce APS. Mice which were cotreated with a thromboxane receptor antagonist had a significant reduction in the fetal resorption rate from 45% to 19.8% and an increase in mean placental and embryo weights. There was also an increased platelet count (from 597,100 to 1,075,000 platelets/mm³) in treated mice, indicating the effect of thrombocyte aggregation in APS.

Inflammatory Responses

During pregnancy, the maternal immune responses undergo immense changes to allow for normal implantation and development of the growing fetus. There is evidence for a dynamic balance between proinflammatory and anti-inflammatory mediators in normal pregnancy. An imbalance towards proinflammatory mediators (complement, tumor necrosis factor, and chemokines) has been linked to aPL-induced fetal loss in animal models.[70] Following fetal resorption due to injection of IgG with aPL activity to pregnant naive mice, histological examination of the decidua has revealed deposition of human IgG with mouse complement, neutrophil infiltration and local TNF secretion. A systemic transient increase in TNF was also noted. Complement involvement in inducing aPL-mediated fetal loss is supported by several lines of evidence.[71–73] Additionally, the protective effect of heparin in a mouse model has been related to the anti-complement rather than anticoagulant activity.[74] A recent study has demonstrated that aPL, by activation of toll-like receptor 4 (TLR4), induce uric acid production response in human trophoblast, which in turn activates the Nalp3/ASC (apoptosis associated speck-like protein) inflammasome complex, leading to IL-1β secretion. This novel mechanism has been suggested to account for the inflammation at the maternal–fetal interface in patients with APS.[75] The anti-inflammatory cytokine, IL-3, is important for the maintenance of normal pregnancy. IL-3 enhances placental and fetal development while increasing the number of megakaryoctes. The serum level of IL-3 in pregnant patients with primary APS or APS secondary to SLE has been found to be lower than in controls.[76] *In vitro* studies have revealed that low dose aspirin (10 mg/microliters) stimulates IL-3 production through its ability to raise leukotriene production while higher doses of aspirin failed to induce IL-3 generation.[76,77] Furthermore, ciprofloxacin treatment significantly decreased the rate of pregnancy loss in BALB/c mice with experimental APS. This effect correlated to an increase in the serum IL-3 level and of bone marrow megakaryocytes.[78] Other cytokines may also be involved. The level of the proinflammatory and prothrombotic cytokine TNF-α, has been shown to be significantly higher in patients with APS than healthy controls.[79] Trophoblast cells express the surface antigen CD1d, bearing PS. In a recent study, anti-β2GP1 antibodies were shown to interact with the PS-bearing CD1d, causing release of IL12 and induction of IFNα production, thus supplying additional evidence that APS-related pregnancy loss involves an inflammatory mechanism.[80]

Defective Endometrial Angiogenesis

The decidua, a newly formed tissue on the maternal side of the placenta, is a place of active angiogenesis and structural modification of the spiral arteries in early pregnancy. Endometrial angiogenesis and decidualization, as well as trophoblast invasion, are crucial for a successful pregnancy. A most important role in the process of basement membrane and matrix degradation, enabling invasion by the trophoblast, is carried out by matrix metalloproteinases (MMP). aPL-mediated inhibition of trophoblast invasion was one of the suggested additional mechanisms for recurrent pregnancy loss in these patients.[81] Several studies have evaluated the effect of aPL on endometrial angiogenesis. aPL may affect the maternal side of the placenta by directly binding human endometrial endothelial cells (HEEC). As a consequence, a significant decrease in both the number and the total length of the capillaries formed in HEEC was observed. In this study, the effect of aPL on HEEC angiogenesis was examined both *in vitro* and *in vivo* in a murine model. The modulation of vascular endothelial growth factor (VEGF) and MMP activity by aPL was associated with a significant reduction in angiogenesis in both the *in vitro* and *in vivo* model. Moreover, aPL was found to reduce both VEGF and MMP production and nuclear factor κB (NFKB) DNA (promoter gene for several MMP) binding activity in a dose-dependent manner.[82] A complementary study demonstrated the beneficial effect of low molecular weight heparin (LMWH) on the aPL inhibited HEEC angiogenesis. The addition of LMWH restored VEGF secretion and MMP activity. This evidence further explains the improved pregnancy outcome seen in aPL patients treated with LMWH.[83] The uterine sonographic characteristics of patients with recurrent aPL-associated miscarriages have been compared to normal fertile women. Parameters such as endometrial thickness, volume, microvessel density (MVD), uterine artery pulsatility index (PI) and resistance index (RI), endometrial vascularization index (VI), flow index (FI), and vascularization flow index (VFI) were measured in the mid-luteal phase of the menstrual cycle. Whereas both groups had similar endometrial thickness, volume, MVD, uterine artery PI and RI, the VI, FI, and VFI were significantly reduced in the aPL group compared to controls.[84]

Alteration of Placental Cell Death

During the course of pregnancy, trophoblast fragments of varying sizes are shed from the placenta into the maternal circulation.[85] In normotensive pregnancy, trophoblast debris is considered the result of mostly programmed cell death. In pregnancies complicated by pre-eclampsia, the process may be more necrotic.[86] Trophoblast debris is partly cleared from the body by endothelial cells. Under normal apoptotic conditions, these endothelial cells in turn become activated, a process not seen when necrotic debris is engulfed by these cells.[87] aPL have been shown to increase the amount of necrotic trophoblast debris from placental explants, which under these conditions do activate endothelial cells. This evidence demonstrates how endothelial cells exhibit different behavior in the presence of aPL.[88] In summary, antiphospholipid antibodies cause increased shedding of necrotic trophoblast debris from the placenta, which contributes to endothelial activation and dysfunction. More recently, antiphospholipid antibodies were also shown to prolong the activation of endothelial cells induced by necrotic trophoblast debris.[89] In a study by Pantham et al., RNA from first trimester placentas treated with aPL was extracted and genomic data analyzed using microarrays. Changes in the transcriptome of placental explants were observed, including the mRNA of multiple genes involved in the regulation of apoptosis.[90]

Further evidence supporting the placental death mechanism in women with APS comes from observation of decreased vasculosyncytial membranes, increased syncytial knots, substantially more fibrosis, hypovascular villi and infarcts from placental histopathological findings in these women.[91] These changes in syncytial membranes may be attributable to thrombosis, although thrombosis could also be secondary to placental damage and cell death, which allows free transplacental passage of maternal aPL. Addition of sera with IgG purified from women with SLE/APS, positive for aCL/anti-DNA antibodies reduced yolk sac and embryonic growth more than sera negative for aPL, but positive for anti-phosphatidylserine and for anti-laminin. The sera of SLE/APS patients has also been shown to inhibit the rate of trophoblastic cell growth and to accelerate the rate of apoptosis of cultured human placental cells.[14,92]

Conclusions

APS is a systemic syndrome whose etiology involves both environmental and genetic factors. Infections may play a highly important part in the etiology of this syndrome, using different mechanisms and predominantly molecular mimicry to induce aPL. Other environmental factors that appear to influence progression of the syndrome are vaccines and other adjuvants, as demonstrated by the ASIA syndrome. aPL exert their pathogenic effects via various mechanisms, including the induction of a hypercoagulable state, inflammatory processes, defective angiogenesis and alterations in placental cell death patterns. In recurrent pregnancy loss the combination of low-molecular-weight heparin and low-dose aspirin is considered to be the treatment of choice. Therapy of APS is traditionally directed towards eliminating the increased thrombotic state, but heparins/LMWH appear to have additional qualities in preventing adverse pregnancy outcome by their anti-inflammatory and proangiogenic properties. However, when therapy fails, other interventions aimed at controlling the levels of autoantibodies rather than their effects should be considered, and immune modulating therapies might theoretically be of value.

REFERENCES

1. Hughes GR. Thrombosis, abortion, cerebral disease, and the lupus anticoagulant. *Br Med J* 1983;287:1088–9.

2. Miyakis S, Lockshin MD, Atsumi T et al. International consensus statement on an update of the classification criteria for definite antiphospholipid syndrome (APS). *J Thromb Haemostasis* 2006;4:295–306.

3. de Carvalho JF, Pereira RM, Shoenfeld Y. The mosaic of autoimmunity: The role of environmental factors. *Front Biosci* 2009;1:501–9.

4. Shoenfeld Y, Zandman-Goddard G, Stojanovich L et al. The mosaic of autoimmunity: Hormonal and environmental factors involved in autoimmune diseases—2008. *Isr Med Assoc J* 2008;10:8–12.

5. Shoenfeld Y, Gilburd B, Abu-Shakra M et al. The mosaic of autoimmunity: Genetic factors involved in autoimmune diseases—2008. *Isr Med Assoc J* 2008;10:3–7.

6. Branch W on behalf of the Obstetric Task Force. Report of the Obstetric APS Task Force: 13th International Congress on Antiphospholipid Antibodies, April 13, 2010. *Lupus* 2011;20:158–64.

7. Ruiz-Irastorza G, Crowther M, Branch W, Khamashta MA. Antiphospholipid syndrome. *Lancet* 2010;376:1498–509.

8. Giannakopoulos B, Passam F, Ioannou Y, Krilis SA. How we diagnose the antiphospholipid syndrome. *Blood* 2009;113:985–94.

9. Cohen D, Berger SP, Steup-Beekman GM et al. Diagnosis and management of the antiphospholipid syndrome. *BMJ* 2010;340:c2541.

10. Meroni PL, Borghi MO, Raschi E, Tedesco F. Pathogenesis of antiphospholipid syndrome: Understanding the antibodies. *Nat Rev Rheumatol* 2011;7:330–9.

11. Blank M, Cohen J, Toder V, Shoenfeld Y. Induction of anti-phospholipid syndrome in naive mice with mouse lupus monoclonal and human polyclonal anti-cardiolipin antibodies. *Proc Natl Acad Sci U S A* 1991;88:3069–73.

12. Bakimer R, Fishman P, Blank M et al. Induction of primary antiphospholipid syndrome in mice by immunization with a human monoclonal anticardiolipin antibody (H-3). *J Clin Invest* 1992;89:1558–63.

13. Ornoy A, Yacobi S, Avraham S, Blumenfeld Z. The effect of sera from women with systemic lupus erythematosus and/or antiphospholipid syndrome on rat embryos in culture. *Reprod Toxicol* 1998;12:185–91.

14. Ornoy A, Yacobi S, Matalon ST et al. The effects of antiphospholipid antibodies obtained from women with SLE/APS and associated pregnancy loss on rat embryos and placental explants in culture. *Lupus* 2003;12:573–8.

15. Cullis PR, Hope MJ, Tilcockn CP. Lipid polymorphism and the roles of lipids in membranes. *Chem Phys Lipids* 1986;40:127–44.

16. Lockwood CJ, Rand JH. The immunobiology and obstetrical consequences of antiphospholipid antibodies. *Obstet Gynecol Surv* 1994;49:432–41

17. Lyden TW, Vogt E, Ng AK et al. Monoclonal antiphospholipid antibody reactivity against human placental trophoblast. *J Reprod Immunol* 1992;22:1–14.

18. Rand JH. The antiphospholipid syndrome. *Annu Rev Med* 2003;54:409–24.

19. Sheng Y, Reddel SW, Herzog H et al. Impaired thrombin generation in beta 2-glycoprotein I null mice. *J Biol Chem* 2001;276:13817–21.

20. Garcia-Carrasco M, Galarza-Maldonado C, Mendoza-Pinto C, Escarcega RO, Cervera R. Infections and the antiphospholipid syndrome. *Clin Rev Allergy Immunol* 2009;36:104–8.

21. Zinger H, Sherer Y, Goddard G et al. Common infectious agents prevalence in antiphospholipid syndrome. *Lupus* 2009;18:1149–53.

22. Cervera R, Asherson RA, Acevedo ML et al. Antiphospholipid syndrome associated with infections: Clinical and microbiological characteristics of 100 patients. *Ann Rheum Dis* 2004;63:1312–7.

23. Eslick GD, Yan P, Xia HH et al. Foetal intrauterine growth restrictions with *Helicobacter pylori* infection. *Aliment Pharmacol Ther* 2002;16:1677–82.

24. Figura N, Piomboni P, Ponzetto A et al. *Helicobacter pylori* infection and infertility. *Eur J Gastroenterol Hepatol* 2002;14:663–9.

25. Blank M, Shoenfeld Y. Beta-2-glycoprotein-I, infections, antiphospholipid syndrome and therapeutic considerations. *Clin Immunol* 2004;112:190–9.

26. Sorice M, Pittoni V, Griggi T et al. Specificity of anti-phospholipid antibodies in infectious mononucleosis: A role for anti-cofactor protein antibodies. *Clin Exp Immunol* 2000;120:301–6.

27. Blank M, Krause I, Fridkin M et al. Bacterial induction of autoantibodies to beta2-glycoprotein-I accounts for the infectious etiology of antiphospholipid syndrome. *J Clin Invest* 2002;109:797–804.

28. Gharavi AE, Pierangeli SS, Espinola RG et al. Antiphospholipid antibodies induced in mice by immunization with a cytomegalovirus-derived peptide cause thrombosis and activation of endothelial cells in vivo. *Arthritis Rheum* 2002;46:545–52.

29. Cruz-Tapias P, Blank M, Anaya JM, Shoenfeld Y. Infections and vaccines in the etiology of antiphospholipid syndrome. *Curr Opin Rheumatol* 2012;24:389–93.

30. Shoenfeld Y. Infections, vaccines and autoimmunity. *Lupus* 2009;18:1127–8.

31. Kivity S, Agmon-Levin N, Blank M, Shoenfeld Y. Infections and autoimmunity—Friends or foes? *Trends Immunol* 2009;30:409–14.

32. Blank M, Faden D, Tincani A et al. Immunization with anticardiolipin cofactor (beta-2-glycoprotein I) induces experimental antiphospholipid syndrome in naive mice. *J Autoimmun* 1994;7:441–55.

33. Pierangeli SS, Harris EN. *In vivo* models of thrombosis for the antiphospholipid syndrome. *Lupus* 1996;5:451–5.

34. Blank M, George J, Barak V et al. Oral tolerance to low dose beta 2-glycoprotein I: Immunomodulation of experimental antiphospholipid syndrome. *J Immunol* 1998;161:5303–12.

35. Inic-Kanada A, Stojanovic M, Zivkovic I et al. Murine monoclonal antibody 26 raised against tetanus toxoid cross-reacts with beta2-glycoprotein I: Its characteristics and role in molecular mimicry. *Am J Reprod Immunol* 2009;61:39–51.

36. Zivkovic I, Stojanovic M, Petrusic V et al. Induction of APS after TTd hyper-immunization has a different outcome in BALB/c and C57BL/6 mice. *Am J Reprod Immunol* 2011;65:492–502.

37. Blank M, Shoenfeld Y, Cabilly S et al. Prevention of experimental antiphospholipid syndrome and endothelial cell activation by synthetic peptides. *Proc Natl Acad Sci U S A* 1999;96:5164–8.

38. de la Torre YM, Pregnolato F, D'Amelio F et al. Anti-phospholipid induced murine fetal loss: Novel protective effect of a peptide targeting the beta2 glycoprotein I phospholipid-binding site. Implications for human fetal loss. *J Autoimmun* 2012;38:J209–15.

39. Shoenfeld Y, Agmon-Levin N. 'ASIA'—Autoimmune/inflammatory syndrome induced by adjuvants. *J Autoimmun* 2011;36:4–8.

40. Orbach H, Agmon-Levin N, Zandman-Goddard G. Vaccines and autoimmune diseases of the adult. *Discovery Med* 2010;9:90–7.

41. Molina V, Shoenfeld Y. Infection, vaccines and other environmental triggers of autoimmunity. *Autoimmunity* 2005;38:235–45.

42. Agmon-Levin N, Paz Z, Israeli E, Shoenfeld Y. Vaccines and autoimmunity. *Nat Rev Rheumatol* 2009;5:648–52.

43. Nancy AL, Shoenfeld Y. Chronic fatigue syndrome with autoantibodies—The result of an augmented adjuvant effect of hepatitis-B vaccine and silicone implant. *Autoimmun Rev* 2008;8:52–5.

44. Satoh M, Kuroda Y, Yoshida H et al. Induction of lupus autoantibodies by adjuvants. *J Autoimmun* 2003;21:1–9.

45. Shaw CA, Petrik MS. Aluminum hydroxide injections lead to motor deficits and motor neuron degeneration. *J Inorg Biochem* 2009;103:1555–62.

46. Toplak N, Avcin T. Vaccination of healthy subjects and autoantibodies: From mice through dogs to humans. *Lupus* 2009;18:1186–91.

47. Blank M, Israeli E, Shoenfeld Y. When APS (Hughes syndrome) met the autoimmune/inflammatory syndrome induced by adjuvants (ASIA). *Lupus* 2012;21:711–4.

48. Zivkovic I, Petrusic V, Stojanovic M et al. Induction of decreased fecundity by tetanus toxoid hyper-immunization in C57BL/6 mice depends on the applied adjuvant. *Innate Immun* 2012;18:333–42.

49. Katzav A, Kivity S, Blank M et al. Adjuvant immunization induces high levels of pathogenic antiphospholipid antibodies in genetically prone mice: Another facet of the ASIA syndrome. *Lupus* 2012;21:210–6.

50. de Groot PG, Horbach DA, Derksen RH. Protein C and other cofactors involved in the binding of antiphospholipid antibodies: Relation to the pathogenesis of thrombosis. *Lupus* 1996;5:488–93.

51. Pengo V, Biasiolo A, Brocco T et al. Autoantibodies to phospholipid-binding plasma proteins in patients with thrombosis and phospholipid-reactive antibodies. *Thromb Haemostasis* 1996;75:721–4.

52. Cuadrado MJ, Lopez-Pedrera C, Khamashta MA et al. Thrombosis in primary antiphospholipid syndrome: A pivotal role for monocyte tissue factor expression. *Arthritis Rheum* 1997;40:834–41.

53. Reverter JC, Tassies D, Font J et al. Effects of human monoclonal anticardiolipin antibodies on platelet function and on tissue factor expression on monocytes. *Arthritis Rheum* 1998;41:1420–7.

54. Forastiero RR, Martinuzzo ME, Broze GJ. High titers of autoantibodies to tissue factor pathway inhibitor are associated with the antiphospholipid syndrome. *J Thromb Haemostasis* 2003;1:718–24.

55. Oosting JD, Derksen RH, Blokzijl L, Sixma JJ, de Groot PG. Antiphospholipid antibody positive sera enhance endothelial cell procoagulant activity—Studies in a thrombosis model. *Thromb Haemostasis* 1992;68:278–84.

56. Kornberg A, Renaudineau Y, Blank M et al. Anti-beta 2-glycoprotein I antibodies and anti-endothelial cell antibodies induce tissue factor in endothelial cells. *Isr Med Assoc J* 2000;2(Suppl):27–31.

57. Meroni PL, Raschi E, Camera M et al. Endothelial activation by aPL: A potential pathogenetic mechanism for the clinical manifestations of the syndrome. *J Autoimmun* 2000;15:237–40.

58. Lellouche F, Martinuzzo M, Said P et al. Imbalance of thromboxane/prostacyclin biosynthesis in patients with lupus anticoagulant. *Blood* 1991;78:2894–9.

59. Jurado M, Paramo JA, Gutierrez-Pimentel M, Rocha E. Fibrinolytic potential and antiphospholipid antibodies in systemic lupus erythematosus and other connective tissue disorders. *Thromb Haemostasis* 1992;68:516–20.

60. Yang CD, Hwang KK, Yan W et al. Identification of anti-plasmin antibodies in the antiphospholipid syndrome that inhibit degradation of fibrin. *J Immunol* 2004;172:5765–73.

61. Cugno M, Cabibbe M, Galli M et al. Antibodies to tissue-type plasminogen activator (tPA) in patients with antiphospholipid syndrome: Evidence of interaction between the antibodies and the catalytic domain of tPA in 2 patients. *Blood* 2004;103:2121–6.

62. Font J, Espinosa G, Tassies D et al. Effects of beta2-glycoprotein I and monoclonal anticardiolipin antibodies in platelet interaction with subendothelium under flow conditions. *Arthritis Rheum* 2002;46:3283–9.

63. Shibata S, Sasaki T, Hirabayashi Y et al. Risk factors in the pregnancy of patients with systemic lupus erythematosus: Association of hypocomplementaemia with poor prognosis. *Ann Rheum Dis* 1992;51:619–23.

64. Wang X, Campos B, Kaetzel MA, Dedman JR. Annexin V is critical in the maintenance of murine placental integrity. *Am J Obstet Gynecol* 1999;180:1008–16.

65. Rand JH, Wu XX, Andree HA et al. Pregnancy loss in the antiphospholipid-antibody syndrome—A possible thrombogenic mechanism. *New Engl J Med* 1997;337:154–60.

66. Matsubayashi H, Arai T, Izumi S et al. Anti-annexin V antibodies in patients with early pregnancy loss or implantation failures. *Fertil Steril* 2001;76:694–9.

67. Carreras LO, Vermylen JG. "Lupus" anticoagulant and thrombosis—Possible role of inhibition of prostacyclin formation. *Thrombosis and Haemostasis* 1982;48:38–40.

68. Robbins DL, Leung S, Miller-Blair DJ, Ziboh V. Effect of anticardiolipin/beta2-glycoprotein I complexes on production of thromboxane A2 by platelets from patients with the antiphospholipid syndrome. *J Rheumatol* 1998;25:51–6.

69. Shoenfeld Y, Blank M. Effect of long-acting thromboxane receptor antagonist (BMS 180,291) on experimental antiphospholipid syndrome. *Lupus* 1994;3:397–400.

70. Meroni PL, Tedesco F, Locati M et al. Anti-phospholipid antibody mediated fetal loss: Still an open question from a pathogenic point of view. *Lupus* 2010;19:453–6.

71. Holers VM, Girardi G, Mo L et al. Complement C3 activation is required for antiphospholipid antibody-induced fetal loss. *J Exp Med* 2002;195:211–20.

72. Girardi G, Berman J, Redecha P et al. Complement C5a receptors and neutrophils mediate fetal injury in the antiphospholipid syndrome. *J Clin Invest* 2003;112:1644–54.

73. Berman J, Girardi G, Salmon JE. TNF-alpha is a critical effector and a target for therapy in antiphospholipid antibody-induced pregnancy loss. *J Immunol* 2005;174:485–90.

74. Girardi G, Redecha P, Salmon JE. Heparin prevents antiphospholipid antibody-induced fetal loss by inhibiting complement activation. *Nat Med* 2004;10:1222–6.

75. Mulla MJ, Salmon JE, Chamley LW et al. A role for uric acid and the Nalp3 inflammasome in antiphospholipid antibody-induced IL-1beta production by human first trimester trophoblast. *PloS One* 2013;8:e65237.

76. Fishman P, Falach-Vaknin E, Sredni B et al. Aspirin-interleukin-3 interrelationships in patients with anti-phospholipid syndrome. *Am J Reprod Immunol* 1996;35:80–4.

77. Fishman P, Falach-Vaknin E, Sredni B et al. Aspirin modulates interleukin-3 production: Additional explanation for the preventive effects of aspirin in antiphospholipid antibody syndrome. *J Rheumatol* 1995;22:1086–90.

78. Blank M, George J, Fishman P et al. Ciprofloxacin immunomodulation of experimental antiphospholipid syndrome associated with elevation of interleukin-3 and granulocyte-macrophage colony-stimulating factor expression. *Arthritis Rheum* 1998;41:224–32.

79. Bertolaccini ML, Atsumi T, Lanchbury JS et al. Plasma tumor necrosis factor alpha levels and the -238*A promoter polymorphism in patients with antiphospholipid syndrome. *Thromb Haemostasis* 2001;85:198–203.

80. Iwasawa Y, Kawana K, Fujii T et al. A possible coagulation-independent mechanism for pregnancy loss involving beta(2) glycoprotein 1-dependent antiphospholipid antibodies and CD1d. *Am J Reprod Immunol* 2012;67:54–65.

81. Pierangeli SS, Chen PP, Raschi E et al. Antiphospholipid antibodies and the antiphospholipid syndrome: Pathogenic mechanisms. *Semin Thromb Hemostasis* 2008;34:236–50.

82. Di Simone N, Di Nicuolo F, D'Ippolito S et al. Antiphospholipid antibodies affect human endometrial angiogenesis. *Biol Reprod* 2010;83:212–9.

83. D'Ippolito S, Marana R, Di Nicuolo F et al. Effect of low molecular weight heparins (LMWHs) on antiphospholipid antibodies (aPL)-mediated inhibition of endometrial angiogenesis. *PloS One* 2012;7:e29660.

84. Chen L, Quan S, Ou XH, Kong L. Decreased endometrial vascularity in patients with antiphospholipid antibodies-associated recurrent miscarriage during midluteal phase. *Fertil Steril* 2012;98:1495–502 e1.

85. Askelund KJ, Chamley LW. Trophoblast deportation part I: Review of the evidence demonstrating trophoblast shedding and deportation during human pregnancy. *Placenta* 2011;32:716–23.

86. Huppertz B, Kingdom J, Caniggia I et al. Hypoxia favours necrotic versus apoptotic shedding of placental syncytiotrophoblast into the maternal circulation. *Placenta* 2003;24:181–90.

87. Chen Q, Stone PR, McCowan LM, Chamley LW. Phagocytosis of necrotic but not apoptotic trophoblasts induces endothelial cell activation. *Hypertension* 2006;47:116–21.

88. Chen Q, Viall C, Kang Y et al. Anti-phospholipid antibodies increase non-apoptotic trophoblast shedding: A contribution to the pathogenesis of pre-eclampsia in affected women? *Placenta* 2009;30:767–73.

89. Chen Q, Guo F, Hensby-Bennett S et al. Antiphospholipid antibodies prolong the activation of endothelial cells induced by necrotic trophoblastic debris: Implications for the pathogenesis of preeclampsia. *Placenta* 2012;33:810–5.

90. Pantham P, Rosario R, Chen Q et al. Transcriptomic analysis of placenta affected by antiphospholipid antibodies: Following the TRAIL of trophoblast death. *J Reprod Immunol* 2012;94:151–4.

91. Out HJ, Kooijman CD, Bruinse HW, Derksen RH. Histopathological findings in placentae from patients with intra-uterine fetal death and anti-phospholipid antibodies. *Eur J Obstet Gynecol Reprod Biol* 1991;41:179–86.

92. Matalon ST, Shoenfeld Y, Blank M et al. Antiphosphatidylserine antibodies affect rat yolk sacs in culture: A mechanism for fetal loss in antiphospholipid syndrome. *Am J Reprod Immunol* 2004;51:144–51.

20

Diagnosis of Antiphospholipid Antibody-Associated Abortions

Marighoula Varla-Leftherioti

Introduction

Antiphospholipid antibodies (aPL) are a heterogeneous group of autoantibodies directed against different antigens, predominantly anionic phospholipids or phospholipid-containing structures. aPL have been associated with pregnancy disorders, including spontaneous miscarriage and recurrent miscarriage. The diagnostic approach of aPL-associated abortions includes the following steps: (i) identification of candidates for investigation, (ii) selection and application of the appropriate diagnostic tests, and (iii) evaluation of the results obtained, in order to choose those women that will benefit from treatment and the kind of treatment to be used.

Identification of Women for Investigation

In 1999 the American Society of Reproductive Immunology defined a broad clinical entity: reproductive autoimmune syndrome (RAS).[1] RAS has been defined as a diagnostic entity to include women having autoimmune clinical symptoms either limited to the reproductive system (reproductive autoimmune failure syndrome—RAFS)[2] or systemic autoimmune disturbances related to the anti-phospholipid syndrome (APS).

The clinical and laboratory findings of APS and RAFS are shown in Table 20.1.

aPL antibodies are recognized to have the strongest association with pregnancy loss among all other factors causing immune-mediated abortions (aPL-associated abortions). There is evidence that 2–20% of women with recurrent pre-embryonic or embryonic pregnancy losses have increased titers of aPL and that these women have an 80–90% pregnancy loss rate with half of their pregnancies lost in the first trimester.

According to the American Society of Reproductive Immunology, an aPL-related etiology should be suspected in women with three or more consecutive pre-embryonic or embryonic pregnancy losses or one or more unexplained fetal deaths above 10 weeks of gestation.[1] Testing should also be considered in women with fewer miscarriages if they have experienced thrombosis or autoimmune thrombocytopenia (criteria of APS) or have a history of endometriosis or unexplained difficulty in conceiving, or even a history of fetal growth retardation, severe pre-eclampsia or other obstetric complications in previous successful pregnancies (criteria of RAFS). Women should also be investigated if histology has revealed thromboses in the placenta of previously missed miscarriages, and should be combined with tests for detecting hereditary thrombophilias.

Diagnostic Tests—Evaluation of the Results

aPL can be detected using sensitive solid-phase immunoassays or coagulation tests. Both assays are easy to perform, but care is required in interpretation of the results. In order to distinguish between those women at risk of abortion and those not at risk, it is important to consider the following parameters:

TABLE 20.1

Clinical and Laboratory Findings in Reproductive Autoimmune Syndrome

	Antiphospholipid Syndrome (APS)	Reproductive Autoimmune Failure Syndrome (RAFS)

Clinical features	• Thrombosis (≥1 unexplained venous or arterial thrombosis, including stroke)
	• Autoimmune thrombocytopenia
	• Recurrent pregnancy loss
	  ≥1 consecutive and otherwise unexplained fetal deaths (≥10 wk)
	  ≥3 consecutive and otherwise unexplained pre-embryonic or embryonic pregnancy losses
		• Fetal growth retardation (<34 week)
		• Severe pre-eclampsia
		• Obstetric complications (abruption placenta, chorea gravidarum, herpes gestationis, HELLP syndrome[a])
		• Unexplained infertility
		• Endometriosis
		• Recurrent pregnancy loss
		  ≥1 consecutive and otherwise unexplained fetal deaths (≥10 wk)
		  ≥3 consecutive and otherwise unexplained pre-embryonic or embryonic pregnancy losses

Laboratory findings	• Anticardiolipin antibodies (ACA) (>20 GPL or MPL units) • Lupus anticoagulant (LAC)	• Antiphospholipid antibodies • Lupus anticoagulant • Gammopathy (usually polyclonal, mostly IgM) • Antinuclear antibodies (including antibodies against histones) • Organ-specific autoantibodies (antithyroid antibodies-ATA, anti-smooth muscle antibodies -ASMA)

[a]Hemolysis, elevated liver enzymes, and low platelet count.

(a) the assays to be used, (b) the type and (c) the isotype of aPL to be identified, (d) the antibody level to be evaluated, (e) the interpretation of the results in relation to the heterogeneity of aPL and clinical data, and (f) the timing for testing.

Assays for the Detection of Antiphospholipid Antibodies

aPL that do not prolong phospholipid-dependent clotting assays can be detected by immunoassays using phospholipid-coated surfaces. Hence, antibodies against cardiolipin (aCL), phosphatidylethanolamine (aPE), phosphatidylserine (aPS), phosphatodylcholine (aPC), phosphatidylglycerol (aPG), phosphatidylinositol (aPI), phosphatidic acid (aPA), and β_2-glycoprotein I (aβ_2GPI) are identified by standardized enzyme-linked immunosorbent assays (ELISA) using surfaces coated with the relevant phospholipid (usually complexed with cofactor proteins). The results are expressed in aPL units, with 1 unit being equivalent to the binding capacity of 1 µg/mL pure phospholipids. Depending on their immunoglobulin isotype (IgG, IgM, IgA), aPL units are defined as GPL, MPL, APL. aPL ELISA tests have high sensitivity, but low specificity, and the interpretation of their results is difficult. For the results to be reliable, the assays must be properly standardized, standard calibrators must be used, and the range of normal values must derive from measurements of aPL levels in a large number of normal individuals.[3]

For the detection of aPL that prolong phospholipid-dependent clotting assays (lupus anticoagulant, LAC), clotting time prolongation assays are used, in which prolongation of clotting is not corrected with normal plasma, but with the addition of phospholipids. The activated partial thromboplastin time (aPTT), and the diluted Russel viper venom time (dRVVT) are the recommended tests.[4]

Type of Antiphospholipid Antibodies

Classically, the work-up for the diagnosis of aPL-associated abortions was limited to the detection of LAC (prolonged time of at least one phospholipid-dependent clotting assay) and the detection of β_2GPI-dependent IgG and IgM aCL antibodies in the serum (aCL-IgG >20 GPL units/mL or/and aCL-IgM >20 MPL units/mL). LAC and increased aCL-IgG antibodies are independently associated with recurrent first and second trimester fetal loss and can be used as prognostic and diagnostic markers.[5] It has been reported that women positive for LAC or aCL have a 16% and 38% rate of pregnancy loss, respectively.[6,7] Studies in women with RPL not receiving anticoagulation, have shown that LAC is most associated with second rather than first trimester miscarriages.[8] Moreover, the presence of aCL in the absence of LAC most likely reduces the chance of live birth by 36–48% compared with the absence of both aCL and LAC,[9] while the detection of aCL before gestation or an increase during gestation are considered as bad prognostic markers for the outcome of pregnancy.[10]

Today, it has become apparent that, although extremely useful, the diagnostic tests for LAC and aCL may not be sufficient for diagnosing all patients with aPL-associated pregnancy loss or to elucidate underlying pathology. A percentage of women experiencing RPL may be negative for aCL but positive for other aPL. Several studies have shown that if only aCL are measured, 10–63% of positive aPL are detected and 37–90% of women with RAFS will have the diagnosis missed.[11,12] It is currently suggested that for the diagnosis of RAFS-related abortions, a full aPL panel should be assessed including:- LAC, aCL, aPE, aPS, aPC, aPG, aPI, aPA, aβ_2GPI.[13] However, the diagnostic value of aPLs other than aCL is extremely controversial.[14] It is thought that the presence of more than one aPL is a more accurate variable than the presence of one aPL in predicting pregnancy loss.[15]

Antibodies against Phosphatidylserine and Phosphatidylethanolamine

Measurement of aPS and aPE antibodies is indicated in women with early recurrent pregnancy losses, since they represent those aPL that affect the cell division during embryogenesis and the normal function of the trophoblast.[16] It has been shown that the trophoblastic layer directly in contact with the maternal circulation is more reactive with aPS than with aCL,[17] and the aPS assay is more sensitive than testing for aCL in RAS-related abortions.[18,19] aPE testing is also advisable, as higher titers of IgG and IgM aPE have been reported in patients with RPL before the 10th week of gestation compared to parous women. Moreover, aPE antibodies appear to be a reliable risk factor for early fetal losses (due to the effect on trophoblast formation), and late pregnancy loss (due to binding to PE-kininogen complexes which results in thrombin-induced platelet aggregation).[20]

Antibodies against Phosphatodylcholine, Phosphatidylglycerol, Phosphatidic Acid, and Phosphatidylinositol

Some studies have shown a predominance of PC, PG, PA, and PI antibodies in women with RPL, but their roles are less clear, and their diagnostic significance has not been established.[21–23]

Antibodies against Cofactor Proteins

Antibodies against cofactor proteins (prothrombin, annexin V, β_2GPI) may be found in women with RPL, but their clinical significance is uncertain. Since these particular antibodies usually coexist with aCL, their effect as independent risk factors for miscarriage is not broadly accepted, and testing for them is not usually included in the investigation. β_2GPI is the main cofactor protein which binds phospholipids.[24] The specific function of β_2GPI remains unclear. However, pathogenic aPLs bind to the first domain of β_2GPI.[25] Consequently anti-β_2GPI antibodies have been included in the revised laboratory criteria for APS.[26] Women with autoantibodies directed against β_2GPI exhibit an increased risk for pregnancy morbidity,[27,28] and testing is considered reasonable in cases where aPL-associated abortions are suspected.[29]

Antibodies against Annexin V

Annexin V is necessary to maintain the integrity of placental structure.[30] Antibodies against Annexin V (aAnxV) are also increased in women with recurrent miscarriage. Although a recent study found no association between aAnxV and the risk of miscarriage,[28] several other studies suggest that aAnxV may be an independent risk factor for early RPL.[31–34] In contrast, anti-prothrombin (aPT) antibodies, although increased in RPL, do not appear to be independently associated with miscarriage and are not usually included in the diagnostic panel.[35]

Isotype of Antiphospholipid Antibodies

Most aPL are of the IgG or IgM class, but a small number, (10%) may be IgA. Some studies report a predominance of IgG antibodies in women with repeated miscarriages,[21] but some others have found that the majority of aPL are of the IgM isotype,[19,36] or that positivity for IgM aCL could be better correlated to pregnancy outcome than IgG aCL positivity.[9,19] In order to avoid misdiagnosis both IgG and IgM isotypes should be assessed. Testing for IgA isotype-specific antibodies is not recommended for women clinically suspected of having aPL-associated abortion.[29]

Titer of Antiphospholipid Antibodies

As low levels of aPL may be found in the normal population, low titers detected in women with RPL should not be considered as risk factors for aPL-associated abortions (above the risk conferred by their medical history), and are of doubtful clinical significance.[37] However, medium and high titers of aCL and/or other aPL antibodies (>40 GPL units) identify the women who would benefit from pharmacological prophylaxis in the next pregnancy. Eighty percent of women with very high levels of aCL (>80 GPL) and a history of previous miscarriage(s) are expected to have fetal death in their next pregnancy.[19,38]

Heterogeneity of Antiphospholipid Antibodies

Depending on type, aPL affect pregnancy through different pathways. aCL, aPE, and aPS target relevant phospholipids on endothelial cells and lead to thrombosis in placental vessels. However, aPE and aPS also target relevant phospholipids on the trophoblast and affect cell division during embryogenesis and the formation of the syncytium.[16] Furthermore, these antibodies and the aPC, aPG, and aPI target relevant phospholipids in pre-embryonic tissues.[39] The above data should be considered in the work-up. In second trimester fetal death where thromboses have been found in the placenta, it is advisable to test for antibodies with an anticoagulant effect (aCL, aPS), However, in women with early pregnancy and pre-embryonic losses, the work-up should include aPL inhibiting trophoblastic cell function (aPS, aPE) and possibly those affecting implantation (aPS, aPE, aPC, aPI, aPG, aPA).

Time of Testing

Since aPL may appear transiently in normal individuals,[40] it is recommended that in order to establish the diagnosis of aPL-associated abortions, increased titers of aPL should be detected in two specimens drawn at an interval of 12 weeks. Furthermore, aPL that are increased during an unsuccessful pregnancy may decrease afterwards. Hence, aPL assays are of diagnostic value if performed during pregnancy or at a time close to pregnancy loss. Occasionally, aCL seem to remain high outside pregnancy.[41]

Epilogue

Because of the various types, the different isotypes, and the heterogeneity of aPL antibodies, a complete investigation expected to provide the maximum sensitivity for the identification of the women with aPL-associated abortions would include more than 10 different tests. To maintain a reasonable cost–benefit ratio, one has to choose the antibodies with the greatest diagnostic accuracy, while taking the clinical features into account. We suggest testing for aCL and aPS antibodies, and, according to the results, to continue by assessing other aPL. Such an algorithm is shown in Figure 20.1.

Finally, in women where an aPL-associated etiology is suspected, it should be borne in mind that other autoantibodies may coexist, which are included in the diagnostic criteria of RAFS (e.g. antinuclear antibodies, antithyroid antibodies). Furthermore, in women found positive for aPL, it is necessary to exclude coexisting infections or recent vaccination, because some infectious pathogens (*Helicobacter pylori*, hepatitis C virus, *Haemophilus influenzae*, *Neisseria gonorrhoeae*, tetanus toxoid) trigger the formation of antibodies targeting not only microbial epitopes but also phospholipid/protein

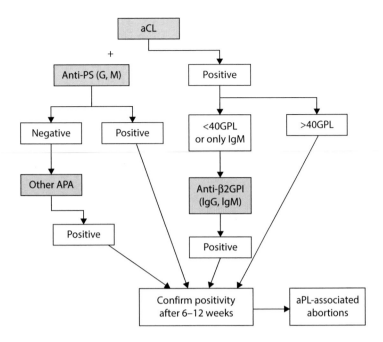

FIGURE 20.1   Algorithm for the diagnosis of aPL-associated abortions.

epitopes (e.g., epitopes of β_2GPI), as a result of molecular mimicry between them.[42,43] Detection of the above antibodies (autoantibodies, cross-reactive antibodies) will help to appropriately treat the women.

REFERENCES

1. Coulam CB, Branch DW, Clark DA et al. American Society for Reproductive Immunology report of the Committee for establishing criteria for diagnosis of reproductive autoimmune syndrome. *Am J Reprod Immunol* 1999;41:121–32.
2. Gleicher N, el-Roeiy A. The reproductive autoimmune failure syndrome. *Am J Obstet Gynecol* 1988;159:223–7.
3. Tincani A, Allegri F, Balestrieri G et al. Minimal requirements for antiphospholipid antibodies ELISAs proposed by the European Forum on antiphospholipid antibodies. *Thromb Res* 2004;114:553–8.
4. Pengo V, Tripodi A, Reber G et al. Update of the guidelines for lupus anticoagulant detection. Subcommittee on lupus anticoagulant/antiphospholipid antibody of the scientific and standardisation committee of the international society on thrombosis and haemostasis. *J Thromb Haemostasis* 2009;7:1737–40.
5. Creagh MD, Malia RG, Cooper SM et al. Screening for lupus anticoagulant and anticardiolipin antibodies in women with fetal loss. *J Clin Pathol* 1991;44:45–7.
6. Pattison NS, Chamley LW, McKay EJ et al. Antiphospholipid antibodies in pregnancy: Prevalence and clinical associations. *Br J Obstet Gynaecol* 1993;100:909–13.
7. Lockwood CJ, Romero R, Feinberg RF et al. The prevalence and biologic significance of lupus anticoagulant and anticardiolipin antibodies in a general obstetric population. *Am J Obstet Gynecol* 1989;161:369–73.
8. Carp HJ, Menashe Y, Frenkel Y et al. Lupus anticoagulant. Significance in habitual first-trimester abortion. *J Reprod Med* 1993;38:549–52.
9. Nielsen HS, Christiansen OB. Prognostic impact of anticardiolipin antibodies in women with recurrent miscarriage negative for the lupus anticoagulant. *Hum Reprod* 2005;20:1720–8.
10. Kwak JY, Barini R, Gilman-Sachs A et al. Down-regulation of maternal antiphospholipid antibodies during early pregnancy and pregnancy outcome. *Am J Obstet Gynecol* 1994;171:239–46.

11. Yetman DL, Kutteh WH. Antiphospholipid antibody panels and recurrent pregnancy loss: Prevalence of anticardiolipin antibodies compared with other antiphospholipid antibodies. *Fertil Steril* 1996;66:540–6.

12. Rote NS. Antiphospholipid antibodies other than lupus anticoagulant and anticardiolipin antibodies in women with recurrent pregnancy loss, fertile controls, and antiphospholipid syndrome. *Obstet Gynecol* 1997;90:642–4.

13. Coulam CB. The role of antiphospholipid antibodies in reproduction: Questions answered and raised at the 18th Annual Meeting of the American Society of Reproductive Immunology. *Am J Reprod Immunol* 1999;41:1–4.

14. Branch DW, Silver R, Pierangeli S et al. Antiphospholipid antibodies other than lupus anticoagulant and anticardiolipin antibodies in women with recurrent pregnancy loss, fertile controls, and antiphospholipid syndrome. *Obstet Gynecol* 1997;89:549–55.

15. Aoki K, Hayashi Y, Hirao Y, Yagami Y. Specific antiphospholipid antibodies as a predictive variable in patients with recurrent pregnancy loss. *Am J Reprod Immunol* 1993;29:82–7.

16. McIntyre JA. Antiphospholipid antibodies in implantation failures. *Am J Reprod Immunol* 2003; 49:221–9.

17. Lyden TW, Vogt E, Ng AK et al. Monoclonal antiphospholipid antibody reactivity against human placental trophoblast. *J Reprod Immunol* 1992;22:1–14.

18. Rote NS, Dostal-Johnson D, Branch DW. Antiphospholipid antibodies and recurrent pregnancy loss: Correlation between the activated partial thromboplastin time and antibodies against phosphatidylserine and cardiolipin. *Am J Obstet Gynecol* 1990;163:575–84.

19. Umehara N, Tanaka T. The incidence of various antiphospholipid antibodies, measured by commercial-based laboratory, with recurrent spontaneous abortion and the impact of their profiles on reproductive outcome with active anticoagulant therapy. *Obstet Gynecol* 2012;2012:819356.

20. Sugi T, Matsubayashi H, Inomo A et al. Antiphosphatidylethanolamine antibodies in recurrent early pregnancy loss and mid-to-late pregnancy loss. *J Obstet Gynecol Res* 2004;30:326–32.

21. Kaider AS, Kaider BD, Janowicz PB et al. Immunodiagnostic evaluation in women with reproductive failure. *Am J Reprod Immunol* 1999;42:335–46.

22. Franklin RD, Kutteh WH. Antiphospholipid antibodies (APA) and recurrent pregnancy loss: Treating a unique APA positive population. *Hum Reprod* 2002;17:2981–5.

23. Ulcova-Gallova Z, Krauz V, Novakova P et al. Anti-phospholipid antibodies against phosphatidylinositol, and phosphatidylserine are more significant in reproductive failure than antibodies against cardiolipin only. *Am J Reprod Immunol* 2005;54:112–7.

24. McNeil HP, Simpson RJ, Chesterman CN et al. Antiphospholipid antibodies are directed against a complex antigen that includes a lipid-binding inhibitor of coagulation: β2-glycoprotein I (apolipoprotein H). *Proc Natl Acad Sci U S A* 1990;87:4120–4.

25. de Laat B, Derksen RH, Urbanus RT et al. IgG antibodies that recognize epitope Gly40-Arg43 in domain I of beta 2-glycoprotein I cause LAC, and their presence correlates strongly with thrombosis. *Blood* 2005;105:1540–5.

26. Miyakis S, Losckin MD, Atsumi T et al. International consensus statement on an update of the classification criteria for definite antiphospholipid syndrome (APS). *J Thromb Haemostasis* 2006;4:295–306.

27. Zammiti W, Mtiraoui N, Kallel C et al. A case-control study on the association of idiopathic recurrent pregnancy loss with autoantibodies against beta2-glycoprotein I and annexin V. *Reproduction* 2006;131:817–22.

28. Alijotas-Reig J, Ferre-Oliveras R, Rodrigo-Anoro MJ et al. Anti-beta(2)-glycoprotein-I and anti-phosphatidylserine antibodies in women with spontaneous pregnancy loss. *Fertil Steril* 2010;93:2330–6.

29. Ortel TL. Antiphospholipid syndrome: Laboratory testing and diagnostic strategies. *Am J Hematol* 2012;87(Suppl 1):S75–81.

30. Wang X, Campos B, Kaetzel MA et al. Annexin V is critical in the maintenance of murine placental integrity. *Am J Obstet Gynecol* 1999;180:1008–16.

31. Matsuda J, Gotoh M, Saitoh N et al. Anti-annexin antibody in the sera of patients with habitual fetal loss or preeclampsia. *Thromb Res* 1994;75:105–6.

32. Matsubayashi H, Arai T, Izumi S et al. Anti-annexin V antibodies in patients with early pregnancy loss or implantation failure. *Fertil Steril* 2001;76:964–9.

33. Bizzaro N, Tonutti E, Villalta D et al. Prevalence and clinical correlation of anti-phospholipid-binding protein antibodies in anticardiolipin-negative patients with systemic lupus erythematosus and women with unexplained recurrent miscarriages. *Arch Pathol Lab Med* 2005;129:61–8.
34. Sater MS, Finan RR, Mustafa FE et al. Anti-annexin V IgM and IgG autoantibodies and the risk of idiopathic recurrent spontaneous miscarriage. *J Reprod Immunol* 2011;89:78–83.
35. Sater MS, Finan RR, Abu-Hijleh FM et al. Anti-phosphatidylserine, anti-cardiolipin, anti-β2 glycoprotein I and anti-prothrombin antibodies in recurrent miscarriage at 8–12 gestational weeks. *Eur J Obstet Gynecol Reprod Biol* 2012;163:170–4.
36. Matzner W, Chong P, Xu G et al. Characterization of antiphospholipid antibodies in women with recurrent spontaneous abortions. *J Reprod Med* 1994;39:27–30.
37. Silver RM, Porter TF, van Leeuwen I et al. Anticardiolipin antibodies: Clinical consequences of "low titers". *Obstet Gynecol* 1996;87:494–500.
38. Reece EA, Garofalo J, Zheng XZ et al. Pregnancy outcome. Influence of antiphospholipid antibody titer, prior pregnancy losses and treatment. *J Reprod Med* 1997;42:49–55.
39. Coulam CB. Antiphospholipid antibody round table report. *Am J Reprod Immunol* 2002;48:262–5.
40. Harris EN, Pierangeli S, Birch D Anticardiolipin wet workshop report. Fifth International Symposium on antiphospholipid antibodies. *Am J Clin Pathol* 1994;101:616–24.
41. Ruiz JE, Cubillos J, Mendoza JC et al. Autoantibodies to phospholipids and nuclear antigens in non-pregnant and pregnant Colombian women with recurrent spontaneous abortions. *J Reprod Immunol* 1995;28:41–51.
42. Harel M, Aron-Maor A, Sherer Y et al. The infectious etiology of the antiphospholipid syndrome: Links between infection and autoimmunity. *Immunobiology* 2005;210:743–7.
43. Cruz-Tapias P, Blank M, Anaya JM et al. Infections and vaccines in the etiology of antiphospholipid syndrome. *Curr Opin Rheumatol* 2012;24:389–93.

21

Management of Antiphospholipid Syndrome in Pregnancy

Alana B. Levine and Michael D. Lockshin

Introduction

Antiphospholipid syndrome (APS) is a systemic autoimmune disorder of vascular thrombosis and/or pregnancy complications. This disease is defined by the presence of both clinical and laboratory criteria.[1] The clinical manifestations of obstetric APS include recurrent early miscarriage, fetal loss, early and/or severe pre-eclampsia, and intrauterine growth restriction (IUGR). Thrombotic APS may include arterial or venous thrombotic events, such as stroke or deep vein thrombosis, or thrombotic microangiopathy. Laboratory criteria include one or more of the following autoantibodies at medium to high titers on more than one occasion at least 12 weeks apart: lupus anticoagulant (LAC), anticardiolipin antibodies (aCL), and/or anti-β_2-glycoprotein-I antibodies (aβ_2GPI).

This chapter outlines the treatment and monitoring of APS pregnancy, beginning with therapeutic options and then describing treatment recommendations in various clinical scenarios.

Specific Therapies in Antiphospholipid Syndrome Pregnancy

Combination heparin and aspirin is standard therapy in pregnant women with a history of obstetric APS. Some treatments used in refractory cases of APS pregnancy include intravenous immunoglobulin (IVIG), hydroxychloroquine (HCQ), and plasma exchange.

Aspirin

Aspirin may affect embryo implantation and placental development by modulating the balance of thromboxane, prostacyclin, and IL-3 production.[2] Aspirin is nearly universally used in the treatment of APS pregnancy, although literature supporting its use is somewhat contradictory. While one observational study demonstrated a lower rate of adverse pregnancy outcomes among patients receiving aspirin at the time of the first study visit,[3] a randomized, placebo-controlled trial of low dose aspirin (LDA) versus placebo in APS patients with recurrent miscarriage failed to show a benefit in the LDA-treated group.[4] This latter result is difficult to interpret as live birth rates in the placebo group exceeded those in published studies. There was also no benefit in a meta-analysis performed by Empson et al. in 2005.[5] However, the results from a recent observational study suggest that patients treated with aspirin had fewer adverse outcomes.[6] LDA is recommended by the American College of Obstetricians and Gynecologists during subsequent pregnancies of APS patients with a history of recurrent pregnancy loss.[7]

Unfractionated Heparin and Low-Molecular-Weight Heparin

The mechanisms of heparin therapy in APS pregnancy include antithrombotic effects, inhibition of complement activation, direct antiphospholipid antibody (aPL) binding, and inhibition of tissue factor-mediated immunopathology in the placental bed.[8] The results of heparin trials in obstetric APS patients are conflicting with regard to heparin's role in improving pregnancy outcomes in APS patients. While several studies demonstrated superior outcomes in aPL-positive patients receiving combination heparin and aspirin therapy,[5,9–13] others found no benefit of combination therapy over aspirin alone.[14,15] In a single-center trial of 50 persistently aCL-positive women, each with at least three consecutive pregnancy losses, Kutteh found significantly improved outcomes in the group receiving unfractionated heparin with LDA compared to the LDA-only group with live birth rates of 80 and 44 percent, respectively.[9] Another study of 90 aPL-positive women with recurrent pregnancy loss also randomized patients to combination heparin and LDA versus LDA alone.[12] In this study, Rai et al. demonstrated live birth rates of 71 percent in the combination therapy group using enoxaparin and 42 percent in the group treated with LDA alone. In contrast, Farquharson et al. failed to find a difference in the outcomes between two similar groups, when dalteparin was used.[14] The study by Farquharson et al.[14] randomized 98 persistently-aPL positive women to receive low molecular weight heparin (LMWH) and LDA or LDA alone, with live birth rates of 72 and 78 percent, respectively, although it should be noted that success rates were high in both groups. Ziakas et al. performed a systematic review and meta-analysis further examining the effect of combination heparin and aspirin therapy on pregnancy outcome in aPL-positive women with recurrent pregnancy loss.[13] Using pooled data from five randomized controlled trials, these authors found heparin therapy to decrease the risk of first trimester losses (OR 0.39, 95% CI 0.24–0.65, number needed to treat six). A recent observational study suggested that heparin may not be effective in patients with lupus anticoagulant.[6]

Both unfractionated heparin (UFH) and LMWH have been shown to be safe and effective in preventing recurrent pregnancy loss.[16,17] Both formulations carry risks of bleeding, osteopenia, and heparin-induced thrombocytopenia, although these risks appear to be lower with LMWH than UFH. There are no comparison studies between LMWH and UFH. They are assumed to be equivalent, but this assertion remains in need of proof.

Warfarin and Other Oral Anticoagulants

Warfarin has been used by some for APS patients requiring therapeutic anticoagulation during late stages of pregnancy. The benefits of switching from heparin to warfarin include lower cost, lower risk of osteoporosis, and respite from self-injection. Warfarin should be avoided during the first trimester (and heparin used instead) due to its potentially teratogenic effects. Anticoagulant therapy should be switched back to heparin toward the end of the third trimester in preparation for labor and delivery.

There are no data regarding the use of oral factor Xa inhibitors, including rivaroxaban and apixaban, in APS patients. Rivaroxaban is considered unsafe in pregnancy and data are insufficient to evaluate the safety of apixaban in pregnancy. We do not recommend the use of either of these drugs in the treatment of APS pregnancy.

Hydroxychloroquine

Evidence for using HCQ in the treatment of APS pregnancy comes from mechanistic studies in which HCQ reversed the effects of aPL on syncytiotrophoblasts by reducing immunoglobulin binding and restoring annexin A5 expression.[18] Long thought to have anti-thrombotic effects, HCQ has been shown to lower the incidence of thrombotic events in lupus patients.[19–23] It is considered safe in both pregnancy and lactation. We suggest the use of HCQ as an adjunctive therapy in those patients who have incidentally been found to have positive aPL (without thrombotic or adverse pregnancy events), aPL-positive lupus patients, and in obstetric APS patients refractory to standard heparin/aspirin combination therapy.

Intravenous Immunoglobulin

Intravenous immunoglobulin (IVIG) has been studied in obstetric APS patients with recurrent fetal loss despite combination heparin and aspirin therapy. An initial case report in 1988 described successful delivery of a live infant at 34 weeks' gestation to a patient treated with two courses of IVIG after nine previous miscarriages.[24] Larger studies have failed to demonstrate improved outcomes in subsequent

APS pregnancies. Two randomized controlled trials comparing combination heparin and aspirin therapy to IVIG alone showed fewer live births and more first trimester miscarriages in the IVIG group.[25,26] Another trial studied the addition of IVIG to standard treatments, comparing combination heparin and aspirin therapy alone with combination heparin, aspirin, and IVIG.[27] There was no significant difference in outcomes between these two groups, although it should be noted that all pregnancies resulted in live birth. Dosing regimens and protocols for IVIG administration vary widely amongst reports and studies; dosing ranged from 400 to 1000 mg/kg daily for one to five consecutive days each month.[27–29] Despite the lack of evidence in favor of its use, IVIG still may serve as adjunctive therapy for patients with refractory disease. Although IVIG does not seem to offer much advantage over standard treatment in terms of live births, there is evidence that the incidence of obstetric complications such as pregnancy induced hypertension, pre-eclampsia, gestational diabetes, intrauterine growth restriction, prematurity and placental abruption [30–33] may be lower. If IVIG is used, anticoagulation continues throughout treatment. Additionally, the cost of IVIG is prohibitive.

Plasma Exchange

Case reports and case series describe the use of plasma exchange in obstetric APS patients who were refractory to treatment with heparin and aspirin combination therapy.[34,35] Plasma exchange regimens varied from one to four sessions per week throughout pregnancy. These reports describe reductions in aPL titers following treatment and rates of successful pregnancy were generally high. Additional studies of plasma exchange in refractory APS pregnancies are warranted.

Glucocorticoids

The literature does not support the use of glucocorticoids in the treatment of APS pregnancy.[36–38] Steroids have been associated with an increased risk of both adverse pregnancy events (pre-eclampsia, IUGR, premature rupture of membranes, premature delivery, and gestational diabetes) as well as maternal complications (osteopenia, avascular necrosis, and infection). In the absence of other indications, we do not recommend the use of glucocorticoids as treatment for APS pregnancy, unless indicated for vasculitis, or other autoimmune phenomena.

Treatment Recommendations by Clinical Scenario

Patients with Prior Thrombosis

APS patients with a history of thrombosis are generally maintained on long-term or lifelong thromboprophylaxis with warfarin. Women of childbearing age should have a thorough understanding of the teratogenic potential of warfarin between weeks six and 12 of gestation[39] and take appropriate contraceptive precautions. Upon confirmation of a positive pregnancy test, warfarin should be replaced with therapeutic doses of heparin, preferably LMWH (such as enoxaparin 1 mg/kg given subcutaneously *twice* daily).[40,41] We generally continue LMWH throughout pregnancy, but if cost or other considerations come into effect, warfarin may be used during mid- to late pregnancy. Warfarin may be restarted at 14 weeks of gestation, then replaced again with LMWH at 36 weeks or two weeks prior to planned delivery. As in the nonpregnant state, the International Normalized Ratio (INR) should be monitored closely and maintained in a range of 2 to 3.[42]

Patients with Recurrent Pregnancy Loss

Patients with a history of recurrent pregnancy loss are generally treated with LDA and prophylactic doses of LMWH. This recommendation comes from several randomized controlled trials showing improved pregnancy outcomes with this strategy.[5,9–13] It should be noted that studies of recurrent pregnancy loss have generally not distinguished between embryonic loss and fetal demise, but instead combined patients into heterogeneous recurrent pregnancy loss groups. We recommend starting treatment with LMWH (such as enoxaparin 1 mg/kg given subcutaneously *once* daily) and LDA upon confirmation of an intrauterine pregnancy.

Patients with a History of Early, Severe Pre-eclampsia

This group has not been well studied. No treatment has been shown to prevent the development of pre-eclampsia in APS patients but LDA and heparin therapy are recommended.[43] However, there are reports that IVIG is associated with a lower incidence.[30,32] The definitive treatment for pre-eclampsia is delivery, regardless of fetal age.

Patients with Asymptomatic Antiphospholipid Antibodies

There are no rigorous studies exploring treatment options for aPL-positive women with no prior thrombotic or pregnancy-related events. Over half of these women will have uneventful pregnancies without any treatment.[44] Treatment options include monitoring and observation alone, LDA alone, LDA with prophylactic heparin, and/or HCQ. When discussing treatment options, physicians should clearly describe the potential risks of these treatments. Patient desires and anxieties should be addressed and taken into account when making treatment decisions.

Preconception Counseling and Monitoring of APS Pregnancy

APS pregnancy is always considered high risk and should be managed by a team comprised of a maternal fetal medicine specialist and a rheumatologist or hematologist with experience in this disease. With proper antenatal care and treatment, APS patients have a 75% chance of live birth.[42]

Preconception Counseling

Prior to becoming pregnant, aPL-positive women should meet with members of their care team to discuss the risks of APS pregnancy to the fetus (fetal loss, intrauterine growth restriction, prematurity) as well as the mother (thrombosis, hypertension, pre-eclampsia). Patients with a history of recent thrombotic events, stroke, and significant pulmonary hypertension are at particularly high risk of death and complications. Alternative methods of expanding a family, such as surrogacy or adoption, should be mentioned, at the very least, ensuring that patients are informed of all possible options.

Preconception laboratory testing should include renal function, liver function, complete blood counts (with particular attention to platelet counts), and quantity of urine protein. Prior aPL results should be reviewed and may be repeated at this time. We generally do not repeat aPL testing during pregnancy as subsequent results and titers are not known to correlate with risk of adverse outcomes.

Additional considerations to optimize pregnancy outcome include:

1. Minimize or eliminate modifiable thrombotic risk factors (i.e., smoking).
2. Ensure that current medications are safe during pregnancy.
3. Initiate prenatal vitamins.
4. Initiate calcium in patients who will be treated with heparin during pregnancy due to osteoporosis risk and consider vitamin D repletion, if necessary.
5. Ask to be notified immediately upon confirmation of a positive pregnancy test.

Monitoring throughout Pregnancy

We recommend initiation of LDA and LMWH in patients with a history of recurrent pregnancy loss upon confirmation of a positive pregnancy test. Obstetric monitoring may include both clinical and ultrasonic assessments of fetal growth in addition to routine antenatal care with monthly office visits to monitor for hypertension, increased urinary protein, and general maternal well-being. The frequency of these visits may need to be increased in late pregnancy, and electronic monitoring added, to assess fetal distress.

Patients should be advised to self-monitor for symptoms of aPL-related pregnancy complications, including venous thromboembolism (VTE) and pre-eclampsia (headache, visual change, and abdominal pain), and should know to seek medical attention immediately if they experience these symptoms. In the event of pregnancy loss, pathologic and genetic evaluation of the abortus may be useful, particularly in patients with loss in the first trimester, to rule out chromosomal anomalies as the reason for the loss. Patients treated with therapeutic doses of LMWH may be monitored using factor Xa levels at periodic intervals.[45]

Labor and Delivery

We recommend scheduled delivery in patients receiving heparin therapy. Heparin should be held 12 hours before invasive procedures (i.e., epidural anesthesia and cesarean delivery) and may be restarted 12 hours after completion of the procedure. Aspirin may be held seven days prior to delivery due to a slightly increased risk of perioperative bleeding, although some recommend simply continuing aspirin in those patients with a history of arterial thrombotic events, including stroke and myocardial infarction.

Postpartum Treatment

Given the increased risk of thrombotic events in the postpartum period, we recommend that obstetric APS patients be treated with thromboprophylaxis for 12 weeks following delivery although data to support this recommendation are lacking. For patients treated with prophylactic doses of heparin and aspirin throughout pregnancy (those with recurrent pregnancy loss or history of pre-eclampsia), we recommend continuing the prophylactic regimen that was used throughout pregnancy for 12 weeks postpartum. This was discussed in great detail by the Obstetric APS Task Force of the 13th International Congress on Antiphospholipid Antibodies in 2010 and was a subject of debate among experts in the field, since the recommendation rests on opinion with no studies presenting valid data either for or against.[45]

For patients with a history of aPL-related thrombosis, we recommended resuming therapeutic anticoagulation as soon as possible after delivery and, in most cases, lifelong anticoagulation. This follows the recommendation of the American College of Chest Physicians Evidence-Based Clinical Practice Guidelines which advises six weeks of prophylactic- or intermediate-dose LMWH or warfarin with a target INR of two to three for women with a history of prior VTE (independent of aPL, lifelong anticoagulation is the recommendation for patients with APS diagnosed because of thrombosis).[40]

All patients should be offered conservative measures in the prevention of thrombosis; these include early ambulation following vaginal delivery and the use of pneumatic compression stockings following cesarean delivery.

Summary and Recommendations

Appropriate management can greatly improve maternal and fetal outcomes in APS pregnancies. The mainstay of treatment for women with a history of thrombotic events is therapeutic dose heparin or LMWH throughout pregnancy; for women with a history recurrent pregnancy loss, IUGR pregnancy, or pre-eclampsia, LDA and prophylactic doses of heparin are recommended. For patients who are refractory to these therapies, IVIG, plasma exchange, and HCG may be considered. Future clinical trials are warranted to guide treatment recommendations.

REFERENCES

1. Miyakis S, Lockshin MD, Atsumi T et al. International consensus statement on an update of the classification criteria for definite antiphospholipid syndrome (APS). *J Thromb Haemostasis* 2006;4:295–306.
2. Fishman P, Falach-Vaknin E, Sredni B et al. Aspirin modulates interleukin-3 production: Additional explanation for the preventive effects of aspirin in antiphospholipid antibody syndrome. *J Rheumatol* 1995;22:1086–90.
3. Lima F, Khamashta MA, Buchanan NM et al. A study of sixty pregnancies in patients with the antiphospholipid syndrome. *Clin Exp Rheumatol* 1996;14:131–6.
4. Pattison NS, Chamley LW, Birdsall M et al. Does aspirin have a role in improving pregnancy outcome for women with the antiphospholipid syndrome? A randomized controlled trial. *Am J Obstet Gynecol* 2000;183:1008–12.
5. Empson M, Lassere M, Craig J et al. Prevention of recurrent miscarriage for women with antiphospholipid antibody or lupus anticoagulant. *Cochrane Database Syst Rev* 2005(2):CD002859
6. Lockshin MD, Kim M, Laskin CA et al. Prediction of adverse pregnancy outcome by the presence of lupus anticoagulant, but not anticardiolipin antibody, in patients with antiphospholipid antibodies. *Arthritis Rheum* 2012;64:2311–8.
7. ACOG Practice Bulletin No. 118: Antiphospholipid syndrome. *Obstet Gynecol* 2010;117:192–9.
8. Salmon JE, Girardi G, Lockshin MD. The antiphospholipid syndrome as a disorder initiated by inflammation: Implications for the therapy of pregnant patients. *Nat Clin Pract Rheumatol* 2007;3:140–7; quiz 1 p following 87.
9. Kutteh WH. Antiphospholipid antibody-associated recurrent pregnancy loss: Treatment with heparin and low-dose aspirin is superior to low-dose aspirin alone. *Am J Obstet Gynecol* 1996;174:1584–9.
10. Empson M, Lassere M, Craig JC et al. Recurrent pregnancy loss with antiphospholipid antibody: A systematic review of therapeutic trials. *Obstet Gynecol* 2002;99:135–44.
11. Mak A, Cheung MW, Cheak AA et al. Combination of heparin and aspirin is superior to aspirin alone in enhancing live births in patients with recurrent pregnancy loss and positive anti-phospholipid antibodies: A meta-analysis of randomized controlled trials and meta-regression. *Rheumatology (Oxford, U K)* 2010;49:281–8.
12. Rai R, Cohen H, Dave M et al. Randomised controlled trial of aspirin and aspirin plus heparin in pregnant women with recurrent miscarriage associated with phospholipid antibodies (or antiphospholipid antibodies). *BMJ* 1997;314:253–7.
13. Ziakas PD, Pavlou M, Voulgarelis M. Heparin treatment in antiphospholipid syndrome with recurrent pregnancy loss: A systematic review and meta-analysis. *Obstet Gynecol* 2010;115:1256–62.
14. Farquharson RG, Quenby S, Greaves M. Antiphospholipid syndrome in pregnancy: A randomized, controlled trial of treatment. *Obstet Gynecol* 2002;100:408–13.
15. Laskin CA, Spitzer KA, Clark CA et al. Low molecular weight heparin and aspirin for recurrent pregnancy loss: Results from the randomized, controlled HepASA Trial. *J Rheumatol* 2009;36:279–87.
16. Noble LS, Kutteh WH, Lashey N et al. Antiphospholipid antibodies associated with recurrent pregnancy loss: Prospective, multicenter, controlled pilot study comparing treatment with low-molecular-weight heparin versus unfractionated heparin. *Fertil Steril* 2005;83:684–90.
17. Stephenson MD, Ballem PJ, Tsang P et al. Treatment of antiphospholipid antibody syndrome (APS) in pregnancy: A randomized pilot trial comparing low molecular weight heparin to unfractionated heparin. *J Obstet Gynaecol Can* 2004;26:729–34.
18. Rand JH, Wu XX, Quinn AS et al. The annexin A5-mediated pathogenic mechanism in the antiphospholipid syndrome: Role in pregnancy losses and thrombosis. *Lupus* 2010;19:460–9.
19. Johnson R, Charnley J. Hydroxychloroquine in prophylaxis of pulmonary embolism following hip arthroplasty. *Clin Orthop Relat Res* 1979:174–7.
20. Wallace DJ. Does hydroxychloroquine sulfate prevent clot formation in systemic lupus erythematosus? *Arthritis Rheum* 1987;30:1435–6.
21. Petri M. Hydroxychloroquine use in the Baltimore Lupus Cohort: Effects on lipids, glucose and thrombosis. *Lupus* 1996;5 Suppl 1:S16–22.
22. Kaiser R, Cleveland CM, Criswell LA. Risk and protective factors for thrombosis in systemic lupus erythematosus: Results from a large, multi-ethnic cohort. *Ann Rheum Dis* 2009;68:238–41.

23. Ruiz-Irastorza G, Egurbide MV, Pijoan JI et al. Effect of antimalarials on thrombosis and survival in patients with systemic lupus erythematosus. *Lupus* 2006;15:577–83.

24. Carreras LD, Perez GN, Vega HR et al. Lupus anticoagulant and recurrent fetal loss: Successful treatment with gammaglobulin. *Lancet* 1988;2:393–4.

25. Triolo G, Ferrante A, Ciccia F et al. Randomized study of subcutaneous low molecular weight heparin plus aspirin versus intravenous immunoglobulin in the treatment of recurrent fetal loss associated with antiphospholipid antibodies. *Arthritis Rheum* 2003;48:728–31.

26. Dendrinos S, Sakkas E, Makrakis E. Low-molecular-weight heparin versus intravenous immunoglobulin for recurrent abortion associated with antiphospholipid antibody syndrome. *Int J Gynaecol Obstet* 2009;104:223–5.

27. Branch DW, Peaceman AM, Druzin M et al. A multicenter, placebo-controlled pilot study of intravenous immune globulin treatment of antiphospholipid syndrome during pregnancy. The Pregnancy Loss Study Group. *Am J Obstet Gynecol* 2000;182:122–7.

28. Spinnato JA, Clark AL, Pierangeli SS, Harris EN. Intravenous immunoglobulin therapy for the antiphospholipid syndrome in pregnancy. *Am J Obstet Gynecol* 1995;172:690–4.

29. Triolo G, Ferrante A, Accardo-Palumbo A et al. IVIG in APS pregnancy. *Lupus* 2004;13:731–5.

30. Vaquero E, Lazzarin N, Valensise H et al. Pregnancy outcome in recurrent spontaneous abortion associated with antiphospholipid antibodies: A comparative study of intravenous immunoglobulin versus prednisone plus low-dose aspirin. *Am J Reprod Immunol* 2001;45:174–9.

31. Branch DW, Peaceman AM, Druzin M et al. A multicenter, placebo-controlled pilot study of intravenous immune globulin treatment of antiphospholipid syndrome during pregnancy. The Pregnancy Loss Study Group. *Am J Obstet Gynecol* 2000;182:122–7.

32. Harris EN, Pierangeli SS. Utilization of intravenous immunoglobulin therapy to treat recurrent pregnancy loss in the antiphospholipid syndrome: A review. *Scand J Rheumatol Suppl.* 1998;107:97–102.

33. Valensise H, Vaquero E, De Carolis C et al. Normal fetal growth in women with antiphospholipid syndrome treated with high-dose intravenous immunoglobulin (IVIG). *Prenatal Diagn.* 1995;15:509–17.

34. Frampton G, Cameron JS, Thom M et al. Successful removal of anti-phospholipid antibody during pregnancy using plasma exchange and low-dose prednisolone. *Lancet* 1987;2:1023–4.

35. Fulcher D, Stewart G, Exner T et al. Plasma exchange and the anticardiolipin syndrome in pregnancy. *Lancet* 1989;2:171.

36. Bramham K, Thomas M, Nelson-Piercy C et al. First-trimester low-dose prednisolone in refractory antiphospholipid antibody-related pregnancy loss. *Blood* 2011;117:6948–51.

37. Cowchock FS, Reece EA, Balaban D et al. Repeated fetal losses associated with antiphospholipid antibodies: A collaborative randomized trial comparing prednisone with low-dose heparin treatment. *Am J Obstet Gynecol* 1992;166:1318–23.

38. Laskin CA, Bombardier C, Hannah ME et al. Prednisone and aspirin in women with autoantibodies and unexplained recurrent fetal loss. *N Engl J Med* 1997;337:148–53.

39. Ginsberg JS, Greer I, Hirsh J. Use of antithrombotic agents during pregnancy. *Chest* 2001;119:122S-31S.

40. Bates SM, Greer IA, Middeldorp S et al. VTE, thrombophilia, antithrombotic therapy, and pregnancy: Antithrombotic Therapy and Prevention of Thrombosis, 9th ed: American College of Chest Physicians Evidence-Based Clinical Practice Guidelines. *Chest* 2012;141:e691S-736S

41. Practice Bulletin No. 132: Antiphospholipid syndrome. *Obstet Gynecol* 2012;120:1514–21.

42. Levy RA, Jesus GR, Jesus NR. Obstetric antiphospholipid syndrome: Still a challenge. *Lupus* 2010;19:457–9.

43. Barton JR, Sibai BM. Prediction and prevention of recurrent preeclampsia. *Obstet Gynecol* 2008;112:359–72.

44. Lockwood CJ, Romero R, Feinberg RF et al. The prevalence and biologic significance of lupus anticoagulant and anticardiolipin antibodies in a general obstetric population. *Am J Obstet Gynecol* 1989;161:369–73

45. Branch W. Report of the Obstetric APS Task Force: 13th International Congress on Antiphospholipid Antibodies, April 13, 2010. *Lupus* 2011;20:158–64.

22

Defects in Coagulation Factors Leading to Recurrent Pregnancy Loss

Aida Inbal and Howard J. A. Carp

Introduction

In recent years, defects in coagulation factors both hereditary and acquired have been widely investigated as causes of pregnancy loss, both sporadic and recurrent. The evidence for pregnancy loss having a thrombotic basis is due to the widely reported association between antiphospholipid antibodies (aPL) and recurrent pregnancy loss (RPL). aPL are thought to cause pregnancy loss by thrombosis in decidual vessels impairing the blood supply to the fetus leading to fetal death. Due to the assumption that aPL induces thrombosis causing pregnancy loss, it has been assumed that any prothrombotic state may also increase the chance of pregnancy loss due to a thrombotic mechanism. Hereditary thrombophilias have been classified into groups.[1] (1) Defects in endogenous inhibitors of the coagulation pathway (antithrombin, protein C, protein S, tissue factor pathway inhibitor, and thrombomodulin deficiency). (2) Increased levels or function of procoagulation factors (factor V Leiden [FVL], prothrombin gene mutation G20210A, dysfibrinogenemia and hyperfibrinogenemia, and increased levels of factors VII, VIII, IX, and XI). (3) Hyperhomocysteinemia, mainly due to C677T homozygosis of the methylenetetrahydrofolate reductase (MTHFR) gene. (4) Defects of the fibrinolytic system, involving plasminogen, tissue plasminogen activator (tPA), plasminogen activator inhibitor (PAI), thrombinactivatable fibrinolysis inhibitor (TAFI), factor XIII, and lipoprotein A. (5) Altered platelet function (platelet glycoproteins GPIb-IX, GPIa-IIa, and GPIIb-IIIa). However, the prevalence of each hereditary thrombophilia varies in different ethnic groups.

In addition, deficiencies of factor XIII (FXIII) and fibrinogen are associated with pregnancy loss. Both of these are bleeding diatheses which become apparent in childhood, and are associated with impaired wound repair in addition to pregnancy loss and excessive bleeding. This chapter deals with the association between decreased or increased levels of coagulation factors and pregnancy loss. The various factors and their association with the trophoblast are shown in Figure 22.1.

Bleeding Diatheses Leading to Pregnancy Loss

Hereditary Factor FXIII Deficiency

Coagulation factor XIII (FXIII) is plasma transglutaminase that participates in the final step of the coagulation cascade. Following activation by thrombin the active form—FXIIIa—cross-links fibrin chains through γ-glutamyl-ε-lysine bonds, creating a stable clot resistant to fibrinolysis.[2] In plasma, FXIII circulates as a heterotetramer (A2B2) composed of two catalytic A subunits (FXIII-A) and two carrier B subunits (FXIII-B).[2] FXIIIa is synthesized by megakaryocytes, monocytes, and monocyte-derived macrophages, whereas FXIII-B is synthesized by hepatocytes. Platelets, monocytes, and macrophages contain only the A subunits of FXIII dimers.[3]

In contrast to factors VII, VIII, IX, X and fibrinogen, which increase during normal pregnancy, the concentration of plasma factor XIII decreases during pregnancy, reaching 50% of normal at term. Likewise, the activity of factor XIIIA is significantly decreased at the time of abortion.[4]

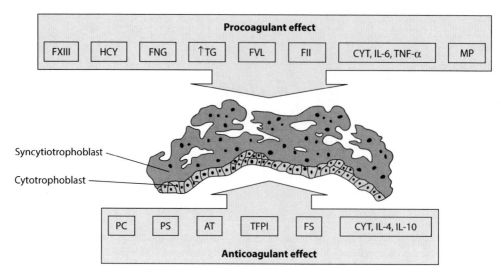

Key: AT = antithrombin, FII = prothrombin gene mutation (G20210A), FNG = fibrinogen, FS = fibrinolytic system, FVL = factor V Leiden, HCY = homocysteine, PC = protein C, PS = protein S, TFPI = tissue factor pathway inhibitor, ↑TG = increased thrombin generation, MP = microparticles

FIGURE 22.1 Procoagulant and anticoagulant balance of trophoblast.

FXIII deficiency is a hereditary bleeding disorder, characterized by severe bleeding manifestations, delay in wound healing and recurrent abortions in homozygous women.[2] Women who are homozygous for FXIII deficiency will not carry the pregnancy until term unless treated with factor XIII concentrate throughout pregnancy.[3,4] The minimal level of FXIIIA required for normal pregnancy is unknown; however, only 0.5% to 2% of FXIIIA is required for normal hemostasis.[5]

The mechanism by which factor XIII supports normal pregnancy is unknown. FXIII is essential for implantation, placental attachment, and further placental development by cross-linking not only between fibrin chains but also between fibronectin and collagen, the major components of connective tissue matrix.[3,6] Hence, FXIII seems to play an essential role in the interaction between the blastocyst and the endometrium at implantation. FXIIIa also cross-links fibrin(ogen) and fibronectin, both of which are important for maintaining the attachment of the placenta to the uterus.[7] FXIII deficiency may result in periplacental hemorrhage and subsequent spontaneous fetal loss. This hypothesis is supported by evidence from a mouse model of FXIII deficiency: Pregnant FXIII A-subunit knock-out mice suffer excessive uterine bleeding followed by embryonic demise.[8] Kobayashi et al.[9] have reported that FXIII-A is present in the extracellular space of the extravillous cytotrophoblast shell adjacent to Nitabuch's layer. FXIII-A has also been colocalized with fibrinogen and fibronectin at Nitabuch's layer.[10] FXIII-A has been reported to be absent from the placenta bed in women with FXIII deficiency, leading to deficient cytotrophoblastic shell formation.[10] Thus, deficiency of FXIII-A at the site of implantation will adversely affect fibrin–fibronectin cross-linking resulting in detachment of the placenta from the uterus and subsequent miscarriage.[8,10] Recent studies have shown FXIII-A to have proangiogenic activity both *in vitro* and *in vivo*.[11] Since embryo implantation requires adequate angiogenesis, FXIII's supportive role in implantation may be partly due to its proangiogenic activity.

Whatever the cause for pregnancy loss in FXIII-deficient women, administration of FXIII throughout pregnancy results in successful outcomes.[3,4,6] A plasma-derived concentrate has been available since 1980. The FXIII concentrate seems have a half-life of 10–12 days.[12] Recently a recombinant FXIII A-subunit protein has become available with a half-life similar to that of the plasma-derived concentrate.[13]

The timing and dose of FXIII replacement for pregnant women and the optimal level of FXIII remain unknown. The level of plasma FXIII generally achieved for successful pregnancy is 10% in women with FXIII deficiency.[12] We treat pregnant women prophylactically with 20 IU/kg of FXIII concentrate every four weeks to achieve a FXIII level of above 3%. A booster dose of 1000 IU is also given before amniocentesis or labor.

Other Alterations in Factor XIII

It is unknown if there is an association between normal or decreased levels of FXIII and RPL. Whereas plasma FXIII-B concentrations increase during pregnancy, FXIII-A tends to decrease resulting in an overall steady reduction in plasma FXIII reaching approximately 50% of normal at term.[14] The A subunit rises with the onset of labor and falls postpartum.[14] This is in contrast to the progressive increase in levels of fibrinogen, factors VII, VIII, IX, and X during pregnancy.[15] Whether the reduction of plasma FXIII during pregnancy represents decreased synthesis of FXIII-A, increased utilization or destruction, or simple dilution by the expanded plasma volume is not clear. In a cohort of non-FXIII deficient women with a history of two or more first trimester miscarriages plasma FXIII levels were not found to be predictive for subsequent pregnancy loss.[16] A substitution of Tyr by Phe at position 204 in exon 5 of the factor XIIIA gene was found in one study to be more prevalent in women suffering three or more miscarriages.[17] The Phe204 Factor XIIIA variant has been associated with lower specific activity. However, in subsequent studies this association has not been confirmed. In a recent study, FXIII-A and FXIII B-subunit (FXIII-B) antigen levels in 264 women with two or more unexplained consecutive miscarriages at or before 21 weeks of gestation or at least one later miscarriage were measured.[18] The control group consisted of 264 women with no history of miscarriage and at least one living child. Overall, there were no differences in FXIII-A and FXIII-B levels between patients and controls. Thus, no associations between FXIII levels and pregnancy loss were observed in this study as well. The findings from these few studies imply that RPL in the general population is not associated with reduced FXIII plasma levels. Whether locally reduced FXIII-A levels or impaired FXIII function in the placenta may contribute to an increased risk of abortion remains to be investigated.

Fibrinogen Deficiency

Fibrinogen, a major blood glycoprotein, is a dimer of three polypeptide chains: Aα, Bβ and γ. It is synthesized by hepatic parenchymal cells and its half-life is 3–4.5 days.[19] Thrombin cleaves fibrinogen to its fibrin monomer, which then polymerizes and is stabilized by FXIII. Fibrin(ogen) is also a target for fibrinolytic factors that dissolve excess fibrin to maintain vascular patency and integrity. Fibrinogen is also a primary bridging molecule, linking activated platelets together via their glycoproteins IIbIIIa.[20]

The three overlapping hereditary abnormalities of fibrinogen: afibrinogenemia, dysfibrinogenemia and hypofibrinogenemia have been associated with RPL. Afibrinogenemia—a defect in hepatic fibrinogen secretion or release—is inherited as an autosomal recessive trait and is associated with bleeding diathesis, impaired wound repair and RPL. A related form of this disorder is hypofibrinogenemia. Hereditary dysfibrinogenemias are characterized by the biosynthesis of structurally and functionally abnormal fibrinogen.

Brenner[21] has reported that women with dysfibrinogenemia are candidates for miscarriage. Of 64 pregnancies in women with dysfibrinogenemia 39% terminated in miscarriage. The mechanisms whereby dysfibrinogenemias are associated with a tendency to thrombosis have been reviewed by Mosesson.[22]

Hypofibrinogenemic women[23] and experimental afibrinogenemic mice[24] show similar features, with regard to bleeding tendency, miscarriage and abnormal scar formation. Based on the mouse model, absence or a significant decrease in maternal fibrinogen is sufficient to cause rupture of the maternal vasculature, thereby affecting embryonic trophoblast infiltration and leading to hemorrhage and subsequent miscarriage.

Cryoprecipitate, fresh-frozen plasma and fibrinogen concentrate are the sources of fibrinogen commercially available. Replacement therapy throughout pregnancy is feasible for patients with pregnancy losses.[25] It has been suggested that the minimal level of normal fibrinogen to maintain pregnancy is about 60 mg/100 mL.[26] A cryoprecipitate infusion of 0.2 bags/kg body weight (approximately 250 mg/bag) will raise the fibrinogen concentration to 100 mg/dL. Since the half-life of fibrinogen is approximately four days, two weekly infusions of cryoprecipitate during the gestational period should be sufficient to keep the fibrinogen level above 60 mg/dL and prevent pregnancy loss.

The benefits of substitution therapy should be weighed against the possibility of inducing thrombosis. Catastrophic thrombosis has been reported during fibrinogen replacement therapy in patients with afibrinogenemia and dysfibrinogenemia.[27] Prophylactic heparin or low-molecular-weight heparin (LMWH) has been advocated for the peripartum period in these patients.[28]

Thrombophilias

The hereditary thrombophilias cause increased tendency to venous thrombosis and comprise a number of conditions such as antithrombin, protein C, protein S deficiency, FVL, prothrombin gene (FII) mutation G20210A, homozygosity for the MTHFR mutation C677T and increased factor VIII. There are also various acquired hypercoagulable states, the most common of which is antiphospholipid syndrome (APS) which is discussed elsewhere. Proteins C and S and antithrombin are physiological anticoagulants. Deficiencies of these anticoagulants are uncommon.[29] FVL is the most common cause of inherited thrombophilia.[29] It results from the substitution of adenine for guanine at nucleotide 1691 of the factor V gene (G1691A), which causes the arginine in residue 506 of the factor V protein to be replaced by glutamine (Arg506Gln). The resulting protein is called FVL. This mutation slows down the proteolytic inactivation of factor Va, by activated protein C (termed activated protein C resistance, APCR), which in turn leads to the augmented generation of thrombin. In the G20210A mutation of the prothrombin gene, adenine is substituted for guanine at the 3′ untranslated part of the prothrombin gene. This mutation leads to more efficient mRNA processing of the prothrombin gene, which in turn is associated with an increased level of prothrombin and generation of thrombin. FVL and the G20210A mutation in the prothrombin gene are common among healthy whites (prevalence of 5% and 1.5%, respectively), but rare in Asians and Africans. Homozygosity for MTHFR (C677T) may lead to hyperhomocysteinemia, mainly when folate storage is decreased, which may also predispose to thrombosis. The mechanism is multifactorial.

Thrombosis in Decidual Vessels

The evidence for pregnancy loss having a thrombotic mechanism rests on three pillars: demonstration of thrombosis in decidual vessels, increased prevalence of thrombophilias in RPL and a higher incidence of pregnancy loss in the presence of thrombophilias. Thrombophilia may be a cause of microembolism in the placenta resulting in miscarriage, fetal death or adverse pregnancy outcome.[30] Placental findings have been compared in women with severe pregnancy complications with and without thrombophilias. The results have not been consistent. The definition of severe pregnancy complications has included numerous conditions such as fetal death, pre-eclampsia, preterm labor, intra-uterine growth restriction (IUGR) or stillbirth. Histopathological examination has revealed lesions due to vascular hypoperfusion. These lesions have included perivillous fibrinoid deposition, subchorionic fibrinoid plaque, subchorial thrombosis, basal intervillous thrombus, intervillous lakes, retroplacental hematomas, maternal surface chorionic villous infarction, and syncytial knots. Many papers have described an increased incidence of placental pathology in hereditary thrombophilias.[30,31] However, the above lesions are common to the above obstetric complications and not to thrombophilia as such. Hence, Mousa and Alfirevic's[32] study could not confirm these results, but found a high incidence of placental infracts (50%) and thrombosis in both women with and without thrombophilias. There are few studies which describe maternal vessel thrombosis as such, making it difficult to confirm thrombosis as the mechanism of the observed pathological changes. A thorough literature search by the author found no reports of placental pathology in recurrent miscarriage as such.

Genetic polymorphisms of the thrombophilic genes of the parents have a 50% likelihood of transmission to the fetus, potentially affecting trophoblast function. Indeed Arias et al.[33] evaluated 13 placentae of women with pre-eclampsia, preterm labor, IUGR or stillbirth. Ten of 13 women (77%) had thrombophilias including aPL, protein C, S and antithrombin deficiencies, APCR, and FVL. Fetal thrombotic vasculopathy is histologically characterized by stem artery thrombosis, which may include occlusive or mural thrombosis sclerotic/avascular terminal villi, hemorrhagic endovasculitis, inflammatory damage to vessels.[34] It is important to note that these histological changes are on the fetal side of the placenta, not the maternal side.

The fact that no specific placental lesion has been found in thrombophilia could have a number of explanations. There may be other thrombophilias as yet unknown, which could explain the high incidence of placental pathology, or that the lesions are the result of inflammatory changes in the placenta associated with the underlying pathology, and unrelated to thrombophilia. Even in APS, thrombosis has not been convincingly demonstrated in decidual vessels. Even in APS, after treatment with monoclonal antiphospholipid antibody, stained placental sections have shown most reactivity to be localized to the cytotrophoblast, suggesting that the trophoblast may be directly damaged by mechanisms unrelated to thrombosis.[35] As in hereditary thrombophilias, these histological changes were on the fetal, rather than maternal side of the placenta. It seems that cell surface-associated membrane receptors rather than soluble factors (such as thrombophilic factors) are the most relevant candidates to affect pregnancy outcome.[36]

The maternal spiral arteries become remodeled by pregnancy hormones and trophoblast into uteroplacental arteries toward the end of the first trimester. In the uteroplacental arteries, the lumen is larger, and the media is replaced by endovascular trophoblast cells. Hereditary thrombophilias predispose to venous thrombosis, and have not been shown to predispose to arterial thrombosis. However, even if there is thrombosis of the maternal uteroplacental arteries, it is by no means certain that thrombosis can also occur in first trimester spiral arteries which are lined by arterial endothelium rather than endovascular trophoblast. It is possible that first trimester miscarriage may be due to failure in the mechanisms governing implantation or due to chromosomal or other abnormalities in the fetus, whereas second trimester losses may be a consequence of thrombotic events in the placenta. However, no study has assessed the placenta in first trimester pregnancy loss in the presence of thrombophilia, and compared the findings to second trimester losses, nor has any study assessed the placenta in the presence of genetic pregnancy loss compared to pregnancy losses with a normal karyotype. Genetic polymorphisms of the thrombophilic genes of the parents have a 50% likelihood of transmission to the fetus, potentially affecting trophoblast function. Thus, to determine the true risk for adverse pregnancy outcome associated with genetic thrombophilias it is necessary to test the fetus for these thrombophilias.

Prevalence of Thrombophilias in Pregnancy Loss

When pregnancy loss is taken as a one condition, and not broken down into subgroups, thrombophilias seem to be more prevalent.[37] Brenner et al.[38] tested women with three or more first trimester losses, two or more second trimester losses or one or more third trimester loss. FVL was more prevalent in the pregnancy loss group than controls; however, neither the MTHFR nor prothrombin mutations were more common in women with pregnancy loss than controls. Forty-nine percent of women with pregnancy loss had a thrombophilia compared to 22% of controls. Rey et al.[39] carried out a meta-analysis of 31 studies in the literature. There was a significant association between hereditary thrombophilias and pregnancy loss. Since the meta-analysis by Rey et al.,[39] a number of papers have appeared assessing the prevalence of one or more thrombophilias in certain population groups. The results have been inconsistent.

The prevalence of hereditary thrombophilias has also been assessed in recurrent miscarriage. The disagreements in the literature have prompted the need for meta-analyses to determine whether the prevalence is increased. Krabbendam et al.[40] have reported a meta-analysis of 11 studies regarding the association between thrombophilias and recurrent miscarriage. There were significantly higher serum homocysteine levels among women with a history of recurrent miscarriage, but no increased prevalence of the MTHFR C667T mutation. No relation was observed for the levels of antithrombin, protein C or protein S. Nelen et al.[41] have performed a meta-analysis to assess the relationship between recurrent early pregnancy loss and hyperhomocyteinemia. Overall, the pooled odds ratios (ORs) for elevated homocysteine were 2.7 (1.5–5.2), for afterload homocysteine 4.2 (2.0–8.8) and for MTHFR 1.4 (1.0–2.0). These data support hyperhomocysteinemia as a risk factor for recurrent early pregnancy loss.

It seems logical that hereditary thrombophilias may be more prevalent in second and third trimester losses rather than first trimester recurrent miscarriage. There are publications which separate early and late pregnancy losses and the prevalence of thrombophilias. Preston et al.[42] reported on hereditary thrombophilias and fetal loss in a cohort of women with FVL or deficiencies of antithrombin, protein C, or protein S. Of 843 women with thrombophilia, 571 had 1524 pregnancies; of 541 control women 395 had 1019 pregnancies. The incidence of miscarriage (fetal loss at or before 28 weeks of gestation), and stillbirth (fetal loss after 28 weeks of gestation) were assessed jointly and separately. The risk of fetal loss was increased in women with thrombophilia, OR 1.35 (95% confidence interval [CI] 1.01–1.82). The OR was higher for stillbirth than for miscarriage 3.6 (CI 1.4–9.4) versus 1.27 (CI 0.94–1.71) respectively. The highest OR for stillbirth was in women with combined defects 14.3 (CI 2.4–86.0) compared with 5.2 (CI 1.5–18.1) in antithrombin deficiency, 2.3 (CI 0.6–8.3) in protein C deficiency, 3.3 (CI 1.0–11.3) in protein S deficiency, and 2.0 (CI 0.5–7.7) with FVL mutation. Sarig et al.[43] evaluated 145 patients with recurrent miscarriage and 145 matched controls. At least one thrombophilic defect was found in 66% of study group patients compared with 28% in controls. Late pregnancy wastage occurred more frequently in women with thrombophilia compared with women without thrombophilia. Grandone et al.[44] investigated the FVL mutation in 43 women with two or more unexplained fetal losses and 118 controls. The FVL mutation was more frequent in women with second trimester loss, but the prevalence of the mutation in women with first trimester loss and controls was similar. A recent meta-analysis[45] reported that the odds of pregnancy loss in women with FVL (absolute risk 4.2%) was 52% higher (OR = 1.52, 95% CI 1.06–2.19) as compared with women without FVL (absolute risk 3.2%).

Prevalence of Thrombophilias in Late Obstetric Complications

Kupferminc et al.[46] first reported that hereditary thrombophilias are more prevalent in pregnant women with fetal growth retardation, pre-eclampsia, abruptio placentae, or stillbirth. A later systematic review of 25 studies by Alfirevic et al.[47] confirmed these findings. In the case-control study by Gris et al.[48] of 232 women with a history of one or more second or third trimester losses, 21.1% of patients and 3.9% of controls had at least one thrombophilia ($p < 0.00001$). The OR for stillbirth associated with any positive thrombophilia was 5.5 (CI 3.4–9.0). Logistic regression analysis showed four risk factors for stillbirth, protein S deficiency, positive anti-beta2 glycoprotein 1 IgG antibodies, positive anticardiolipin IgG antibodies and the FVL mutation. The conclusion was that late fetal loss, might sometimes be the consequence of a maternal multifactorial prothrombotic state involving placental thrombosis. The systematic review by Alfirevic et al.[47] has shown that placental abruption was more often associated with homozygous and heterozygous FVL, heterozygous G20210A and hyperhomocysteinemia. Women with pre-eclampsia/eclampsia were more likely to have heterozygous FVL mutation, heterozygous G20210A prothrombin gene mutation, homozygous MTHFR, protein C deficiency, protein S deficiency or activated protein C resistance. Stillbirth was more often associated with FVL, protein S deficiency and activated protein C resistance. Women with intrauterine growth restriction had a higher prevalence of G20210A, MTHFR or protein S deficiency. However, they concluded that "Women with adverse pregnancy outcome are more likely to have a positive thrombophilia screen but studies published so far are too small to adequately assess the true size of this association."

Infante-Rivarde et al.[49] were the first to dispute the increased prevalence of hereditary thrombophilias in late obstetric complications. Silver et al.,[50] investigated the prevalence of the prothrombin gene mutation (G20210A), in a multicenter, prospective, observational cohort of 5188 unselected singleton gestations. There was no association between the prothrombin G20210A mutation and pregnancy loss, pre-eclampsia, abruption, or small for gestational age (SGA) neonates in a low-risk, prospective cohort. A similar study by Kjellberg et al.[51] showed that FVL carriership did not influence pregnancy-induced hypertension, birthweight, or prematurity but raised the risk of venous thromboembolism

The different results could reflect heterogeneity of study design, inclusion criteria, sample size and population studied, outcome definition and diagnostic criteria, as well as the prevalence of thrombophilias studied. Nevertheless, there may be an association, between some thrombophilias and some adverse pregnancy outcomes.

Cohort Studies

Case control studies can only show associations between thrombophilias and pregnancy losses. In order to infer cause and to come to conclusions about treatment, cohort studies are necessary. In the case of miscarriage, Ogasawara et al[16] have reported that the subsequent miscarriage rate was not different for patients with decreased protein C or S activity, or antithrombin. Carp et al.[52] found the live birth rate to be similar to that expected in recurrent miscarriage, whether the patient had FVL, G20210A, MTHFR, protein C or S or antithrombin deficiencies. Salomon et al.[53] have followed up 191 thrombophilic patients who attended an ultrasound clinic to prospectively assess obstetric complications. The blood flow to the fetus was not compromised.

In the case of late obstetric complications, Sanson et al.[54] investigated women with deficiencies of antithrombin, protein S and protein C. In the 60 deficient subjects, 22.3% of the 188 pregnancies resulted in miscarriage or stillbirth as compared to 11.4% of the 202 pregnancies in the 69 nondeficient subjects. The relative risk of abortion and stillbirth per pregnancy for deficient women as compared to nondeficient women was 2.0 (C.I. 1.2–3.3). However, a recent meta-analysis[45] has suggested otherwise. Rodger et al.[45] analyzed 10 prospective cohort studies that examined the association between FVL and the prothrombin gene mutation (G20210A), and placenta-mediated pregnancy complications and that met their predefined criteria. Neither FVL nor prothrombin gene mutation (PGM) increased a woman's risk of pre-eclampsia or of giving birth to a SGA infant.

Treatment

This chapter only gives an outline of the treatment options, as the chapter is followed by a debate on the place of treatment. Suffice to say, there are isolated reports that the presence of hereditary thrombophilias warrants thromboprophylaxis. The presumed benefit of antithrombotic therapy, and the absence of side effects has led many clinicians to prescribe LMWH, aspirin, or both to women with recurrent miscarriage and late pregnancy loss based on the presence of thrombophilia. However, the role of treatment can only be determined in well-designed randomized trials where the effect of treatment is compared to untreated, or placebo-treated patients. High-quality evidence for the beneficial effect of LMWH is still absent, as there are no such trials. There has been a prospective study by Gris et al.[55] comparing enoxaparin to aspirin in patients with thrombophilia and one pregnancy loss. Enoxaparin was found to be superior to low dose aspirin. However, several methodological issues were raised, and the results of this single study have neither been confirmed by other trials nor were they implemented in the American College of Clinical Pharmacy (ACCP) guidelines.[56] Carp et al.[57] have reported a comparative cohort study comparing enoxaparin to no treatment in women with hereditary thrombophilias and recurrent miscarriage. In all, 26 of the 37 pregnancies in treated patients (70.2%) terminated in live births, compared to 21 of 48 (43.8%) in untreated patients (OR 3.03, 95% CI 1.12–8.36). The beneficial effect was mainly seen in primary aborters, that is women with no previous live births (OR 9.75, 95% CI 1.59–52.48). This benefit was also found in patients with a poor prognosis for a live birth (five or more miscarriages), where the live birth rate was increased from 18.2% to 61.6%. However, the trial was neither randomized nor blinded. There are three randomized trials of anticoagulants in the literature which compared the live birth rate in women receiving anticoagulants for unexplained pregnancy loss.[58–60] Two of these[58,60] assessed hereditary thrombophilias. If the results of these two trials are summarized together with the trial by Carp et al.[57] there was a statistically significant 21% improvement in the live birth rate (Figure 22.2) (OR 2.45, CI 1.24–4.85). However, the subgroup analyses in the two randomized trials were insufficiently powered to address the effect of antithrombotic treatment in thrombophilic women. In the ALIFE[58] study, a nonsignificant increase in live birth was observed in the two active treatment arms for women with inherited thrombophilia (relative risk for live birth 1.22; 95% CI 0.69–2.16 for aspirin, and 1.31; 95% CI 0.74–2.33 for aspirin combined with nadroparin, as compared to placebo), highlighting the urgent need for new randomized controlled trials. This is the only evidence available for a beneficial effect of thromboprophylaxis in women with hereditary thrombophilias and RPL. There has been no trial of anticoagulants comparing the effects of treatment to untreated patients regarding late obstetric complications. Recently, the ALIFE2 study (www.trialregister.nl, NTR 3361)

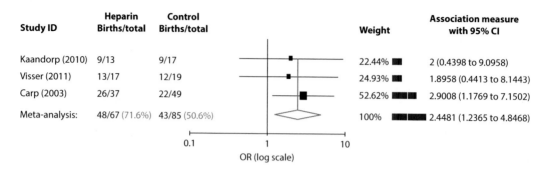

FIGURE 22.2 Meta-analysis of anticoagulants and live birth rate in hereditary thrombophilias.

has started recruiting, in which women with inherited thrombophilia and RPL will be randomized to either treatment with LMWH plus standard pregnancy surveillance or standard pregnancy surveillance only. The optimal dose of anticoagulants has not yet been determined. In a randomized prospective study, no difference was found between 40 mg and 80 mg of enoxaparin (Clexane, Sanofi Aventis Ltd. France) in women with thrombophilia and pregnancy losses.[61]

Other Prothrombotic Mechanisms of Pregnancy Loss

There are other mechanisms which may induce thrombosis, or may allow thrombosis to become apparent in patients with genetic predispositions to thrombosis.

Cytokines

Cytokines are low molecular weight peptides or glycopeptides, produced by lymphocytes, monocytes/macrophages, mast cells, eosinophils, and blood vessel endothelial cells. Two cytokines have been associated with initiation of coagulation in infections; TNFα and IL-6 upregulate the expression of tissue factor, which initiates the extrinsic phase of the coagulation cascade and subsequent thrombin generation. Additionally, interferon γ has been described as detrimental to thrombus resolution.[62]

Cytokine imbalances have been described in RPL,[63] antiphospholipid syndrome,[64,65] pre-eclampsia,[66] preterm births,[67] and intrauterine growth restriction.[68] The predominance of prothrombotic cytokines may well lead to placental thrombosis in genetically susceptible individuals.

Microparticles

Placental apoptosis has been described as a salient feature of pregnancy loss.[69] Following apoptosis and cell activation, the cell membrane is remodeled with the release of microparticles. The microparticles express procoagulant phospholipids, such as phosphotidylserine on their external surface. These phospholipids are normally found inside the cell membrane. Microparticles lead to increased expression of adhesion molecules, thus amplifying the procoagulant and/or inflammatory response on the endothelial cell surface. Microparticles have been found in increased numbers in normal pregnancy, when there is constant deportation of trophoblast into the maternal circulation. Shetty et al.[70] have analyzed nine papers reporting the prevalence of microparticles in RPL. The majority of studies have found an increased prevalence. However, it has not been determined whether endothelial microparticles may cause pregnancy loss through subsequent thrombotic mechanisms, or may be a consequence of embryonic death. Twenty-nine to 60 percent of recurrent first trimester miscarriages are due to chromosomal aberrations, which are incompatible with life and lead to miscarriage irrespective of other associations or causes of pregnancy loss including the presence of microparticles. Even in missed abortion due to chromosomal aberrations, the trophoblast undergoes apoptosis with subsequent microparticle formation and thrombosis. Microparticles may by themselves result in adverse conditions or they may be additive factors to an already existing prothrombotic state in addition to the pre-existing hypercoagulable status of pregnancy.

Hormones and Thrombosis

The hormones of pregnancy, estrogen, progesterone and hCG, all affect thrombosis. Estrogen may alter the concentrations of clotting factors to a prothrombotic profile, for example, raising factor VII[71] and plasminogen activator (PAI-1)[72] and reducing antithrombin III.[72] In mice, estrogen sulfotransferase (a cytosolic enzyme which catalyzes the sulfoconjugation of estrogens) has a critical role in modulating estrogen activity in the mouse placenta during mid-gestation.[73] Inactivation of estrogen sulfotransferase caused local and systemic estrogen excess and an increase in tissue factor leading to placental thrombosis and fetal loss. Additionally, estrogen can either stimulate or inhibit the production of IL-1 and TNF cytokines.[74]

Progesterone, however, seems to have opposing effects. Progesterone has prothrombotic effects including upregulation of tissue factor expression,[75] but progesterone also induces the production of cytokines such as IL-4 which upregulates protein S, which inhibits coagulation.[76]

In addition to its endocrine luteotrophic role, hCG could also have a local role within the uterine environment. Specific binding sites for hCG have been shown in various cells of the endometrium and decidua. The local role of hCG in the endometrium has not been fully elucidated. Uzumcu et al.[77] have assessed endometrial production of cytokines when stimulated by hCG. Increasing doses of hCG caused a dose-dependent increase in TNFα and IL-6 secretion both of which have been reported to be thrombogenic.

Single Nucleotide Polymorphisms in Coagulation Factors and Pregnancy Loss

The beta-fibrinogen -455G/A polymorphism (A/A genotype) and homozygosity for plasminogen activator inhibitor (PAI)-1, -675 4G/5G polymorphism were found to be associated with RPL; however, the association is actually very slight.[78–80]

Control of thrombin generation is essential for normal hemostasis and is achieved by the physiological anticoagulants. One such anticoagulant is tissue factor pathway inhibitor (TFPI), an endothelial-associated protein that downregulates the initial phase of coagulation by inhibiting tissue factor–factor VIIa and factor Xa complex.[81] Another anticoagulant is antithrombin (AT), a multi-functional serpin (serine protease inhibitor) that inhibits essentially almost all the active coagulation factors A recent study[82] analyzed the association of SNPs in TFPI and antithrombin genes with RPL in 117 nonpregnant women with three or more consecutive losses prior to 20 weeks of pregnancy without a previous history of carrying a fetus to viability, and 264 healthy fertile nonpregnant women who had at least two term deliveries and no known pregnancy losses.[83] The results of the study showed that antithrombin 786G > A variant increases the risk for RPL, while TFPI T-287C variant is protective. Further studies are required to confirm these findings.

Fetal Thrombophilia

As placental histology usually shows a fetal vasculopathy rather than maternal thrombosis, fetal thrombophilia may explain the pathological changes. The hemostatic balance in the placenta may be determined by both maternal and fetal factors cooperatively regulating coagulation at the feto-maternal interface.[84] Humans have an almost unique placentation in which trophoblast cells line the maternal blood lakes rather than endothelial cells. Using genomewide expression analysis, Sood et al.[36] identified a panel of genes that determine the ability of fetal trophoblast cells to regulate hemostasis at the feto-maternal interface. Additionally, the trophoblast was shown to sense the presence of activated coagulation factors via the expression of protease activated receptors. Engagement of these receptors was reported to result in specific changes in gene expression. Hence, fetal genes might modify the risks associated with maternal thrombophilia. Additionally, coagulation activation at the feto-maternal interface might affect trophoblast physiology and alter placental function in the absence of frank thrombosis.

The author has seen fetal deaths *in utero* in which sonograms have shown complete occlusion of the umbilical blood vessels. However, it is impossible to say whether the thromboses caused fetal death or whether the changes occurred post mortem.

REFERENCES

1. Crowther MA, Kelton JG. Congenital thrombophilic states associated with venous thrombosis: A qualitative overview and proposed classification system. *Ann Intern Med* 2003;138:128–34.
2. Lorand L, Losowsky MS, Miloszewski KJ. Human factor XIII fibrin stabilizing factor. *Prog Thromb Haemostasis* 1980;5:245–90.
3. Muszbek L, Adany R, Mikkola H. Novel aspects of blood coagulation factor XIII. I. Structure, distribution, activation, and function. *Crit Rev Clin Lab Sci* 1996;33:357–421.
4. Schubring C, Grulich-Henn J, Burkhard PAT et al. Fibrinolysis and factor XIII in women with spontaneous abortion. *Eur J Obstet Gynecol Reprod Biol* 1990;35:215–21.
5. Burrows RF, Ray JG, Burrows EA. Bleeding risk and reproductive capacity among patients with factor XIII deficiency: A case presentation and review of the literature. *Obstet Gynecol Surv* 2000;55:103–7.
6. Mosher DF, Schad PE, Kleinman HK. Cross-linking of fibronectin to collagen by blood coagulation factor XIII. *J Clin Invest* 1979;64:781–7.
7. Wartiovaara J, Leivo I, Virtanen I et al. Cell surface and extracellular matrix glycoprotein fibronectin. Expression in embryogenesis and in teratocarcinoma differentiation. *Ann NY Acad Sci* 1978;312:132–41.
8. Koseki-Kuno S, Yamakawa M, Dickneite G et al. Factor XIII A subunit deficient mice developed severe uterine bleeding events and subsequent spontaneous miscarriages. *Blood* 2003;102:4410–2.
9. Kobayashi T, Asahina T, Okada Y et al. Studies on the localization of adhesive proteins associated with the development of extravillous cytotrophoblast. *Trophoblast Res* 1999;13:35–53.
10. Asahina T, Kobayashi T, Okada Y et al. Maternal blood coagulation factor XIII is associated with the development of cytotrophoblastic shell. *Placenta* 2000;21:388–93.
11. Dardik R, Loscalzo J, Inbal A. Factor XIII (FXIII) and angiogenesis. *J Thromb Haemostasis* 2005;4:19–25.
12. Anwar T, Miloszewski K. Factor XIII deficiency. *Br J Haematol* 1999;107:468–84.
13. Reynolds TC, Butine MD, Visich JE et al. Safety, pharmacokinetics, and immunogenicity of single-dose rFXIII administration *J Thromb Haemostasis* 2005;3:922–8.
14. Hayano Y, Ima N, Kasaraura T. Studies on the physiologic changes of blood coagulation factor XIII during pregnancy and their significance. *Acta Obstet Gynaecol Jpn* 1982;34:469–77.
15. Stirling Y, Woolf L, North WRS et al. Haemostasis in normal pregnancy. *Thromb Haemostasis* 1984;52:176.
16. Ogasawara MS, Aoki K, Katano K et al. Factor XII but not protein C, protein S, antithrombin III, or factor XIII is a predictor of recurrent miscarriage. *Fertil Steril* 2001;75:916–9.
17. Anwar R, Gallivan L, Edmonds SD et al. Genotype/phenotype correlations for coagulation factor XIII: Specific normal polymorphisms are associated with high or low factor XIII specific activity. *Blood* 1999;93:897–905.
18. Pasquier E, De Saint Martin I, Kohler HP, Schroeder V. Factor XIII plasma levels in women with unexplained recurrent pregnancy loss. *J Thromb Haemostasis* 2012;10:723–5.
19. Galanakis DK. Fibrinogen anomalies and disease. A clinical update. *Hematol Oncol Clin North Am* 1992;6:1171–87.
20. Doolittle, RF. The molecular biology of fibrin. In: Stamatoyannopoulos GS, Nienhuis AW, Majerus PW, Harmus H. eds. *The Molecular Basis of Blood Diseases*. Philadelphia, PA: WB. Saunders Co; 1994. p. 701–23.
21. Brenner B. Inherited thrombophilia and fetal loss. *Curr Opin Hematol* 2000;7:290–5.
22. Mosesson MW. Dysfibrinogenemia and thrombosis. *Semin Thromb Hemostasis* 1999;25:311–9.
23. Ridgway, HJ, Brennan, SO, Faed, JM et al. Fibrinogen Otago: A major α chain truncation associated with severe hypofibrinogenaemia and recurrent miscarriage. *Br J Haematol* 1997;98:632–9.
24. Suh TT, Holmback K, Jensen N et al. Resolution of spontaneous bleeding events but failure of pregnancy in fibrinogen-deficient mice. *Genes Dev* 1995;9:2020–33.

25. Inamoto Y, Terao T. First report of a case of congenital afibrinogenemia with successful delivery. *Am J Obstet Gynecol* 1985;153:803–4.

26. Gilabert J, Reganon E, Vila V et al. Congenital hypofibrinogenemia and pregnancy: Obstetric and hematological management. *Gynecol Obstet Invest* 1987;24:271–6.

27. MacKinnon HH, Fekete JF. Congenital afibrinogenemia: Vascular changes and multiple thromboses induced by fibrinogen infusions and contraceptive medication. *Can Med Assoc* 1971;140:597–9.

28. Beck EA. Congenital abnormalities of fibrinogen. *Clin Haematol* 1979;8:169–81.

29. Seligsohn U, Lubetsky A. Genetic susceptibility to venous thrombosis. *New Engl J Med* 2001;344:1222–31.

30. Many A, Schreiber L, Rosner S et al. Pathologic features of the placenta in women with severe pregnancy complications and thrombophilia. *Obstet Gynecol* 2001;98:1041–4.

31. Sedano S, Gaffney G, Mortimer G, Lyons M, Cleary B, Murray M, Maher M. Activated protein C resistance (APCR) and placental fibrin deposition. *Placenta* 2008;29:833–7.

32. Mousa HA, Alfirevic Z. Do placental lesions reflect thrombophilia state in women with adverse pregnancy outcome? *Hum Reprod* 2000;15:1830–3.

33. Arias F, Romero R, Joist H et al. Thrombophilia: A mechanism of disease in women with adverse pregnancy outcome and thrombotic lesions in the placenta. *J Matern–Fetal Med* 1998;7:277–86.

34. Raspollini MR, Oliva E, Roberts DJ. Placental histopathologic features in patients with thrombophilic mutations. *J Matern Fetal–Neonatal Med* 2007;20:113–23.

35. Lyden TW, Vogt E, Ng AK et al. Monoclonal antiphospholipid antibody reactivity against human placental trophoblast. *J Reprod Immunol* 1992;22:1–14.

36. Sood R, Kalloway S, Mast AE et al. Fetomaternal cross talk in the placental vascular bed: Control of coagulation by trophoblast cells. *Blood* 2006;107:3173–80.

37. Kupferminc MJ. Thrombophilia and pregnancy. *Reprod Biol Endocrinol* 2003;1:111.

38. Brenner B, Sarig G, Weiner Z et al. Thrombophilic polymorphisms are common in women with fetal loss without apparent cause. *Thromb Haemostasis* 1999;82:6–9.

39. Rey E, Kahn SR, David M et al. Thrombophilic disorders and fetal loss: A meta-analysis. *Lancet* 2003;361:901–8.

40. Krabbendam I, Franx A, Bots ML et al. Thrombophilias and recurrent pregnancy loss: A critical appraisal of the literature. *Eur J Obstet Gynecol Reprod Biol* 2005;118:143–53.

41. Nelen WL, Blom HJ, Steegers EA et al. Hyperhomocysteinemia and recurrent early pregnancy loss: A meta-analysis. *Fertil Steril* 2000;74:1196–9.

42. Preston FE, Rosendaal FR, Walker ID et al. Increased fetal loss in women with heritable thrombophilia. *Lancet* 1996;348:913–6.

43. Sarig G, Younis JS, Hoffman R et al. Thrombophilia is common in women with idiopathic pregnancy loss and is associated with late pregnancy wastage. *Fertil Steril* 2002;77:342–7.

44. Grandone E, Margaglione M, Colaizzo D et al. Factor V Leiden is associated with repeated and recurrent unexplained fetal losses. *Thromb Haemostasis* 1997;77:822–4.

45. Rodger MA, Betancourt MT, Clark P et al. The association of factor V Leiden and prothrombin gene mutation and placenta-mediated pregnancy complications: A systematic review and meta-analysis of prospective cohort studies. *PLoS Med* 2010;7:e1000292. doi: 10.1371.

46. Kupferminc MJ, Eldor A, Steinman N et al. Increased frequency of genetic thrombophilias in women with complications of pregnancy. *N Engl J Med* 1999;340:9–13.

47. Alfirevic Z, Roberts D, Martlew V. How strong is the association between maternal thrombophilia and adverse pregnancy outcome? A systematic review. *Eur J Obstet Gynecol Reprod Biol* 2002;101:6–14.

48. Gris JC, Quere I, Monpeyroux F et al. Case-control study of the frequency of thrombophilic disorders in couples with late fetal loss and no thrombotic antecedent. The Nimes obstetricians and haematologists study (NOHA). *Thromb Haemostasis* 1999;81:891–9.

49. Infante-Rivard C, Rivard GE, Yotov WV et al. Absence of association of thrombophilia polymorphisms with intrauterine growth restriction. *N Engl J Med* 2002;347:19–25.

50. Silver RM, Zhao Y, Spong CY et al. Eunice Kennedy Shriver National Institute of Child Health and Human Development Maternal-Fetal Medicine Units (NICHD MFMU) Network. Prothrombin gene G20210A mutation and obstetric complications. *Obstet Gynecol* 2010;115:14–20.

51. Kjellberg U, van Rooijen M, Bremme K et al. Factor V Leiden mutation and pregnancy-related complications. *Am J Obstet Gynecol* 2010;203:469.

52. Carp HJA, Dolitzky M, Inbal A. Hereditary thrombophilias are not associated with a decreased live birth rate in women with recurrent miscarriage. *Fertil Steril* 2002;78:58–62.

53. Salomon O, Seligsohn U, Steinberg DM et al. The common prothrombotic factors in nulliparous women do not compromise blood flow in the feto-maternal circulation and are not associated with preeclampsia or intrauterine growth restriction. *Am J Obstet Gynecol.* 2004;191:2002–9.

54. Sanson BJ, Friederich PW, Simioni P et al. The risk of abortion and stillbirth in antithrombin-, protein C-, and protein S-deficient women. *Thromb Haemostasis* 1996;75:387–8.

55. Gris JC, Mercier E, Quere I et al. Low-molecular-weight heparin versus low-dose aspirin in women with one fetal loss and a constitutional thrombophilic disorder. *Blood* 2004;103:3695–9.

56. Bates SM, Greer IA, Middeldorp S et al. Venous thromboembolism, thrombophilia, antithrombotic therapy and pregnancy: ACCP evidence-based clinical practice guidelines (Ninth Edition). *Chest* 2012;2(Suppl): E691S–736S

57. Carp HJA, Dolitzky M, Inbal A. Thromboprophylaxis improves the live birth rate in women with consecutive recurrent miscarriages and hereditary thrombophilia. *J Thromb Hemostasis* 2003;1:433–8.

58. Kaandorp SP, Goddijn M, van der Post JA et al. Aspirin plus heparin or aspirin alone in women with recurrent miscarriage. *N Engl J Med* 2010;362:1586–96.

59. Clark P, Walker ID, Langhorne P et al. Scottish Pregnancy Intervention Study (SPIN) collaborators. SPIN (Scottish Pregnancy Intervention) study: A multicenter, randomized controlled trial of low-molecular-weight heparin and low-dose aspirin in women with recurrent miscarriage. *Blood* 2010;115:4162–7.

60. Visser J, Ulander VM, Helmerhorst FM et al. Thromboprophylaxis for recurrent miscarriage in women with or without thrombophilia. HABENOX: A randomised multicentre trial. *Thromb Haemostasis* 2011;105:295–301.

61. Brenner B, Hoffman R, Carp HJA et al. The Live-Enox Investigators. Efficacy and safety of two doses of enoxaparin in women with thrombophilia and recurrent pregnancy loss: The LIVE-ENOX study. *J Thromb Haemostasis* 2005;3:227–9.

62. Nosaka M, Ishida Y, Kimura A et al. Absence of IFN-γ accelerates thrombus resolution through enhanced MMP-9 and VEGF expression in mice. *J Clin Invest* 2011;121:2911–20.

63. Carp HJA, Torchinsky A, Fein A et al. Hormones, Cytokines and fetal anomalies in habitual abortion. *J Gynecol Endocrinol* 2002;15:472–83.

64. Krause I, Blank M, Levi Y et al. Anti-idiotype immunomodulation of experimental anti-phospholipid syndrome via effect on Th1/Th2 expression. *Clin Exp Immunol* 1999;117:190–7.

65. Kowalska MA, Rauova L, Poncz M. Role of the platelet chemokine platelet factor 4 (PF4) in hemostasis and thrombosis. *Thromb Res* 2010;125:292–6.

66. Darmochwal-Kolarz D, Rolinski J, Leszczynska-Goarzelak B et al. The expressions of intracellular cytokines in the lymphocytes of preeclamptic patients. *Am J Reprod Immunol* 2002;48:381–6.

67. Maymon E, Ghezzi F, Edwin SS et al. The tumor necrosis factor alpha and its soluble receptor profile in term and preterm parturition. *Am J Obstet Gynecol* 1999;181:1142–8.

68. Hahn-Zoric M, Hagberg H, Kjellmer I et al. Aberrations in placental cytokine mRNA related to intrauterine growth retardation. *Pediatr Res* 2002;51:201–6.

69. Brill A, Torchinsky A., Carp HJA et al. The role of apoptosis in normal and abnormal embryonic development. *J Assist Reprod Genet* 1999;16:512–9.

70. Shetty S, Patil R, Ghosh K. Role of microparticles in recurrent miscarriages and other adverse pregnancies: A review. *Eur J Obstet Gynecol Reprod Biol* 2013;169:123–9.

71. Meilahn EN, Kuller LH, Matthews KA et al. Hemostatic factors according to menopausal status and use of hormone replacement therapy. *Ann Epidemiol* 1992;2:445–55.

72. Cosman F, Baz-Hecht M, Cushman M et al. Short-term effects of estrogen, tamoxifen and raloxifene on hemostasis: A randomized-controlled study and review of the literature. *Thromb Res* 2005;116:1–13.

73. Tong MH, Jiang H, Liu P et al. Spontaneous fetal loss caused by placental thrombosis in estrogen sulfotransferase-deficient mice. *Nat Med* 2005;11:153–9.

74. Polan ML, Daniele A, Kuo A. Gonadal steroids modulate human monocyte interleukin-1 (IL-1) activity. *Fertil Steril* 1988;49:964–8.

75. Schatz F, Krikun G, Caze R et al. Progestin-regulated expression of tissue factor in decidual cells: Implications in endometrial hemostasis, menstruation and angiogenesis. *Steroids* 2003;68:849–60.
76. Smiley ST, Boyer SN, Heeb MJ et al. Protein S is inducible by interleukin 4 in T cells and inhibits lymphoid cell procoagulant activity. *Proc Natl Acad Sci U.S.A* 1997;94:11484–9.
77. Uzumcu M, Coskun S, Jaroudi K et al. Effect of human chorionic gonadotropin on cytokine production from human endometrial cells in vitro. *Am J Reprod Immunol* 1998;40:83–8.
78. Jeddi-Tehrani M, Torabi R, Zarnani AH et al. Analysis of plasminogen activator inhibitor-1, integrin beta3, beta fibrinogen, and methylenetetrahydrofolate reductase polymorphisms in Iranian women with recurrent pregnancy loss. *Am J Reprod Immunol* 2011;66:149–56.
79. Ticconi C, Mancinelli F, Gravina P, Federici G, Piccione E, Bernardini S. Beta-fibrinogen G-455A polymorphisms and recurrent miscarriage. *Gynecol Obstet Invest* 2011;71:198–201.
80. Yenicesu GI, Cetin M, Ozdemir O et al. A prospective case-control study analyzes 12 thrombophilic gene mutations in Turkish couples with recurrent pregnancy loss. *Am J Reprod Immunol* 2010; 63:126–36.
81. Dahlbäck B. Advances in understanding pathogenic mechanisms of thrombophilic disorders. *Blood* 2008;112:19–27.
82. Segers O, van Oerle R, ten Cate H et al. Thrombin generation as an intermediate phenotype for venous thrombosis. *Thromb Haemostasis* 2010;103:114–22.
83. Guerra-Shinohara EM, Bertinato JF, Tosin Bueno C et al. Polymorphisms in antithrombin and in tissue factor pathway inhibitor genes are associated with recurrent pregnancy loss. *Thromb Haemostasis* 2012;108:693–700.
84. Rosing J. Mechanisms of OC related thrombosis. *Thromb Res.* 2005;115:Suppl 1:81–3.

23

Debate: Should Thromboprophylaxis Be Used in Hereditary Thrombophilias with Recurrent Pregnancy Loss? Yes

Benjamin Brenner

Introduction

Normal pregnancy is characterized by a prothrombotic phenotype, which may be relevant to implantation success and the hemostatic challenges of delivery, but also to the development of pregnancy complications. As pregnancy progresses, a marked increase in thrombin generation is observed[1] along with elevation in procoagulant factors and decrease in natural anticoagulants.[2] In *in vivo* models, targeting tissue factor (TF), tissue factor pathway inhibitor (TFPI), thrombomodulin (TM) and endothelial protein C receptor (EPCR) was found to cause placental thrombosis and early embryonic lethality in mice.[3] Treatment with heparin appeared to extend survival of EPCR−/− embryos,[4] but not of TM−/− embryos.[5]

Recurrent miscarriage, late pregnancy loss, fetal growth restriction (FGR), placental abruption (PA), and pre-eclampsia (PE) are common gestational pathologies, often sharing pathophysiological features. Collectively, these disorders present in 10–20% of pregnancies and are potentially associated with severe maternal and fetal outcome. Recurrent pregnancy loss (RPL) is a health problem affecting 1–5% of women at the reproductive age, which has significant emotional, social and economical impact. The hemostatic system plays an important role in these pathologies. For instance, coagulation activation is observed and fibrin deposition is found in small vessels in patients with pre-eclampsia and PA and in placentas of women with intrauterine fetal death.

Thrombophilic Risk Factors

Some case control and cohort studies have suggested an association between inherited thrombophilia and RPL.[6–8] Thrombophilic risk factors are frequent and can be observed in 15–25% of Caucasian populations. Since pregnancy is an acquired hypercoagulable state, women harboring thrombophilia may present with clinical symptoms of vascular complications for the first time during gestation.[9] Several meta-analyses support an association between pregnancy loss and maternal factor V Leiden (FVL), and factor II G20210A genotypes.[10–12] Findings from the "NOHA first" study, a large carefully designed case control study nested in a cohort of nearly 32,700 women, 18% of whom had pregnancy loss with first gestation, demonstrate in a multivariate analysis an association between unexplained first pregnancy loss after 10 weeks of gestation and the two thrombophilic risks factors (odds ratio, OR = 3.46 and OR = 2.60, respectively).[13]

Likewise, pre-eclampsia was found to be associated with FVL or prothrombin mutation (PTM) and homozygous MTHFR677T with mean OR around two.[14] A large Finnish study of 100,000 consecutive pregnancies reported that the risk of late preterm birth was three times higher in the FVL carriers, but not in women with prothrombin polymorphism.[15] Similarly, the Danish nested case-cohort study of pregnant women showed that FVL elevated the risk of late pregnancy complications.[16]

Finally, a meta-analysis of prospective cohort studies demonstrated the likelihood of pregnancy loss in FVL women to be around 50% higher. Notably, even this meta-analysis lacked power to detect increased risks in women with PTM.[17] Thus, the current notion is that, while thrombophilias are not the primary cause of pregnancy complications, they may still contribute to the miscarriage potential.

Women with antiphospholipid syndrome (APS) frequently present with RPL and/or late pregnancy complications. A modest association has been found between the thrombophilic risk factors and pregnancy complications.[17,18] Antithrombotics have been suggested to be beneficial in preventing late pregnancy loss in this clinical setting.[18]

Intervention with Antithrombotics

Documentation of thrombophilic risk factors in women with pregnancy complications may have therapeutic implications since recent clinical studies have demonstrated the potential efficacy of prophylaxis with low-molecular-weight heparin (LMWH) in these settings.[19,20] Gris et al.[21] performed a prospective randomized study in 160 women with thrombophilia and one previous pregnancy loss after 10 weeks of gestation. They reported that enoxaparin given throughout gestation at a dose of 40 mg daily, resulted in a significantly better live-born rate than low-dose aspirin (LDA) (86% vs. 29%, respectively). These differences were found in women with FVL and factor II G20210A mutations as well as in women with protein S deficiency. Moreover, thrombophilic women with copresence of protein Z deficiency or antibodies to protein Z had a reduced live birth rate following enoxaparin prophylaxis.[21]

In the LIVENOX study[19,20] (a randomized control study of 160 women comparing thromboprophylaxis with either 40 mg/day or 80 mg/day of enoxaparin), the incidence of pre-eclampsia in the 40 mg/day and 80 mg/day groups was 6.7% and 14.3%, respectively, and the incidence of PA was 13.5% and 8.8%, respectively. Approximately a quarter of the women in both groups had intrauterine growth restriction (IUGR) in previous gestations (22.5% and 24.2%, respectively). The live birth rate before the study was only 28%. During the study, the live birth rates were 84% for the 40 mg/day group, and 78% for the 80 mg/day group. Late gestational complications decreased after enoxaparin treatment. The incidence of pre-eclampsia in the enoxaparin 40 mg/day and 80 mg/day groups was 3.4% and 4.4%, respectively. Similarly, the incidence of PA in the enoxaparin 40 mg/day and 80 mg/day groups was 4.5% and 3.3%, respectively.[20]

In view of the lack of any effective alternative treatment and based on the safety of LMWH in pregnancy,[22,23] some obstetricians introduced thromboprophylaxis in women with recurrent miscarriage without thrombophilia.

In addition to pregnancy loss, a favorable local hemostatic milieu seems to be a prerequisite for successful implantation.[24] While procoagulant factors remain stable, impaired activity of the protein C pathway can be observed in implantation failure.[25,26] Based on the potential influence of heparin on implantation through various mechanisms,[27] various studies suggest that LMWH may improve the implantation rate.[28]

Several mechanisms have been implied in placental hemostasis. The procoagulant nature of placental trophoblasts may reflect the physiological requirement of hemostatic control in the intervillous space and preventing PA. TFPI is highly expressed in the placenta starting with the late first trimester of gestation up to term.[29,30] Heparanase has been reported to upregulate TF expression and interact with TFPI on endothelial cells, leading to elevated cell-surface coagulation activity.[31] This effect on TFPI and TFPI-2 in trophoblasts suggests potential involvement of heparanase in pregnancy complications.[32]

It was recently shown that microparticles (MPs), membrane vesicles shed from vascular and blood cells, take part in the placental and maternal crosstalk in normal pregnancies as well as in pregnancy complications[33] and occur with increased frequency in RPL.[34,35] A hemostatic balance, manifested by the TF/TFPI ratio on MPs originating from maternal and placental cells, has been suggested to reflect thrombogenicity in normal and pathological pregnancies.[36]

LMWHs stimulate expression, synthesis, and release of TFPI in endothelial cells and may exert their effect in pregnant women at risk for gestational vascular complications (GVC) by modulating local hemostasis at the syncytiotrophoblast (STB) surface, and affect trophoblast apoptosis, angiogenesis, and complement activation.[30,37] LMWH also promotes sflt1 release from first trimester placental villi. These effects are mediated in part by an interaction between heparin and cytotrophoblasts.[38]

The safety of LMWH in pregnancy has been reviewed in about 2800 treated pregnancies,[22] with the main indications being venous thromboembolism (VTE) prophylaxis and late pregnancy loss prevention.

The minor bleeding rate was low, thrombocytopenia was uncommon without heparin-induced thrombocytopenia, or clinically significant osteoporosis.

Low-Molecular-Weight Heparin for (Early) Miscarriage Prevention

Three recently published randomized controlled studies demonstrate that antithrombotic interventions are not effective in nonthrombophilic women with two or more miscarriages.[39–41] Notably, SPIN,[39] ALIFE,[40] and HABENOX[41] also recruited a small number of thrombophilic women (6%, 15.6%, and 24.6%, respectively). However, these trials were not powered to detect differences in particular settings, such as inherited thrombophilia and three or more recurrent miscarriages. In addition, an Italian multicenter observational study evaluated the efficacy of LMWH with/without aspirin on pregnancy outcome in a large number of women with FVL or PTM, compared to no treatment.[42] While a protective effect of LMWH on miscarriage rate was observed, LDA appeared to be ineffective.

Antithrombotics for Pregnancy Complications

Several randomized controlled trials (RCTs) have assessed the role of antithrombotics in women with placenta-mediated complications,[43–47] with only one study addressing this issue in thrombophilic women.[48] The majority of these studies showed a beneficial effect of LMWH. In the FRUIT study, adding LMWH to aspirin reduced recurrent early-onset pre-eclampsia, with no impact on general recurrence rate.[48] A recent meta-analysis of these six RCTs compared LMWH versus no LMWH for the prevention of recurrent placenta-mediated pregnancy complications, including 848 pregnant women with previous complications. Prophylactic LMWH was associated with a significantly lower recurrence of a composite outcome (pre-eclampsia, birth of a small for gestational age [SGA] newborn [<10th percentile], PA, or pregnancy loss >20 weeks) of pregnancy complications (19% versus 43%). The conclusions of this meta-analysis were that LMWH may be a promising therapy for recurrent, especially severe, placenta-mediated pregnancy complications but further research is required. Finally, a recent Cochrane review[49] found that antithrombotic intervention was associated with a statistically significant reduction in risk of perinatal mortality (RR 0.40; 95% CI 0.20–0.78), preterm birth before 34 (RR 0.46; 95% CI 0.29–0.73), and 37 weeks (RR 0.72; 95% CI 0.58–0.90) of gestation and birth weight below the 10th percentile for gestational age (RR 0.41; 95% CI 0.27–0.61), when compared with no treatment in women with previous pregnancy complications. The effect of LMWH may be particularly relevant in RPL where the incidence of pregnancy complications is higher (see Chapter 37).

Future studies should focus on examining antithrombotic interventions versus placebo (or suitable controls) in thrombophilic women with well characterized pregnancy complications, stratified by disease mechanism severity and pathological findings, such as a severely infarcted placenta.

Practical Considerations

Current available data suggest that thrombophilia is associated with recurrent and late pregnancy loss and also severe placenta-mediated complications. Early intervention with LMWH has the potential to improve maternal, fetal, and neonatal outcome. However, further studies focusing on subgroups of patients defined according to the disease pathology, such as specific thrombophilias or placental pathological findings, need to be conducted. In the meantime, risk assessment analysis is recommended, in terms of maternal age, comorbidities, personal and family history of VTE, pregnancy complications, and type of thrombophilia. In women at increased risk, thromboprophylaxis should be considered.

REFERENCES

1. McLean KC, Bernstein IM, Brummel-Ziedins KE. Tissue factor-dependent thrombin generation across pregnancy. *Am J Obstet Gynecol* 2012;207:135–6.
2. Szecsi PB, Jorgensen M, Klajnbard A et al. Haemostatic reference intervals in pregnancy. *Thromb Haemostasis* 2010;103:718–27.

3. Gu JM, Crawley JT, Ferrell G et al. Disruption of the endothelial cell protein C receptor gene in mice causes placental thrombosis and early embryonic lethality. *J Biol Chem* 2002;277:43335–43.

4. Li W, Zheng X, Gu JM et al. Extraembryonic expression of EPCR is essential for embryonic viability. *Blood* 2005; 106:2716–22.

5. Isermann B, Sood R, Pawlinski R et al. The thrombomodulin-protein C system is essential for the maintenance of pregnancy. *Nat Med* 2003; 9:331–7.

6. Grandone E, Margaglione M, Colaizzo D et al. Factor V Leiden is associated with repeated and recurrent unexplained fetal losses. *Thromb Haemostasis* 1997; 77:822–4.

7. Ridker PM, Miletich JP, Buring JE et al. Factor V Leiden mutation as a risk factor for recurrent pregnancy loss. *Ann Intern Med* 1998; 128:1000–3.

8. Brenner B, Sarig G, Weiner Z et al. Thrombophilic polymorphisms are common in women with fetal loss without apparent cause. *Thromb Haemostasis* 1999; 82:6–9.

9. Brenner B. Clinical management of thrombophilia-related placental vascular complications. *Blood* 2004;103:4003–9.

10. Rey E, Kahn SR, David M et al. Thrombophilic disorders and fetal loss: A meta-analysis. *Lancet* 2003;361:901–8.

11. Kovalevsky G, Gracia CR, Berlin JA et al. Evaluation of the association between hereditary thrombophilias and recurrent pregnancy loss: A meta-analysis. *Arch Intern Med* 2004;164:558–63.

12. Dudding TE, Attia J. The association between adverse pregnancy outcomes and maternal factor V Leiden genotype: A meta-analysis. *Thromb Haemostasis* 2004;91:700–11.

13. Lissalde-Lavigne G, Fabbro-Peray P, Cochery-Nouvellon E et al. Factor V Leiden and prothrombin G20210A polymorphisms as risk factors for miscarriage during a first intended pregnancy: The matched case-control 'NOHA first' study. *J Thromb Haemostasis* 2005;3:2178–84.

14. Robertson L, Wu O, Langhorne P et al. Thrombophilia in pregnancy: A systematic review. *Br J Haematol* 2006;132:171–96.

15. Hiltunen LM, Laivuori H, Rautanen A et al. Factor V Leiden as risk factor for unexplained stillbirth—A population-based nested case-control study. *Thromb Res* 2010;125:505–10.

16. Lykke JA, Bare LA, Olsen J et al. Thrombophilias and adverse pregnancy outcomes: Results from the Danish National Birth Cohort. *J Thromb Haemostasis* 2012;10:1320–5.

17. Rodger MA, Betancourt MT, Clark P et al. The association of factor V Leiden and prothrombin gene mutation and placenta-mediated pregnancy complications: A systematic review and meta-analysis of prospective cohort studies. *PLoS Med* 2010;7:e1000292.

18. Bates SM, Greer IA, Middeldorp S et al. VTE, thrombophilia, antithrombotic therapy, and pregnancy: Antithrombotic therapy and prevention of thrombosis, 9th ed: American College of Chest Physicians Evidence-Based Clinical Practice Guidelines. *Chest* 2012;141(2 Suppl):e691S–736S.

19. Brenner B, Bar J, Ellis M et al. Effects of enoxaparin on late pregnancy complications and neonatal outcome in women with recurrent pregnancy loss and thrombophilia: Results from the Live-Enox study. *Fertil Steril* 2005;84:770–3.

20. Brenner B, Hoffman R, Carp H et al. Efficacy and safety of two doses of enoxaparin in women with thrombophilia and recurrent pregnancy loss: The LIVE-ENOX study. *J Thromb Haemostasis* 2005;3:227–9.

21. Gris JC, Mercier E, Quere I et al. Low-molecular-weight heparin versus low-dose aspirin in women with one fetal loss and a constitutional thrombophilic disorder. *Blood* 2004;103:3695–9.

22. Greer IA, Nelson-Piercy C. Low-molecular-weight heparins for thromboprophylaxis and treatment of venous thromboembolism in pregnancy: A systematic review of safety and efficacy. *Blood* 2005;106:401–7.

23. Nelson-Piercy C, Powrie R, Borg JY et al. Tinzaparin use in pregnancy: An international, retrospective study of the safety and efficacy profile. *Eur J Obstet Gynecol Reprod Biol* 2011;159:293–9.

24. Lockwood CJ, Krikun G, Rahman M et al. The role of decidualization in regulating endometrial hemostasis during the menstrual cycle, gestation, and in pathological states. *Semin Thromb Hemostasis* 2007;33:111–7.

25. Knol HM, Kemperman RF, Kluin-Nelemans HC et al. Haemostatic variables during normal menstrual cycle. A systematic review. *Thromb Haemostasis* 2012;107:22–9.

26. van Vliet HA, Rodrigues SP, Snieders MN et al. Sensitivity to activated protein C during the menstrual cycle in women with and without factor V Leiden. *Thromb Res* 2008;121:757–61.

27. Nelson SM, Greer IA. The potential role of heparin in assisted conception. *Hum Reprod Update* 2008;14:623–45.

28. Qublan H, Amarin Z, Dabbas M et al. Low-molecular-weight heparin in the treatment of recurrent IVF-ET failure and thrombophilia: A prospective randomized placebo-controlled trial. *Hum Fertil (Camb)* 2008;11:246–53.

29. Edstrom CS, Calhoun DA, Christensen RD. Expression of tissue factor pathway inhibitor in human fetal and placental tissues. *Early Hum Dev* 2000;59:77–84.

30. Aharon A, Lanir N, Drugan A et al. TFPI is decreased in gestational vascular complications and can be restored by maternal enoxaparin treatment. *J Thromb Haemostasis* 2005;3:2355–7.

31. Nadir Y, Brenner B, Gingis-Velitski S et al. Heparanase induces tissue factor pathway inhibitor expression and extracellular accumulation in endothelial and tumor cells. *Thromb Haemostasis* 2008;99:133–41.

32. Nadir Y, Kenig Y, Drugan A et al. Involvement of heparanase in vaginal and cesarean section deliveries. *Thromb Res* 2010;126:444–50.

33. Shomer E, Katzenell S, Zipori Y et al. Microvesicles of women with gestational hypertension and pre-eclampsia affect human trophoblast fate and endothelial function. *Hypertension* 2013;62:893–8.

34. Laude I, Rongieres-Bertrand C, Boyer-Neumann, C. et al. Circulating procoagulant microparticles in women with unexplained pregnancy loss: A new insight. *Thromb Haemostasis* 2001;85:18–2 1.

35. Carp H, Dardik R, Lubetsky A et al. Prevalence of circulating procoagulant microparticles in women with recurrent miscarriage: A case-controlled study. *Hum Reprod* 2004;19:191–5.

36. Aharon A, Katzenell S, Tamari T et al. Microparticles bearing tissue factor and tissue factor pathway inhibitor in gestational vascular complications. *J Thromb Haemostasis* 2009;7:1047–50.

37. Sarig G, Blumenfeld Z, Leiba R et al. Modulation of systemic hemostatic parameters by enoxaparin during gestation in women with thrombophilia and pregnancy loss. *Thromb Haemostasis* 2005;94:980–5.

38. Drewlo S, Levytska K, Sobel M et al. Heparin promotes soluble VEGF receptor expression in human placental villi to impair endothelial VEGF signaling. *J Thromb Haemostasis* 2011;9:2486–97.

39. Clark P, Walker ID, Langhorne P et al. SPIN (Scottish Pregnancy Intervention) study: A multicenter, randomized controlled trial of low-molecular-weight heparin and low-dose aspirin in women with recurrent miscarriage. *Blood* 2010;115:4162–7.

40. Kaandorp SP, Goddijn M, van der Post JA et al. Aspirin plus heparin or aspirin alone in women with recurrent miscarriage. *N Engl J Med* 2010;362:1586–96.

41. Visser J, Ulander VM, Helmerhorst FM et al. Thromboprophylaxis for recurrent miscarriage in women with or without thrombophilia. HABENOX: A randomised multicentre trial. *Thromb Haemostasis* 2011;105:295–301.

42. Tormene D, Grandone E, De Stefano V et al. Obstetric complications and pregnancy-related venous thromboembolism: The effect of low-molecular-weight heparin on their prevention in carriers of factor V Leiden or prothrombin G20210A mutation. *Thromb Haemostasis* 2012;107:477–84.

43. Mello G, Parretti E, Fatini C et al. Low-molecular-weight heparin lowers the recurrence rate of pre-eclampsia and restores the physiological vascular changes in angiotensin-converting enzyme DD women. *Hypertension* 2005;45:86–91.

44. Rey E, Garneau P, David M et al. Dalteparin for the prevention of recurrence of placental-mediated complications of pregnancy in women without thrombophilia: A pilot randomized controlled trial. *J Thromb Haemostasis* 2009;7:58–64.

45. Gris JC, Chauleur C, Faillie JL et al. Enoxaparin for the secondary prevention of placental vascular complications in women with abruptio placentae. The pilot randomised controlled NOH-AP trial. *Thromb Haemostasis* 2010;104:771–9.

46. Gris JC, Chauleur C, Molinari N et al. Addition of enoxaparin to aspirin for the secondary prevention of placental vascular complications in women with severe pre-eclampsia. The pilot randomised controlled NOH-PE trial. *Thromb Haemostasis* 2011;106:1053–61.

47. Martinelli I, Ruggenenti P, Cetin I et al. Heparin in pregnant women with previous placenta-mediated pregnancy complications: A prospective, randomized, multicenter, controlled clinical trial. *Blood* 2012;119:3269–75.

48. de Vries JI, van Pampus MG, Hague WM et al. Low-molecular-weight heparin added to aspirin in the prevention of recurrent early-onset pre-eclampsia in women with inheritable thrombophilia: The FRUIT-RCT. *J Thromb Haemost* 2012;10:64–72.

49. Dodd JM, McLeod A, Windrim RC et al. Antithrombotic therapy for improving maternal or infant health outcomes in women considered at risk of placental dysfunction. *Cochrane Database Syst Rev* 2013;7:CD006780.

24

Debate: Should Thromboprophylaxis Be Used in Hereditary Thrombophilias with Recurrent Pregnancy Loss? No

Pelle G. Lindqvist

Habitual abortion is usually defined as at least three consecutive fetal losses. It affects 0.3% of the pregnant population in proportion to a 75% live birth rate after three consecutive fetal losses.[1,2] Recurrent fetal loss often has a broader definition of at least three first trimester fetal losses and/or ≥two second trimester fetal losses. It affects between 1% and 2% of the pregnant population. Factors that are major determinants of the risk of miscarriage are; increasing maternal age, the number of prior fetal losses, and if cardiac activity had been detected or not.[2] The pathogenesis of recurrent fetal loss in the majority of cases is still unclear. Several causes have been suggested: chromosome aberrations, thrombophilias, thyroid abnormality, microparticles, and complement activation.[3]

Treatment of recurrent fetal loss with low-molecular-weight heparin (LMWH) is mainly based on a supposed causative relationship between thrombophilias and recurrent fetal loss. Such a link is not established and still disputed. Since more than 90% of women with heritable thrombophilias in Caucasian populations are carriers of either coagulation factor V Leiden (FVL) or the prothrombin gene mutation G20210A (FII), the analysis below will focus on these factors which are present in between 7% and 13% in European populations. First trimester fetal loss has not been related to hereditary thrombophilia, neither in large cohorts[4,5] nor in the largest case-control studies.[6,7] Studies of early recurrent fetal loss show no increased risk in the largest case-control studies.[6,8] However, meta-analysis and systematic reviews have reported an increased prevalence of thrombophilias in miscarriages.[9,10] Meta-analyses may not be a sound method of amassing evidence from retrospective, uncontrolled, underpowered studies, which are subject to several types of bias and the reviews failed to identify large studies. In addition, the conclusions drawn from case-control studies tend to overestimate risk assessments as compared to cohort studies. With regard to second trimester (or >10 gestational weeks) or third trimester fetal loss, there seems to exist an increased risk.[7,11,12]

Both FVL and FII are single gene mutations that appear first to have occurred 25,000 years ago.[13] A strong relation between these thrombophilias and fetal loss would have had a strong negative impact on the respective gene pool. Instead, the number of carriers of FVL have gone from one person 25,000 years ago to about 50 million carriers of Caucasian descent today.[14] Thus, in an evolutionary perspective it is unlikely that a large increase in risk of fetal loss in the general population has been caused by these thrombophilias. However, this does not exclude the possibility of a relationship to small subgroups, that is, second or third trimester fetal losses or habitual abortions. Thus, a causative link between fetal loss and rare mutations such as antithrombin, protein C, and protein S deficiencies is more likely, as compared to FVL and FII.[12]

There have been some treatment studies published using a "before and after" design.[15,16] This design lacks a control group and the result is conditioned by the phenomenon of "regression toward the mean."[17,18] Therefore, in this type of design one should expect the group of women with a high rate of recurrent fetal loss to have a lower rate in the following pregnancies by natural causes, independent of medical intervention. Therefore, no conclusions may be drawn from the results. From our prospective cohort study of FVL and pregnancy complications,[5] we have compiled data on the magnitude of "regression toward the mean" (see data in Table 24.1).[19] Our untreated women with recurrent fetal

TABLE 24.1

Pregnancy Outcome in Different Subgroups of Women with Prior Fetal Loss

	Prior Live Birth Rate (%)	Present Live Birth Rate (%)
Recurrent fetal loss		
Enoxaparin 40 or 80 mg (*n* = 50) (Brenner et al., 2000[15])[a]	20%	75%
Enoxaparin 40 mg (*n* = 89) (Brenner et al., 2005[16])[a]	28%	84%
Enoxaparin 80 mg (*n* = 91) (Brenner et al., 2005[16])[a]	28%	78%
No treatment (*n* = 37) (Lindqvist and Merlo, 2006[17])[b]	28%	89%
Second trimester fetal loss		
1 prior (*n* = 43) No treatment (Lindqvist and Merlo, 2006[17])	49%	98%
≥2 prior (*n* = 10) No treatment (Lindqvist and Merlo, 2006[17])	30%	80%
Nulliparous women with one prior fetal losses and carriers of FVL		
Low-dose aspirin (*n* = 36) (Gris et al., 2004[20])	0%	29%
Enoxaparin 40 mg (*n* = 36) (Gris et al., 2004[20])	0%	94%
No treatment (*n* = 20) (Lindqvist and Merlo, 2006[17])[c]	0%	95%
No treatment (*n* = 52) (Lindqvist and Merlo, 2006[17])[d]	40%	98%

Recurrent fetal loss ≥3 first trimester and/or ≥2 second trimester fetal loss.

[a] Includes or/and ≥1 stillbirth.

[b] Includes women with and without thrombophilia.

[c] Nulliparous carriers of FVL with at least 1 prior fetal loss.

[d] FVL carriers with at least 1 prior fetal loss.

loss have a similar outcome as those treated with enoxaparin.[15,16] Moreover, our untreated FVL carriers with prior fetal loss had similar outcomes as the subgroup with FVL carriers with a single prior fetal loss who were treated with enoxaparin (Table 24.1).[19,20] Since, low-dose aspirin has not been shown to be effective in recurrent pregnancy loss due to hereditary thrombophilia, comparisons must be made with no treatment or placebo and not with low-dose aspirin.[19,21] Two randomized controlled trials were recently published on thromboprophylaxis for recurrent miscarriage.[21,22] These were not designed for comparison of hereditary thrombophilias but data are given. In these studies, 13% and 16% of women tested positive for hereditary thrombophilia, that is, somewhat higher than expected. However, there were no differences in the live birth rate between the study groups.

Regarding first trimester recurrent fetal loss there are presently no data suggesting increased prevalence of thrombophilias, which was the basis for LMWH treatment for this group. In addition, future studies must deal with the high prevalence of abnormal embryonic karyotype (25–57%) in early miscarriage.[23]

Regarding second and third trimester recurrent fetal losses there seems to be a slightly increased prevalence of thrombophilias. However, in the absence of studies specifically designed to address the issue at hand, we have as yet no evidence to recommend treatment with LMWH for recurrent fetal loss due to thrombophilia. Thus, adopting anticoagulant prophylaxis to prevent late recurrent fetal loss should be considered experimental.

REFERENCES

1. Warburton D, Fraser FC. On the probability that a woman who has had a spontaneous abortion will abort in subsequent pregnancies. *J Obstet Gynaecol Br Emp* 1961;68:784–8.

2. Brigham SA, Conlon C, Farquharson RG. A longitudinal study of pregnancy outcome following idiopathic recurrent miscarriage. *Hum Reprod* 1999;14:2868–71.

3. Carp H, Dardik R, Lubetsky A et al. Prevalence of circulating procoagulant microparticles in women with recurrent miscarriage: A case-controlled study. *Hum Reprod* 2004;19:191–5.

4. Roque H, Paidas MJ, Funai EF et al. Maternal thrombophilias are not associated with early pregnancy loss. *Thromb Haemostasis* 2004;91:290–5.

5. Lindqvist PG, Svensson PJ, Marsaal K et al. Activated protein C resistance (FV:Q506) and pregnancy. *Thromb Haemostasis* 1999;81:532–7.

6. Rai R, Shlebak A, Cohen H et al. Factor V Leiden and acquired activated protein C resistance among 1000 women with recurrent miscarriage. *Hum Reprod* 2001;16:961–5.

7. Lissalde-Lavigne G, Fabbro-Peray P, Cochery-Nouvellon E et al. Factor V Leiden and prothrombin G20210A polymorphisms as risk factors for miscarriage during a first intended pregnancy: The matched case-control "NOHA first" study. *J Thromb Haemostasis* 2005;3:2178–84.

8. Carp H, Salomon O, Seidman D et al. Prevalence of genetic markers for thrombophilia in recurrent pregnancy loss. *Hum Reprod* 2002;17:1633–7.

9. Kovalevsky G, Gracia CR, Berlin JA et al. Evaluation of the association between hereditary thrombophilias and recurrent pregnancy loss: A meta-analysis. *Arch Intern Med* 2004;164:558–63.

10. Robertson L, Wu O, Langhorne P et al. Thrombophilia in pregnancy: A systematic review. *Br J Haematol* 2006;132:171–96.

11. Rodger MA, Betancourt MT, Clark P et al. The association of factor V Leiden and prothrombin gene mutation and placenta-mediated pregnancy complications: A systematic review and meta-analysis of prospective cohort studies. *PLoS Med* 2010;7:e1000292.

12. Preston FE, Rosendaal FR, Walker ID et al. Increased fetal loss in women with heritable thrombophilia. *Lancet* 1996;348:913–6.

13. Zivelin A, Mor-Cohen R, Kovalsky V et al. Prothrombin 20210G>A is an ancestral prothrombotic mutation that occurred in whites approximately 24,000 years ago. *Blood* 2006;107:4666–8.

14. Lindqvist PG, Zöller B, Dahlbäck B. Improved hemoglobin status and reduced menstrual blood loss among female carriers of activated protein C resistance (FV Leiden). An evolutionary advantage? *Thromb Haemostasis* 2001;86:1122–3.

15. Brenner B, Hoffman R, Blumenfeld Z et al. Gestational outcome in thrombophilic women with recurrent pregnancy loss treated by enoxaparin. *Thromb Haemostasis* 2000;83:693–7.

16. Brenner B, Hoffman R, Carp H et al. Efficacy and safety of two doses of enoxaparin in women with thrombophilia and recurrent pregnancy loss: The LIVE-ENOX study. *J Thromb Haemostasis* 2005;3:227–9.

17. Lindqvist PG, Merlo J. Low molecular weight heparin for repeated pregnancy loss: Is it based on solid evidence? *J Thromb Haemostasis* 2005;3:221–3.

18. Regression toward the mean. December 21, 2005. [cited; Available from: http://en.wikipedia.org/wiki/Regression_toward_the_mean].

19. Lindqvist PG, Merlo J. The natural course of women with recurrent fetal loss. *J Thromb Haemostasis* 2006;4;896–7.

20. Gris JC, Mercier E, Quere I et al. Low-molecular-weight heparin versus low-dose aspirin in women with one fetal loss and a constitutional thrombophilic disorder. *Blood* 2004;103:3695–9.

21. Visser J, Ulander VM, Helmerhorst FM et al. Thromboprophylaxis for recurrent miscarriage in women with or without thrombophilia. HABENOX: A randomised multicentre trial. *Thromb Haemostasis* 2011;105:295–301.

22. Kaandorp SP, Goddijn M, van der Post JA et al. Aspirin plus heparin or aspirin alone in women with recurrent miscarriage. *N Engl J Med* 2010;362:1586–96.

23. Sugiura-Ogasawara M, Ozaki Y, Katano K et al. Abnormal embryonic karyotype is the most frequent cause of recurrent miscarriage. *Hum Reprod* 2012;27:2297–303.

25

Opinion: Can Recurrent Pregnancy Loss Be Prevented by Antithrombotic Agents?

Howard J. A. Carp

The association between inherited thrombophilic disorders and miscarriage was first detected in family studies of probands diagnosed with venous thromboembolus (VTE).[1–3] Many studies have subsequently assessed the relationship between inherited thrombophilia and pregnancy complications.[4–6] A presumed benefit of antithrombotic therapy, and lack of side effects has led many clinicians to prescribe low-molecular-weight heparins (LMWH), aspirin, or both to women with recurrent miscarriage and unexplained pregnancy loss, even in the absence of thrombophilia. The aim is entirely laudable, to prevent women with recurrent pregnancy losses from suffering additional miscarriages. The rationale is that aspirin may act on hitherto unrecognized thrombophilias, and that both aspirin and heparins have anti-inflammatory effects in addition to anticoagulant effect. Indeed, there are additional throbmophilas which are not usually assessed in the clinical setting. Endothelial microparticles and Protein Z are just two. Aspirin selectively irreversibly acetylates the hydroxyl group of one serine residue in cyclooxgenase (COX) leading to COX inhibition.[7] Aspirin and other antiplatelet agents have also been reported to have a role in the inhibition of the proinflammatory cytokines TNFα and IL-8 in stroke.[8] TNFα induces thrombin generation.[9,10] IL-8 causes polymorph accumulation.[11] Polymorphs react with fibrin and damaged tissues to form clots. In addition, aspirin is capable of stimulating IL-3 production *in vitro*.[12] Hence aspirin may also modify cytokine-mediated thrombosis. The maintenance of pregnancy has been widely reported to be dependent on a shift of the proinflammatory to anti-inflammatory cytokines.[13]

Heparins also have anti-inflammatory actions. Heparin increases serum TNF binding protein, protecting against systemic harmful manifestations of tumor necrosis factor (TNF).[14] LMWH inhibit TNFα production.[15]

Thrombosis results in an inflammatory response in the vein wall. Both heparin and LMWT limit the anti-inflammatory response,[16] including neutrophil extravasation and decreasing vein wall permeability. Heparin also has direct effects on the trophoblast. It has been reported to restore the invasive properties of the trophoblast in antiphospholipid syndrome (APS),[17] and to enhance placental human chorionic gonadotrophin (hCG) production.

However, the high-quality evidence for the beneficial effect of aspirin or LMWH is still absent. Aspirin and LMWH will be examined separately.

Aspirin

Except in APS, there is only one randomized trial of aspirin for the prevention of miscarriage.[18] The authors concluded that low dose aspirin is ineffective in the prevention of miscarriage in recurrent spontaneous abortion. Rai et al.[19] carried out a prospective observational study to assess the value of low dose aspirin (75 mg daily) in improving the subsequent live birth rate in women with either unexplained recurrent early miscarriage (<13 weeks gestation; $n = 805$) or unexplained late pregnancy loss ($n = 250$). There was no significant difference in the live birth rate between women with early pregnancy losses who took aspirin compared to women who did not take aspirin (odds ratio [OR] 1.24; 95% confidence interval [CI] 0.93–1.67). In contrast, women with a previous late miscarriage who took aspirin had a significantly higher live birth rate than those who did not take aspirin (OR 1.88; 95% CI

TABLE 25.1

Aspirin in Unexplained Recurrent Pregnancy Loss

	Aspirin	Control	RR (CI)
Tulppala et al.[18]	22/27 (81.5%)	22/27 (81.5%)	1.0 (0.78–1.29)
Rai et al.[19]	373/556 (67.1%)	308/449 (61.7%)	1.26 (0.92–1.64)
Kaandorp et al.[23]	42/82 (51.2%)	47/81 (58.0%)	0.90 (0.66–1.22)
Visser et al.[27] (aspirin and enoxaparin vs. enoxaparin and placebo)	32/48 (66.7%)	35/51 (68.3%)	0.96 (0.62–1.46)

Note: Proportion of live births are shown in parentheses.

TABLE 25.2

Heparins in Unexplained Recurrent Pregnancy Loss

	Heparin	Controls	RR (CI)
Badawey et al.[20] (enoxaparin and folic acid vs. folic acid alone)	161/170 (94.7%)	151/170 (88.8%)	1.07 (1.00–1.14)
Dolitzky et al.[21] (enoxaparin vs. aspirin)	44/54 (81.5%)	42/50 (84.0%)	0.92 (0.58–1.46)
Clark et al.[22] (heparin and aspirin vs. surveillance alone)	111/143 (77.6%)	111/140 (79.3%)	0.95 (0.73–1.25)
Kaandorp et al.[23] (nandoparin and aspirin vs. placebo)	45/92 (48.9%)	47/81 (58.0%)	0.84 (0.64–1.11)
Visser et al.[27] (enoxaparin and placebo vs. aspirin)	35/51 (68.2%)	34/57 (59.6%)	1.24 (0.79–1.92)

1.04–3.37). The authors concluded that empirical use of low dose aspirin in women with unexplained recurrent early miscarriage is not justified. Table 25.1 shows the various series in the literature from which the effect of aspirin could be deduced. No trial showed a statistically significant effect.

Heparins

A randomized control trial (RCT) by Badawey et al.[20] suggests that heparins may raise the live birth rate in women with unexplained RPL. However, since the trial by Badawey et al.,[20] there have been a number of additional trials which are very heterogeneous in their nature. Dolitzky et al.[21] compared enoxaparin to aspirin in women with unexplained RPL loss in whom thrombophilas had been excluded. There was no difference in the live birth rate. In the SPIN study,[22] 294 women with two or more unexplained pregnancy losses were randomized to enoxaparin 40 mg combined with aspirin, 75 mg plus standard surveillance or standard surveillance only. No effect of the medical intervention was observed. In the ALIFE study,[23] 364 women with two or more unexplained pregnancy losses were randomized to nadroparin 2850 IU combined with aspirin 80 mg, aspirin 80 mg only, or placebo (for aspirin) before conception or at a maximum gestational age of six weeks. The chance of live birth did not differ between the treatment groups. The various trials have been summarized in Table 25.2. No trial shows any benefit from the use of heparins. Based on the updated available evidence various guidelines recommend against the use of antithrombotic agents in women with unexplained RPL.[24,25]

In conclusion, none of the abovementioned intervention studies have clearly and unequivocally shown the benefit of LMWH with or without the addition of aspirin in women with unexplained recurrent pregnancy loss. These gaps should be filled by multinational collaborative studies.[26]

REFERENCES

1. Sanson BJ, Friederich PW, Simioni P et al. The risk of abortion and stillbirth in antithrombin-, protein C-, and protein S-deficient women. *Thromb Haemostasis* 1996;3:387–8.
2. Preston FE, Rosendaal FR, Walker ID et al. Increased fetal loss in women with heritable thrombophilia. *Lancet* 1996;348:913–6.

3. Meinardi JR, Middeldorp S, de Kam PJ et al. Increased risk for fetal loss in carriers of the factor V Leiden mutation. *Ann Int Med* 1999;9:736–9.

4. Rey E, Kahn SR, David M, Shrier I. Thrombophilic disorders and fetal loss: A meta-analysis. *Lancet* 2003;361:901–8.

5. Robertson L, Wu O, Langhorne P et al. Thrombophilia in pregnancy: A systematic review. *Br J Haematol* 2006;2:171–96.

6. Rodger MA, Betancourt MT, Clark P et al. The association of factor V Leiden and prothrombin gene mutation and placenta-mediated pregnancy complications: A systematic review and meta-analysis of prospective cohort studies. *PLoS Med* 2010;6:e1000292.

7. Vane JR, Botting RM. The mechanism of action of aspirin. *Thromb Res* 2003;110:255–258.

8. Al-Bahrani A, Taha S, Shaath H et al. TNF-alpha and IL-8 in acute stroke and the modulation of these cytokines by antiplatelet agents. *Curr Neurovasc Res* 2007;4:31–7.

9. Levi M, Ten Cate H. Disseminated intravascular coagulation. *N Engl J Med*, 1999;341:586–92.

10. Yan SB, Helterbrand J, Hartman DL et al. Low levels of protein C are associated with poor outcome in severe sepsis. *Chest* 2001;120: 915–22.

11. Schraufstatter IU, Trieu K, Zhao M et al. IL-8-mediated cell migration in endothelial cells depends on cathepsin B activity and transactivation of the epidermal growth factor receptor. *J Immunol* 2003;171:6714–22.

12. Fishman P, Falach-Vaknin E, Sredni B et al. Aspirin-interleukin-3 interrelationships in patients with anti-phospholipid syndrome. *Am J Reprod Immunol* 1996;35:80–4

13. Carp HJA. Cytokines in recurrent miscarriage. *Lupus* 2004;13:630–4.

14. Lantz M, Thysell H, Nilsson E et al. On the binding of tumor necrosis factor (TNF) to heparin and the release *in vivo* of the TNF-binding protein I by heparin. *J Clin Invest* 1991;88:2026–31.

15. Baram D, Rashkovsky M, Hershkoviz R et al. Inhibitory effects of low molecular weight heparin on mediator release by mast cells: Preferential inhibition of cytokine production and mast cell-dependent cutaneous inflammation. *Clin Exp Immunol* 1997;110:485–91.

16. Downing LJ, Strieter RM, Kadell AM et al. Low-dose low-molecular-weight heparin is anti-inflammatory during venous thrombosis. *J Vasc Surg* 1998;28:848–54.

17. Bose P, Black S, Kadyrov M et al. Adverse effects of lupus anticoagulant positive blood sera on placental viability can be prevented by heparin in vitro. *Am J Obstet Gynecol* 2004;191:2125–31

18. Tulppala M, Marttunen M, Soderstrom-Anttila V et al. Low dose aspirin in the prevention of miscarriage in women with unexplained or autoimmune related recurrent miscarriage: Effect on prostacyclin and thromboxane A2 production. *Hum Reprod* 1997;12:1567–72.

19. Rai R, Backos M, Baxter N et al. Recurrent miscarriage—An aspirin a day? *Hum Reprod* 2000;15:2220–3.

20. Badawey AM, Khiary M, Sherif LS et al. Low-molecular weight heparin in patients with recurrent early miscarriages of unknown aetiology. *J Obstet Gynaecol* 2008;28:280–4.

21. Dolitzky M, Inbal A, Segal Y et al. A randomized study of thromboprophylaxis in women with unexplained consecutive recurrent miscarriages. *Fertil Steril* 2006;86:362–6.

22. Clark P, Walker ID, Langhorne P et al. SPIN: The Scottish Pregnancy Intervention Study: A multicentre randomised controlled trial of low molecular weight heparin and low dose aspirin in women with recurrent miscarriage. *Blood* 2010;21:4162–7.

23. Kaandorp SP, Goddijn M, van der Post JA et al. Aspirin plus heparin or aspirin alone in women with recurrent miscarriage. *N Engl J Med* 2010;17:1586–96.

24. Bates SM, Greer IA, Middeldorp S et al. Venous thromboembolism, thrombophilia, antithrombotic therapy and pregnancy: ACCP evidence-based clinical practice guidelines (Ninth Edition). *Chest* 2012;2(Suppl):e691S–736S.

25. Royal College of Obstetricians and Gynaecologists. The investigation and treatment of couples with recurrent first-trimester and second-trimester miscarriage. *Green-top Guideline no 17* 2011;1–18.

26. Middeldorp S. Thrombosis in women: What are the knowledge gaps in 2013? *J Thromb Haemostasis* 2013;11(s1):180–91.

27. Visser J, Ulander VM, Helmerhorst FM et al. Thromboprophylaxis for recurrent miscarriage in women with or without thrombophilia. HABENOX: A randomised multicentre trial. *Thromb Haemostasis* 2011;105:295–301.

26

Uterine Anomalies and Recurrent Pregnancy Loss

Daniel S. Seidman and Mordechai Goldenberg

Introduction

Although uterine anomalies have been associated with recurrent miscarriage, it is frustrating to realize how little is known about the pathophysiology underlying uterine anomalies and fetal wastage. Additionally, the prevalence and impact of uterine malformations have not been conclusively determined.[1] Even the true incidence of congenital uterine anomalies in the general population is unknown. A review of the available literature reveals a wide range of reported incidences, from 0.2% to 10.0%.[2] Using newer imaging modalities, it is currently estimated that the incidence of uterine anomalies in the general population is approximately 1%, and it is about three-fold higher in women with recurrent pregnancy loss and poor reproductive outcomes.[2] Below, we will discuss in detail the new modes of imaging that have been introduced over the last two decades and which may modify the previously reported data on the incidence.

In addition to pregnancy loss, uterine malformations predispose women to other reproductive difficulties including infertility, preterm labor, and abnormal fetal presentation. These poor reproductive outcomes are often attributed to the presence of a uterine septum, intrauterine adhesions, polyps, and fibroids, all of which are amenable to surgical correction. Therefore, an accurate diagnosis is essential in order to offer appropriate treatment.

In this chapter, we will review the common congenital and acquired uterine anomalies associated with recurrent pregnancy losses, and discuss contemporary diagnosis and treatment options.

Development and Classification of Mullerian Tract Defects

Uterine anomalies are commonly classified as congenital or acquired. The classification of congenital uterine defects is largely based on the understanding of Mullerian duct development. The two-paired Mullerian ducts of the embryo ultimately develop into the female reproductive tract. The cephalic ends of the Mullerian ducts form the fallopian tubes and the caudal portions fuse to form the uterus, cervix, and the upper two-thirds of the vagina. The ovaries and lower one third of the vagina have separate embryologic origins. The Mullerian ducts grow caudally and become enclosed in peritoneal folds that later develop into the round and ovarian ligaments. In the female embryo, sexual differentiation is marked by degeneration of the Wolffian ducts in the absence of fetal testes and testosterone. Absence of Mullerian-inhibiting substance, allows the Mullerian ducts to fully mature. At 9 weeks of gestation, the uterine cervix is recognizable and by 17 weeks, the formation of the myometrium is complete. Vaginal development begins at approximately 9 weeks. The uterovaginal plate forms between the caudal buds of the Mullerian ducts and the dorsal wall of the urogenital sinus. These cells will degenerate, thereby increasing the distance between the uterus and urogenital sinus. Hence, the upper two thirds of the vagina derives from Mullerian ducts while the remainder derives from the urogenital sinus. Complete formation and differentiation of the Mullerian ducts into the segments of the female reproductive tract depend on completion of the following three phases of development: organogenesis, fusion both laterally and vertically, and resorption.

In failure of organogenesis, one or both Mullerian ducts may not develop fully, resulting in abnormalities such as uterine agenesis or hypoplasia (bilateral) or unicornuate uterus (unilateral). In lateral fusion

TABLE 26.1

Classification of Mullerian Duct Anomalies

1	Class I—Uterine agenesis or hypoplasia
2	Class II—Unicornuate uterus
3	Class III—Didelphys uterus
4	Class IV—Bicornuate uterus
5	Class V—Septate uterus
6	Class VI—Arcuate uterus
7	Class VII—Diethystilbestrol (DES) exposed uterus

defects, the process by which the lower segments of the paired Mullerian ducts fuse to form the uterus, cervix, and upper vagina fails. Failure of fusion results in anomalies, such as bicornuate or didelphys uterus. Vertical fusion refers to fusion of the ascending sinovaginal bulb with the descending Mullerian system (i.e., fusion of the lower one third and upper two thirds of the vagina). Complete vertical fusion forms a normal patent vagina, while incomplete vertical fusion results in an imperforate hymen.

After the lower Mullerian ducts fuse, a central septum is present, which subsequently must be resorbed to form a single uterine cavity and cervix. Failure of resorption results in a septate uterus.

Mullerian tract anomalies occur throughout development, although the etiology of these defects remains poorly understood. The most commonly used classification of mullerian anomalies is that of the American Fertility Society (AFS) (now named the American Society for Reproductive Medicine, ASRM),[3] which is shown in Table 26.1.

Subseptate Uterus

Subseptate uterus is considered to be the most common major uterine anomaly in women with recurrent pregnancy loss,[4] and recurrent first trimester pregnancy loss.[5] Indeed the subseptate uterus accounted for 70–90% of major anomalies found in low risk women with uterine anomalies.[6–8] A recent study has suggested that pregnancy outcome is poor if a septate uterus is incidentally diagnosed in the early stage of a viable intrauterine pregnancy.[9]

The association between repeated pregnancy loss and subseptate uterus has been attributed to the decreased amount of connective tissue in the relatively avascular septum resulting in poor decidualization and placentation. In addition, the increased amount of muscle tissue in the septum can cause miscarriage by the production of local uncoordinated myometrial contractility. The view that inadequate blood supply to the developing embryo accounts for the fetal losses is supported by histological evaluation of the septum showing a significantly reduced vascular supply relative to the rest of the uterus.[10,11] If this theory is correct, then the likelihood of miscarriage caused by septal implantation should increase with the severity of the disruption of uterine morphology.[6]

Salim et al.[6] showed that the degree of distortion of the uterine cavity in subseptate uterus was higher in women with recurrent miscarriage, compared with low risk women. The uterine cavity was mainly distorted due to the reduced length of the unaffected cavity, rather than increased septum length. The greater degree of uterine cavity distortion in recurrent pregnancy loss supports the hypothesis of septal implantation as a potential cause of miscarriage, as the likelihood of septal implantation increases with an increasing ratio of septal size to functional cavity.

Arcuate Uterus

An arcuate uterus has, by definition, an intrauterine indentation of <1 cm. The AFS has classified the arcuate uterus as a minor malformation with a benign clinical behavior. Using three-dimensional (3D) ultrasound, Salim et al.[6] found that the prevalence of arcuate uterus was 17% in women with recurrent miscarriage, which is significantly higher than the 3.2% prevalence in low risk women.[8] In addition, it has been shown that distortion of uterine cavity is greater in women with recurrent first trimester loss as with the subseptate uterus.

The diagnosis of arcuate uterus is difficult when conventional diagnostic methods are used such as hysteroscopy or laparoscopy, as the diagnostic criteria are far from clear.[12] As a result, little is known about the prevalence and clinical significance. Although many believe that the arcuate uterus has little or no impact on reproduction and obstetrical outcomes,[13] some studies have reported an increase in adverse reproductive outcomes, mostly second trimester loss.[9,14,15] Gergolet at al.[15] followed women with at least one early miscarriage and a subseptate or arcuate uterus undergoing hysteroscopic metroplasty. The miscarriage rates after metroplasty were similar between the women with subseptate and arcuate uterus (14.0% and 11.1%, respectively). Before metroplasty, the miscarriage rates were significantly higher in subseptate uterus group, as well as in the arcuate uterus group. The authors therefore concluded that the arcuate uterus had a similar effect on reproductive outcome as the subseptate uterus both before and after surgical correction.[15]

Unicornuate Uterus

A unicornuate uterus is the result of complete, or almost complete, arrest of development of one of the Mullerian ducts (Figure 26.1). When the arrest is incomplete (in 90% of patients with unicornuate uterus), a rudimentary horn with or without functioning endometrium may be present. If the rudimentary horn is obstructed, it may present as an enlarging pelvic mass, with unilateral cyclical pelvic pain secondary to hematometra. Pregnancies can occur in the rudimentary horn with an estimated incidence of 2%. These cases may be difficult to diagnose, and may result in rupture of the rudimentary horn.

The incidence of unicornuate uterus has been estimated to be 6.3% of uterine anomalies, and may be associated with urinary tract and renal anomalies. Urinary tract anomalies should be suspected in all women with a unicornuate uterus.[16] Unicornuate uterus has been associated with the worst reproductive outcome.[17] About one third of all pregnancies result in miscarriage.[9,18,19] The high miscarriage rate is mostly attributed to abnormal uterine vasculature and decreased muscle mass. Increased cesarean section rates are a result of fetal malpresentation and irregular uterine contractions during labor.

There are no surgical procedures to correct the unicornuate uterus. Prophylactic cervical cerclage has been suggested for the prevention of miscarriage in patients with unicornuate uterus, although there is no clear evidence of cervical incompetence.[20] However, with little data to support the use of cerclage, most clinicians prefer to use careful follow-up with frequent clinical and sonographic evaluation of cervical length. Resection of the cavitated rudimentary horn is often recommended in symptomatic

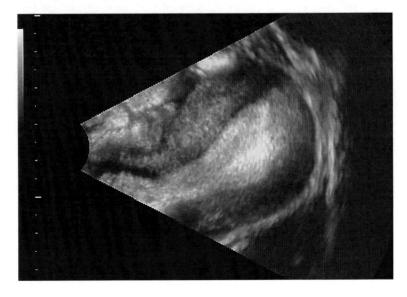

FIGURE 26.1 Three-dimensional (3D) transvaginal ultrasound of a unicornuate uterus using volume contrast imaging in plane C (VCIC). (Courtesy of Prof. Yaron Zalael MD, Sheba Medical Center, Tel-Hashomer, Israel.)

patients with unicornuate uterus, suffering from dysmenorrhea and hematometra. Laparoscopic excision of the rudimentary horn has been shown to be an effective surgical approach.[21]

Uterus Didelphis

A double uterus results from the complete failure of the two Mullerian ducts to fuse (Figures 26.2 and 26.3). Therefore, each duct develops into a separate uterus each of which is narrower than a normal uterus and has only a single horn. The two uteri may each have a cervix or may share a cervix. In 67% of cases, uterus didelphis is associated with two vaginas separated by a thin wall. Didelphic

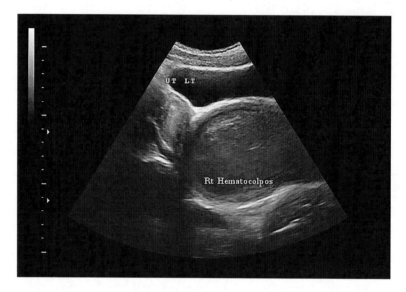

FIGURE 26.2   Two-dimensional (2D) transvaginal ultrasound of a didelphys uterus with obstructed right vagina (hematocolpus). (Courtesy of Prof. Yaron Zalael MD, Sheba Medical Center, Tel-Hashomer, Israel.)

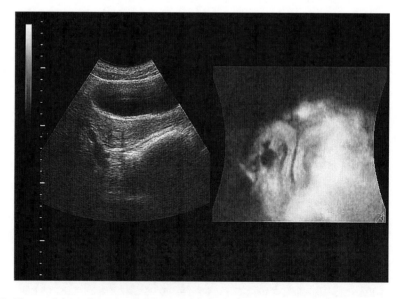

FIGURE 26.3   Two- and three-dimensional (2D and 3D) transvaginal ultrasound of a didelphis uterus (using volume contrast imaging in plane C [VCIC]). (Figure courtesy of Prof. Yaron Zalael MD, Sheba Medical Center, Tel-Hashomer, Israel.)

uteri are relatively uncommon with an estimated incidence of 6.3% of uterine anomalies.[6] The two uteri do not always function normally and are associated with a miscarriage rate of 20.9% and a preterm delivery rate of 24.4%.[6,22] A long-term follow-up of 49 Finnish women with didelphic uteri and a longitudinal vaginal septum reported an obstructed hemivagina in nine women (18%). Eight of these nine women also had ipsilateral renal agenesis.[22] Cesarean section rates are higher due to uterine dystocia and malpresentation.[23] In addition, didelphic uterus is commonly associated with a patent or obstructed vaginal septum. Fertility in women with didelphic uterus is not notably impaired. However, endometriosis is more commonly associated with a didelphic uterus possibly because of retrograde menstruation.[22]

Bicornuate Uterus

A bicornuate uterus results from partial nonfusion of the Mullerian ducts (Figure 26.4). The central myometrium may extend to the level of the internal cervical os (bicornuate unicollis) or external cervical os (bicornuate bicollis). The latter is distinguished from uterus didelphis as there is some degree of fusion between the two horns, while in uterus didelphis, the two horns and cervices are separated completely. In addition, the horns of the bicornuate uteri are not fully developed; typically, they are smaller than those of didelphys uteri. Bicornuate uteri are probably the most common uterine anomaly after septate and arcuate uterus.[23] The reproductive outcome seems to be directly correlated with the severity of fundal indentation. It is generally considered that the bicornuate uterus does not directly affect infertility, but may be linked with recurrent miscarriages. Bicornuate uterus can be corrected surgically by metroplasty.

T-Shaped Uterus and Diethylstilbestrol Exposure

Diethylstilbestrol (DES) is a synthetic estrogen that was used from 1948 up to its ban in 1971 to prevent further pregnancy losses in women with recurrent pregnancy loss. However, approximately two thirds of embryos exposed *in utero* developed uterine abnormalities, including a characteristic small, incompletely formed uterus with a T-shaped cavity and a hypoplastic cervix. The spontaneous incidence of T-shaped uterus is unknown in the general population. In addition, approximately half of DES exposed women have structural cervical defects, including an incompletely formed cervix. The mechanism by

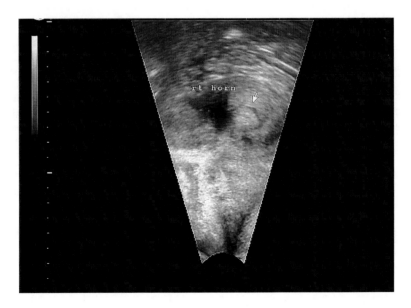

FIGURE 26.4 Three-dimensional (3D) transvaginal ultrasound of a bicornuate uterus. (Courtesy of Prof. Yaron Zalael MD, Sheba Medical Center, Tel-Hashomer, Israel.)

which DES disrupts normal uterine development is not known. Diethylstilbestrol exposed women are less likely than unexposed women to have a full term live birth, and are more likely to have premature births, spontaneous pregnancy losses, or ectopic pregnancies.[24] Women exposed to DES *in utero* are also at increased risk for breast cancer and clear cell adenocarcinoma of the vagina and cervix.[25]

The molecular mechanism through which DES exposure induces vaginal adenosis has recently been attributed to inhibition of BMP4/Activin A-regulated vaginal cell fate decision through a downregulation of RUNX1.[26] It has been suggested that BMP4 and Activin A produced by vaginal mesenchyme synergistically activates the expression of ΔNp63, thus deciding vaginal epithelial cell fate in the Müllerian duct epithelial cells via direct binding of SMADs on the highly conserved 5′ sequence of ΔNp63.[26]

Goldberg and Falcone,[27] in a metaanalysis of DES-exposed subjects, found a 9-fold increase in ectopic pregnancy, a 2-fold increase in miscarriage rate, and a 2-fold increase in preterm delivery compared with a matched control population. Pregnancy rates were similar between DES-exposed women and controls, 72% and 79%, respectively. The poor obstetric outcomes are caused not only by the uterine anomaly, but also by an antiestrogenic effect at the level of the endometrium.[25] The clinical significance of DES exposure is rapidly diminishing as those affected women pass their reproductive years.[25]

Myomas

Myomas are considered the most common acquired anomaly of the uterus. It has been shown[28] that infertile women with fibroids have a lower pregnancy rate when undergoing assisted reproduction than age-matched women with no fibroids. Submucous myomas deform the uterine cavity; the overlying endometrium is usually thin and inadequate for normal implantation. Submucous fibroids can also be associated with pregnancy loss.[29] The case is less clear with intramural and subserosal fibroids.[30] In these locations, the size and the number of fibroids may be significant. Significantly lower implantation and pregnancy rates have been found in patients with intramural or submucosal fibroids undergoing *in vitro* fertilization and intracytoplasmic sperm injection (IVF/ICSI) even when there was no uterine cavity deformation.[28] Furthermore, the pregnancy rate observed within one year of myomectomy is higher than that observed in couples with unexplained infertility and no treatment.[31,32] A recent large retrospective study reaffirmed the observation that while non cavity-distorting fibroids did not affect IVF/ICSI outcomes, intramural fibroids greater than 2.85 cm in size significantly impaired the delivery rate of patients undergoing IVF/ICSI.[33]

Polyps

Polyps are benign hyperplastic endometrial growths that have also been associated with adverse pregnancy outcomes. It is postulated that polyps and fibroids with intracavitary extension may act like foreign bodies within the endometrial cavity.[34] It has also been proposed that polyps and fibroids might induce chronic inflammatory changes in the endometrium that make it unfavorable for pregnancy. A recent case-control study suggested a molecular mechanism to support the clinical findings of diminished pregnancy rates in women with endometrial polyps.[35] The effect of hysteroscopically identified endometrial polyps on the endometrium has been evaluated using HOXA10 and HOXA11, expression, HOXA10 and HOXA11 are molecular markers of endometrial receptivity. Uteri with endometrial polyps demonstrated a marked decrease in HOXA10 and HOXA11 messenger RNA levels, which may impair implantation.[35]

As the presence of polyps has been associated with a worse prognosis for pregnancy, polypectomy is usually considered if no other explanation for the recurrent loss is found.[34,36]

Intrauterine Adhesions

Intrauterine synechiae may not be a frequent cause of recurrent miscarriage, but may lead to secondary infertility. Intrauterine adhesions develop as a result of surgical procedures, typically curettage, or endometritis. Intrauterine scars can probably interfere with normal implantation and may be responsible for pregnancy loss. A recent systematic review estimated that intrauterine adhesions are encountered in one in five women after miscarriage.[37] However, in more than half of these women, the severity and extent of the adhesions was mild, with unknown clinical relevance. The authors' identified recurrent miscarriage and dilatation and curettage procedures as risk factors for adhesion formation. Congenital and acquired intrauterine abnormalities, such as polyps or fibroids, were frequently identified. The authors failed to identify studies associating intrauterine adhesions and long-term reproductive outcome after miscarriage. Nevertheless, they noted that similar pregnancy outcomes were reported subsequent to conservative, medical or surgical management.[37] Intrauterine adhesions are expected to be more common among patients with recurrent miscarriage, since the formation of adhesions may even follow a simple manual vacuum aspiration for early pregnancy loss.[38]

Investigation of Uterine Integrity

In patients with recurrent pregnancy loss, imaging studies are important during the initial work-up in order to assess the integrity of the uterus. The guidelines of the Royal College of Obstetricians and Gynaecologists[39] for investigating recurrent miscarriage, recommend an ultrasound scan of the pelvis, but this recommendation is based solely on the clinical experience of the guideline development group, rather than on published evidence. A cross-sectional study if 875 women who had two or more consecutive miscarriages found a uterine anomaly in 169 (19.3%) of the patients.[40] It was further shown that recurrent miscarriage patients with a prior viable birth were less likely to have a uterine anomaly than those who had never given birth. The authors concluded that their results support diagnostic imaging of the uterus after two losses in women with secondary recurrent miscarriage as well as for women with primary recurrent miscarriage.[40]

Transvaginal sonography (TVS) is usually the initial investigation, but can be enhanced by 3D ultrasound. TVS allows accurate and rapid characterization of the uterus including its size and position, as well as the presence of anomalies such as a duplicated cervix, duplicated uterus, uterine septum or unicornuate uterus. TVS is also useful in determining the size and location of uterine myomas, as well as the presence of intrauterine polyps and endometrial irregularities that might suggest adhesions.

Reports on two-dimensional (2D) and 3D transvaginal ultrasound, as well as saline contrast sonohysterography, appear promising for the diagnosis and classification of congenital uterine anomalies. It was recently suggested that current advances in ultrasound technology, specifically 3D ultrasound, achieve the same benefits of magnetic resonance imaging (MRI) in being accurate and noninvasive, but also offer the advantages of being office available, cost effective and providing immediate results.[41]

The ability to visualize both the uterine cavity and the fundal uterine contour on a 3D scan facilitates the diagnosis of uterine anomalies and enables differentiation between septate and bicornuate uteri. The additional use of color Doppler ultrasound may also allow visualization of intraseptal vascularity and may help in distinguishing the avascular from the vascular septum.

Intravenous pyelogram is recommended during the work-up of congenital anomalies. Defects in the urinary tract are commonly seen when a uterine anomaly is diagnosed.[16]

Hysterosalpingography

Hysterosalpingography (HSG) has long been used to evaluate the contour of the uterine cavity, cervical canal, and fallopian tube.[42] The radio-opaque contrast medium fills the cavity allowing the accurate identification of filling defects, scarring, or a septum. However, HSG alone cannot differentiate between a septate uterus and a bicornuate uterus. Furthermore, HSG cannot determine the myometrial extension or the size of intra-uterine lesions. Therefore, HSG is primarily used to assess tubal patency and has a limited role in the imaging of uterine malformations.

Three-Dimensional Ultrasound

Three-dimensional ultrasound is an accurate and reproducible means of diagnosing congenital uterine anomalies[41] (Figures 26.1 and 26.5); 3D ultrasound has a clear advantage over HSG, hysteroscopy and laparoscopy for the diagnosis of congenital uterine anomalies, as it is a noninvasive method currently available in most out-patient settings. The results of 3D ultrasound have been shown to concur with

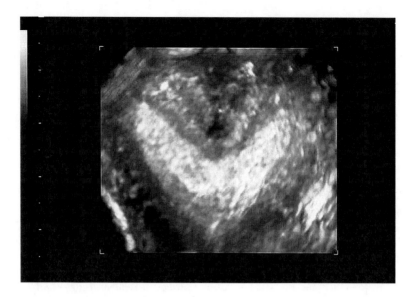

FIGURE 26.5   Three-dimensional (3D) transvaginal ultrasound of a septated uterus (3D rendering). (Courtesy of Prof. Yaron Zalael MD, Sheba Medical Center, Tel-Hashomer, Israel.)

HSG in all cases of arcuate uterus and major congenital anomalies.[8] It has been suggested that the ability to visualize both the uterine cavity and the myometrium on a 3D scan facilitates the diagnosis of uterine anomalies and enable easy differentiation between subseptate and bicornuate uteri.

Salim et al.[6] have examined the differences in the morphology of uterine anomalies found in 509 women with a history of unexplained recurrent miscarriage and 1976 low risk women that were examined for the presence of congenital uterine anomalies by 3D ultrasound. Salim et al.[6] detected 121 anomalies in the recurrent miscarriage group and 105 among low risk women. Surprisingly there was no significant difference in relative frequency of various anomalies or the depth of fundal distortion between the two groups. However, with both arcuate and subseptate uteri, the length of the remaining uterine cavity was significantly shorter and the distortion ratio was significantly higher in the recurrent miscarriage group. Salim et al.[6] therefore concluded that the distortion of uterine anatomy is more severe in congenital uterine anomalies found in women with a history of recurrent first trimester miscarriage.

Woelfer et al.[14] tried to determine the reproductive outcomes in women with congenital uterine anomalies detected incidentally by 3D ultrasound. One thousand and eighty-nine women with no history of infertility or recurrent miscarriage, undergoing a transvaginal ultrasound scan were screened for uterine abnormalities. Nine hundred and eighty-three women had a normally shaped uterine cavity, 72 an arcuate, 29 a subseptate, and five a bicornuate uterus. Women with a subseptate uterus had a significantly higher proportion of first-trimester loss compared with women with a normal uterus. Women with an arcuate uterus had a significantly greater proportion of second-trimester loss and preterm labor. Woelfer et al.'s[14] study demonstrated the potential value of 3D ultrasound and contributed evidence to the proposed association between congenital uterine anomalies and adverse pregnancy outcomes.

Sonohysterography

The diagnostic value and usefulness of transvaginal sonohysterography (SHG) in the detection of uterine anomalies, compared with other diagnostic methods is now well established.[43] SHG was able to detect all uterine anomalies found in a study of 54 patients with primary or secondary infertility or repeated spontaneous miscarriage and a clinically or sonographically suspected abnormal uterus. SHG was carried out by the intrauterine infusion of an isotonic saline solution. The sensitivity and specificity of SHG were similar to hysteroscopy. However, there was no significant difference between the diagnostic capabilities of the methods analyzed. With the proper set-up and training, transvaginal SHG with saline solution is a low-cost, easy, and helpful method of diagnosing uterine malformations.

It is now possible to combine 3D ultrasound with SHG. Sylvestre et al.[44] carried out a study of 209 infertile patients suspected to have an intrauterine lesion on 3D SHG. Ninety-two patients with a lesion underwent hysteroscopy. In these 92 patients, polyps were found in 48 women, submucous or intramural myomas in 35 cases, both polyps and myomas in three cases, four mullerian anomalies, one thick endometrium, and one patient had intrauterine synechiae. It was concluded that 3D SHG allowed precise recognition and localization of lesions. It was further suggested that if 2D and 3D SHG are normal, invasive diagnostic procedures such as hysteroscopy could be avoided.

Alborzi et al.[45] performed a prospective study to determine whether SHG can differentiate septate from bicornuate uterus, in 20 patients with a history of recurrent pregnancy loss and an HSG diagnosis of septate or bicornuate uterus. SHG was found to effectively differentiate septate and bicornuate uterus and may eliminate the need for laparoscopy in order to differentiate between these anomalies.

The diagnostic accuracy of SHG has been evaluated prospectively and compared to HSG and TVS in a study comprising of 65 infertile women.[46] Hysteroscopy was used as the gold standard. SHG was found to have the same diagnostic accuracy, and to sometimes even be markedly superior to hysteroscopy with respect to polypoid lesions and endometrial hyperplasia. In the diagnosis of intrauterine adhesions, SHG had limited accuracy, similar to that obtained by HSG, with a high false-positive diagnosis rate.[46]

Magnetic Resonance Imaging

MRI is an accurate noninvasive technique for the evaluation of uterine anomalies. MRI has been shown to be a valuable tool in the diagnosis of selected cases of Mullerian duct anomalies.[47] Although most anomalies will be initially diagnosed at HSG and SHG, further imaging will often be required for definitive diagnosis and elaboration of secondary findings.[48] At this time, MRI is justified only in special cases where its high accuracy and detailed elaboration of uterovaginal anatomy is needed.

The use of MRI remains limited due to its cost. However, in selected cases careful use of MRI to delineate the pelvic soft tissues may greatly aid in precise definition of the anomaly and in planning the most appropriate corrective surgery.[49]

Diagnostic Hysteroscopy

Hysteroscopy offers the best and the most direct assessment of the uterine cavity. During the procedure, intracavitary structures can be directly visualized and directed biopsies can be obtained when indicated. A retrospective study by Zuppi et al.[50] found an association between the hysteroscopic findings in 344 women with recurrent spontaneous abortion and major, or even minor, uterine anomalies. The anomalies were shown to correlate with an increased risk of recurrent miscarriage.[50]

Weiss et al.[51] performed hysteroscopy on 165 women referred for recurrent pregnancy loss: 67 after two and 98 after three or more consecutive miscarriages. The prevalence of uterine anomalies did not differ significantly and was 32% and 28%, respectively. Weiss et al.[51] concluded that hysteroscopy may be justified following two spontaneous pregnancy losses.

The intramyometrial extension of fibroids cannot be assessed, however, and therefore the estimate of size remains imprecise. Hysteroscopy alone cannot differentiate between a septate uterus and a bicornuate uterus; laparoscopy or SHG is required to complete the evaluation.

Diagnostic Laparoscopy

Laparoscopy allows the surgeon to assess the outer surface of the uterus and other pelvic structures. It is used to establish the precise diagnosis of the various congenital and acquired anomalies. Laparoscopy is also used for the removal of subserosal and intramural fibroids.[52,53] Currently, laparoscopy is rarely used just to clarify uterine anatomy and is generally reserved for women in whom interventional therapy is likely to be undertaken.

Choice of Method for Imaging Uterine Morphology

Ultrasonography is currently the most readily available and least invasive mode of imaging in cases of suspected uterine abnormalities (Table 26.2); 2D sonography allows excellent assessment of myometrial morphology, and is especially useful for determining the number, size, and location of myomas. Filling the uterine cavity with fluid facilitates the use of SHG for accurate delineation of intrauterine polyps, and improves the accuracy of identifying submucous myomas encroaching on the cavity and to assess the size of uterine septa. Three-dimensional sonography greatly enhances our ability to differentiate between a uterine septum and a bicornuate uterus (Figures 26.2 through 26.5). Hysterosalpingography can help delineate the integrity of the uterine cavity, but due to its invasive nature and the associated exposure to radiation, is limited to infertility investigation where evaluation of tubal patency is required.

Hysteroscopy can be performed today with 2–3 mm scopes without the need for speculum, tenaculum, or anesthesia.[54] This simple outpatient procedure provides an accurate assessment of the uterine cavity. It remains the method of choice for assessment of the presence and extent of intrauterine adhesions. It is also the optimal method to evaluate the size and extension of polyps and submucous myomas. However, hysteroscopy cannot fully differentiate between a uterine septum and a bicornuate uterus. A recent study found that patients with two, three, and four or more consecutive miscarriages have a similar prevalence of uterine anatomical abnormalities. It was thus concluded that diagnostic hysteroscopy should be carried out after two miscarriages.[55]

The role of MRI is limited due to its cost. However, in selected and complicated cases MRI may help to clarify the details of soft tissue anatomy and may be especially useful when planning surgical correction.[47] Laparoscopy used to be the gold standard for differentiating between a uterine

TABLE 26.2

Imaging Modalities for Assessing Uterine Anomalies in Women with Recurrent Pregnancy Loss

Imaging Modalities	Advantages	Disadvantages	Cost
Ultrasonography	Readily available Least invasive Excellent assessment of the myometrial morphology	Poor demonstration of uterine contour Uterine cavity not clearly demonstrated	Low
Hysterosalpingography	Shows the contour of the uterine cavity, cervical canal, and tubal lamina	Exposure to radiation Iodine sensitivity risk Painful Pelvic inflammatory disease (PID) risk High false positive rates	Moderate
3D sonography	Allows visualizion of both uterine cavity and myometrium Enables easy differentiation between subseptate and bicornuate uteri	Equipment not readily available Requires experienced operator	Moderate
Sonohysterography	Good evaluation of uterine cavity Tubal patency assessed	Time consuming High false-positive diagnosis rate for intrauterine adhesions	Low
Diagnostic Hysteroscopy	Most accurate assessment of the uterine cavity Simple outpatient procedure	Limited efficiency of differentiating between uterine septum and bicornuate uterus No information on tubal patency Invasive Risk of infection, perforation	Moderate
Magnetic resonance imaging	Useful in clarifying details of soft tissue anatomy	No information on tubal patency Not easy to interpret results	High
Diagnostic Laparoscopy	Accurate for differentiating between a uterine septum and a bicornuate uterus	Invasive Requires general anesthesia Low postoperative morbidity	High

septum and a bicornuate uterus, but with modern imaging modalities, it is rarely needed for determination of uterine anatomy and is usually only used when a decision has been made to attempt surgical correction.

Treatment

As stated above, little evidence can be found in the current literature demonstrating that uterine factors, including intrauterine adhesions, septa, myomas and endometrial polyps, are causally linked with reproductive loss. However, there are reports suggesting that treatment of these abnormalities may improve the fertility outcome.[56,57] The published evidence includes several observational series that demonstrate successful fertility, with term pregnancy rates ranging from 32% to 87% following hysteroscopic division of intrauterine adhesions. The evidence supporting a direct link between a septate uterus and reproductive loss is derived from the results of metroplasty. Several case series have demonstrated a reduction in the spontaneous abortion rate, from 91% to 17%, after hysteroscopic metroplasty. Furthermore, following metroplasty, the mean pregnancy rate in previously infertile patients is 47%. However, there are no prospective controlled trials that have provided conclusive evidence that the correction of uterine anatomic abnormalities benefits the next pregnancy.[57] Furthermore, the above data is mostly based on observational, retrospective studies with small sample sizes and heterogeneous patient populations, and is therefore a far cry from the type of evidence required for current treatment guidelines. A review of all published large randomized controlled trials and metaanalyses undertaken by the ESHRE Special Interest Group for Early Pregnancy (SIGEP) protocol for the investigation and medical management of recurrent miscarriage concluded that the only interventions that do not require more randomized controlled trials are tender loving care and health advice.[58]

Surgery is the main course of treatment offered to patients with uterine anomalies (Table 26.3). However, not all anatomic defects can be surgically corrected and not all anomalies require surgical intervention. The most crucial step before making any treatment decision is accurate imaging in order to determine the exact anomaly. Currently endoscopic procedures are the main approach used to correct most uterine defects. Operative hysteroscopy currently allows a technically straightforward method of correcting intrauterine pathology such as septum, fibroids or polyps. Laparotomy currently has a very limited role in the management of congenital uterine anomalies in women with recurrent miscarriage.

There are many questions regarding the optimal management of patients with recurrent miscarriage and uterine anomalies such as the indications for resection of a uterine septum, and whether small intrauterine polyps significantly influence reproductive performance. It is debatable whether surgical reconstruction such as Strassman's metroplasty should be performed for bicornuate uterus. When should myomectomy be performed? What is the role of nonsurgical management of myomas? When should cervical cerclage be offered? We will try to discuss these questions in the light of currently available data.

TABLE 26.3

Role of Surgical Intervention in Women with Uterine Anomalies and Recurrent Pregnancy Loss

Study	Postoperative Morbidity	Technical Difficulty	Likelihood of Benefit	Cost
Hysteroscopic polypecomy	+	+	++	+
Hysteroscopic adhesiolysis	+	+—++	+++	+
Hysteroscopic myomectomy	+—++	++—+++	++	+—++
Hysteroscopic metroplasty for septate uterus	+	+	++	+—++
Hysteroscopic metroplasty for hypoplastic/diethystilbestrol (DES)-exposed uterus	+	++	+	++
Abdominal metroplasty	+++	+++	++	+++
Cervical cerclage	++	++	+	++
Interruption of a fallopian tube with hydrosalpinx	++	++	++?	++

Low: +; high +++.

Should Intrauterine Polyps Be Excised?

Although the association between endometrial polyps and pregnancy loss has not been proven, polyps are more common in patients with recurrent spontaneous abortion.[59] Surgical excision is usually recommended,[2] as there is data suggesting that hysteroscopic polypectomy can increase fertility.[34,36] A prospective, randomized study in 215 infertile women scheduled to undergo intrauterine insemination (IUI) showed that hysteroscopic polypectomy improved the likelihood of conception, with a relative risk of 2.1 (95% confidence interval [CI] 1.5–2.9).[36] Pregnancies in the patients who underwent polypectomy were obtained before the first IUI in 65% of cases. A subsequent study from Athens also proposed that hysteroscopic polypectomy of any size may improve fertility in women with otherwise unexplained infertility.[60] Hence, a Cochrane database systematic review suggested that hysteroscopic polypectomy after ultrasound detection in women prior to IUI might increase the clinical pregnancy rate.[57]

Hysteroscopy resection is probavly the optimal method of performing polypectomy. Hysteroscopic polypectomy can be performed by excision with forceps or gentle curettage. A study that assessed 240 cases of hysteroscopic polypectomy concluded that resectoscopic polypectomy required more operating time, had more glycine absorption and complications, but had a lower recurrence rate than other hysteroscopic techniques.[61] The resectoscope had a 0% recurrence rate and that grasping forceps had a 15% recurrence rate.[61] The introduction of bipolar electrodes may increase the safety of hysteroscopic endometrial polypectomy in an outpatient setting.[62]

Does the Resection of a Uterine Septum Improve Pregnancy Outcome?

Septate uterus is more prevalent in women with repeated pregnancy loss.[63] However, it may be difficult to differentiate between a "normal" arcuate uterus and a septate uterus (Figures 26.6 and 26.7). In order to justify metroplasty, reliable diagnosis is required.

Although no randomized controlled studies are available, observational studies have reported impressive results following incision of a septum in patients with recurrent abortion.[57] Fedele et al.[64] studied the reproductive outcome in 102 patients with a complete ($n = 23$) or partial septate uterus ($n = 79$) and infertility or recurrent miscarriage. Following hysteroscopic metroplasty the cumulative pregnancy and birth rates at 36 months were 89% and 75%, respectively, in the septate uterus group and 80% and 67% in the subseptate uterus group. Fedele et al.[64] concluded that after hysteroscopic metroplasty the reproductive prognosis was favorable and not influenced by the malformation subclass. Dalal et al.[65]

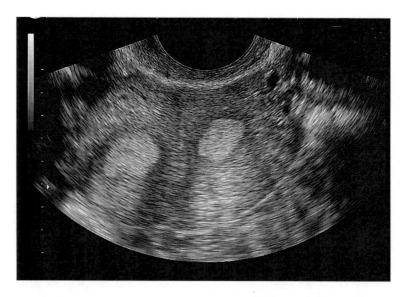

FIGURE 26.6   Two-dimensional (2D) transvaginal ultrasound of a septated uterus. (Courtesy of Prof. Yaron Zalael MD, Sheba Medical Center, Tel-Hashomer, Israel.)

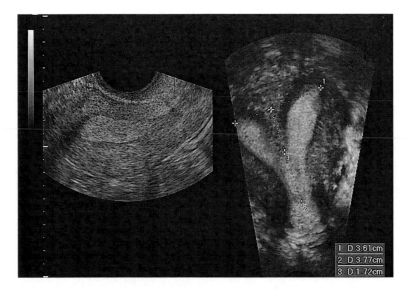

FIGURE 26.7   Two and three-dimensional (2D and 3D) transvaginal ultrasound of a septated uterus of the same patient in Figure 26.6 (using volume contrast imaging in plane C [VCIC]). (Courtesy of Prof. Yaron Zalael MD, Sheba Medical Center, Tel-Hashomer, Israel.)

reported on 72 women with unexplained primary infertility who underwent hysteroscopic septal resection. Thirty-three women (45.8%) conceived within one year of surgery. Only four women (12%) had spontaneous abortions and five (15%) had preterm delivery.

A recent Cochrane systemic review assessed the efficiency of metroplasty versus expectant management for women with recurrent miscarriage and a septate uterus.[63] The authors note that only noncontrolled studies were available for assessment. Metroplasty was found to have a possible positive effect on pregnancy outcomes. However, these noncontrolled studies were all biased as the participants with recurrent miscarriage treated by hysteroscopic metroplasty served as their own controls. The effectiveness and possible complications of hysteroscopic metroplasty have never been evaluatd in a randomised controlled trial. Such studies are urgently needed.[63]

Grimbizis et al.[66] summarized the results of a highly selected group of symptomatic patients drawn from a large number of reports. The patients had previously had a term delivery and live birth rates of only 5%. After hysteroscopic septum resection, the outcome was remarkable, in that the subsequent term delivery rate was approximately 75% and the live birth rates about 85%.[66] However, Grimbizis et al.'s trial[66] was not randomized.

Transabdominal surgical techniques, such as the modified Tompkins metroplasty, are still occasionally used to repair uterine septa.[67] However, in light of the low morbidity associated with hysteroscopic resection and the possibility of performing the procedure on an ambulatory basis, abdominal surgery seems to be rarely, if ever, indicated.[56] However, hysteroscopic metroplasty is associated with a substantial and as yet non quantified, increased risk of uterine rupture during subsequent pregnancies.[68] This is especially significant when the risk of uterine rupture after hysteroscopic metroplasty is compared to that of women undergoing uncomplicated hysteroscopic resection of submucous myomas or endometrial polyps.[68] Uterine perforation and/or the use of electrosurgery increase this risk, but are not considered independent risk factors.[68]

Pang et al.[69] have suggested that a septate uterus per se is not an indication for surgical intervention, because it is not always associated with a poor obstetric outcome. This approach is supported by a retrospective study of 67 patients who had a complete septate uterus including the cervix and a longitudinal vaginal septum.[70] There was no association with primary infertility and pregnancy was reported to progress successfully without surgical treatment. The results did not support elective hysteroscopic incision of the septum in asymptomatic patients before the first pregnancy.[70] In women with one miscarriage, the situation remains controversial, and a conservative approach has been suggested since it is expected that after a single miscarriage 80–90% will have a live birth in the next pregnancy.[63] However, a more liberalized approach to treatment is currently advocated by most authorities in light of the simplicity, minimal postoperative sequelae, and improved reproductive outcome associated with hysteroscopic metroplasty.[63,66] A recent study pointed out that hysteroscopic septotomy seems to significantly improve pregnancy outcomes in women with a history of recurrent spontaneous abortion, while no conclusive influence on reproductive outcomes was demonstrated in women with no history of poor pregnancy outcomes.[69]

Should the Cervical Portion of the Septum Be Spared in Patients with a Complete Septate Uterus?

It was previously believed that patients with a complete septate uterus, the cervical portion of the septum, should be spared and the dissection started at the level of the internal os to avoid secondary cervical incompetence. However, a multicenter, randomized, controlled clinical trial by Parsanezhad et al.[71] examined whether division of the cervical portion of a uterine septum is associated with intraoperative bleeding, cervical incompetence, or secondary infertility. Twenty-eight women with complete uterine septum and a history of pregnancy wastage or infertility were randomized to undergo metroplasty including division of the cervical portion of the septum or the same procedure with preservation of the cervical portion. Resection of the cervical portion was reported to make the procedure safer, easier, and less complicated than preservation of the cervical septum.[71]

Management of Myomas in Recurrent Pregnancy loss

Myomas are frequently found in women of reproductive age, and are more prevalent in women over 35 years of age. Although myomas are more prevalent in women with recurrent spontaneous abortion,[59] the causal association remains poorly established. It is therefore still undetermined which women will benefit most from myomectomy. Evidence, mostly from IVF literature, suggests that only those myomas that distort the endometrial cavity impair fertility.[33,72] Patients with distorted uterine cavities due to submucous fibroids of more than 2 cm have higher pregnancy rates following hysteroscopic resection. As submucous myomas are easily treatable in recurrent pregnancy loss, it has been suggested that these patients should be identified early after other potential causes of recurrent pregnancy loss are eliminated.[33]

The location and size of the myomas are the two parameters that influence the success of a future pregnancy.[72] At present, it seems that subserosal myomas have little, if any, effect on reproductive outcome, especially if they are up to 5 to 7 cm in diameter. The impact of intramural myomas on the outcome of pregnancy is still disputed.[73,74] However, intramural myomas that do not encroach upon the endometrium also can be considered to be relatively harmless to reproduction, if they are smaller than 4 to 5 cm in diameter. Myomectomy is therefore currently recommended for intramural myomas that compress the uterine cavity and submucous myomas significantly reduce pregnancy rates.[33,73]

Hysteroscopic myomectomy is the gold standard for the treatment of submucous myomas. Size and intramural extension can limit the success, although this greatly depends on the operator's experience. The removal of larger fibroids may require a two-stage procedure in order to avoid intraoperative complications. Fibroids with significant intramural extension present a challenge during the procedure.

Conservative myomectomy is the gold standard for the removal of most intramural and subserosal uterine myomas in women who desire to preserve their uterus, and laparoscopic excission is gradually replacing laparotomy as the procedure of choice.[52] Pregnancy rates following myomectomy, are in the 50–60% range, with most having good outcomes.[53] It should be noted that spontaneous uterine rupture during pregnancy has been reported following laparoscopic myomectomy.[75]

Laparoscopic-assisted myomectomy (LAM) is another new approach that is often a very convenient and less invasive form of surgery.[76] By decreasing the technical demands, and thereby the operative time, LAM may be more widely offered to patients. In carefully selected patients, LAM is a safe and efficient alternative to both laparoscopic myomectomy and myomectomy by laparotomy. Indications include numerous large or deep intramural myomas. LAM allows easier repair of the uterus and rapid morcellation of the myomas. In women who desire a future pregnancy, LAM may be a better approach because it allows meticulous suturing of the uterine wall in layers and thereby eliminates excessive electrocoagulation.[76]

Laparoscopy is also being expanded to include such techniques as laparoscopic uterine artery ligation and directed laparoscopic cryomyolysis. However, many of these treatment options are still associated with significant concerns regarding future reproductive performance. Additional nonsurgical techniques introduced to treat myomas include uterine artery embolization and transabdominal interventional MRI cryoablation.[52] Furthermore, MRI guided focused ultrasound surgery has been approved by the U.S. FDA to treat myomas. It is apparent the physician's skills and experience, as well as local availability of these new techniques, will largely determine patient assignment to therapy.[52]

Uterine fibroid embolization is an increasingly popular, minimally invasive technique that has been successfully used in the management of symptomatic myomas.[53,77] This procedure is not without risk however, for women desiring to enhance their reproductive outcome. Following uterine fibroid embolization, transient ovarian failure has been reported, as has permanent amenorrhea associated with endometrial atrophy. Amenorrhea seems to occur after the procedure in approximately 1% of the patients and is highly age dependent with a reported incidence of 3% (range: 1% to 7%) in women under 40 years of age and 41% (range: 26% to 58%) in women over 50.

The pregnancy rate has not been established following uterine artery embolization. However, higher rates of pregnancy complications have been reported following uterine artery embolization compared to myomectomy.[53] These complications include: preterm delivery (odds ratio [OR] 6.2, 95% CI 1.4–27.7), malpresentations (OR 4.3, 95% CI 1.0–20.5), spontaneous abortion, abnormal placentation, and postpartum hemorrhage.

A recent prospective cohort study the followed 66 women who desired a future pregnancy and were treated with uterine artery embolization for symptomatic fibroids has resulted in an alarming observation.[77] Although uterine artery embolization was effective in improving bleeding, bulking and pain symptoms, and in sparing the ovarian reserve, no woman in this study delivered successfully after uterine artery embolization.[77] These poor reproductive outcomes could be explained in part by the high rate of associated infertility in the study population and the high prevalence of previous surgery. However, neither preexisting infertility, nor previous surgery sufficiently account for the total absence of ongoing pregnancy. Torre et al.[77] suggest that embolization might have a negative impact on fertility, which may not be related to ovarian function. The poor reproductive outcomes indicate that uterine artery embolization should not be performed routinely in young women of childbearing age with extensive fibroids.[77] At present, it seems that although most pregnancies following uterine artery embolization are expected to have good outcomes, myomectomy should still be recommended as the treatment of choice over uterine artery embolization in most patients desiring future fertility.[53,77]

Is Cervical Cerclage Indicated in Women with Uterine Anomalies?

Cervical incompetence has been associated with uterine anomalies, as well as following *in utero* exposure to DES. Furthermore, cervical incompetence is of special concern in women with recurrent pregnancy losses as weakening of the cervix may occasionally be due to repeated trauma to the cervix, following excessive dilatation at repeated curettage.

Seidman et al.[78] have studied the effect of cervical cerclage on the survival rate of the fetus in 86 pregnancies in women with congenital uterine anomalies and a random group of 106 pregnancies in women with normal shaped uteri. The uterine morphology was determined by HSG, and if necessary, by additional hysteroscopy and laparoscopy. The incidence of cervical incompetence diagnosed by HSG (23%) was similar in both groups.[78] Sixty-seven and 29 pregnancies were managed with cervical cerclage in each group, respectively. The fetal outcome was stratified by cervical incompetence and obstetric history. The proportion of viable live births was significantly higher in women with malformed uteri who underwent cerclage (88%) compared to those without cerclage (47%). No statistically significant beneficial effect of cerclage was found for normal uteri, even when only those patients with a history of recurrent fetal loss were considered.[78]

The precise indications for cervical cerclage remain controversial. The Cervical Incompetence Prevention Randomized Cerclage Trial (CIPRACT) found that therapeutic cerclage with bed rest reduces preterm delivery before 34 weeks of gestation and compound neonatal morbidity in women with risk factors and/or symptoms of cervical incompetence and a cervical length of <25 mm before 27 weeks of gestation.[79] Risk factors for cervical incompetence included in this included, DES exposure and uterine anomaly.

Levine and Berkowitz[80] studied the effect of conservative management on pregnancy outcome in 120 DES-exposed women with and without gross structural lesions of the genital tract. Cerclage was limited to two women with a history of cervical incompetence or acute cervical change in the second trimester. Women with cervical change occurring after 25 weeks' gestation were managed with bed rest. It was found that the majority of pregnancy losses in DES-exposed patients occurred in the first trimester. Patients exposed *in utero* to DES, who had conservative management, had good pregnancy outcomes.[80]

Cervical incompetence is a challenging clinical diagnosis and is an infrequent cause of pregnancy loss even in patients with gross structural abnormalities of the genital tract. Prophylactic cerclage for patients with uterine anomalies and DES-exposure should be recommended only when other risk factors, such as three or more midtrimester pregnancy losses or preterm deliveries, are present.[78,80]

Does Strassman Metroplasty Still Have a Role in Patients with a Bicornuate Uterus?

The Strassman procedure involves the unification of the two uterine horns of a bicornuate uterus and is carried out via laparotomy. This procedure often leaves a small cavity with scarring, which makes implantation difficult, and may also cause pelvic adhesions resulting in secondary infertility. However, the postmetroplasty reproductive capacity of women with a bicornuate uterus has been reported to be good.[81,82] Furthermore, the role of abdominal metroplasty has been suggested as a valid approach[82] (using Jones' or Strassman's techniques) in patients with bicornuate, T-shaped or septate uteri, when associated with other pelvic lesions not amenable to transcervical hysteroscopic surgery. However, surgical correction of a bicornuate uterus is poorly supported by data and rarely seems to be warranted for pregnancy maintenance. As a bicornuate uterus is usually associated with third trimester complications, the procedure should be limited to very few well-selected cases with recurrent second- and third-trimester complications. The development of a laparoscopic approach to metroplasty for bicornuate uterus needs further study, as laparoscopy may be associated with less postoperative morbidity.

Does Hydrosalpinx Affect Pregnancy Outcome after Early Recurrent Miscarriage?

Hydrosalpinx is known to have a detrimental effect on the outcome of IVF. A Cochrane systematic review identified five randomized controlled trials involving 646 women.[83] Four studies assessed salpingectomy versus no treatment, two of which also included a tubal occlusion arm. One trial assessed aspiration versus no treatment. No trials reported on the primary outcome: live birth. The odds of ongoing pregnancy (Peto OR 2.14, 95% CI 1.23 to 3.73) and of clinical pregnancy (Peto OR 2.31, 95% CI 1.48 to 3.62) were increased with laparoscopic salpingectomy for hydrosalpinges prior to IVF. Comparison of tubal occlusion to salpingectomy did not show a significant advantage of either surgical procedure in terms of ongoing pregnancy or clinical pregnancy. The authors concluded that surgical treatment should be considered for all women with hydrosalpinges prior to IVF. The updated review provides evidence that laparoscopic tubal occlusion is an alternative to laparoscopic salpingectomy in improving IVF pregnancy rates in women with hydrosalpinges. It still remains unclear whether aspiration of hydrosalpinges prior to, or during IVF is warranted and whether tubal restorative surgery should still be considered as an alternative to IVF.[83]

A prospective randomized controlled trial[84] enrolled 13 patients with a history of unexplained recurrent early spontaneous abortion and a unilateral hydrosalpinx diagnosed by sonography or HSG and in whom other causes of miscarriage had been excluded. The patients were randomized to undergo laparoscopic unilateral tubal fulguration or no surgical intervention. Six of the seven patients in the treatment group and five of the six in the control group conceived. Five patients in the treatment group and none in the control group had a pregnancy progress beyond the first trimester. The progressing pregnancies in the treatment group reached 36–40 weeks of gestation, a statistically significant difference. The authors concluded that laparoscopic tubal fulguration improves pregnancy outcome in selected patients with previous recurrent early miscarriage and a unilateral hydrosalpinx. This study clearly needs further confirmation in a larger patient sample.[84]

Is Hysteroscopic Metroplasty Indicated in DES Exposed Women?

Hysteroscopic metroplasty has been reported as a safe and feasible method to improve the reproductive performance in patients with DES-exposed and hypoplastic malformed uteri suffering from severe infertility, recurrent pregnancy loss, or implantation failures.[85–87] In one series,[85] eight patients with infertility, recurrent pregnancy loss, or both, and an abnormal uterine contour at HSG underwent hysteroscopic metroplasty. Each patient served as their own control. Three of five patients with secondary infertility and recurrent pregnancy losses had live births as did a patient with secondary infertility.[85]

In a larger study,[86] with a similar design 24 patients with hypoplastic uterus and/or uterine deformity, at HSG underwent hysteroscopic metroplasty. Postoperative HSG showed an improved uterine cavity in 23 of the 24 cases. The final result was considered to be excellent in terms of anatomical correction in fifteen patients. Eleven pregnancies occurred, the abortion rate decreased from 88% in previous pregnancies to 12.5%, and the incidence of term deliveries increased from 3% to 87.5%.[86] Ten patients delivered healthy infants after 30 weeks' gestation and one patient delivered more prematurely. Six deliveries were normal and four required Cesarean section.[86]

Uteri affected by DES exposure are no longer prevalent, yet T-shaped uteri seem to be often diagnosed in patients with recurrent spontaneous abortion and their surgical correction remains controversial.[88] A recent study reported that among 97 women with a T-shaped uterus almost half (49.5%) became pregnant after metroplasty.[89] The overall live birth rate per pregnancy before surgery was 0%; for these patients, it increased to 73%, and their miscarriage rate fell from 78 to 27%. It was suggested the hysteroscopic metroplasty may improve the live birth rate for women with a T-shaped uterus and a history of primary infertility, recurrent abortion or preterm delivery.[89] Another study reporting on the results of hysteroscopic metroplasty in patients with recurrent spontaneous abortion concluded that term delivery rates were about 10-fold higher after surgery.[88] Moreover, T-shaped uterus surgery yielded the best term delivery rate.[88]

At present, it seems that hysteroscopic metroplasty, with its simplicity and minimal post-operative sequelae, seems to be the operation of choice in women with a hypoplastic malformed uterus and a history of severe infertility and/or recurrent pregnancy loss.[87,88] However, the previously quoted series used historical controls. Larger series with a better study design are necessary before hysteroscopic metroplasty can be recommended for all women with DES-exposed, T-shaped, or hypoplastic malformed uterus and recurrent miscarriage.

Conclusions

The prevalence and impact of uterine malformations on reproduction are still not clearly established in spite of the wide use of modern imaging modalites.[13] Consequently, the investigation of women with recurrent abortion should be limited in most cases to screening with ultrasonography, preferably utilizing 3D techniques and in selected cases benefiting from the application of hydrosonography (Table 26.2).[41] More invasive and expensive imaging modalities, including hysteroscopy, laparoscopy and MRI, should be reserved for inconclusive cases with a suspected uterine deformity.

Surgical intervention for uterine malformations remains poorly supported by randomized controlled trials (Table 26.3). It is generally agreed that adhesions, polyps, and protruding submucous myomas should be hysteroscopically resected. However, the need for hysteroscopic division of a uterine septum remains debatable, although it may be indicated in a patient with two or more pregnancy losses, as its associated morbidity is low. Abdominal metroplasty for the bicornuate uteri is even more difficult to support in light of its significant associated morbidity and lack of controlled data. Abdominal metroplasty is currently recommended only in selected cases with recurrent severe problems in the second and third-trimesters. Cervical cerclage is only indicated in women with uterine anomalies in the presence of a clinical diagnosis of cervical incompetence or additional risk factors. In women with hydrosalpinges and early recurrent abortion, laparoscopic salpingectomy or proximal tubal occlusion should be considered.

Miscarriages seem to be the inevitable by-product of the mechanism of human reproduction and do not always point to the presence of a correctable defect. Thus, surgical intervention should be carefully considered and based on the patient's clinical history, and not merely be an attempt to correct all anatomical uterine defects now more commonly diagnosed by modern imaging modalities.

REFERENCES

1. Chan YY, Jayaprakasan K, Zamora J et al. The prevalence of congenital uterine anomalies in unselected and high-risk populations: A systematic review. *Hum Reprod Update* 2011;17:761–71.
2. Devi Wold AS, Pham N, Arici A. Anatomic factors in recurrent pregnancy loss. *Semin Reprod Med* 2006;24:25–32.
3. The American Fertility Society classifications of adnexal adhesions, distal tubal occlusion, tubal occlusion secondary to tubal ligation, tubal pregnancies, mullerian anomalies and intrauterine adhesions. *Fertil Steril* 1988;49:944–55.
4. Homer HA, Li TC, Cooke ID. The septate uterus: A review of management and reproductive outcome. *Fertil Steril* 2000;73:1–4.
5. Proctor JA, Haney AF. Recurrent first trimester pregnancy loss is associated with uterine septum but not with bicornuate uterus. *Fertil Steril* 2003;80:1212–5.
6. Salim R, Regan L, Woelfer B et al. A comparative study of the morphology of congenital uterine anomalies in women with and without a history of recurrent first trimester miscarriage. *Hum Reprod* 2003;18:162–6.
7. Simon C, Martinez L, Pardo F et al. Mullerian defects in women with normal reproductive outcome. *Fertil Steril* 1991;56:1192–3.
8. Jurkovic D, Geipel A, Gruboeck K et al. Three-dimensional ultrasound for the assessment of uterine anatomy and detection of congenital anomalies: A comparison with hysterosalpingography and two-dimensional sonography. *Ultrasound Obstet Gynecol* 1995;5:233–7.
9. Ghi T, DeMusso F, Maroni E et al. The pregnancy outcome in women with incidental diagnosis of septate uterus at first trimester scan. *Hum Reprod* 2012;27:2671–5.
10. Dabirashrafi H, Bahadori M, Mohammad K et al. Septate uterus: New idea on the histologic features of the septum in this abnormal uterus. *Am J Obstet Gynecol* 1995;172:105–7.
11. Valle RF, Ekpo GE. Hysteroscopic metroplasty for the septate uterus: Review and meta-analysis. *J Minim Invasive Gynecol.* 2013;20:22–42.
12. Pundir J, Pundir V, Omanwa K et al. Hysteroscopyprior to the first IVF cycle: A systematic review and meta-analysis. *Reprod Biomed Online* 2014;28:151–61.
13. Jayaprakasan K, Chan YY, Sur S et al. Prevalence of uterine anomalies and their impact on early pregnancy in women conceiving after assisted reproduction treatment. *Ultrasound Obstet Gynecol.* 2011;37:727–32.
14. Woelfer B, Salim R, Banerjee S et al. Reproductive outcomes in women with congenital uterine anomalies detected by three-dimensional ultrasound screening. *Obstet Gynecol* 2001;98:1099–103.
15. Gergolet M, Campo R, Verdenik I et al. No clinical relevance of the height of fundal indentation in subseptate or arcuate uterus: A prospective study. *Reprod Biomed Online* 2012;24:576–82.
16. Fedele L, Bianchi S, Agnoli B et al. Urinary tract anomalies associated with unicornuate uterus. *J Urol* 1996;155:847–8.
17. Heinonen PK, Saarikoski S, Pystynen P. Reproductive performance of women with uterine anomalies. An evaluation of 182 cases. *Acta Obstet Gynecol Scand* 1982;61:157–62.
18. Fedele L, Bianchi S, Tozzi L et al. Fertility in women with unicornuate uterus. *Br J Obstet Gynaecol* 1995;102:1007–9.
19. Heinonen PK. Unicornuate uterus and rudimentary horn. *Fertil Steril* 1997;68:224–30.
20. Chifan M, Tîrnovanu M, Grigore M et al. Cervical incompetence associated with congenital uterine malformations. *Rev Med Chir Soc Med Nat Iasi* 2012;116:1063–8.
21. Fedele L, Bianchi S, Zanconato G et al. Laparoscopic removal of the cavitated noncommunicating rudimentary uterine horn: Surgical aspects in 10 cases. *Fertil Steril* 2005;83:432–6.

22. Heinonen P. Clinical implications of the didelphic uterus: Long-term follow-up of 49 cases. *Eur J Obstet Gynecol Reprod Biol* 2000;91:183–90.

23. Lin PC. Reproductive outcomes in women with uterine anomalies. *J Womens Health (Larchmt)* 2004;13:33–9.

24. Kaufman RH, Adam E, Hatch EE et al. Continued follow-up of pregnancy outcomes in diethylstilbestrol-exposed offspring. *Obstet Gynecol* 2000;96:483–9.

25. Veurink M, Koster M, Berg LT. The history of DES, lessons to be learned. *Pharm World Sci* 2005;27:139–43.

26. Laronda MM, Unno K, Ishi K et al. Diethylstilbestrol induces vaginal adenosis by disrupting SMAD/RUNX1-mediated cell fate decision in the Müllerian duct epithelium. *Dev Biol.* 2013;381:5–16.

27. Goldberg JM, Falcone T. Effect of diethylstilbestrol on reproductive function. *Fertil Steril* 1999;72:1–7.

28. Eldar-Geva T, Meagher S, Healy DL et al. Effect of intramural, subserosal, and submucosal uterine fibroids on the outcome of assisted reproductive technology treatment. *Fertil Steril* 1998;70:687–91.

29. Casini ML, Rossi F, Agostini R et al. Effects of the position of fibroids on fertility. *Gynecol Endocrinol* 2006;22:106–9.

30. Oliveira FG, Abdelmassih VG, Diamond MP et al. Impact of subserosal and intramural uterine fibroids that do not distort the endometrial cavity on the outcome of *in vitro* fertilization-intracytoplasmic sperm injection. *Fertil Steril* 2004;81:582–7.

31. Ribeiro SC, Reich H, Rosenberg J et al. Laparoscopic myomectomy and pregnancy outcome in infertile patients. *Fertil Steril* 1999;71:571–4.

32. Rossetti A, Sizzi O, Soranna L et al. Long-term results of laparoscopic myomectomy: Recurrence rate in comparison with abdominal myomectomy. *Hum Reprod* 2001;16:770–4.

33. Yan L, Ding L, Li C et al. Effect of fibroids not distorting the endometrial cavity on the outcome of *in vitro* fertilization treatment: A retrospective cohort study. *Fertil Steril* 2014;101:716–21.

34. Neuwirth RS, Levin B, Keltz MD. Pregnancy rates after hysteroscopic polypectomy and myomectomy in infertile women. *Obstet Gynecol* 1999;94:168–71.

35. Rackow BW, Jorgensen E, Taylor HS. Endometrial polyps affect uterine receptivity. *Fertil Steril* 2011;95:2690–2.

36. Perez-Medina T, Bajo-Arenas J, Salazar F et al. Endometrial polyps and their implication in the pregnancy rates of patients undergoing intrauterine insemination: A prospective, randomized study. *Hum Reprod* 2005;20:1632–5.

37. Hooker AB, Lemmers M, Thurkow AL et al. Systematic review and meta-analysis of intrauterineadhesions after miscarriage: Prevalence, risk factors and long-term reproductive outcome. *Hum Reprod Update* 2014;20:262–78.

38. Iton VK, Saunders NA, Harris LH et al. Intrauterine adhesions after manual vacuum aspiration for early pregnancy failure. *Fertil Steril* 2006;85:1823.

39. Royal College of Obstetricians and Gynaecologists. *The Investigation and Treatment of Recurrent Miscarriage. Guideline No 17*. London: RCOG Press; 2011.

40. Jaslow CR, Kutteh WH. Effect of prior birth and miscarriage frequency on the prevalence of acquired and congenital uterine anomalies in women with recurrent miscarriage: A cross-sectional study. *Fertil Steril* 2013;99:1916–22.

41. Berger A, Batzer F, Lev-Toaff A et al. Diagnostic imaging modalities for mullerian anomalies: The case for a new gold standard. *J Minim Invasive Gynecol* 2013:S1553–4650.

42. Baramki TA. Hysterosalpingography. *Fertil Steri* 2005;83:1595–606.

43. Bhaduri M, Tomlinson G, Glanc P. Likelihood ratio of sonohysterographic findings for discriminating endometrial polyps from submucosalfibroids. *J Ultrasound Med* 2014;33:149–54.

44. Sylvestre C, Child TJ, Tulandi T et al. A prospective study to evaluate the efficacy of two- and three-dimensional sonohysterography in women with intrauterine lesions. *Fertil Steril* 2003;79:1222–5.

45. Alborzi S, Dehbashi S, Parsanezhad ME. Differential diagnosis of septate and bicornuate uterus by sonohysterography eliminates the need for laparoscopy. *Fertil Steril* 2002;78:176–8.

46. Soares SR, Barbosa dos Reis MM et al. Diagnostic accuracy of sonohysterography, transvaginal sonography, and hysterosalpingography in patients with uterine cavity diseases. *Fertil Steril* 2000;73:406–11.

47. Marcal L, Nothaft MA, Coelho F et al. Mullerian duct anomalies: MR imaging. *Abdom Imaging* 2011;36:756–64.

48. Troiano RN, McCarthy SM. Mullerian duct anomalies: Imaging and clinical issues. *Radiology* 2004;233:19–34.

49. Pui MH. Imaging diagnosis of congenital uterine malformation. *Comput Med Imaging Graph* 2004;28:425–33.

50. Zupi E, Marconi D, Vaquero E et al. Hysteroscopic findings in 344 women with recurrent spontaneous abortion. *J Am Assoc Gynecol Laparosc* 2001;8:398–401.

51. Weiss A, Shalev E, Romano S. Hysteroscopy may be justified after two miscarriages. *Hum Reprod* 2005;20:2628–31.

52. Seidman DS, Nezhat CH, Nezhat F et al. Minimally invasive surgery for fibroids. *Infert Reprod Med Clin N Am* 2002;13:375–91.

53. Goldberg J, Pereira L. Pregnancy outcomes following treatment for fibroids: Uterine fibroid embolization versus laparoscopic myomectomy. *Curr Opin Obstet Gynecol* 2006;18:402–6.

54. Sagiv R, Sadan O, Boaz M et al. A new approach to office hysteroscopy compared with traditional hysteroscopy: A randomized controlled trial. *Obstet Gynecol* 2006;108:387–92.

55. Seckin B, Sarikaya E, Oruc AS et al. Office hysteroscopic findings in patients with two, three, and four or more, consecutive miscarriages. *Eur J Contracept Reprod Health Care* 2012;17:393–8.

56. Alijotas-Reig J, Garrido-Gimenez C. Current concepts and new trends in the diagnosis and management of recurrent miscarriage. *Obstet Gynecol Surv* 2013;68:445–66.

57. Bosteels J, Kasius J, Weyers S et al. Hysteroscopy for treating subfertility associated with suspected major uterine cavity abnormalities. *Cochrane Database Syst Rev.* 2013;1:CD009461.

58. Jauniaux E, Farquharson RG, Christiansen OB et al. On behalf of ESHRE special interest group for early pregnancy (SIGEP). Evidence-based guidelines for the investigation and medical treatment of recurrent miscarriage. *Hum Reprod* 2006;21:2216–22.

59. Valli E, Zupi E, Marconi D et al. Hysteroscopic findings in 344 women with recurrent spontaneous abortion. *J Am Assoc Gynecol Laparosc* 2001;8:398–401.

60. Kalampokas T, Tzanakaki D, Konidaris S et al. Endometrial polyps and their relationship in the pregnancy rates of patients undergoing intrauterine insemination. *Clin Exp Obstet Gynecol* 2012;39:299–302.

61. Preutthipan S, Herabutya Y. Hysteroscopic polypectomy in 240 premenopausal and postmenopausal women. *Fertil Steril* 2005;83:705–9.

62. Marsh F, Rogerson L, Duffy S. A randomised controlled trial comparing outpatient versus day case endometrial polypectomy. *BJOG* 2006;113:896–901.

63. Kowalik CR, Goddijn M, Emanuel MH et al. Metroplasty versus expectant management for women with recurrent miscarriage and a septate uterus. *Cochrane Database Syst Rev* 2011:CD008576.

64. Fedele L, Arcaini L, Parazzini F et al. Reproductive prognosis after hysteroscopic metroplasty in 102 women: Life-table analysis. *Fertil Steril* 1993;59:768–72.

65. Dalal RJ, Pai HD, Palshetkar NP et al. Hysteroscopic metroplasty in women with primary infertility and septate uterus: Reproductive performance after surgery. *J Reprod Med* 2012;57:13–6.

66. Grimbizis GF, Camus M, Tarlatzis BC et al. Clinical implications of uterine malformations and hysteroscopic treatment results. *Hum Reprod Update* 2001;7:161–74.

67. Patton PE, Novy MJ, Lee DM et al. The diagnosis and reproductive outcome after surgical treatment of the complete septate uterus, duplicated cervix and vaginal septum. *Am J Obstet Gynecol* 2004;190:1669–75.

68. Sentilhes L, Sergent F, Roman H et al. Late complications of operative hysteroscopy: Predicting patients at risk of uterine rupture during subsequent pregnancy. *Eur J Obstet Gynecol Reprod Biol* 2005;120:134–8.

69. Pang LH, Li MJ, Li M et al. Not every subseptate uterus requires surgical correction to reduce poor reproductive outcome. *Int J Gynaecol Obstet* 2011;115:260–3.

70. Heinonen PK. Complete septate uterus with longitudinal vaginal septum. *Fertil Steril* 2006;85:700–5.

71. Parsanezhad ME, Alborzi S, Zarei A et al. Hysteroscopic metroplasty of the complete uterine septum, duplicate cervix, and vaginal septum. *Fertil Steril* 2006;85:1473–7.

72. Kolankaya A, Arici A. Myomas and assisted reproductive technologies: When and how to act? *Obstet Gynecol Clin North Am* 2006;33:145–52.

73. Oliveira FG, Abdelmassih VG, Diamond MP et al. Impact of subserosal and intramural uterine fibroids that do not distort the endometrial cavity on the outcome of *in vitro* fertilization-intracytoplasmic sperm injection. *Fertil Steril* 2004;81:582–7.

74. Benecke C, Kruger TF, Siebert TI et al. Effect of fibroids on fertility in patients undergoing assisted reproduction. A structured literature review. *Gynecol Obstet Invest* 2005;59:225–30.

75. Seidman DS, Nezhat CH, Nezhat FR et al. Spontaneous uterine rupture in pregnancy 8 years after laparoscopic myomectomy. *J Am Assoc Gynecol Laparosc* 2001;8:333–5.

76. Seidman DS, Nezhat FR, Nezhat CH et al. The role of laparoscopic-assisted myomectomy (LAM). *JSLS* 2001;5:299–303.

77. Torre A, Paillusson B, Fain V et al. Uterinearteryembolization for severe symptomaticfibroids: Effects on fertility and symptoms. *Hum Reprod* 2014;29:490–501.

78. Seidman DS, Ben-Rafael Z, Bider D et al. The role of cervical cerclage in the management of uterine anomalies. *Surg Gynecol Obstet* 1991;173:384–6.

79. Althuisius SM, Dekker GA, Hummel P et al. Final results of the Cervical Incompetence Prevention Randomized Cerclage Trial (CIPRACT): Therapeutic cerclage with bed rest versus bed rest alone. *Am J Obstet Gynecol* 2001;185:1106–12.

80. Levine RU, Berkowitz KM. Conservative management and pregnancy outcome in diethylstilbestrol-exposed women with and without gross genital tract abnormalities. *Am J Obstet Gynecol* 1993;169:1125–9.

81. Lolis DE, Paschopoulos M, Makrydimas G et al. Reproductive outcome after Strassman metroplasty in women with a bicornuate uterus. *J Reprod Med* 2005;50:297–301.

82. Khalifa E, Toner JP, Jones HW Jr. The role of abdominal metroplasty in the era of operative hysteroscopy. *Surg Gynecol Obstet* 1993;176:208–12.

83. Johnson N, vanVoorst S, Sowter MC et al. Surgical treatment for tubal disease in women due to undergo *in vitro* fertilisation. *Cochrane Database Syst Rev.* 2010;1:CD002125.

84. Zolghadri J, Momtahan M, Alborzi S et al.Pregnancy outcome in patients with early recurrent abortion following laparoscopic tubal corneal interruption of a fallopian tube with hydrosalpinx. *Fertil Steril* 2006;86:149–51.

85. Nagel TC, Malo JW. Hysteroscopic metroplasty in the diethylstilbestrol- reproductive performance; a preliminary report. *Fertil Steril* 1993;59:502–6.

86. Garbin O, Ohl J, Bettahar-Lebugle K et al. Hysteroscopic metroplasty in diethylstilboestrol-exposed and hypoplastic uterus: A report on 24 cases. *Hum Reprod* 1998;13:2751–5.

87. Barranger E, Gervaise A, Doumerc S et al. Reproductive performance after hysteroscopic metroplasty in the hypoplastic uterus: A study of 29 cases. *BJOG* 2002;109:1331–4.

88. Giacomucci E, Bellavia E, Sandri F et al. Term delivery rate after hysteroscopic metroplasty in patients with recurrent spontaneous abortion and T-shaped, arcuate and septate uterus. *Gynecol Obstet Invest* 2011;71:183–8.

89. Fernandez H, Garbin O, Castaigne V et al. Surgical approach to and reproductive outcome after surgical correction of a T-shaped uterus. *Hum Reprod.* 2011;26:1730–4.

27

The Immunobiology of Recurrent Miscarriage

Marighoula Varla-Leftherioti

Introduction

Initially, recurrent spontaneous abortions (RSA) were considered to be due to either chromosomal aberrations of the fetus that are incompatible with its development or to maternal causes such as uterine anatomical abnormalities, hormonal or metabolic disturbances, hereditary thrombophilias, and infectious agents. When all the above causes of miscarriages were excluded, the miscarriages were characterized as "unexplained miscarriages." During the last 25 years, it has become clear that a large percentage of unexplained RSA may be due to immunological causes.[1] About 50% of preclinically lost embryos and 95% of those clinically lost in women with RSA have a normal karyotype and most of these losses may be of immune etiology.[2] Immune-mediated abortions are characterized by either autoimmune or alloimmune disturbances.[3] In autoimmune abortions, the development of the placenta and the embryo is affected by maternal autoantibodies and autoreactive cells, which target decidual and trophoblastic molecules. In alloimmune abortions, the maternal immune system reacts against the embryo and damages the trophoblast through allogeneic, rejection-type reactions. Clinically, the two categories of auto- and alloimmune-mediated abortions cannot be distinguished as both of them represent a broad immunological imbalance that leads to pregnancy loss.[4] However, the classification helps to better understand underlying mechanisms, to identify candidates for immune testing, and select immunological treatment.

Autoimmune Abortions

Maternal autoimmune disturbances may be the cause of a high percentage of hitherto-unexplained miscarriages. Approximately 30% of women with "unexplained" RSA have increased serum levels of autoantibodies, with antiphospholipid antibodies (aPL) predominating.[5]

Autoimmune Abortions Associated with Antiphospholipid Antibodies

The pathogenic antiphospholipid antibodies (aPL) are those that target the first domain (epitope comprising Gly40 and Arg43) of β_2-GPI, the main protein which binds PLs. Kuwana et al.[6] were able to detect β_2-GPI-specific CD4(+) and human leukocyte antigen (HLA) class II restricted autoreactive T-cells, which preferentially recognize the antigenic peptide containing the major phospholipid-binding site and have the capacity to stimulate B-cells to produce pathogenic anti-β_2-GPI antibodies. Interestingly, epitopes of some bacteria (*Haemophilus influenzae*, *Neisseria gonorrhoeae*, *Helicobacter pylori* or *tetanus toxoid*) have homology with β_2-GPI, and can induce pathogenic anti-β_2GPI antibodies along with APS manifestations, including pregnancy loss.[7] Similar mechanisms of molecular mimicry may involve various viruses (HIV-1, hepatitis A, B, C viruses). However, most of the antibodies induced by viral infections are not pathogenic, as they are not β_2-GPI-dependent but recognize phospholipids directly.[8]

Because of the different methods by which they are induced, aPL are a heterogeneous group of autoantibodies.[9] aPL that bind to PL, present in unique hexagonal phases either alone or complexed with prothrombin or β_2-GPI, prolong PL-dependent clotting assays and are known as Lupus anticoagulants

(LAC). The subgroup of aPL that bind to PL/protein complexes and may or may not prolong PL-dependent clotting assays includes antibodies against cardiolipin (aCL), phosphatidylethanolamine (aPE), phosphatidylserine (aPS), phosphatidyl-choline (aPC), phosphatidylglycerol (aPG), phosphatidylinositol (aPI), and phosphatidic acid (aPA).

Today, it is clear that inflammation, inhibition of trophoblast functions, and shift to Th1-type response, are responsible for fetal loss[10,11] and probably the basis for the subsequent placental thrombosis and vasoconstriction. Complement activation by aPL leads to the generation of C5a anaphylatoxin, which can induce thrombosis and inflammation-mediated placental tissue damage. By interacting with its receptor (C5aR) on various cells, C5α induces expression of TF on endothelial cells, neutrophils and monocytes, and a prothrombotic phenotype in mast cells.[12] Moreover, cells activated by C5α release inflammatory mediators, including reactive oxidants, proteolytic enzymes, cytokines, chemokines and complement factors, which lead to oxidative damage and trophoblast injury. Cytokines, such as tumor necrosis factor-α (TNFα) and interleukin-6 (IL-6) may be responsible for placental thromboses,[13] while membrane attack complex (MAC) triggers endothelial cell and platelet activation, and causes lysis of placental cells.[14,15] Depending on the extent of damage, either death *in utero* or fetal growth restriction ensues. In addition, some aPL directly target trophoblastic cells, and may affect pregnancy by inhibiting normal PL functions related to trophoblastic cell division, intertrophoblastic fusion, hormonal secretion, and trophoblast invasion.[16] Antibodies against phosphatidylethanolamine (aPE) may affect implantation and cell division during embryogenesis.[17] Antibodies against phosphatidylserin (aPS) may inhibit syncytialization by blocking PS, which normally acts as an adhesion molecule for the fusion of cytotrophoblast cells,[18] and reduce the secretion of human chorionic gonadotrophin (hCG), possibly by inhibiting signal transduction of factors inducing its production.[19] Finally, anti-β2GPI antibodies may reduce gonadotropin release, hormone dependent hCG mRNA expression, and protein synthesis.[20,21]

Effect on cytokine production—shift to Th1-type response: aPL may cause abortion by altering the production of cytokines. Decreased levels of immunotrophic placental cytokines (IL-3 and granulocyte-macrophage colony-stimulating factor [GM-CSF]) have been found in mice with experimental APS.[22] Moreover, the inflammatory reactions against PLs modified by oxidative events may promote a Th1-type immune response at the fetomaternal interface, which do not favor pregnancy. Buttari et al.[23] have shown that *in vitro* oxidized β$_2$-GPI interacts with dendritic cells (DC) and stimulates them to secrete cytokines that support T-cell responses (IL-12, IL-1β, IL-6, IL-8, tumor necrosis factor α (TNF-α, and IL-10). Among these, IL-12, a proinflammatory cytokine that forms a link between innate and adaptive immunity, induces the production of interferon γ (IFN-γ), and favors differentiation of Th1 cells. Th1 profile of β$_2$-GPI autoreactive CD4+ T cells has been determined in the peripheral blood of patients with APS and histories of thromboses or fetal loss.[24]

Clarification of the immunological mechanisms of action of aPL have resulted in novel forms of treatment for the prevention of aPL-associated abortions. Immunomodulation and neutralization of aPL intravenous administration of immunoglobulin G (IVIg) is one such teatment, and recently treatment with statins (HMG-CoA reductase inhibitors) has been suggested for the modulation of inflammatory reaction caused by aPL.

Autoimmune Abortions not Associated with aPL

Finally, a genetic background may predispose to fetal loss in women with autoimmune-mediated abortions. Beer et al.[25] have reported an increase of the HLA-DQA1*0501 allele (now classified as 05:05) in women with recurrent pregnancy losses who are aPL positive. They have suggested that fetuses compatible with their mothers for this allele, are autoimmune unacceptable to the mother and they trigger her to develop aPL when the pregnancy fails and to be most prone to miscarriage in subsequent pregnancies.[26] However, the author could not confirm these findings.[27]

Alloimmune Abortions

The observations that, in some cases of abortion, the embryo is infiltrated by lymphocytes and the lesions found to the placenta resemble the allogeneic reactions found in transplanted grafts indicate that in these cases the embryo is "rejected" by the mother.[28] To assess the mechanisms leading to such miscarriages, it is necessary to know the nature of the immune response in normal pregnancy, since it is the disturbances in normal pregnancy immunological mechanisms that result in allogeneic antifetal reactions.

Immune Response in Normal Pregnancy

The conseptus is a *semiallogeneic graft*, as it has genetic and antigenic contributions from both the mother and the father. Although fetal alloantigens encoded by genes inherited from the father should provoke a maternal response and lead to fetal loss. Normally this does not happen. This *immunological paradox of pregnancy* is considered to be the result of a particular immune response of the pregnant woman, and for more than 50 years it has been a challenge for reproductive immunologists to attempt to elucidate the underlying immunological mechanisms.

Facilitation Reaction

The first reliable explanation for fetal tolerance suggested that in allogeneic reactions such as transplantation and pregnancy, the immune response is bipolar, which can be either harmful or favorable to the target cells expressing alloantigens. The harmful effect (rejection reaction observed in transplantation) is characterized by cytotoxic antibodies and cytotoxic cells that damage the antigenic target. The enhancing effect (facilitation reaction) is characterized by a predominance of humoral responses, which may counteract the rejection reaction and have a beneficial effect on the antigenic target.[29] Predominance of this facilitation reaction over the rejection reaction appears in pregnancy, where enhancing non-complement-fixing antibodies and suppressor cells favor the acceptance of the embryos; they prevent complement-mediated cell lysis, while they block allogeneic reactions, either by covering the alloantigens or through the function of an idiotype-anti-idiotype antibody network.[30] If the coexisting but suppressed rejection reaction is up regulated, the embryo is rejected. The suggestion that the facilitation reaction prevails over the rejection reaction and results in fetal tolerance has been followed by a plethora of studies that have focused on the mechanisms mediating this specific response.

Th2-Type Immune Response

In 1987, Wegmann[31] presented the "immunotrophic" theory, according to which the normal development of the placenta is the result of the influence of cytokines (placenta immunotrophic cytokines, such as granulocyte macrophage colony stimulating factor [GM-CSF], transforming growth factor [TGF-β], and interleukin-3 [IL-3]). In 1993, Wegman et al.[32] suggested that during pregnancy there is a change of the T-h1 (Th1)//Th2 equilibrium so that Th2-type cytokines (IL-4, IL-5, IL-10) predominate over Th1-type cytokines (IL-2, interferon γ [IFN-γ]) and benefit the developing embryo by enhancing placental growth and function as well as by preventing inappropriate anti-trophoblast cytotoxic reactions.

The role of cytokines in maternal–fetal symbiosis has been well documented. However, the trophoblastic antigenic stimulus, the maternal cells that are stimulated for the initiation of the enhancing response and the exact factors modulating the Th2 shift remain unclarified. Several antigenic systems, that are expressed on trophoblast (molecules of the major histocompatibility complex [MHC], erythrocyte antigens, complement regulatory proteins, Fc receptors, various isoenzymes, adhesion molecule, R80K protein, etc.), have been assessed, but no specific antigen has been identified.[33] Nevertheless, specific trophoblastic molecules as well as various proteins produced by the trophoblast appear to modulate the cytokine pattern towards preferential expression of Th2 cytokines. Heat shock proteins (HSP), pregnancy specific β_1-glycoprotein and increased expression of the non-classical MHC class I HLA-G molecule have been suggested as stimulants of endometrial macrophages for IL-10 production which enhances a Th2 shift.[34] Decidual cells may also produce high levels of Th2-type cytokines after interacting with trophoblastic CD1d molecules, which present glycolipid antigens to specific cell populations bearing T and natural killer (NK) cell receptors.[35] Moreover, binding of leukemia inhibitory factor (LIF) (produced by decidual cells) to its receptor (LIF-R) on the syncytiotrophoblast, may enhance placental growth and differentiation and a Th2 shift.[36] Finally, hCG produced by the tropho-blast, induces the production of progesterone by the corpus luteum. Through an immunoregulatory protein known as progesterone induced blocking factor (PIBF), progesterone may induce the production of IL-4 by γδ T lymphocytes and, thus, enhance a Th2 response.[37]

Cytokine and Hormone Network

The theory of the Th2 shift alone, is a simplification of the cytokine-mediated mechanisms enhancing pregnancy at the fetomaternal interface, as both Th1 and Th2 cytokines are necessary during specific stages of fetal development: Th1 pro-inflammatory cytokines are required in early pregnancy and at the end of pregnancy, Th2 anti-inflammatory cytokines are required in mid-pregnancy.[38] IFN-γ, a Th1 ctyokine, has a beneficial role in promoting implantation contributing to the vascular development and remodeling of uterine spiral arteries required for implantation and successful gestation.[39] Different cell populations are potentially involved in the production not only of Th2 cytokines, but also of Th1 cyto-kines as well as other cytokines (i.e., IL-12, -15, -18), chemokines and growth factors that control the differentiation and the activation of immune cells locally. A cytokine that controls the shift to Th1 response (i.e., IL-12) coexists with one enhancing the Th2 response (IL-10), and all these are possibly controlled by primary regulatory factors on a competitive basis. This regulatory and competitive role was initially attributed to homones (i.e., hCG, progesterone, relaxin), the secretion of which is induced by cytokines at the same time that the hormones themselves control the production of cytokines.

Regulatory T Cells and Th17 Inflammtory Cells

Our understanding of the cytokine network and the regulation of the Th1/Th2 balance has changed immensely with the recognition of the important role of two other immune factors at the fetomaternal interface: regulatory T-cells (Treg) and Th17 cells.[40] Treg cells are a subset of immunoregulatory T lym-phocytes (CD4+CD25+Foxp3+), which derive either from the thymus or by activation of naïve CD4+ T-cells following antigen stimulation under the influence of TGF-β.[41] These cells play central role in the induction of tolerance as they can inhibit the proliferation of and cytokine production by CD4+, CD8+ T-cells, antibody production by B-cells, cytotoxic activity of natural killer (NK) cells and maturation of dendritic cells (DC).[42] A unique property of Treg cells is their ability to induce infectious tolerance by conferring upon the cells they target suppressive capabilities and the ability to inhibit down stream steps in the immune cascade (bystander suppression phenomenon).[43]

The first data suggesting that pregnancy-induced Treg cells play a vital role in maternal tolerance to the allogeneic murine and human fetus appeared in 2004. Aluvihare et al.[44] demonstrated that during murine pregnancy there is a systemic expansion of Treg cells, which can suppress aggressive allogeneic responses directed against the fetus. Sasaki et al.[45] showed that early human pregnancy decidua contains an abundance of CD4+CD25[bright] T-cells that can inhibit the proliferation of autologous CD4+ T-cells, and are significantly lower in specimens from spontaneous abortions compared to those from specimens from induced abortions. Somerset et al.[46] found that CD25+ CD4+ (Foxp3 mRNA+) Treg cells, which inhibit *in vitro* the induction of T lymphocyte proliferation by a third-party allogeneic stimulus, are increased in the peripheral blood during early pregnancy, peak during the second trimester, and decline postpartum. Consequently, Zenclussen et al.[47] were able to prevent fetal rejection in a murine abortion model (CBA/JxDBA/2) by adoptive transfer of Treg cells from normal pregnant mice, and showed that the transfer increased the expression of progesterone receptors on decidual cells.

Studies in mice and humans have revealed that decidual Tregs derive either from activation and pro-liferation of regulatory cells of thymic origin in the draining lymph nodes of the uterus,[48] or by selective recruitment of fetus-specific CD4+CD25[bright] from the peripheral blood.[49] Before implantation (possibly during the follicular phase), a hormone-dependant accumulation of Treg cells takes place in the lymph nodes. At the outset of pregnancy there is an expansion of Tregs from naïve CD4+ cells in response to paternal antigens delivered from the seminal fluid.[50] During pregnancy, a peripheral expansion and/or conversion from Foxp3[-] into Foxp3[+] cells is induced by fetal allogeneic antigens.[51] Saito et al.[40] have suggested a model for paternal antigen-specific Treg cell expansion, proliferation, and mobilization from the vagina to the pregnant uterus. DCs take up paternal antigens from the seminal plasma after coitus, and they present them to naïve Treg cells of thymic origin, which become paternal antigen-specific, they proliferate and migrate to the pregnant uterus by chemokine,[52,53] and hCG-induced[54] chemoattractant mechanisms. Up-regulation of the transcription factor Foxp3, allows decidual Treg cells to begin their suppressive effect on decidual immune cells and transfer suppressive capabilities and the ability to inhibit down stream steps in the maternal anti-fetal immune cascade. However, the mechanism is not well defined. Based on our existing knowledge of the mode of action of Tregs, decidual Tregs are expected to control effector cells by cytokine-mediated mechanisms and mechanisms mediated by direct cell-to-cell contact with target cells. By secretion of inhibitory cytokines (TGF-β, IL-10, and IL-35), and consumption of γc-family cytokines (IL-2, IL-4, IL-7, IL-15), decidual Treg cells may suppress activation and expansion of conventional T lymphocytes, inhibit the release of proinflammatory cytokine, increase T-cell apoptotic rates, and modulate the functions of decidual DCs.[55,56] IL-10 inhibits the up-regulation of the expression of MHC and costimulatory molecule on DC (attenuation of interaction with T cells and decreased antigen-presenting capacity), suppresses release of pro-inflammatory cytokines such as IL-1β, IL-6, TNF-α, and IL-12, and up-regulates the expression of inhibitory molecules. Tregs may also have cytolytic effects on target decidual T cells and on DCs, through the secretion of granzymes and perforin.[57] Contact-mediated suppression results from ligation of a range of Treg surface molecules to effector cells: Galectin-1 promotes apoptosis of activated T cells,[57] lymphocyte activation gene 3 (LAG-3) modulates DC phenotype and function,[58] programmed death ligand 1 (PDL-1) promotes apoptosis of maternal antigen-specific activated cells, and prevents the accumulation of fetal antigen-specific CD8+ T cells in the lymph nodes,[59] cytotoxic T lymphocyte antigen 4 (CTLA-4) down-regulates the expression of costimulatory molecules (CD80, CD86) on DCs and enhances immunosuppressive tryptophan catabolism in decidual cells.[60] It is suggested that the ligation of CTLA-4 is important for generating an immunosuppressive milieu at the fetomaternal interface, since it induces the expression of the tryptophan-degrading enzyme indoleamine 2,3-dioxygenase (IDO) on DCs, and controls the balance between Treg and Th1 cells responses.[61] IDO is a potent regulatory molecule known to inhibit T-cell activation by inducing the production of pro-apoptotic metabolites from the catabolism of tryptophan and suppression of T-cells.[62] Therefore, bi-directional signaling between Treg cells and DCs may be one means of infectious tolerance, since Treg cells can condition DCs to express IDO and thereby exert a suppressive influence over neighboring T-cells.

An emerging area of interest is the relationship between Treg cells and pro-inflammatory IL-17-producing T (Th17) cells.[40,63] Th17 cells have recently been described as a key effector T-cell subset, which has changed our understanding of immune regulation, immune pathogenesis and host defense. They represent the third member of the T-cell trilogy having probably evolved to enhance host clearance of a range of pathogens distinct from those targeted by Th1 and Th2.[64] In humans, Th17 are differentiated from naïve T-cells in response to a combination of cytokine signals distinct from, and antagonized by, cytokines of the Th1 and Th2 lineages (TGF-β, IL-1β, and IL-23).[65] They express CCR6, IL-23R, and also IL-12Rβ2 and CD161. They are characterized by the production of a distinct profile of effector cytokines, including IL-17 (or IL-17A), IL-17F, IL-21, and can be induced to produce IFN-γ in addition to IL-17A in the presence of IL-12.[66]

Little data is available on the allogeneic pregnancy model. However, Th17 expansion appears to present a barrier for establishing maternal tolerance because of mutual antagonism and plasticity between Treg cells and Th17 cells. These two cell subsets appear to share a common lineage with their relative abundance influenced dramatically by the cytokine environment (particularly the ratio of IL-6 to TGF-β) in which T-cell priming occurs.[67] In the absence of IL-6, TGF-β suppress the conversion of naïve T-cells to Th17 cells, while in the presence of IL-6 naïve T-cells are converted to Th17 cells, and existing Treg cells can function as inducers of Th17 cells and themselves convert to Th17 cells. Apart from TGF-β and IL-6, other factor can also influence the antagonism between Treg cells and Th-17 cells. IL-1 can induce Th17 cells as opposed to Treg cells,[68] and IDO has been shown to block the conversion of Tregs into Th-17 cells.[69] A recent study[70] has found that IL17+ were significantly higher in patients with inevitabile abortion, compared to normal pregnancy, but not in asymptomatic missed abortion. Therefore, IL-17 expression might be the mechanism of expulsion of the fetus rather than the cause of miscarriage.

Although the Th1/Th2 paradigm provides the framework for understanding immune mechanisms and maternal tolerance in pregnancy, the mutual antagonism and plasticity between Treg cells and Th17 cells illustrates the fine balance between a suppressive or pro-inflammatory immune outcome at the fetomaternal interface and the major importance of the cytokine environment for the success of pregnancy.

Other Mechanisms Enhancing Fetal Tolerance

Th2 cytokines and Treg cells characterize the immune response in normal pregnancy, but many different mechanisms acting locally or at distance ensure tolerance to the semiallogeneic graft by the maternal natural and adaptive immune defences. Thus, tolerance is modulated by the cumulative effect of preimplantation factors, molecules expressed on the trophoblast as well as decidual immune cells. Changes in metabolic factors, hormones, and cytokines during ovulation, coitus and fertilization result in local immunosuppression within the maternal genital tract and prepare the uterus for the implantation of the blastocyst.[71] Trophoblastic molecules may be specifically recognized by maternal immune cells as alloantigens or may act as antigen-presenting molecules or have a suppressive or immunomodulatory function. Decidual immune cells may regulate the immune response not only by producing cytokines and growth factors, but also by specific recognition of trophoblastic molecules, suppression of cytotoxic reactions, and NK-cell toxicity.

Several specific immunosuppressive and cytotoxicity-blocking mechanisms have been suggested to contribute to fetal tolerance. Sperm may promote local immunosuppression via prostaglandins, while TGF-β contained in seminal plasma may provide the necessary antigenic and environmental signals for the accumulation of Treg cell in the uterus, the production of growth factors (GM-CSF) by the uterine epithelium and the initiation of an appropriate maternal immune response to the conceptus if pregnancy is achieved.[72] The trophoblast may prevent activation of placental immune cells or induce apoptosis of activated cells. The maternal innate immune system, which is the first to confront the embryo, actively reacts by developing an inflammatory response mediated by Toll-like receptors (TLR) expressed on trophoblast cells. This response enhances decidual and trophoblast development, and may induce tolerance.[38,54] IDO expressed by trophoblastic cells may catabolize tryptophane in maternal T cells and prevent them from activating lethal antifetal immune responses.[73] The expression of the CD95-L (FasL) molecule on the trophoblast and its interaction with CD95 (Fas) expressed on decidual cells protects trophoblastic cells by inducing apoptosis of activated CD95+ T lymphocytes.[74] Modulation of local placental immunity during pregnancy has been also ascribed to HLA-G, which is expressed in extravillous cytotrophoblast that invade decidual tissue and maternal spiral arteries as well as villous cytotrophoblast (soluble form). Soluble HLA-G1 isoforms might play an important role in implantation, while HLA-G induces apoptosis of activated CD8+ T-cells, down-regulates the proliferation of T-helper cells and modulates cytokine secretion by NK cells upon interaction with specific receptors.[75] Under the control of Treg cells, decidual antigen presenting cells express their activation by the production of anti-inflammatory rather than proinflammatory cytokines, and have an immunosuppressive action and a limited antigen presenting capacity.[76]

The Role of NK Cells in the Maintenance of Pregnancy

NK cells are part of the inate immune system and have a variable set of receptors belonging to five families: KIR (killer immunoglobulin-like receptors), NCR (natural cytotoxicity receptors), ILT/LIR (immunoglobulin-like transcripts), CD94/NKGs, and NKG2D.[77–79] The proportions of immunosoppressive NK subset (NK3 and NKr1) are suppressed in miscarriages compared to normal pregnancy. Progesterone, prolactin, HCG and soluble HLA-G1 could contibute to fetal tolerance by inducing the production of immunosoppressive NK subsets.[80]

Decidual NK (dNK) cells (CD3-CD16-CD56+[bright]) are the dominant decidual cell population from the first stages of pregnancy through the first trimester. Due to their increased presence and direct contact with invading trophoblast, they have been considered as important for the establishment of normal pregnancy. There is evidence that, coincident with blastocyst implantation and decidualization, when uterine NK cells become activated, they produce IFN-γ, perforin, and other molecules, including angiogenetic factors. In this way, they can control trophoblast invasion through their cytotoxic activity, and they also initiate vessel instability and remodeling of decidual arteries to increase the blood supply to the fetoplacental unit.[44] Furthermore, dNK may be involved in cytokine-mediated immunoregulation of the maternal immune response producing Th2-type cytokines and growth factors, which result in placental augmentation and local immunosuppression and immunomodulation.[81,82] Through their receptors, dNK cells may recognize selected epitopes on HLA-class I molecules expressed on invading trophoblast. It is interesting that the specific ligands for most of the receptors are the non-classical HLA class I molecules G and E as well the classical HLA class I antigen C, which are the only HLA molecules expressed on the extravillous trophoblast. Moreover, some of the receptors recognizing HLA-G and HLA-C epitopes are selectively expressed on dNK cells. The specific interaction of the NK-cell receptors with trophoblastic antigens led to the concept of an embryo recognition model through an "NK-cell allorecognition system." High-affinity interactions of NK receptors with their ligands may provide self-signals to either cytotoxic NK activation (Th1 response) or inhibition of activation and protection of the trophoblast (Th2 response). Which one of the two responses will predominate depends on the action of the inhibitory receptors, which prevails over the action of the activating ones. Consequently, if the inhibitory dNK receptors recognize their specific ligands on the trophoblast, they are expected to inhibit dNK activation for trophoblast damage, otherwise dNK are allowed to develop anti-trophoblast activity.[83] Most studies that have investigated the effect of dNK receptors in the maintenance of pregnancy have specifically focused on the interactions involving HLA-G molecules, because of their restricted distribution to placental tissues. HLA-G has been shown to be the ligand for at least three inhibitory receptors, and the expression of some HLA-G isoforms has been shown to protect trophoblastic cells from lysis by activated cytotoxic cell clones.[84] Nevertheless, the control of the anti-trophoblast activity of dNK cells is probably the result of the cumulative interaction of several receptors on maternal dNK with different self and non-self class-I molecules appearing on the HLA haplotypes expressed on the trophoblast. Among the different NK-cell receptor interactions with their specific counterparts on the trophoblast, the interactions between inhibitory receptors of the KIR family (inhKIR) and their ligands HLA-C molecules appear to be those mainly involved in the function of an NK-cell-mediated allorecognition system in pregnancy.[85] Given the differences in both the inhKIR repertoire and the HLA-C allotypes among unrelated individuals, each pregnancy presents a different combination of maternal inhKIR receptors on dNK and self and non-self HLA-C allotypes on the trophoblast. This combination is expected to ensure the appropriate receptor–ligand interactions to inhibit dNK anti-trophoblast activity, thus favoring pregnancy.

A recent pilot randomized control trial (RCT)[86] assessed the possibility of "screening and treating " women with recurrent miscarriage. One hundred and sixty women underwent endometrium sampling 5–9 days after the LH surge. Seventy-two were found to have a high uterine NK density (>5%), Several other studies have suggested that peripheral blood NK levels are elevated in women aborting karyotypically normal embryos.[87,88]

Immunopathology of Alloimmune Abortion

In contrast to normal pregnancy, a predominant Th1-type response or defective production of Th2-type cytokines appears in spontaneous abortion.[89] In response to the conceptus or other antigens, decidual lymphocytes secrete proinflammatory Th1-type cytokines such as IL-2, IFN-γ, TNF-α, which adversely affect the development of the embryo. Fetal rejection occurs through immune-induced inflammation (delayed-type hypersensitivity reactions which result in lymphocyte infiltration of the trophoblast), tissue degradation (cytotoxic reactions which result in damage of the trophoblast by NK cells and cytotoxic antibodies produced by specific subpopulations of B lymphocytes) and coagulation (upregulation of a novel prothrombinase fgl2, which results in vasculitis affecting the maternal blood supply to the implanted embryo).[34,81] In addition to the Th1-type response, disturbances of other mechanisms thought to be involved in the response to normal pregnancy, may contribute to abortion (e.g., disturbances in tryptophane catabolism[90] or reduced apoptosis.[91]

Unfortunately, the specific mechanism causing fetal rejection is as yet undefined, since no relevant single specific mechanism has been recognized as essential for a successful pregnancy. We speculate that the disruption of one or more of the mechanisms leading to tolerance in normal pregnancy may occur in stress situations and can lead to rejection. These disturbances may include (a) absence of immunosuppressive proimplantation factors in the genital tract; (b) absence of immuno-dependant specific suppression at the fetomaternal interface; and (c) inappropriate expression or defective recognition of trophoblastic and immunoregulatory molecules by decidual cells, including disturbances in the NK allorecognition system. Alone or in combination, the above disturbances seem to deregulate the sensitive balance of maternal tolerance to the embryo and lead to its "rejection" (Figure 27.1).

Preimplantation factors cause local immunosuppression in the genital tract and prepare the endometrium to accept the semiallogeneic embryo.

- In an environment of hormone-dependant maternally and fetally derived immunosuppression (including predominance of Treg cells over Th17 cells), specific decidual cells recognize specific molecules on the trophoblast.
- Activated, decidual cells secrete growth factors (GM-CSF, TGF-β, IL-3) that enhance placental growth (immunotrophism).
- Specific lymphocytes of the pregnant woman are also activated and secrete anti-inflammatory cytokines (IL-4, IL-10, IL-13), so that a Th2-type immune response is developed.
- Produced antibodies block cytotoxic reactions that would harm the embryo.

In miscarriage (Figure 27.2), tolerance enhancing preimplantation factors may be absent, trophoblastic antigens may be inappropriately expressed, and the recognition of trophoblastic antigens and/or immunoregulatory molecules may be defective. Treg cell function is inhibited, Th1 cells produce proinflammatory cytokines (IL-2, IFN-γ, and TNF-α), which generate a Th1-type response. In the absence of blocking factors, cytotoxic antibodies and cytotoxic cells (mainly NK cells) damage the trophoblast.

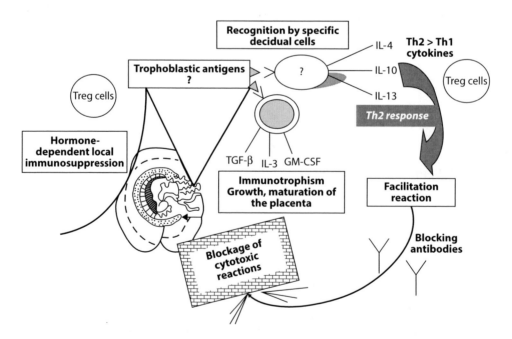

FIGURE 27.1   Immunologic mechanisms in normal pregnancy. IL: interleukin; Th: T-helper; TGF-β: transforming growth factor β; GM-CSF: granulocyte-macrophage colony-stimulating factor; Treg: regulatory T cell.

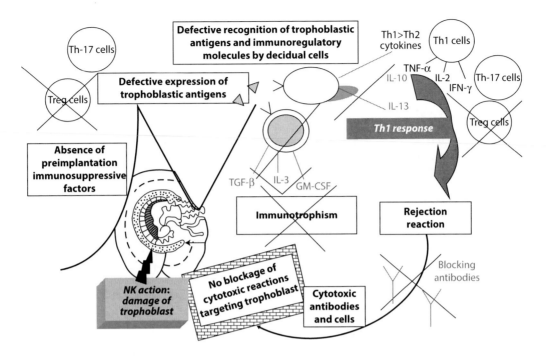

FIGURE 27.2 Immunologic mechanisms in abortion.

Factors Inducing a Th1 Response in Abortion

Although the immunopathology underlying Th1 preponderance in abortion is unknown, it is widely accepted that situations such as stress, infection, and autoimmunity, as well as genetic factors may cause Th1 cytokine-triggered abortions.

Stress may affect the endocrine system (corticotropin releasing hormone [CRH], adrenocorticotropin [ACTH], and progesterone), which triggers an immune bias towards an abortogenic Th1 cytokine profile.[92] Tometten et al.[93] have studied stress-triggered abortion in the murine CBA/J × DBA/2 J model and found that fetal loss is the result of a neurogenic inflammatory response and Th1 cytokine profile in decidua. They suggest that stress provokes tachykinin 1 (formerly known as substance P) release at the fetomaternal interface, which mediates the local and endothelial increase of nerve growth factor β (NGFB) which mediates a neurogenic inflammatory response. Subsequently, increased expression of NGFB in the uterus skews the immune system toward an inflammatory Th1 response via upregulation of adhesion molecules.

Th1 cytokine-triggered abortions may also be affected by bacterial endotoxins (LPS).[94] The Th1 response is induced by infectious agents when they are recognized by specific decidual T cells bearing $V\delta_2$ receptors, which when activated secrete abortogenic cytokines. Barakonyi et al.[95] have shown that peripheral blood $\gamma\delta^+$ T cells from women with RSA preferentially express the $V\gamma_9 V\delta_2$ TcR combination. $V\gamma_9 V\delta_2$ T cells are known to recognize non-peptide organophosphate and alkylamine antigens and eliminate bacteria and parasites. We have investigated the bias towards these cells in women with unexplained pregnancy losses and have found that the majority had undiagnosed genital tract or even systematic bacterial infections.[96]

The cytokine balance is determined by maternal genes, which regulate the response to stress, LPS and paternally inherited trophoblastic antigens.[34] Furthermore, cytokine gene polymorphisms (i.e., TNF, IFN-γ) have been associated with recurrent miscarriage in women with Th1 immunity to the trophoblast. However, several studies investigating the relationship between cytokines, angiogenic mediators, hormones, gene polymorphisms, and RSA have produced contradictory results.[97]

As mentioned above, one of the mechanisms by which aPL antibodies damage the embryo is the development of an inflammatory response involving TNF-α, the main factor for the induction of

Th1-type response. Furthermore, the presence of ATA combines with changes in the profile of endometrial T cells, which results in the hypersecretion of Th1 cytokines, such IFN-γ.

Treg Cell and Th17 cells in Women with RSA

Sasaki et al.[45] first reported that decidual CD4+CD25[bright] T-cells that can inhibit the proliferation of autologous CD4+ T-cells are significantly lower in specimens from spontaneous abortions compared to induced abortions. Many other studies have shown similar findings in women with RSA Treg cells do not show any significant fluctuation during the menstrual cycle, their number is as low as that observed in postmenopausal women, and their suppressive functions are lower than those of fertile controls, The proportion of Treg cells in the decidua and peripheral blood is significantly lower in unexplained recurrent spontaneous abortion than in control women.[98,99] The abnormal performance of Treg cells in mediating feto-maternal tolerance in cases of abortion has been associated with alteration in the IL-6 trans-signaling pathway, decrease of TGF-β and IL-2 as well down-regulation of IL-2-STAT-5 signaling.[100]

Increased Th17 cells and Th17 cyokines (e.g., IL-17, and IL-23) have been shown in unexplained RSA patients.[101,102] Nakashima et al.[103] found a correlation between the number of decidual IL-17+ cells and the number of neutrophils in women with miscarriage, and suggested that these cells may be involved in the induction of inflammation in the late stage of abortion. The excessive Th17 activity in RSA patients may reflect the suppressed function of Treg cells, but may also be stimulated by IL-6 produced during subclinical uterine infections and inflammation.[104] Immunotherapy may reverse the decreased number and function of Treg cells. Adoptive transfer of CD4+CD25+ regulatory T from normal pregnant females[47,65] or expanded in vitro[105] was shown to significantly reduce the fetal resorption rates in the CBA/JxDBA/2 murine abortion model. In women with RSA, lymphocyte immunotherapy (LIT) with paternal or third-party lymphocytes has been demonstrated to increase Treg cells.[106] Additionally, an *in vitro* study has shown that the suppressive activity of Treg cells from healthy individuals can increase when they are cocultured with intravenous immunoglobulin G (IVIg).[107]

Role of NK Cells in Abortion

Decidual NK cells appear to be the main cell population involved in alloimmune abortion. Under the influence of Th1-type cytokines, they are stimulated to become classical NK cells expressing CD16 (CD3-CD16+CD56+), which can damage the trophoblast either directly by releasing cytolytic substances or indirectly by producing inflammatory cytokines.[108] Clinical studies have demonstrated that women who tend to abort have increased numbers of NK cells of the conventional CD3-CD56+CD16+ type in the uterus[109] as well as increased blood NK-cell subsets and NK-cell activity, all of which have been associated with abortion of chromosomally normal embryos.[110]

A direct increase in numbers and/or activation of maternal NK cells may be either infection-related or related to the NK allorecognition system. Thomas et al.[111] have suggested that subclinical herpes virus viraemia may be an important cause of peripheral blood NK cell stimulation in women with fertility problems, and they associated antiviral treatment with a decrease of NK cell levels. Alternatively, rejection of the embryo may be the result of a defect in the NK allorecognition system. Our studies in RSA couples as well as in cases of sporadic abortion have suggested that aborting women have a limited repertoire of inhKIR receptors or an imbalance of KIR receptors in favor of activating KIRs.[112,113] Furthermore, many women with miscarriages lack the appropriate inhKIRs to interact with trophoblastic HLA-C molecules (lack of maternal inhKIR-fetal HLA-C epitope matching) or were found to possess inhKIRs that do not bind strongly their ligands (HLA-C), in order to sufficiently inhibit NK toxicity.[27,43] The contribution of the predominance of an activating state in the balance between inhibitory and activating KIR receptors as well as in the KIR/HLA-C interactions to pregnancy loss has also been found by other authors.[114–116] Vargas et al.[114] have reported that women carrying a high content of activating KIR genes have a threefold increased probability of developing recurrent miscarriage. Finally, a higher activating potential resulting from particular maternal KIR/fetal HLA-C combinations was shown in a study by Keramitsoglou et al.,[117] that was performed on the abortus and HLA-C ligands were directly genotyped on trophblast cells. All the above data suggest that in RSA women the triggering signals that the dNK cells may receive to attack the trophoblast may be not be inhibited.

Because of the critical role of NK in trophoblast damage, the diagnostic approach to alloimmune abortions is almost limited to the study of these cells. The diagnostic value of various tests that have been used (partner's HLA typing for the detection of increased HLA sharing between them, detection of lymphocytotoxic antibodies against paternal cells (antipaternal antibodies-APCA), mixed lymphocyte cultures for the detection of bocking antibodies, Th1/Th2 cytokine balance for detection of predominance of Th1 response) is of doubtful value. Therefore, the detection of NK cell disturbances (increase of CD3-CD16+CD56+ cells) in the peripheral blood of unexplained RSA women is often used as a marker of an underlying alloimmune mechanism for miscarriage. Furthermore, monitoring of NK cells is used for the estimation of the effect of immunotherapy.

Epilogue

The two categories of auto- and alloimmune-mediated pregnancy loss do not describe distinct immunological entities. Antiphospholipid antibodies may induce a Th1 shift through cytokines and complement activation. Cytotoxic cytokines or NK cells, which play a role in alloimmune abortions, may also mediate those with an autoimmune pathology. The disturbances in the two types of abortion are now suggested to associate with a misdirection of the immune response that is characterized by exaggerated inflammation and breakdown of tolerance to autoantigens or fetal alloantigens. The classification of the immunological disturbances as autoimmune or alloimmune helps explain a number of miscarriages that were previously considered as "unexplained," to identify candidates for immune testing, and to offer immunologic treatments. In autoimmune pregnancy loss, especially when associated with antiphospholipid antibodies, the immunopathology is better defined, the diagnosis is relatively simple and the therapy has been widely described to be beneficial. In alloimmune abortions, the pathophysiology is far less clear, the diagnostic value of tests uncertain, and the effectiveness of immunotherapy remains controversial.

REFERENCES

1. McIntyre JA, Coulam CB, Faulk WP. Recurrent Spontaneous Abortion. *Am J Reprod Immunol* 1989;21:100–4.
2. Coulam CB, Stephenson M, Stern JJ et al. Immunotherapy for recurrent pregnancy loss: Analysis of results from clinical trials. *Am J Reprod Immunol* 1996;35:352–9.
3. Stern JJ, Coulam CB. Current status of immunologic recurrent pregnancy loss. *Curr Opin Obstet Gynecol* 1993;5:252–9.
4. Gleicher N. Some thoughts on the reproductive autoimmune failure syndrome (RAFS) and Th-1 versus Th-2 immune responses. *Am J Reprod Immunol* 2002;48:252–4.
5. Matzner W, Chong P, Xu G et al. Characterization of antiphospholipid antibodies in women with Recurrent Spontaneous Abortions. *J Reprod Immunol* 1994;33:31–9.
6 Kuwana M, Matsuura E, Kobayashi K et al. Binding of beta 2-glycoprotein I to anionic phospholipids facilitates processing and presentation of a cryptic epitope that activates pathogenic autoreactive T cells. *Blood* 2005;105:1552–7.
7. Blank M, Krause I, Fridkin M et al. Bacterial induction of autoantibodies to beta2-glycoprotein-I accounts for the infectious etiology of antiphospholipid syndrome. *J Clin Invest* 2002;109:797–804.
8. Guglielmone H, Vitozzi S, Elbarcha O et al. Cofactor dependence and isotype distribution of anticardiolipin antibodies in viral infections. *Ann Rheum Dis* 2001;60:500–4.
9. Lockwood CJ, Rand JH. The immunobiology and obstetrical consequences of antiphospholipid antibodies. *Obstet Gynecol Surv* 1994;49:432–41.
10. Meroni PL, Borghi MO, Raschi E et al. Pathogenesis of antiphospholipid syndrome: Understanding the antibodies. *Nat Rev Rheumatol* 2011;7:330–9.

11. Girardi G, Mackman N. Tissue factor in antiphospholipid antibody-induced pregnancy loss: Thrombosis versus inflammation. In: Cervera R, Reverter JC, Khamashta M, eds. *Handbook of Systemic Autoimmune Diseases*. Volume 10. Oxford: Elsevier; 2009. p. 69–79.

12. Girardi G. Role of tissue factor in the maternal immunological attack of the embryo in the antiphospholipid syndrome. *Clin Rev Allergy Immunol* 2010;39:160–5.

13. Carp H. Cytokines in recurrent miscarriage. *Lupus* 2004;13:630–4.

14. Salmon J, Girargi G. Antiphospholipid antibodies and pregnancy loss: A disorder of inflammation. *J Reprod Immunol* 2008;77:51–6.

15. Cohen D, Buurma A, Goemaere NN et al. Classical complement activation as a footprint for murine and human antiphospholipid antibody-induced fetal loss. *J Pathol* 2011;225:502–11.

16. Lyden TW, Vogt E, Ng AK et al. Monoclonal antiphospholipid antibody reactivity against human placental trophoblast. *J Reprod Immunol* 1992;22:1–14.

17. Emoto K, Kobayashi T, Yamaji A et al. Redistribution of phosphatidylethanolamine at the cleavage furrow of dividing cells during cytokinesis. *Proc Natl Acad Sci USA* 1996;93:12867–72.

18. Adler RR, Ng AK, Rote NS. Monoclonal antiphosphatidylserine antibody inhibits intercellular fusion of the choriocarcinoma line JAR. *Biol Reprod* 1995;53:905–10.

19. Di Simone N De Carolis S, Lanzone A et al. *In vitro* effect of antiphospholipid antibody-containing sera on basal and gonadotrophin releasing hormone-dependent human chorionic gonadotrophin release by cultured trophoblast cells. *Placenta* 1995;16:75–83.

20. Di Simone N, Raschi E, Testoni C et al. Pathogenic role of anti-beta 2-glycoprotein I antibodies in antiphospholipid associated fetal loss: Characterisation of beta 2-glycoprotein I binding to trophoblast cells and functional effects of anti-beta 2-glycoprotein I antibodies in vitro. *Ann Rheum Dis* 2005;64:462–7.

21. Shurtz-Swirski R, Inbar O, Blank M et al. *In vitro* effect of anticardiolipin autoantibodies upon total and pulsatile placental hCG secretion during early pregnancy. *Am J Reprod Immunol* 1993;29:206e10.

22. Fishman P, Bakimer R, Blank M et al. The putative role of cytokines in the induction of primary antiphospholipid syndrome in mice. *Clin Exp Immunol* 1992;90:266–70.

23. Buttari B, Profumo E, Mattei V et al. Oxidized beta2-glycoprotein I induces human dendritic cell maturation and promotes a T helper type 1 response. *Blood* 2005;106:3880–7.

24. Visvanathan S, McNeil HP. Cellular immunity to beta 2-glycoprotein-1 in patients with the antiphospholipid syndrome. *J Immunol* 1999;162:6919–25.

25. Beer AE, Kwak JY, Ruiz JE. Immunophenotypic profiles of peripheral blood lymphocytes in women with recurrent pregnancy losses and in infertile women with multiple failed *in vitro* fertilization cycles. *Am J Reprod Immunol* 1996;35:376–82.

26. Beer AE, Kwak JYH, Gilman-Sacks A et al. New horizons in the evaluation and treatment of recurrent pregnancy loss. In: Hunt, JS, ed. *Immunobiology of Reproduction*. New York: Serono Symposia USA; 1994. p. 316–34.

27. Varla-Leftherioti M, Keramitsopoulou T, Parapanissiou E et al. HLA-DQA1*0505 sharing and killer immunoglobulin-like receptors in sub fertile couples: Report from the 15th International Histocompatibility Workshop. *Tissue Antigens* 2010;75:668–72.

28. Labarrere CA. Allogeneic recognition and rejection reactions in the placenta. *Am J Reprod Immunol* 1989;21:94–9.

29. Voisin GA. Immunological facilitation, a broadening of the concept of the enhancement phenomenon. *Prog Allergy* 1971;15:328–485.

30. Chaouat G, Voisin GA, Escalier D et al. Facilitation reaction (enhancing antibodies and suppressor cells) and rejection reaction (sensitized cells) from the mother to the paternal antigens of the conceptus. *Clin Exp Immunol* 1979;35:13–24.

31. Wegmann TG. Placental immunotrophism: Maternal T cells enhance placental growth and function. *Am J Reprod Immunol* 1987;15:67–9.

32. Wegmann TG, Lin H, Guilbert L et al. Bidirectional cytokine interactions in the maternal-fetal relationship: Is successful pregnancy a TH2 phenomenon? *Immunol Today* 1993;14:353–6.

33. Clark DA. Immunobiological characterization of the trophoblast-decidual interface in human pregnancy. In: Kurpisz, M, Fernandez, N, eds. *Immunology of Human Reproduction*. Oxford: BIOS Scientific Publishers Limited; 1995. p. 301–11.

34. Clark DA, Arck PC, Chaouat G. Why did your mother reject you? Immunogenetic determinants of the response to environmental selective pressure expressed at the uterine level. *Am J Reprod Immunol* 1999;41:5–22.

35. Boyson JE, Rybalov B, Koopman LA et al. CD1d and invariant NKT cells at the human maternal-fetal interface. *Proc Natl Acad Sci* 2002;99:13741–6.

36. Kojima K, Kanzaki H, Iwai M et al. Expression of leukaemia inhibitory factor (LIF) receptor in human placenta: A possible role for LIF in the growth and differentiation of trophoblasts. *Hum Reprod* 1995;10:1907–11.

37. Szekeres-Bartho J, Barakonyi A, Polgar B et al. The role of γ/δ T cells in progesterone-mediated immunomodulation during pregnancy. A Review. *Am J Reprod Immunol* 1999;42:44–8.

38. Koga K, Aldo PB, Mor G. Toll-like receptors and pregnancy: Trophoblast as modulators of the immune response. *J Obstet Gynecol Res* 2009;35:191–202.

39. Ashkar AA, Di Santo JP, Croy BA. Interferon gamma contributes to initiation of uterine vascular modification, decidual integrity, and uterine natural killer cell maturation during normal murine pregnancy. *J Exp Med* 2000;192:259–70.

40. Saito S, Nakashima A, Shima T et al. Th1/Th2/Th17 and regulatory T-cell paradigm in pregnancy. *Am J Reprod Immunol* 2010;63:601–10.

41. Bluestone JA, Abbas AK. Natural versus adaptive regulatory T cells. *Nat Rev Immunol* 2003;3:253–7.

42. Sakaguchi S. Naturally arising CD4+ regulatory T cells for immunologic self-tolerance and negative control of immune responses. *Annu Rev Immunol* 2004;22:531–62.

43. Jonuleit H, Schmitt E, Kakirman H et al. Infectious tolerance: Human CD25(+) regulatory T cells convey suppressor activity to cobnventional CD4(+) T helper cells. *J Exp Med* 2002;196:255–60.

44. Aluvihare VR, Kallikourdis M, Betz AG. Regulatory T cells mediate maternal tolerance to the fetus. *Nat Immunol* 2004;5:288–71.

45. Sasaki Y, Sakai M, Miyazaki S et al. Decidual and peripheral blood CD4+CD25+ regulatory T cells in early pregnancy subjects and spontaneous abortion cases. *Mol Hum Reprod* 2004;10:347–53.

46. Somerset DA, Zheng Y, Kilby MD et al. Normal human pregnancy is associated with an elevation in the immune suppressive CD25+ CD4+ regulatory T-cell subset. *Immunology* 2004;112:38–43.

47. Zenclussen AC, Gerlof K, Zenclussen ML et al. Abnormal T-cell reactivity against paternal antigens in spontaneous abortion: Adoptive transfer of pregnancy-induced CD4+CD25+ T regulatory cells prevents fetal rejection in a murine abortion model. *Am J Pathol* 2005;166:811–22.

48. Arruvito L, Sanz M, Banham AH et al. Expansion of CD4+CD25+ and FOXP3+ regulatory T cells during the follicular phase of the menstrual cycle: Implications for human reproduction. *J Immunol* 2007;178:2572–8.

49. Tilburg T, Roelen DL, van der Mast BJ et al. Evidence for a selective migration of fetus-specific CD4+CD25[bright] regulatory T cells from the peripheral blood to the decidua in human pregnancy. *J Immunol* 2008;180:5737–45.

50. Robertson SA, Guerin LR, Bromfield JJ et al. Seminal fluid drives expansion of the CD4[+]CD25[+] T regulatory cell pool and induces tolerance to paternal alloantigens in mice. *Biol Reprod* 2009;80:1036–45.

51. Zhao J, Zeng Y, Liu YF et al. Alloantigen is responsible for the expansion of the CD4[+]CD25[+] regulatory T cell pool during pregnancy. *J Reprod Immunol.* 2007;75:71–81.

52. Kallikourdis M, Andersen KG, Welch KA et al. Alloantigen-enhanced accumulation of CCR5+ effector regulatory T cells in the gravid uterus. *Proc Natl Acad Sci USA* 2007;104:594–9.

53. Guerin LR, Moldenhauer LM, Prins JR et al. Seminal fluid regulates accumulation of FOXP3+ regulatory T cells in the preimplantation mouse uterus through expanding the FOXP3+ cell pool and CCL19-mediated recruitment. *Biol Reprod* 2011;85:397–408.

54. Schumacher A, Heinze K, Witte J et al. Human chorionic gonadotropin as a central regulator of pregnancy immune tolerance. *J Immunol* 2013;190:2650–8.

55. Schumacher A, Wafula PO, Bertoja AZ et al. Mechanisms of action of regulatory T cells specific for paternal antigens during pregnancy. *Obstet Gynecol* 2007;110:1137–45.

56. Rochman Y, Spolski R, Leonard WJ. New insights into the regulation of T cells by gamma(c) family cytokines. *Nat Rev Immunol* 2009;9:480–90.

57. Garin MI, Chu CC, Golshhayan D et al. Galectin-1: A key effector of regulation mediated by CD4+CD25+ T cells. *Blood* 2007;109:2058–65.

58. Huang CT, Workman CJ, Flies D et al. Role of LAG-3 in regulatory T cells. *Immunity* 2004;21:503–13.

59. Habicht A, Dada S, Jurewicz M et al. A link between PDL1 and T regulatory cells in fetomaternal tolerance. *J Immunol.* 2007;179:5211–9.

60. Oderup C, Cederbom L, Makowska A et al. Cytotoxic T lymphocyte antigen-4-dependent down-modulation of costimulatory molecules on dendritic cells in CD4 + CD25+ regulatory T-cell-mediated suppression. *Immunology* 2006;118, 240–9.

61. Kornete M, Piccirillo CA. Functional crosstalk between dendritic cells and Foxp3+ regulatory T cells in the maintenance of immune tolerance. *Front Immunol* 2012;3:165.

62. Mellor AL, Baban B, Chandler P et al. Cutting edge: Induced indoleamine 2,3 dioxygenase expression in dendritic cell subsets suppresses T cell clonal expansion. *J Immunol* 2003;171:1652–5.

63. Lee SK, Kim JY, Lee M et al. Th17 and regulatory T cells in women with recurrent pregnancy loss. *Am J Reprod Immunol* 2012;67:311–8.

64. Harrington LE, Mangan PR, Weaver CT. Expanding the effector CD4 T-cell repertoire: The Th17 lineage. *Curr Opin Immunology* 2006;18:349–56.

65. Weaver CT, Harrington LE, Mangan PR et al. Th17: An effector CD4 T cell lineage with regulatory T cell ties. *Eur J Onstet Gynecol Reprod Biol* 2012;161:177–81.

66. Romagnani S, Maggi E, Liotta F et al. Properties and origin of human Th17 cells. *Mol Immunology* 2009;7:3–7.

67. Bettelli E, Carrier Y, Gao W et al. Reciprocal developmental pathways for the generation of pathogenic effector TH17 and regulatory T cells. *Nature* 2006;441:235–8.

68. Yang XO, Nurieva R, Martinez GJ et al. Molecular antagonism and plasticity or regulatory and inflammatory T cell programs. *Immunity* 2008;29:44–56.

69. Baban B, Chandler PR, Sharma MD et al. IDO activates regulatory T cells and blocks their conversion into Th17-like T cells. *J Immunol* 2009;183:2475–83.

70. Nakashima A, Ito M, Yoneda S et al. Circulating and decidual TH17 cell levels in healthy pregnancy. *Am J Reprod Immunol* 2010;63:104–9.

71. Mellor AL, Munn DH. Immunology at the maternal-fetal interface: Lessons for T cell tolerance and suppression. *Annu Ren Immunol* 2000;18:367–91.

72. Robertson SA. Seminal plasma and male factor signalling in the female reproductive tract. *Cell Tissue Res* 2005;322:43–52.

73. Munn DH, Zhou M, Attwood JT et al. Prevention of allogeneic fetal rejection by tryptophan catabolism. *Science* 1998;281:1191–3.

74. Jerzak M, Bischof P. Apoptosis in the first trimester human placenta: The role in maintaining immune privilege at the maternal-fetal interface and in the trophoblast remodeling. *Eur J Obstet Gynecol* 2002;100:138–42.

75. Le Bouteiller P. HLA-G and local placental immunity. *Gynecol Obstet Fertil* 2003;31:782–5.

76. Laskarin G, Kammerer U, Rukavina D et al. Antigen-presenting cells and materno-fetal tolerance: An emerging role for dendritic cells. *Am J Reprod Immonol* 2007;58:255–67.

77. O'Connor GM, Hart Om, Gardiner CM. Putting the natural killer cell in its place. *Immunology* 2008;77:14–22.

78. Hornung V, Rothenfusser S, Britsch S et al. Quantitative expression of Toll-like receptor 1–10mRNA in cellular subset of human peripheral blood mononuclear cells and sensivity to CpG oligodeoxynucleotides. *J Immunol* 2002;168:4531–7.

79. Beaman KD, Ntrivalas E, Mallers TM et al. Immune etiology of recurrent pregnancy loss and its diagnosis. *Am J Reprod Immunol* 2012;67:319–25.

80. Nakashima A, Shima T, Inada K et al. The balance of the immune system between T cells and NK cells in miscarriages. *Am J Reprod Immunol* 2012;67:304–10.

81. Clark D, Arck PC, Jallili R et al. Psycho-Neuro-Cytokine/Endocrine pathways in immunoregulation during pregnancy. *Am J Reprod Immunol* 1996;35:330–7.

82. Chaouat G, Tranchot Diallo J, Volumenie JL et al. Immune suppression and Th1/Th2 balance in pregnancy revisited: A (very) personal tribute to Tom Wegmann. *Am J Reprod Immunol* 1997;37:427–34.

83. Varla-Leftherioti M. The significance of women's NK cell receptors' repertoire in the maintenance of pregnancy. *Chem Immunol Allergy* 2005;89:84–95.

84. Menier C, Riteau B, Dausset J et al. HLA-G truncated isoforms can substitute for HLA-G1 in fetal survival. *Hum Immunol* 2000;61:1118–25.

85. Varla-Leftherioti M. Role of a KIR/HLA-C allorecognition system in pregnancy. *J Reprod Immunol* 2004;62:19–27.

86. Tang AW, Alfirevic Z, Turner MA et al. A feasibility trial of screening women with idiopathic recurrent miscarriage for high uterine natural killer cell density and randomizing to prednisolone or placebo when pregnant. *Hum Reprod* 2013;28:1743–52.

87. Clark DA, Coulam CB. Is there an immunological cause of repeated pregnancy wastage? *Adv Obstet Gynecol* 1995;3:321–42.

88. Coulam CB, Stephenson M, Stern JJ et al. Immunotherapy for recurrent pregnancy loss: Analysis of results from clinical trials. *Am J Reprod Immunol* 1996;35:352–9.

89. Raghupathy R. TH1-Type immunity is incompatible with successful pregnancy. *Immunol Today* 1997;18:478–82.

90. Ban Y, Chang Y, Dong B et al. Indoleamine 2,3-dioxygenase levels at the normal and recurrent spontaneous abortion fetal-maternal interface. *J Int Med Res* 2013;41:1135–49.

91. Kokawa K, Shikone T, Nakano R. Apoptosis in human chorionic villi and eciduas during normal embryonic development and spontaneous abortion in the first trimester. *Placenta* 1998;19:21–2.

92. Arck PC. Stress and pregnancy loss: Role of immune mediators, hormones and neurotransmitters. *Am J Reprod Immunol* 2001;46:117–23.

93. Tometten M, Blois S, Kuhlmei A et al. Nerve growth factor translates stress response and subsequent murine abortion via adhesion molecule-dependent pathways. *Biol Reprod* 2006;74:674–83.

94. Clark DA, Chaouat G, Gorczynski RM. Thinking outside the box: Mechanisms of environmental selective pressures on the outcome of the materno-fetal relationship. *Am J Reprod Immunol* 2002;47:275–82.

95. Barakonyi A, Polgar B, Szekeres-Bartho J. The role of gamma/delta T-cell receptor-positive cells in pregnancy: Part II. *Am J Reprod Immunol* 1999;42:83–7.

96. Bouloukos K, Tsekoura C, Chioti A et al. Association of increased peripheral Vgamma9/delta2 TCR lymphocytes with genital track infections in women with recurrent abortions. *Am J Reprod Immunol* 2007;58:203(abstract).

97. Daher S, Mattar R, Gueuvoghlanian-Silva BY et al. Genetic polymorphisms and recurrent spontaneous abortions: An overview of current knowledge. *Am J Reprod Immunol* 2012;67:341–7.

98. Yang H, Qiu L, Chen G et al. Proportional change of CD4+CD25+ regulatory T cells in decidua and peripheral blood in unexplained recurrent spontaneous abortion patients. *Fertil Steril* 2008;89:656–61.

99. Jin LP, Chen QY, Zhang T et al. The CD4+CD25 bright regulatory T cells and CTLA-4 expression in peripheral and decidual lymphocytes are down-regulated in human miscarriage. *Clin Immunol* 2009;133:402–10.

100. Arruvito L, Sotelo AL, Billordo A et al. A physiological role for inducible FOXP3(+) Treg cells. Lessons from women with reproductive failure. *Clin Immunol* 2010;136:432–41.

101. Wang WJ, Hao CH, Yi-Lin GJ et al. Increased prevalence of T helper 17 (Th17) cells in peripheral blood and decidua in unexplained recurrent spontaneous abortion patients. *J Reprod Immunol* 2010;84:164–70.

102. Liu YS, Wu L, Tong XH et al. Study on the relationship between Th17 cells and unexplained recurrent spontaneous abortion. *Am J Reprod Immunol* 2011;65:503–11.

103. Nakashima A, Ito M, Shima T et al. Accumulation of IL-17-positive cells in decidua of inevitable abortion cases. *Am J Reprod Immunol* 2010;64:4–11.

104. Basal AS. Joining the immunological dots in recurrent miscarriage. *Am J Reprod Immunology* 2010;64:307–15.

105. Yin Y, Han X, Shi Q et al. Adoptive transfer of CD4+CD25+ regulatory T cells for prevention and treatment of spontaneous abortion. *Eur J Obstet Gynecol Reprod Biol* 2012;161:177–81.

106. Yang H, Qiu L, Di W, Zhao A et al. Proportional change of CD4 + CD25+ regulatory T cells after lymphocyte therapy in unexplained recurrent spontaneous abortion patients. *Fertil Steril* 2009;92:301–5.

107. Kessel A, Ammuri H, Peri R et al. Intravenous immunoglobulin therapy affects T regulatory cells by increasing their suppressive function. *J Immunol* 2007;179:5571–5.

108. King A, Wheeler R, Carter NP et al. The response of human decidual leukocytes to IL-2. *Cell Immunol* 1992;141:409–42.

109. Kwak JY, Beer AE, Kim SH et al. Immunopathology of the implantation site utilizing monoclonal antibodies to natural killer cells in women with recurrent pregnancy losses. *Am J Reprod Immunol* 1999;41:91–8.

110. Aoki K, Kajiura S, Matsumoto Y et al. Preconceptual natural killer cell activity as a predictor of miscarriage. *Lancet* 1995;345:1340–2.

111. Thomas D, Michou V, Tegos V et al. The effect of valacyclovir treatment on natural killer cells of infertile women. *Am J Reprod Immunol* 2004;51:248–55.

112. Varla-Leftherioti M, Spyropoulou-Vlachou M, Niokou D et al. Natural killer (NK) cell receptors' repertoire in couples with recurrent spontaneous abortions. *Am J Reprod Immunol* 2003;49:183–91.

113. Varla-Leftherioti M, Spyropoulou-Vlachou M, Keramitsoglou T et al. Lack of the appropriate natural killer cell inhibitory receptors in women with spontaneous abortion. *Hum Immunol* 2005;66:65–71.

114. Vargas RG, Bompeixe EP, Franca PP et al. Activating killer cell immunoglobulin-like receptor genes' association with recurrent miscarriage. *Am J Reprod Immunol* 2009;62:34–43.

115. Faridi RM, Das V, Tripthi G et al. Influence of activating and inhibitory killer immunoglobulin-like receptors on predisposition to recurrent miscarriages. *Hum Reprod* 2009;24:1758–64.

116. Faridi RM, Agrawal S. Killer immunoglobulin-like receptors (KIRs) and HLA-C allorecognition patterns implicative of dominant activation of natural killer cells contribute to recurrent miscarriages. *Human Reprod* 2011;26:491–7.

117. Keramitsoglou T, Dempegioti F, Dinou A et al. Maternal KIR repertoire and KIR/HLA-C recognition model in early pregnancy and implantation failure. *Adv Neuroim Biol* 2011;2:99–103.

28

Debate: Should Immunotherapy Be Used?
Lymphocyte Immunization Therapy—Yes

Edward E. Winger and Jane L. Reed

In a field not without controversy, lymphocyte immunization therapy (LIT) has arguably generated the most intense debate. LIT is an immunologic treatment for miscarriage involving the immunization of the prospective mother with paternal mononuclear cells. In January of 2002, the U.S. Food and Drug Administration (FDA) posted a letter limiting LIT to the terms of an investigational new drug application, an "IND." Two reasons were given for the restriction: first, the FDA claimed LIT involved unsafe administration of a human blood product. Second, a randomized controlled trial published in the *Lancet* concluded that LIT does not work.[1] Citing these two concerns, the FDA restricted use of the therapy in the United States.[2] Despite the U.S. restriction, many practitioners continue to utilize the therapy elsewhere in the world, claiming (a) LIT is effective; (b) LIT can be administered within legal blood transfusion guidelines; and (c) the study reported in the *Lancet*, the "Ober study," was fatally compromised by poor design and execution. We will show that the study results were rendered uninterpretable by a number of methodological problems. Supporters claim that, when used in accordance with procedures advocated by Beer on appropriately selected patients,[3] LIT is both safe and effective. We will argue for the need for larger prospective trials to overcome flaws of the study if we are to fairly judge LIT's efficacy.

Perhaps the earliest description of lymphocyte immunization was made by Billingham et al.[4] They observed that skin grafts between fraternal twins were accepted while grafts between non-twin siblings were not. This led them to hypothesize that blood cells exchanged through the twins' placentas persisted and maintained a state of immunologic tolerance. Studies from the 1970s reported that pretransplant transfusion decreased the immunologic rejection of the transplanted organ.[5–9] Observations that parental MHC antigen sharing might be associated with adverse pregnancy outcomes suggested that inadequate maternal recognition of paternal alloantigens could cause deficient tolerogenesis.[10–12] Influenced by these observations, Beer reasoned that immunization with paternal mononuclear cells might enhance maternal recognition of paternal alloantigen allowing patients suffering from recurrent spontaneous abortion to carry a pregnancy to term.[13] Mowbray et al. conducted the first randomized controlled trial of LIT in unexplained recurrent spontaneous abortion (RSA) patients and reported a striking increase in the success rate in those who rapidly achieved pregnancy after treatment.[14] Subsequently Mowbray reported that protection waned after 80 days in women who failed to make anti-paternal HLA antibodies, but persisted in those who had made such antibodies. He found that, in antibody-negative patients, protection could be restored by reimmunization within 40 days prior to conception.[15] A prospective, collaborative observational study and meta-analysis confirmed efficacy in women with primary RSA lacking anti-paternal antibodies. Inefficacy was reported in women with preexisting paternal antibodies, prior live birth with their partner, and reduced live birth rate in women testing positive for anti-cardiolipin or anti-nuclear antibodies.[16] A subsequent meta-analysis[17] on the same cohort of patients showed a 16% absolute benefit in the live birth rate in primary aborters lacking anti-paternal antibodies at initial testing. There was a significantly decreased live birth rate in women with a history of three or more spontaneous abortions. A third meta-analysis[18] was performed on women with five or more miscarriages. This criterion was chosen as the prognosis is poorer after five miscarriages, and the possibility of confounding the results due to genetic factors is reduced. In this study, there was a significantly increased chance of a live birth following LIT. Three primary aborters required treatment in order to achieve an extra live birth. Immunization had no effect on the secondary aborters.

Several allospecific mechanisms have been proposed to explain the protective effects of LIT. A number of studies have suggested that diminished allo-immune recognition prevents development of a protective anti-paternal antibody response. Properties of the antibody response have been quantified in several assays: those measuring cytotoxic antibodies, asymmetric antibodies and mixed lymphocyte reaction blocking antibodies.[19–21] In aggregate, these antibodies have been described as "blocking" antibodies because of the effect attributed to them. LIT appears to enhance the development of "blocking" antibodies in pregnancy by intentional exposure of the mother's immune system to living cells expressing paternal antigen.[22] Malan et al. showed that pregnant women express much higher levels of asymmetric antibodies than nonpregnant women.[23] Asymmetric antibodies were described by Margni in the 1970s.[24] These antibodies exhibit posttranslational high mannose glycosylation of one of the two Fab regions which sterically hinders binding by the modified Fab. The functionally univalent antibody is unable to form complexes, thereby, inhibiting complement activation, efficient Fc-binding, and phagocytosis. However, because the unmodified Fab fragment retains its full antigen-binding capacity, it competes efficiently with unmodified, symmetric antibody. Margni demonstrated enhanced production of asymmetric antibody when antigen was presented as particulate or cellular antigen.[25] Barrientos and others demonstrated that women suffering pregnancy loss had significantly lower levels of asymmetric antibody than their healthy counterparts.[26] Zenclussen et al. demonstrated that asymmetric antibody levels increased following lymphocyte immunotherapy.[27]

Skin functions as an immunologic barrier comprising a network rich in immunologic sensor cells. These sensor cells interact with both environmental and self-antigen subsequently presenting antigen to the immune system for response. These cells consist of a diverse group of cells together known as "dendritic cells" due to their dendrite-like processes. These dendrite-like processes extend through the local environment enhancing antigen-capturing capacity. Upon antigen capture, dendritic cells mature and undergo morphologic transformation into migratory cells that find their way to regional lymph nodes. Depending on the nature of antigen and local factors encountered during antigen contact, the matured dendritic cell delivers an immunogenic or tolerogenic signal upon subsequent interactions in the lymph node.[28–30]

The injection of sufficient numbers of paternal lymphocytes into the dermis is essential to ensure adequate physical interaction with dendritic cells. Interactions with macrophages and mast cells may also generate nonspecific suppressive responses. Nonspecific suppressive responses include reduction in the ratio of Th1 to Th2 cells, increase in T regulatory cells, suppression of *in vitro* natural killer cell cytotoxicity as well as reduction in the number of CD3$^-$/CD56$^+$ cells.[31–39] As occasionally practiced, mononuclear cells are delivered by intramuscular and intravenous routes. These routes do not result in an interaction with a barrier type immune structure replete with dendritic cells as found in the skin. Though permitted in the Ober trial, it is doubtful that such routes are capable of generating tolerogenic interactions with dendritic cells.

Mononuclear cells should be maintained for no more than a few hours at room temperature. Clark and Chaouat have shown that cold (4°C) exposure results in a loss of CD200 expression and tolerogenesis.[40,41] In addition, apoptotic material is rapidly cleared *in vivo*, resulting in a profound anti-inflammatory effect on the phagocytosing cell. Cold storage instead promotes a continuous process of transformation that has been dubbed "aponecrosis." Aponecrotic cellular material is pro-inflammatory when infused.[42] While simple in principle, apoptosis requires functional cellular machinery. Aged, and in particular, cold-shocked cells have diminished apoptotic capacity. These cells may preferentially undergo necrosis or follow various pathways leading to aponecrosis or necroptosis that is pro-inflammatory and potentially counterproductive for purposes of the therapy. Pandey, in contrast to Ober, reported a high rate of successful live births in an intention-to-treat analysis of LIT where the cells were maintained at 37°C before use.[20,39]

While the mechanics of LIT are relatively simple, its consistent and successful practice calls for an understanding of the immune response in healthy pregnancy as well as the response of the skin barrier immune system upon exposure to injected antigen. The arrival of the embryo at a receptive endometrial surface, in natural, healthy pregnancy, is preceded by a period of tolerogenic immunologic response to paternal antigen.[43,44] As with all adaptive immune responses, their development requires time. In the case of LIT, optimal response may require several weeks.[3] LIT performed just prior to conception, may not provide sufficient time for the development of the maximum protective response.[45] The Ober study permitted LIT just two weeks prior to conception. Pandy and Beer recommended 4 weeks.[3,20] Further, the Ober study did not measure antibody development confirming response. The preferred LIT protocol utilizes intradermal inoculation, similar to Pandey and Beer.[3,46,47] Inoculations should be repeated until a sufficient immunological response has developed before conception. An adequate immunological response usually takes several weeks to develop and should be monitored. Ober permitted alternative methods of paternal cell delivery including intramuscular and intravenous routes that do not result in encounter with a high density of dendritic cells.[1] The Ober study failed to adhere to a common LIT protocol, including lack of monitoring for immunologic response.

Immunologic response to LIT is most commonly quantified in a flow cytometric assay using paternal antigen-expressing lymphocytes as solid phase. However, in primary recurrent spontaneous abortion (RSA), any woman who has not carried a pregnancy to term with the prospective father, would not be expected to express antibodies to his lymphocyte-expressed antigens. However, in those patients treated with LIT, a rapid rise in antibody level would be anticipated. Mowbray found that, in the absence of such a response, an additional boost of LIT was beneficial if the patients failed to become pregnant within 90 days.[15]

The decision to perform LIT, however, should not only rely upon initial quantification. Clinical history should be taken into account as well. Patients with chromosomal, structural, endocrine, and certain autoimmune causes of miscarriage would not be expected to benefit from LIT.[48] In addition, various investigators have shown that patients with primary RSA may benefit more from LIT than patients with secondary RSA.[18,49,50] However, much of the literature combines both groups.[51-53] The development of more effective testing, possibly including asymmetric antibody testing, as well as taking into account other clinical and immunologic abnormalities, would likely improve the accuracy of our patient selection process.[23,54,55]

Because LIT involves the administration of live allogeneic mononuclear cells, its use has also raised certain safety issues in the past. One of these was the potential for transmission of infectious agents. However, LIT correctly performed, requires both the donor and recipient to be tested for a panel of serologic tests for infectious agents. It should be noted, in almost all cases, the donor and recipient are a married couple, so would have already been exposed to transmissible agents. In 2006, Kling led two large European trials each involving over 4000 patients over a 3-year time span using LIT techniques similar to those used in this study, and no anaphylaxis, autoimmune or graft versus host disease were detected.[56,57]

In summary, the literature is plagued by studies providing contradictory results where widely varying protocols self-described as "LIT" have been used. Agreement upon a common protocol that recognizes well-understood principles is a step that must precede a study designed to judge its efficacy. LIT, when used correctly on a well-selected patient population, still holds much potential as a safe and effective treatment approach for reproductive patients who have failed with less aggressive protocols. Controversies have arisen due to studies that practice poor patient selection and incorrect LIT procedure. Prohibition in the United States has resulted in a flow of patients to countries where LIT continues to be practiced. In the future, large prospective trials should be designed that select appropriate patient groups for treatment. These trials should use correct LIT procedures and monitor treatment progress with appropriate immunological testing and patient selection. This is essential if we are to fairly judge efficacy.

REFERENCES

1. Ober C, Karrison T, Odem RR et al. Mononuclear-cell immunisation in prevention of recurrent miscarriages: A randomised trial. *Lancet* 1999;354:365–9.
2. U.S. Food and Drug Administration. Lymphocyte immune therapy (LIT) letter. Published online at www.fda.gov/BiologicsBloodVaccines/SafetyAvailability/ucm105848.htm (accessed September 16, 2013).
3. Kwak JY, Gilman-Sachs A, Moretti M et al. Natural killer cell cytotoxicity and paternal lymphocyte immunization in women with recurrentspontaneous abortions. *Am J Reprod Immunol* 1998;40:352–8.

4. Billingham RE, Brent L, Medawar PB. 'Actively acquired tolerance' of foreign cells. 1953. *J Immunol* 2010;184:5–8.

5. Halasz NA, Orloff MJ, Hirose F. Increased survival of renal homografts in dogs after injection of graft donor blood. *Transplantation* 1964;2:453–8.

6. Jenkins AM, Woodruff MA. The effect of prior administration of donor strain blood or blood constituents on the survival of cardiac allografts in rats. *Transplantation* 1972;12:57–60.

7. Febre JW, Morris PJ. The effect of donor strain blood pretreatment on renal allograft rejection in rats. *Transplantation* 1972;14:608–17.

8. Opelz G, Sengar DPS, Mickey MR et al. Effect of blood transfusion on subsequent kidney transplants. *Transplat Proc* 1973;V:253–9.

9. Tiwari, JL. Review: Kidney transplantation and transfusion. In: Terasaki PI, ed. *Clinical Kidney Transplants*. Los Angeles: UCLA Tissue Typing Laboratory; 1985. p. 257–71.

10. Beer AE. Immunology of reproduction. In: Samter M, Talmage DW, Frank MM et al., eds. *Immunological Diseases*. Boston: Little, Brown & Co.; 1988: p. 329–60.

11. Faulk WP, Coulam CB, McIntyre JA. Recurrent pregnancy loss. In: Machelle M, ed. *Infertility: A comprehensive text*. Norwalk: Appleton & Lange; 1990: p. 273–84.

12. Ober, CL, Hauck WW, Kostyu DD et al. Adverse effects of human leukocyte antigen-DR sharing on fertility: A cohort study in a human isolate. *Fertil Steril* 1985;44:227–32.

13. Beer AE, Semprini AE, Zhu XY et al. Pregnancy outcome in human couples with recurrent spontaneous abortions: HLA antigen profiles; HLA antigen sharing; female serum MLR blocking factors; and paternal leukocyte immunization. *Exp Clin Immunogenet* 1985;2:137–53.

14. Mowbray JF, Gibbings C, Liddell H et al. Controlled trial of treatment of recurrent spontaneous abortion by immunisation with paternal cells. *Lancet* 1985;1(8435):941–3.

15. Mowbray JF. Immunology of early pregnancy. *Hum Reprod* 1988;3:79–82.

16. Recurrent Miscarriage Immunotherapy Trialists Group. Worldwide collaborative observational study and meta-analysis on allogenic leukocyte immunotherapy for recurrent spontaneous abortion. *Am J Reprod Immunol* 1994;32:55–72.

17. Daya S, Gunby J. The effectiveness of allogeneic leucocyte immunization in unexplained primary recurrent spontaneous abortion. *Am J Reprod Immunol* 1994;32:294–302.

18. Carp HJA, Toder V, Torchinsky A et al. Allogeneic leucocyte immunization in women with five or more recurrent abortions. *Hum. Reprod* 1997;12: 250–5.

19. Pandey MK, Thakur S, Agrawal S. Lymphocyte immunotherapy and its probable mechanism in the maintenance of pregnancy in women with recurrent spontaneous abortion. *Arch Gynecol Obstet* 2004;269:161–72.

20. Ito K, Tanaka T, Tsutsumi N et al. Possible mechanisms of immunotherapy for maintaining pregnancy in recurrent spontaneous aborters: Analysis of anti-idiotypic antibodies directed against autologous T-cell receptors. *Hum Reprod* 1999;14:650–5.

21. Kishore R, Agarwal S, Halder A et al. HLA sharing, anti-paternal cytotoxic antibodies and MLR blocking factors in women with recurrent spontaneous abortion. *J Obstet Gynaecol Res* 1996;22:177–83.

22. Pandey MK, Agrawal S. Induction of MLR-Bf and protection of fetal loss: A current double blind randomized trial of paternal lymphocyte immunization for women with recurrent spontaneous abortion. *Int Immunopharmacol* 2004;4:289–98.

23. Gentile T, Malan Borel Y, Angelucci J et al. Preferential synthesis of asymmetric antibodies rats immunized with paternal particulate antigens. Effect on pregnancy. *J Reprod Immunol* 1992;2:173–83.

24. Margni RA, Paz CB, Cordal ME. Immunochemical behavior of sheep non-precipitating antibodies isolated by immunoadsorption. *Immunochemistry* 1976;13:209–14.

25. Margni RA, Perdigon G, Gentile T et al. IgG precipitating and non-precipitating antibodies in rabbits repeatedly injected with soluble and particulate antigens. *Vet Immunol Immunopathol* 1986;13: 51–61.

26. Barrientos G, Fuchs D, Schröcksnadel K et al. Low levels of serum asymmetric antibodies as a marker of threatened pregnancy. *J Reprod Immunol* 2009;79:201–10.

27. Zenclussen AC, Gentile T, Kortebani G et al. Asymmetric antibodies and pregnancy. *Am J Reprod Immunol* 2001;45:289–94.

28. Steinman RM, Nussenzweig MC. Avoiding horror autotoxicus: The importance of dendritic cells in peripheral T cell tolerance. *Proc Natl Acad Sci USA* 2002;99:351–8.

29. Inaba K, Inaba M, Romani N et al. Generation of large numbers of dendritic cells from mouse bone marrow cultures supplemented with granulocyte/macrophage colony-stimulating factor. *J Exp Med* 1992;176:1693–702.

30. Lenz A, Heine M, Schuler G et al. Human and murine dermis contain dendritic cells. Isolation by means of a novel method and phenotypical and functional characterization. *J Clin Invest* 1993;92:2587–96.

31. Yokoo T, Takakuwa K, Ooki I et al. Alteration of TH1 and TH2 cells by intracellular cytokine detection in patients with unexplained recurrent abortion before and after immunotherapy with the husband's mononuclear cells. *Fertil Steril* 2006;85:1452–8.

32. Szpakowski A, Malinowski A, Głowacka E et al. [The influence of paternal lymphocyte immunization on the balance of Th1/Th2 type reactivity in women with unexplained recurrent spontaneous abortion] *Ginekol Pol* 2000;71:586–92. [In Polish].

33. Hayakawa S, Karasaka-Suzuki, Ishii M et al. Effects of paternal lymphocyte immunization on peripheral Th1/Th2 balance and TCR Vβ and VΓ repertoire usage of patients with recurrent spontaneous sbortions. *Am J Repro Immunol* 2000;43:107–15.

34. Gafter U, Sredni B, Segal J et al. Suppressed cell-mediated immunity and monocyte and natural killer cell activity following allogeneic immunization of women with spontaneous recurrent abortion. *J Clin Immunol* 1997;17:408–19.

35. Gilman-Sachs A, Luo SP, Beer AE et al. Analysis of anti-lymphocyteantibodies by flow cytometry or microlymphocytotoxicity in women with recurrent spontaneous abortions immunized with paternal leukocytes. *J Clin Lab Immunol* 1989;30:53–9.

36. Liang P, Mo M, Li GG et al. Comprehensive analysis of peripheral blood lymphocytes in 76 women with recurrent miscarriage before and after lymphocyte immunotherapy. *Am J Reprod Immunol* 2012;68:164–74.

37. Kheshtchin N, Gharagozloo M, Andalib A et al. The expression of Th1- and Th2-related chemokine receptors in women with recurrent miscarriage: The impact of lymphocyte immunotherapy. *Am J Reprod Immunol* 2010;64:104–12.

38. Yang H, Qiu L, Di W et al. Proportional change of CD4 + CD25+ regulatory T cells after lymphocyte therapy in unexplained recurrentspontaneous abortion patients. *Fertil Steril* 2009;92:301–5.

39. Ob Liang P, Mo M, Li GG et al. Comprehensive analysis of peripheral blood lymphocytes in 76 women with recurrent miscarriage before and after lymphocyte immunotherapy. *Am J Reprod Immunol* 2012;68:164–74.

40. Clark DA, Chaouat G. Loss of surface CD200 on stored allogeneic leukocytes may impair anti-abortive effect in vivo. *Am J Reprod Immunol* 2005;53:13–20.

41. Clark DA, Banwatt D. Altered expression of cell surface CD200 tolerance-signaling molecule on human PBL stored at 4°C or 37°C correlates with reduced or increased efficacy in controlled trials of treatment of recurrent miscarriages. *Am J Reprod Immunol* 2006;55:392–93.

42. Kaczmarek A, Vandenabeele P, Krysko DV. Necroptosis: The release of damage-associated molecular patterns and its physiological relevance. *Immunity* 2013;38:209–23.

43. Guerin LR, Prins JR, Robertson SA. Regulatory T-cells and immune tolerance in pregnancy: A new target for infertility treatment? *Hum Reprod Update* 2009;15:517–35.

44. Arruvito L, Sanz M, Banham AH et al. Expansion of CD4+ CD25+ and FOXP3+ regulatory T cells during the follicular phase of the menstrual cycle: Implications for human reproduction. *J Immunol* 2007;178:2572–8.

45. Kwak JY, Gilman-Sachs A, Beaman KD et al. Reproductive outcome in women with recurrent spontaneous abortions of alloimmune and autoimmune causes: Preconception versus postconception treatment. *Am J Obstet Gynecol* 1992;166:1787–95.

46. Pandey K, Halder A, Agarwal, S et al. Immunotherapy in recurrent spontaneous abortion: Randomized and nonrandomized trials. *Internet Journal of Gynecology and Obstetrics* 2003;2:rsa/xml. Available at: http://ispub.com/IJGO/2/1/12411 (accessed September 25, 2013).

47. Lubinski J, Vrdoljak VJ, Beaman KD et al. Characterization of antibodies induced by paternal lymphocyte immunization in couples with recurrent spontaneous abortion. *J Reprod Immunol* 1993;24:81–96.

48. Coulam CB, Stephenson M, Stern JJ et al. Immunotherapy for recurrent pregnancy loss: Analysis of results from clinical trials. *Am J Reprod Immunol* 1996;35:352–9.

49. Gharesi-Fard B, Zolghadri J, Foroughinia L et al. Effectiveness of leukocyte immunotherapy in primary recurrent spontaneous abortion (RSA). *Iran J Immunol* 2007;4:173–8.

50. Carp HJ, Toder V, Mashiach S. Immunotherapy of habitual abortion. *Am J Reprod Immunol* 1992;28:281–4.

51. Peña RB, Cadavid AP, Botero JH et al. The production of MLR-blocking factors after lymphocyte immunotherapy for RSA does not predict the outcome of pregnancy. *Am J Reprod Immunol* 1998;39:120–4.

52. Bermas BL, Hill JA. Proliferative responses to recall antigens are associated with pregnancy outcome in women with a history of recurrent spontaneous abortion. *J Clin Invest* 1997;100:1330–4. Erratum: *J Clin Invest* 1998;101:513.

53. Hwang JL, Ho HN, Yang YS et al. The role of blocking factors and antipaternal lymphocytotoxic antibodies in the success of pregnancy in patients with recurrent spontaneous abortion. *Fertil Steril* 1992;58:691–6.

54. Agrawal S, Pandey MK, Mandal S et al. Humoral immune response to an allogenic foetus in normal fertile women and recurrent aborters. *BMC Pregnancy Childbirth* 2002;2:6.

55. Kotlan B, Fülöp V, Padányi A et al. High anti-paternal cytotoxic T-lymphocyte precursor frequencies in women with unexplained recurrent spontaneous abortions. *Hum Reprod* 2001;16:1278–85.

56. Kling C, Steinnmann J, Flesch B et al. Transfusion-related risks of intradermal allogeneic lymphocyte immunotherapy: Single cases in a large cohort and review of the literature. *Am J Reprod Immunol* 2006;56:157–71.

57. Kling C, Steinnmann J, Westpahl E et al. Adverse effects of intradermal allogeneic lymphocyte immunotherapy: Acute reactions and role of autoimmunity. *Hum Reprod* 2006;21:429–35.

29

Debate: Should Immunotherapy Be Used?
Intravenous Immunoglobulin—Yes

Carolyn B. Coulam

Does immunotherapy, specifically intravenous immunoglobulin (IVIg), for treatment of reproductive failure enhance live births? The answer to this question has been controversial. The reason for the controversy lies in the problem of patient selection for a particular treatment. A treatment is more likely to work if it is given to those with a physiologic abnormality that the treatment can correct, and, if the treatment in fact corrects it.[1] Not all pregnancies fail for the same reason. Causes for recurrent pregnancy loss have included chromosomal, anatomic, hormonal, immunologic, and thrombophilic abnormalities.[2] Thus, one cannot use obstetrical history alone to determine whether immunotherapy will be useful. Only patients experiencing reproductive failure with an immunologic cause would be expected to respond to immunotherapy. The following paragraphs will discuss how to identify those individuals most likely to respond to treatment with IVIg, describe published success rates of IVIg therapy, and present alternative treatments to IVIg.

How to Identify Those Individuals Most Likely to Respond to Treatment with IVIg

Of all of the causes of recurrent pregnancy loss, the ones that would be expected to respond to IVIg treatment are the etiologies that involve a mechanism that can be modulated by IVIg. The mechanisms by which IVIg are believed to enhance live birth rates include[3]:

- IVIg decreases killing activity of natural killer (NK) cells.
- IVIg decreases expression of proinflammatory T cell cytokines.
- IVIg increases the activity of regulatory T cells.
- IVIg suppresses B cell production of autoantibody.
- IVIg contains antibodies to antibodies or anti-idiotypic antibodies.
- IVIg actions on Fc receptors including binding of complement by the Fc component of IgG.

Based upon these mechanisms, IVIg would be expected to enhance live birth rates in individuals who had elevated circulating NK cells or elevated NK cytotoxicity, activated T cell activity, excess of proinflammatory Th1-type cytokines, diminished regulatory T cells, elevated production of autoantibodies that can cause endothelial damage and clotting, and increase activation of complement. Indeed, all of these findings have been reported among women experiencing recurrent pregnancy loss.[4–14] Proinflammatory cytokines at the maternal–fetal surface can cause clotting of the placental vessels and subsequent pregnancy loss. One source of these cytokines is the NK cell. Biopsies of the lining of the uterus from women experiencing recurrent pregnancy loss reveal an increase in activated NK cells.[15] Peripheral blood NK cells are also elevated in women with recurrent pregnancy loss compared with women without a history of pregnancy loss.[16] Measurement of NK cells in peripheral blood of women with a history of recurrent pregnancy loss has shown a significant elevation associated with loss of a normal karyotypic pregnancy and a normal level associated with loss of embryos that are karyotypically abnormal.[17,18] Furthermore, increased NK activity in the blood of nonpregnant women is predictive of recurrence of pregnancy loss.[6] Th1 cytokine expression has been shown to be increased in circulating T lymphocytes of women experiencing recurrent pregnancy loss.[7] Regulatory T cells (Tregs) suppress immune responses of other cells including T effector cells, thus helping to avoid unrestricted expansion of T cell proinflammatory response. IVIg has been shown to decrease Th1/Th2 cytokine ratios[12] and enhance T reg cells[19] as well as to decrease NK cell killing activity.[9–11] All of these events are necessary for pregnancy to be successful.

IVIg would *not* be expected to be effective in enhancing live birth rates in women who had chromosomally abnormal pregnancies or anatomic, hormonal, or thrombotic risk factors contributing to their losses. Therefore, to select the person most likely to respond to IVIg treatment would require documentation of an immunologic risk factor and the absence of nonimmunologic risk factors. Laboratory evaluations to determine the presence of an immunologic risk factor could include:

- Blood drawn for antiphospholipid antibodies, antinuclear antibodies, antithyroid antibodies, lupus-like anticoagulant, reproductive immunophenotype, NK activation assay, TH1/Th2 ratios in peripheral lymphocytes, and T reg cells, as well as tests for circulating embryotoxins (embryotoxicity assay) including TH1 cytokines.

Examples of testing for risk factors not responsive to treatment with IVIg include:

- Chromosome analysis of previous pregnancy losses or both partners.
- Hysterosonogram, hysterosalpingogram, or hysteroscopy.
- Thrombophilia panel.

Success Rates of IVIg Therapy

Originally, IVIg therapy was used to treat women with post-implantation pregnancy losses who had not been successful in pregnancies previously treated with aspirin and prednisone or heparin.[20–25] The rationale for the use of IVIG in the original studies was the suppression of the lupus anticoagulant in a woman being treated for severe thrombocytopenia. IVIg was often given with prednisone or heparin plus aspirin. The estimated success rate of 71% for women at very high risk for failure with a history of previous treatment failures suggested IVIg treatment was effective.[20–24] More recently, IVIg therapy alone has been used to successfully treat women with antiphospholipid antibodies as well as women who become refractory to conventional autoimmune treatment with heparin or prednisone and aspirin.[25] IVIg has been reported to successfully treat women with elevated circulating levels of NK cells with live birth rates between 80% and 90%.[26]

IVIg has also been used to treat women with unexplained recurrent pregnancy loss. Ten controlled trials of IVIg for treatment of recurrent pregnancy loss have been published.[27–35] Four of these report significant enhancement in the live birth rate with IVIg treatment and six were unable to show benefit of treatment. The number of patients participating in each trial, the time of first IVIg administration (preconception or postconception), whether the patients were selected for treatment with IVIg based on obstetrical history alone or obstetrical history and immunologic test results and whether the trial showed benefit or no benefit from treatment are summarized in Table 29.1. Five trials gave IVIG before conception and four of the five showed significant benefit in enhancing live birth rates, whereas five trials delayed treatment until pregnancy was established and of these none demonstrated benefit of treatment ($p = 0.04$, Fisher's exact test). Among the trials showing benefit of treatment with IVIg, three out of four used immune test results to select patients for IVIG treatment, and among trials showing no benefit from treatment, zero out of six selected patients for treatment using immune testing ($p = 0.03$). By waiting until 5–8 weeks of pregnancy to begin treatment, women with pathology occurring earlier would have been excluded and those pregnancies destined to succeed would be included, leading to selection bias. Indeed, a negative correlation with delay in treatment is significant. Only one study

TABLE 29.1

Classification of Outcome of Controlled Trials of Intravenous Immunoglobulin (IVIg) in Recurrent Pregnancy Loss

Trial	*n*	IVIg Started	Selection	Outcome Benefit (*p* < 0.05)
Moraru et al.[26]	157	Preconception	Immune testing	Yes
Coulam et al.[28]	95	Preconception	Ob history	Yes
Kiprov et al.[31]	35	Preconception	Immune testing	Yes
Strickler et al.[32]	47	Preconception	Immune testing	Yes
Stevenson et al.[30]	39	Preconception	Ob history	No
Mueller-Eckhart et al.[27]	64	Postconception	Ob history	No
Christiansen et al.[29]	34	Postconception	Ob history	No
Christiansen et al.[33]	58	Postconception	Ob history	No
Perino et al.[34]	46	Postconception	Ob history	No
Jablonowska et al.[35]	41	Postconception	Ob history	No

Ob: Obstetric.

TABLE 29.2

Summary of Published Meta-Analyses of Efficacy of Intravenous Immunoglobulin (IVIg) for Treatment of Unexplained Recurrent Reproductive Failure

Study	No. Trials	No. Patients	OR (95% CI) Overall	OR (95% CI) Primary Ab	OR (95% CI) Secondary Ab
Hutton et al.[38]	8	442	1.28 (0.78–2.10)	0.66 (0.35–1.20)	2.71 (1.09–6.77)*
Daya et al.[39]	6	240	1.08 (0.63–1.86)	1.04 (0.54–2.01)	1.18 (0.43–3.21)
Ata et al.[40]	6	272	0.92 (0.55–1.54)	0.67 (0.32–1.39)	1.15 (0.47–2.84)
Clark[41]	5	210			2.10 (1.06–4.49)*
Li et al.[42]	10	8207	1.62 (1.24–2.1)*		

OR: odds ratio; CI: confidence interval; Ab: aborters. *p < 0.05.

took into account the pregnancies lost as a result of chromosomal abnormalities.[29] Approximately 70% of the pregnancies lost in the clinical trials including all unexplained pregnancy losses would be expected to have chromosomal or other nonimmunologic abnormalities that would not be corrected by IVIg.[36] Furthermore, it has also been shown that some brands of IVIG can be as much as eight times less potent in suppressing NK cells than others (that were used in "negative" trials).[37]

The aforementioned clinical trials have been included in four published meta-analyses summarized in Table 29.2.[38–41] None of the meta-analyses showed benefit of treatment with IVIg for primary aborters. Two of the analyses demonstrated significant benefit for only secondary aborters (Table 29.2) (39 = 8.40). None of the studies included in the meta-analysis selected patients for inclusion based on immunologic testing. All were included based on reproductive history alone. How can the effect of an immunomodulatory treatment be evaluated if the subjects receiving the treatment were not determined to have any detectable immune abnormalities that would merit their inclusion into the study? The sample size required to show an effect would depend on the prevalence of immunologic problems among the unselected patients. Indeed IVIg was shown to increase the success rate in patients undergoing IVF for treatment of unexplained infertility based on meta-analysis with a sample size of over 8000 patients.[42] A number of clinical trials have demonstrated increased live birth rates after treatment with IVIg when patients are selected based on immunologic testing provided treatment is given prior to conception.[3,11,26,36,37]

Alternative Treatment to IVIg in Patients with Elevated NK Cells

As IVIg has been associated with significant cost and potential side effects, an alternative treatment has been sought. Evidence from both animal[43] and human[36,44,45] studies suggest that intralipid administered intravenously may enhance implantation and maintenance of pregnancy. Intralipid is a 20% intravenous fat emulsion used routinely as a source of fat and calories for patients requiring parental nutrition. It is composed of 10% soybean oil, 1.2% egg yolk phospholipids, 2.25% gylcerine, and water. Intralipid has been shown to decrease NK cytotoxicity both *in vitro*[44] and *in vivo*.[45] While the mechanism by which intralipids suppresses NK function is not known, effects of fatty acids have been demonstrated to be mediated through receptors such as peroxisome proliferator-activated receptors (PPARs),[46] G-protein-coupled receptors[47] and CD1 receptors.[48] Furthermore, intralipids have been shown to stimulate the reticulo-endothelial system and remove "danger signals" that can lead to pregnancy loss.[49] Sedman et al.[50] have found a significant fall of NK activity and lymphokine-activated killer activity after total parenteral nutrition regimens with long-chain triglycerides. Parenteral fat emulsions are known to accumulate in macrophages and to impair various functions of macrophages and those of the reticuloendothelial system. It was shown that the administration of fat emulsion, intralipid 20%, to recipient mice can suppress NK cell activity, probably through the impairment of macrophage function.[51]

When the pregnancy outcomes of women with a history of reproductive failure and elevated NK cell cytotoxicity treated with intralipid were compared with age and indication matched women treated with IVIg, no significant differences were seen.[36] The overall livebirth/ongoing pregnancy rate per cycle of treatment was 61% for women treated with intralipid and 56% with IVIg.[36] The appeal of intralipid lies in the fact that it is relatively inexpensive and is not a blood product.

Conclusion

IVIg is effective treatment for women experiencing recurrent pregnancy loss, if the patients who are treated actually have a condition that IVIG is expected to correct, as evidenced by immunologic testing. Patients not demonstrating an immunologic risk factor are not expected to respond to IVIg therapy. Intralipid is an alternative treatment in women experiencing recurrent pregnancy loss who express elevated NK cell cytoxicity as live birth rates are the same following treatment.

REFERENCES

1. Clark DA. The power of observation. *Am J Reprod Immunl* 2011;66:71–5.
2. Ford HB, Schust D. Recurrent pregnancy loss: Etiology, diagnosis, and therapy. *Rev Obstet Gynecol* 2009;2:76–83.
3. Sewell WAC, Jolles S. Immunomodulatory action of intravenous immunoglobulins. *Immunol* 2002;107:387–93.
4. Coulam CB, Roussev RG. Correlation of NK cell activation and inhibition markers with NK cytotoxicity among women experiencing immunological implantation failure after *in vitro* fertilization and embryo transfer. *J Assist Reprod Genet* 2003;20:58–62.
5. Coulam CB, Roussev RG. Increasing circulating T-cell activation markers are linked to subsequent implantation failure after transfer of *in vitro* fertilized embryos. *Am J Reprod Immunol* 2003;50:340–5.
6. Aoki K, Kajijura S, Matsumoto Y et al. Preconceptional natural killer cell activity as a predictor of miscarriage. *Lancet* 1995;135:1340–2.
7. Yamada H, Morikawa M, Kato EH et al. Preconceptional natural killer cell activity and percentage as predictors of biochemical pregnancy and spontaneous abortion with a normal karyotype. *Am J Reprod Immunol* 2003;50:351–4.
8. Kwak-Kim JY, Chung-Bang HS, Ng SC et al. Increased T helper 1 cytokine responses by circulating T cells are present in women with recurrent pregnancy losses and in infertile women with multiple implantation failures after IVF. *Hum Reprod* 2003;18:767–73.
9. Ruiz JE, Kwak JY, Baum L et al. Intravenous immunoglobulins inhibits natural killer activity *in vivo* in women with recurrent spontaneous abortion. *Am J Reprod Immunol* 1996;35:370–5.
10. Kwak JY, Kwak FM, Ainbinder SW et al. Elevated peripheral blood natural killer cells are effectively downregulated by immunoglobulin G infusion in women with recurrent spontaneous abortions. *Am J Reprod Immunol* 1996;35:363–9.
11. Ruiz JE, Kwak JY, Baum L et al. Effects of intravenous immunoglobulin G on natural killer cell cytotoxicity *in vitro* in women with recurrent spontaneous abortion. *J Reprod Immunol* 1996;31:125–41.

12. Graphou O, Chioti A, Pantazi A et al. Effect of intravenous immunoglobulins treatment on the Th1/Th2 balance in women with recurrent spontaneous abortions. *Am J Reprod Immunol* 2003;49:21–9.

13. Saito S, Nakashima A, Shima T et al. Th1/Th2/Th17 and regulatory T-cell paradigm in pregnancy. *Am J Reprod Immunol* 2000;63:601–10.

14. Lee SK, Kim JY, Lee M et al. Th17 and regulatory T cells in women with recurrent pregnancy loss. *Am J Reprod Immunol* 2012;67:311–5.

15. Lachapelle MH, Miron P, Hemmings R et al. Endometrial T, B, and NK cells in patients with recurrent spontaneous abortion. *J Immunol* 1996;158:4886–91.

16. Yamada H, Morikawa M, Kato EH et al. Preconceptional natural killer cell activity and percentage as predictors of biochemical pregnancy and spontaneous abortion with a normal karyotype. *Am J Reprod Immunol* 2003;50:351–4.

17. Coulam CB, Stephenson M, Stern JJ et al. Immunotherapy for recurrent pregnancy loss: Analysis of results from clinical trials. *Am J Reprod Immunol* 1996;35:352–9.

18. Clark DA, Daya S, Coulam CB et al. Implications of abnormal human trophoblast karyotype for the evidence-based approach to the understanding, investigation, and treatment of recurrent spontaneous abortion. *Am J Reprod Immunol* 1996;35:495–8.

19. Kessel A, Ammuri H, Peri R et al. Intravenous immunoglobulin therapy affects T regulatory cells by increasing their suppressive function. *J Immunol* 2007;179:5571–5.

20. Lubbe WF, Liggins CG. Lupus anticoagulant and pregnancy. *Am J Obstet Gynecol* 1985;153:322–7.

21. Carreras KO, Perez GN, Vega HR et al. Lupus anticoagulant and recurrent fetal loss: Successful treatment with gammaglobulin. *Lancet* 1988;2:393.

22. Francois A, Freund M, Reym P. Repeated fetal losses and the lupus anticoagulant. *Ann Int Med* 1988;109:933–4.

23. Scott JR, Branch DW, Knochenour NK et al. Intravenous treatment of pregnant patients with recurrent pregnancy loss caused by antiphospholipid antibodies and Rh immunization. *Am J Obstet Gynecol* 1988;159:1055–6.

24. Parke A, Maier D, Wilson D et al. Intravenous immunoglobulin, antiphospholipid antibodies, and pregnancy. *Ann Int Med* 1989;110:495–6.

25. Mac Lachlan NA, Letsky E, De Sweit M. The use of intravenous immunoglobulin therapy in the management of antiphospholipid antibody associated pregnancies. *Clin Exp Rheumatol* 1990;8:221–4.

26. Moraru M, Carbone J, Alecsandru D et al. Intervenous immunoglobulin treatment increased live birth rate ina Apanish cohort of women with recurrent reproductive failure and expanded CD56+ cells. *Am J Reprod Immunol* 2012;68:75–84.

27. Mueller-Eckhart G, Mallmann P, Neppert J et al. Immunogenetic and serological investigations of non-pregnancy and pregnant women with a history of recurrent spontaneous abortion. German RSA/IVIG Trialist Group. *J Reprod Immunol* 1994;27:95–109.

28. Coulam CB, Krysa LW, Stern JJ et al. Intravenous immunoglobulin for treatment of recurrent pregnancy loss. *Am J Reprod Immunol* 1995;34:333–7.

29. Christiansen OB, Pedersen B, Rosgaard A et al. A randomized, double-blind, placebo controlled trial of intravenous immunoglobulin in the prevention of recurrent miscarriage: Evidence for a therapeutic effect in women with secondary recurrent miscarriage. *Hum Reprod* 2002;17:809–16.

30. Stephenson MD, Dreher K, Houlihan E et al. Prevention of unexplained recurrent spontaneous abortion using intravenous immunoglobulin: A prospective, randomized, double-blinded, placebo-controlled trial. *Am J Reprod Immunol* 1998;39:82–8.

31. Kiprov DD, Nachtigall RD, Weaver RC et al. The use of intravenous immunoglobulin in recurrent pregnancy loss associated with combined alloimmune and autoimmune abnormalities. *Am J Reprod Immunol* 1996;36:228–34.

32. Stricker RB, Steinleitner A, Bookoff CN et al. Successful treatment of immunological abortion with low-dose intravenous immunoglobulin. *Fertil Steril* 2000;73:536–40.

33. Chriatiansen OB, Mathiesen O, Husth M et al. Placebo-controlled trial of treatment of unexplained secondary recurrent spontaneous abortions and recurrent late spontaneous abortions with i.v. immunoglobulin. *Hum Reprod* 1995;10:2690–5.

34. Perino A, Vassiliadis A, Vucetich A et al. Short-term therapy for recurrent abortion using intravenous immunoglobulins: Results of a double-blind placebo-controlled Italian study. *Hum Reprod* 1997;12:2388–92.

35. Jablonowska B, Selbing A, Palfi M et al. Prevention of recurrent spontaneous abortion by intravenous immunoglobulin: A double-blind placebo-controlled study. *Hum Reprod* 1999;14:838–41.

36. Coulam CB, Acacio B. Does immunotherapy for treatment of reproductive failure enhance live births? *Am J Reprod Immunol* 2012;67:296–303.

37. Clark DA, Coulam CB, Stricker RB. Is intravenous immunoglobulins (IVIG) efficacious in early pregnancy failure? A critical review and meta-analysis for patients who fail *in vitro* fertilization and embryo transfer (IVF). *J Assist Reprod Genet* 2006;23:383–96.

38. Hutton B, Sharma R, Fergusson D et al. Use of intravenous immunoglobulin for treatment of recurrent miscarriage: A systematic review. *BJOG* 2007;114:134–42.

39. Daya S, Gunby J, Claark DA. Intrvenous immunoglobulin for treatment of recurrent spontaqneous abortion: A meta-analysis. *Am J Reprod Immunol* 1998;39:69–76.

40. Ata B, Tan SL, Shehata F et al. A systematic review of intravenous immunoglobulin for treatment of enexplained recurrent miscarriage. *Fertil Steril* 2011:95:1080–5.

41. Clark DA. Intravenous immunoglobulin and idiopathic secondary recurrent miscarriages methodological problems. *Hum Reprod* 2011;25:2586–7.

42. Li J, Chen Y, Liu C et al. Intravenous immunoglobulin treatment for repeated IVF/ICSI failure and unexplained infertility: A systematic review and a meta-analysis. *Am J Reprod Immunol* 2013;70:434–7.

43. Clark DA. Intralipid as treatment for recurrent unexplained abortion? *Am J Reprod Immunol* 1994;32:290–3.

44. Roussev RG, Ng SC, Coulam CB. Natural killer cell functional activity suppression by intravenous immunoglobulin, intralipid and soluble human leukocyte antigen G. *Am J Reprod Immunol* 2007;57:262–6.

45. Roumen RG, Acacio B, Ng SC et al. Duration of intralipid's suppressive effect on NK cell's functional activity. *Am J Reprod Immunol* 2008;60:258–63.

46. Khan SA, Vanden-Heuvel JP. Role of nuclear receptors in the regulation of gene expression by dietary fatty acids (review). *J Nutr Biochem* 2003;14:554–67.

47. Kostenis E. A glance a G-protein-coupled receptors for lipid mediators: A growing receptor family with remarkable diverse ligands. *Pharmacol Ther* 2004;102:243–257.

48. Leslie D, Dascher CC, Cembrola K et al. Serum lipids regulate dendritic cell CD1 expression and function. *Immunology* 2008;125:289–301.

49. Clark DA. Intralipid as a treatment for recurrent unexplained abortion? *Am J Reprod Immunol* 1994;32:290–3.

50. Sedman PC, Somers SS, Ramsden CW et al. Effects of different lipid emulsions on lymphocyte function during total parenteral nutrition. *Br J Surg* 1991;78:1396–9.

51. Tezuka H, Sawada H, Sakoda H et al. Suppression of genetic resistance to bone marrow grafts and natural killer activity by administration of fat emulsion. *Exp Hematol* 1988;12:609–12.

30

Debate: Should Immunotherapy Be Used? Granulocyte Colony Stimulating Factor—Yes

Fabio Scarpellini and Marco Sbracia

Introduction

Cytokines and growth factors, produced by trophoblast and endometrial immune-cells, are involved in implantation and pregnancy development.[1] These substances play a relevant role in regulating trophoblast cell growth and migration, as well as trophoblast differentiation, promoting its invasiveness and decreasing its survival rate. In order to balance these functions, a large number of cytokines and growth factors are involved in regulating the paracrine and autocrine mechanisms of trophoblast-decidual cell crosstalk.[2] Some of these proteins have been thoroughly investigated and colony stimulating factors (CSFs), macrophage colony stimulating factor (M-CSF or CSF1), granulocyte-macrophage stimulating factor (GM-CSF or CSF2), and granulocyte colony stimulating factor (G-CSF or CSF3) have gained particular interest due to their possible use in the treatment of reproductive disorders.

The CFSs are a group of glycoproteins that bind to specific receptors on hemopoietic stem cells, promoting cell proliferation and differentiation into macrophages and granulocytes. They show different structures and gene location, and also have different receptors. M-CSF is a cytokine of 554 amino acids with a molecular weight of 60,179 kDa, the gene is located on the short arm of chromosome 1, region 1p13.3.[3] It binds to a specific receptor, the M-CSFR or CD115, encoded by a gene located on the long arm of chromosome 5, region 5q32; this gene codes for a protein of 972 amino acids and is 107,984 kDa in molecular weight, a receptor related to the tyrosin kinase protein family.[4] M-CSF is a hematopoietic growth factor that is involved in the proliferation and differentiation of monocytes, macrophages, and bone marrow progenitor cells, and is involved in bone reabsorption.[5] GM-CSF is a protein of 14,435 kDa in molecular weight, consisting of 144 amino acids, encoded by a gene located on the long arm of chromosome 5, region 5q31, in a cluster of genes associated with the 5q-syndrome and acute myelogenous leukemia.[6] GM-CSF binds to a specific receptor, the GM-CSFR or CD116, whose gene is located in the Xp22.32 and Yp11.3 regions encoding for a protein consisting of 400 amino acids and is 46,207 kDa in molecular weight.[7] GM-CSFR consists of two subunits, α and β chain, phosphorylated by one of the JAK family. G-CSF is a glycoprotein of 174–180 amino acids long and with a molecular weight of 19,600 kDa: its gene is located on the long arm of chromosome 17, region 17q11.2-q12.[8] It binds to a specific receptor, the G-CSF R or CD114, encoded by a gene on the short arm of chromosome 1 region 1p35–34.3, a protein 836 amino acids long and of 92,156 in molecular weight.[9] GCSF-R is associated with signal transduction through the JAK-STAT3 pathways. G-CSF stimulates bone marrow to produce granulocytes and stem cells released into the bloodstream.

All CSFs are involved in the reproductive process from ovulation to implantation and pregnancy. M-CSF and its receptor are expressed in the human endometrial epithelium and in the placenta.[10,11] It is expressed in follicular fluid and lactating mammary glands in both humans and mice.[12,13] This cytokine seems to be involved in the pathogenesis of endometriosis.[14] GM-CSF and its receptor have been found expressed in human trophoblast cells and in the decidua and human endometrium.[15,16] GM-CSF stimulates trophoblast growth and hCG production, whereas null mutant mice for GM-CSF showed aberrant placental development.[17] Preimplantation embryos express the GM-CSF receptor, and culture medium for embryos supplemented with GM-CSF has beneficial effects on embryo development.[18] G-CSF and its receptor have been found on trophoblasts and in the decidua of several mammals, including human placenta.[19,20] An anti-abortive role has been demonstrated for G-CSF in the animal models, and its depletion is indirectly involved in miscarriages.[21,22] It has also been shown that G-CSF has a positive effect on trophoblast metabolism.[23] Furthermore, G-CSF is secreted in follicular fluid and its levels correlated with oocyte competence and the implantation potential of corresponding embryos.[24]

G-CSF and Recurrent Miscarriage

We have evaluated the role of G-CSF in early pregnancy and its use in the treatment of recurrent miscarriage (RM) and recurrent implantation failure (RIF).[25,26] More than 40% of RM cases remain unexplained[27] and for them several causes have been proposed, including the allo-immune response. RM could be due to an imbalance in the Th1/Th2 systems, with a preponderance of Th1 cytokine production instead of Th2 cytokine production (with an immuno-suppression role).[28] Several treatment modalities have been proposed for RM, but all have showed controversial results.[29]

We started using G-CSF in RM in 1997, successfully treating a woman after five consecutive miscarriages. We used this treatment in several other women with encouraging results. The results of a pilot study were first presented in 1998 at the Annual ASRM Meeting. We followed up with a randomized controlled study, the results of which were published in 2009.[25] We selected a group of patients fulfilling these inclusion criteria: age <39 years, more than four previous miscarriages, failure of previous treatments for RM, and they had to be negative for all of the known causes of RM, including normal karyotyping of embryonic tissues in the previous miscarriage. Sixty-eight patients were included in the study: 35 women underwent daily administration of recombinant G-CSF (Filgastrim) 1 µg (100,000 IU)/kg/day from the sixth day after ovulation until the occurrence of menstruation or to the end of 9 weeks of gestation. The control group consisted of 33 subjects who were treated with saline solution. The live births in women treated with G-CSF were 82.8%, whereas in the controls they were 48.5% ($p = 0.0061$). The number of patients needed to treat for one additional live birth was 2.9. None of the newborns showed any major or minor abnormalities. This study showed that G-CSF is a promising tool for the treatment of selected cases of RM. The use of G-CSF during pregnancy is safe since in our experience as well as in the literature no adverse effects have been reported.[30,31]

Subsequently data have been reported on the use of G-CSF in women with RIF, showing good results in an uncontrolled study.[26] G-CSF seems to increase the chance of pregnancy in patients with RIF. Therefore, we have started a controlled trial on RIF patients that is due to terminate in 2014. The preliminary data seem to be encouraging (presented at the ASRM Annual Meeting in 2011). Other investigators are also assessing G-CSF in RM and RIF, and a multicenter controlled trial is required in order to establish the potential of G-CSF, and in which patients it may be beneficial.

There is circumstantial evidence regarding the interaction of G-CSF with the trophoblast and immune system. G-CSF activates and mobilizes stem cells; it is used to increase the number of stem cells after organ transplant, or to activate the reconstruction of the vascular bed after heart ischemia, and in neurology, to treat patients with severe degenerative diseases. In our study we observed a significant increase of β-hCG levels in the ongoing pregnancies from the fifth through the ninth gestational week in G-CSF treated pregnancies compared to normal pregnancies.[25] These data show a direct effect of this G-CSF on the trophoblast, with the mobilization and activation of placental stem cells. Another mechanism of action may be the effect of G-CSF on lymphocytes, several studies have shown that G-CSF promotes the mobilization and proliferation of several lymphocyte and dendritic cells, in particular Treg and DC2 cells.[32,33] Our unpublished data show that women with RM treated with G-CSF had a remarkable increase of peripheral blood levels of Treg cells compared to normal pregnancy. Furthermore, in women with RM treated with G-CSF who subsequently miscarried again due to embryonic aneuploidy, there was still an increase of Treg cells in the decidua compared to the controls. These data suggest that G-CSF may mobilize stem cells and immune cells enhancing trophoblast function.

Conclusion

In the evaluation of the effectiveness of any treatment in RM there are several difficulties: several factors play a confounding role, maternal age, number of previous miscarriages, and the causes of previous miscarriages. Additionally, the incidence of embryo aneuploidy increases with maternal age.[27,34] Furthermore, it has been shown that the spontaneous resolution of RM occurs in 40–60% of cases, depending on the number of previous miscarriages.[30,31] A controlled randomized study is now required, which accounts for these covariates. Such a study would need to recruit a large number of patients, and would need to be multicenter.

Although there are effective treatments for RM with clear immunologic origin, such as in antiphospholipid syndrome, where heparin plus aspirin is generally used for treatment,[34] in idiopathic RM there is no evidence of effective treatment. In these cases, G-CSF may be effective, even though more studies are needed to confirm the effectiveness of this treatment in idiopathic RM.

REFERENCES

1. Sykes L, MacIntyre DA, Yap XJ et al. The Th1:Th2 dichotomy of pregnancy and preterm labour. *Mediators Inflamm* 2012;2012:967629.
2. Oreshkova T, Dimitrov R, Mourdjeva M. A cross-talk of decidual stromal cells, trophoblast, and immunecells: A prerequisite for the success of pregnancy. *Am J Reprod Immunol* 2012;68:366–73.
3. Saltman DL, Dolganov GM, Hinton LM et al. Reassignment of the human macrophage colony stimulating factor gene to chromosome 1p13–21. *Biochem Biophys Res Commun* 1992;182:1139–43.
4. Galland F, Stefanova M, Lafage M et al. Localization of the 5' end of the MCF2 oncogene to human chromosome 15q15 → q23. *Cytogenet Cell Genet* 1992;60:114–6.
5. Stanley ER, Berg KL, Einstein DB et al. Biology and action of colony—Stimulating factor 1 *Mol Reprod Dev* 1997;46:4–10.
6. Cantrell MA, Anderson D, Cerretti DP et al. Cloning, sequence, and expression of a human granulocyte/macrophage colony-stimulating factor. *Proc Natl Acad Sci U S A* 1985;82:6250–4.
7. Rappold G, Willson TA, Henke A et al. Arrangement and localization of the human GM-CSF receptor alpha chain gene CSF2RA within the X-Y pseudoautosomal region. *Genomics* 1992;14:455–61.
8. Nagata S, Tsuchiya M, Asano S et al. Molecular cloning and expression of cDNA for human granulocyte colony-stimulating factor. *Nature* 1986;319:415–8.
9. Tweardy DJ, Anderson K, Cannizzaro LA et al. Molecular cloning of cDNAs for the human granulocyte colony-stimulating factor receptor from HL-60 and mapping of the gene to chromosome region 1p32–34. *Blood* 1992;79:1148–54.
10. Pollard JW, Bartocci A, Arceci R et al. Apparent role of the macrophage growth factor, CSF-1, in placental development. *Nature* 1987;330:484–6.
11. Kauma SW, Aukerman SL, Eierman D et al. Colony-stimulating factor-1 and c-fms expression in human endometrial tissues and placenta during the menstrual cycle and early pregnancy. *J Clin Endocrinol Metab* 1991;73:746–51.
12. Pollard JW, Hennighausen L. Colony stimulating factor 1 is required for mammary gland development during pregnancy. *Proc Natl Acad Sci U S A* 1994;91:9312–6.
13. Witt BR, Pollard JW. Colony stimulating factor-1 in human follicular fluid. *Fertil Steril* 1997;68:259–64.
14. Aligeti S, Kirma NB, Binkley PA et al. Colony-stimulating factor-1 exerts direct effects on the proliferation and invasiveness of endometrial epithelial cells. *Fertil Steril* 2011;95:2464–6.
15. Armstrong DT, Chaouat G. Effects of lymphokines and immune complexes on murine placental cell growth in vitro. *Biol Reprod* 1989;40:466–74.
16. Giacomini G, Tabibzadeh SS, Satyaswaroop PG et al. Epithelial cells are the major source of biologically active granulocyte macrophage colony-stimulating factor in human endometrium. *Hum Reprod* 1995;10:3259–63.
17. Robertson SA, Roberts CT, Farr KL et al. Fertility impairment in granulocyte-macrophage colony-stimulating factor-deficient mice. *Biol Reprod* 1999;60:251–61.
18. Robertson SA, Sjöblom C, Jasper et al. Granulocyte-macrophage colony-stimulating factor promotes glucose transport and blastomere viability in murine preimplantation embryos. *Biol Reprod* 2001;64:1206–15.
19. Uzumaki H, Okabe T, Sasaki N et al. Identification and characterization of receptors for granulocyte colony-stimulating factor on human placenta and trophoblastic cells. *Proc Natl Acad Sci U S A* 1989;86:9323–6.

20. McCracken SA, Grant KE, MacKenzie IZ et al. Gestational regulation of granulocyte-colony stimulating factor receptor expression in the human placenta. *Biol Reprod* 1999;60:790–6.

21. Novales JS, Salva AM, Modanlou HD et al. Maternal administration of granulocyte colony-stimulating factor improves neonatal rat survival after a lethal group B streptococcal infection. *Blood* 1993;81:923–7.

22. Sugita K, Hayakawa S, Karasaki-Suzuki M et al. Granulocyte colony stimulation factor (G-CSF) suppresses interleukin (IL)-12 and/or IL-2 induced interferon (IFN)-gamma production and cytotoxicity of decidual mononuclear cells. *Am J Reprod Immunol* 2003;50:83–9.

23. Marino VJ, Roguin LP. The granulocyte colony stimulating factor (G-CSF) activates Jak/STAT and MAPK pathways in a trophoblastic cell line. *J Cell Biochem* 2008;103:1512–23.

24. Lédée N, Lombroso R, Lombardelli L et al. Cytokines and chemokines in follicular fluids and potential of the corresponding embryo: The role of granulocyte colony-stimulating factor. *Hum Reprod* 2008;23:2001–9.

25. Scarpellini F, Sbracia M. Use of granulocyte colony-stimulating factor for the treatment of unexplained recurrent miscarriage: A randomised controlled trial. *Hum Reprod* 2009;24:2703–8.

26. Würfel W, Santjohanser C, Hirv K et al. High pregnancy rates with administration of granulocyte colony-stimulating factor in ART-patients with repetitive implantation failure and lacking killer-cell immunglobulin-like receptors. *Hum Reprod* 2010;25:2151–2.

27. Carrington B, Sacks G, Regan L. Recurrent miscarriage: Pathophysiology and outcome. *Curr Opin Obstet Gynecol* 2005;17:591–7.

28. Michimata T, Sakai M, Miyazaki S et al. Decrease of T-helper 2 and T-cytotoxic 2 cells at implantation sites occurs in unexplained recurrent spontaneous abortion with normal chromosomal content. *Hum Reprod* 2003;18:1523–8.

29. Porter TF, LaCoursiere Y, Scott JR. Immunotherapy for recurrent miscarriage. *Cochrane Database Syst Rev* 2006;CD000112.

30. Dale DC, Cottle TE, Fier CJ et al. Severe chronic neutropenia: Treatment and follow-up of patients in the Severe Chronic Neutropenia International Registry. *Am J Hematol* 2003;72:82–93.

31. Pessach I, Shimoni A, Nagler A. Granulocyte-colony stimulating factor for hematopoietic stem cell donation from healthy female donors during pregnancy and lactation: What do we know? *Hum Reprod Update* 2013;19:259–67.

32. Condomines M, Quittet P, Lu ZY et al. Functional regulatory T cells are collected in stem cell autografts by mobilization with high-dose cyclophosphamide and granulocyte colony-stimulating factor. *J Immunol* 2006;176:6631–9.

33. Rossetti M, Gregori S, Roncarolo MG. Granulocyte-colony stimulating factor drives the in vitro differentiation of human dendritic cells that induce anergy in naïve T cells. *Eur J Immunol* 2010;40:3097–106.

34. Rai RS, Regan L. Recurrent miscarriage. *Lancet* 2006;368:601–11.

31

Debate: Should Immunotherapy Be Used? No

Raj Rai

The investigation and treatment of women with recurrent miscarriage (RM) has historically been based on anecdotal evidence, personal bias of physicians, and the results of small uncontrolled studies.[1] This has led to the situation where women have been subjected to treatments of no proven benefit, some of which have subsequently been demonstrated to be harmful.[2] This is unacceptable. Indeed, in the current climate in which patient demands and expectations for a "treatment/cure" of their reproductive failure is ever increasing, it is incumbent upon clinicians to reject previous practice and embrace an evidence-based approach to the management of RM.

The concept of immune dysfunction as a basis for miscarriage is an attractive one. Whilst pregnancy has traditionally been viewed as a battle between the semi-allogenic fetus and the mother, in which the fetus and surrounding trophoblast have to evade an immune response if that response is not suppressed, an immune attack on the pregnancy has never been demonstrated. From an evolutionary viewpoint, it seems that the maternal immune cells and trophoblast cooperate rather than compete.[3] Indeed, there is no evidence of a classic graft versus host response in pregnancy. It is now recognized that pregnancy itself is not an immune-suppressed state but one in which the maternal immune system is modulated without suppression.

Much of the data pertaining to immune responses to the trophoblast have been obtained from murine models, and the same mechanisms have been assumed to be relevant in humans. Although the modulation of the immune system into a cooperative response probably developed once in the evolution of mammalian reproduction, there may be wide differences in the subsequent development of immune modulation in different orders of mammals. Therefore, caution has to be applied to the extrapolation of data from murine pregnancies to the human. Additionally, the observed immune aberrations in pregnancy failure may be a consequence rather than the cause of pregnancy loss.

Regardless, immunotherapy has been introduced into clinical practice, as a treatment for RM based on the hypotheses that either alloimunity or autoimmunity is responsible for pregnancy failure. In order to critically evaluate the use of paternal or third party white cell immunization (active immunization), intravenous immunoglobulin (passive immunization), or cytokine modulation as treatment for RM, it is necessary to examine the rationale for their use, and the results which are currently available.

Rationale (or not) for Immunotherapy

Paternal White Cell Immunization

There have been a number of concepts suggested to explain the mechanism of action of active immunization; none have stood the test of thorough investigation. The first concept of an alloimmune basis for RM was based on an increased sharing of human leukocyte antigens (HLA) between both partners that prevents the maternal production of a "blocking" antibody that protects the fetus against immunological attack.[4] Women with successful pregnancies were thought to produce this "blocking" antibody and those whose pregnancy ends in miscarriage do not. White cell immunization has been reported to induce production of the "blocking" antibody.[5] However, the "blocking antibody" hypothesis has never been validated and an increased sharing of HLA Class I alleles between partners has been refuted in a number of articles and in the meta-analysis of Beydoun et al.[6] Further, (a) production of "blocking" antibody is usually not evident until after 28 weeks of gestation and may disappear between pregnancies[7]; (b) miscarriage occurs despite the presence of "blocking" antibody[8,9]; and (c) women who exhibit no production of "blocking" antibodies do experience successful pregnancies. Leucocyte immunization has also been reported to reduce natural killer cell numbers,[10] and modulate cytokine levels in favor of a Th-2 response. These mechanisms have also not been confirmed in large studies and have not been shown to be relevant to human pregnancies.

Intravenous Immunoglobulin (IVIg)/Intralipid

Current concepts on the etiology of RM focus on autoimmune mediated pregnancy loss (such as antiphospholipid syndrome); natural killer (NK) cells; a disordered cytokine balance at the feto-maternal interface; Th-17 cells; and the role of T regulatory cells. IVIg has a number of immuno-modulatory effects on cytokine production, antigen neutralization, Fc receptor blockade, alteration in the distribution and function of T-cell subsets, antibodies, and autoantigens that may potentially ameliorate a dysregulated immune response causal of pregnancy loss. However, the role of autoantibodies, apart from antiphospholipid antibodies, in the pathogenesis of RM is unproven.[2]

The relationship between peripheral blood NK (PBNK) cells and reproductive failure is one of the most controversial fields in reproductive immunology. The levels and activation of NK cells is dependent on other variables such as whether whole blood or fractionated mononuclear cells are used in the assay, the time of day a sample is taken, whether any physical exercise has been performed, the parity of the patient, and whether the samples have been previously frozen.[11–15] Different NK assays have also been employed and results may vary depending on whether the chromium-51 release cytotoxicity assay or CD69 expression is assayed. Importantly, it is not known which *in vitro* assay most accurately reflects *in vivo* function, and indeed what biological relevance such activity has. Furthermore, it is unclear what an abnormal NK cell number is. Whilst traditionally a peripheral NK cell level greater than 12% of all lymphocytes has been regarded as the cut-off between a raised and a normal level,[16] this figure is well within the normal range (up to 29%) published by others.[17] Hence, individuals with entirely normal results are being labelled as have raised NK cell numbers. A fascinating study has cast further doubt on the validity of PBNK cell testing in women with RM.[18] The authors reported that immediately after insertion of an intravenous cannula for blood withdrawal, women with RM show an increased proportion of NK cells within lymphocytes, elevated blood NK cell concentrations and augmented NK activity per milliliter of blood compared to control women who have no known fertility problems. However, these differences disappear after 20 minutes, when blood is drawn again from the same cannula. The authors concluded that the elevated NK indices previously observed in women with RM are due to a transient increase in NK cell numbers, rather than a chronic state.

Despite the above caveats and amidst much publicity, PBNK cell testing is being promoted as a useful diagnostic test to guide the initiation of a variety of immunosuppressive therapies amongst patients with either recurrent miscarriage or infertility. Indeed, several small observational studies reported enhanced PBNK cell activity with subsequent failure to conceive or miscarry.[16,19–24] However, the largest single observational study of 552 women with a history of between two and six miscarriages reported that PBNK cell cytotoxic activity was not correlated with subsequent pregnancy outcome and a meta-analysis of 22 studies reported no relationship between either PBNK cell numbers or activity and pregnancy outcome[25]

Uterine natural killer cells (uNK), which are phenotypically and functionally different to PBNK cell, and the numbers of which are maximal during the window of implantation are perhaps of more interest. Whilst intra-cycle variation in uNK cell numbers has been documented,[26] several studies have reported that women with RM have a raised uNK cell level.[27–29] The largest reported prospective study reported no correlation between uNK cell numbers and pregnancy outcome.[27] In addition, a prospective randomized study designed to assess the efficacy of prednisolone suppression of "raised" uNK cell numbers reported no significance in live birth rate between those treated with prednisolone compared to those receiving placebo.[29] Is this surprising? Perhaps not. It is clear that interactions between HLA-C and killer-immunoglobulin-like receptors (KIR) on decidual NK cells can influence the success of early pregnancy events after implantation has occurred.[30] Both genetic and functional studies support the view that in fact, activation of decidual NK cells by MHC ligands on trophoblast has beneficial effects on pregnancy outcome.[30]

As an alternative to IVIg, intralipid, which is a 20% intravenous fat emulsion is usually used and consists of soybean oil, as well as egg yolk phospholipids, glycerin, and water, has been introduced into the clinical arena. A single small non-randomized study, presented only in abstract form, reported a 50% pregnancy rate and 46% clinical pregnancy rate amongst women with recurrent implantation failure who had an elevated TH1 cytokine response. There are no published results in RM. The mechanism by which intralipid modulates the immune system is still unclear. It has been proposed that fatty acids within the emulsion serve as ligands to activate peroxisome proliferator-activated receptors expressed by the NK cells. Activation of such nuclear receptors has been shown to decrease NK cytotoxic activity, enhancing implantation.[31] Clearly large randomized studies are needed.[32]

Efficacy of Immunotherapy

The patient with RM is interested in the results regarding her subsequent pregnancy rather than the theoretical basis. If the results of treatment show evidence of effect, the mechanism will eventually be clarified. However, it is important that when evaluating the effect of any intervention proposed as a treatment for RM to be cognizant of the fact that the two most important determinants of the outcome of a particular pregnancy are the mother's age and the number of miscarriages she has previously experienced. The rate of sporadic fetal aneuploidy is in the region of 50% amongst women between 40 and 44 years of age, rising to 75% amongst those older than 45 years. On the basis of a 15% clinical miscarriage rate, 35% of women with three consecutive miscarriages will have done so purely by chance alone. Amongst such women aged less than 39 years, a live birth rate of between 65% and 70% with supportive care alone can be expected.[33] However, 30–35% of women with a recurring cause will miscarry again. It is against this high spontaneous resolution rate that the efficacy of any putative treatment for RM has to be judged. It has been claimed that immunotherapy may be effective in certain subgroups of women with RM, rather than in all women with RM as a whole. However, these subgroups have not been well defined.

Paternal White Cell Immunization

A number of studies have examined the efficacy of paternal white cell immunization as a treatment for RM. These studies, which have used differing methodologies, entry criteria and analyses, have reported conflicting results. The largest study (183 women), which was a double-blind, multicenter, randomized clinical trial, reported that on an intention to treat basis, the success rate was 36% in the treatment group versus 48% in the control group (odds ratio [OR] 0.60; 95% confidence interval [CI] 0.33–1.12).[34] If analysis was restricted to only those who conceived, the corresponding success rates were 46% with immunization but 65% with placebo saline injections (OR 0.45; 95% CI 0.22 0.91), suggesting that immunization may *increase* the rate of clinically recognized pregnancy loss. Partly on the basis of this large study and the lack of scientific validity underlying paternal white cell immunization, the FDA issued guidance in 2002 highlighting the lack of efficacy of this treatment and reminding clinicians that it should only be offered in the context of therapeutic studies and will require investigational new drug approval (http://www.fda.gov/CBER/ltr/lit013002.htm) for use in the U.S.

The conclusions of several published meta-analyses have also been conflicting. A Cochrane review published in 2006, based on 12 trials (641 women), reported an OR of 1.23 (95% CI 0.89–1.70) amongst those administered paternal white cells compared with controls.[35] Intention to treat analysis did not result in a significant difference between treatment and controls (4 trials; 350 women; OR 1.35; 95% CI 0.89–2.05).

Intravenous Immunoglobulin

Studies using IVIg have used different preparations, doses, starting times, frequency and duration of administration. In addition, differing entry criteria have been used. Some studies included those with an auto-immune disturbance only, whilst others have included those with "unexplained" RM. Hence, at present, the only reasonable basis for assessment of the efficacy of IVIg as a treatment for RM would be to examine the results of meta-analyses. The Cochrane review[35] reports that irrespective of whether analysis is performed on an intention to treat basis (OR 1.18; 95% CI 0.72–1.93) or not (0.98; 0.61–1.58), IVIg does not improve pregnancy outcome amongst women with RM. The results of this analysis are supported by two more recent publications that report, irrespective of the dose of IVIg, the time of administration (prepregnancy, early pregnancy) or whether primary or secondary recurrent miscarriage is examined, IVIg administration is not associated with an increase in the live birth rate.[36,37]

Other Immunomodulators

Other agents have also been used to try to improve the live birth rate in RPL. G-CSF and anti-TNF-α agents are two examples. There is one trial of G-CSF and none on anti-TNF-α agents. Trials have to be performed and evidence needs to accumulate before any other agents can be recommended for routine use.

Conclusion

The lack of scientific rationale for immunotherapy has not stopped its introduction into clinical practice. However, despite the limitations of meta-analyses, the use of either paternal white cell immunization or IVIg as a treatment for RM has not been shown to be of benefit. The use of these immunomodulatory agents should be resisted until adequately powered prospective randomized placebo controlled studies in defined populations of those with a specified immune disturbance have been conducted.

REFERENCES

1. Rai R, Clifford K, Regan L. The modern preventative treatment of recurrent miscarriage. *Br J Obstet Gynaecol* 1996;103:106–10.
2. Rai R, Regan L. Recurrent miscarriage. *Lancet* 2006;368:601–11.
3. Parham P. NK cells and trophoblasts: Partners in pregnancy. *J Exp Med* 2004;200:951–5.
4. Rocklin RE, Kitzmiller JL, Carpenter CB et al. Maternal-fetal relation. Absence of an immunologic blocking factor from the serum of women with chronic abortions. *N Engl J Med* 1976;295:1209–13.
5. Takakuwa K, Kanazawa K, Takeuchi S. Production of blocking antibodies by vaccination with husband's lymphocytes in unexplained recurrent aborters: The role in successful pregnancy. *Am J Reprod Immunol Microbiol* 1986;10:1–9.
6. Beydoun H, Saftlas AF. Association of human leucocyte antigen sharing with recurrent spontaneous abortions. *Tissue Antigens* 2005;65:123–35.
7. Regan L, Braude PR, Hill DP. A prospective study of the incidence, time of appearance and significance of anti-paternal lymphocytotoxic antibodies in human pregnancy. *Hum Reprod* 1991;6:294–8.
8. Peña RB, Cadavid AP, Botero JH et al. The production of MLR-blocking factors after lymphocyte immunotherapy for RSA does not predict the outcome of pregnancy. *Am J Reprod Immunol* 1998;39:120–4.
9. Jablonowska B, Palfi M, Ernerudh J et al. Blocking antibodies in blood from patients with recurrent spontaneous abortion in relation to pregnancy outcome and intravenous immunoglobulin treatment. *Am J Reprod Immunol* 2001;45:226–31.
10. Kwak JY, Gilman-Sachs A, Moretti M et al. Natural killer cell cytotoxicity and paternal lymphocyte immunization in women with recurrent spontaneous abortions. *Am J Reprod Immunol*. 1998;40:352–8.
11. Pross HF, Maroun JA. The standardization of NK cell assays for use in studies of biological response modifiers. *J Immunol Methods* 1984;68:235–49.
12. Plackett TP, Boehmer ED, Faunce DE et al. Aging and innate immune cells. *J Leukoc Biol* 2004;76:291–9.
13. Reichert T, DeBruyere M, Deneys V et al. Lymphocyte subset reference ranges in adult Caucasians. *Clin Immunol Immunopathol* 1991;60:190–208.
14. Porzsolt F, Gaus W, Heimpel H. The evaluation of serial measurements of the NK cell activity in man. *Immunobiology* 1983;165:475–84.

15. Strong DM, Ortaldo JR, Pandolfi F et al. Cryopreservation of human mononuclear cells for quality control in clinical immunology. I. Correlations in recovery of K- and NK-cell functions, surface markers, and morphology. *J Clin Immunol* 1982;2:214–21.

16. Beer AE, Kwak JY, Ruiz JE. Immunophenotypic profiles of peripheral blood lymphocytes in women with recurrent pregnancy losses and in infertile women with multiple failed *in vitro* fertilization cycles. *Am J Reprod Immunol* 1996;35:376–82.

17. Eidukaite A, Siaurys A, Tamosiunas V. Differential expression of KIR/NKAT2 and CD94 molecules on decidual and peripheral blood CD56bright and CD56dim natural killer cell subsets. *Fertil Steril* 2004;81 (Suppl 1):863–8.

18. Shakhar K, Rosenne E, Loewenthal R et al. High NK cell activity in recurrent miscarriage: What are we really measuring? *Hum Reprod* 2006;21:2421–5.

19. Aoki K, Kajiura S, Matsumoto Y et al. Preconceptional natural-killer-cell activity as a predictor of miscarriage. *Lancet* 1995;345(8961):1340–2.

20. Emmer PM, Nelen WL, Steegers EA et al. Peripheral natural killer cytotoxicity and CD56(pos) CD16(pos) cells increase during early pregnancy in women with a history of recurrent spontaneous abortion. *Hum Reprod* 2000;15:1163–9.

21. Fukui A, Fujii S, Yamaguchi E et al. Natural killer cell subpopulations and cytotoxicity for infertile patients undergoing *in vitro* fertilization. *Am J Reprod Immunol* 1999;41:413–22.

22. Ntrivalas EI, Kwak-Kim JY, Gilman-Sachs A et al. Status of peripheral blood natural killer cells in women with recurrent spontaneous abortions and infertility of unknown aetiology. *Hum Reprod* 2001;16:855–61.

23. Putowski L, Darmochwal-Kolarz D, Rolinski J et al. The immunological profile of infertile women after repeated IVF failure (preliminary study). *Eur J Obstet Gynecol Reprod Biol* 2004;112:192–6.

24. Yamada H, Morikawa M, Kato EH et al. Pre-conceptional natural killer cell activity and percentage as predictors of biochemical pregnancy and spontaneous abortion with normal chromosome karyotype. *Am J Reprod Immunol* 2003;50:351–4.

25. Katano K, Suzuki S, Ozaki Y et al. Peripheral natural killer cell activity as a predictor of recurrent pregnancy loss: A large cohort study. *Fertil Steril* 2013;100:1629–34.

26. Mariee N, Tuckerman E, Ali A et al. The observer and cycle-to-cycle variability in the measurement of uterine natural killer cells by immunohistochemistry. *J Reprod Immunol* 2012;95:93–100.

27. Tuckerman E, Laird SM, Prakash A et al. Prognostic value of the measurement of uterine natural killer cells in the endometrium of women with recurrent miscarriage. *Hum Reprod* 2007;22:2208–13.

28. Clifford K, Flanagan AM, Regan L. Endometrial CD56+ natural killer cells in women with recurrent miscarriage: A histomorphometric study. *Hum Reprod* 1999;14:2727–30.

29. Quenby S, Kalumbi C, Bates M et al. Prednisolone reduces preconceptual endometrial natural killer cells in women with recurrent miscarriage. *Fertil Steril* 2005;84:980–4.

30. Colucci F, Boulenouar S, Kieckbusch J et al. How does variability of immune system genes affect placentation? *Placenta* 2011;32:539–45.

31. Roussev RG, Acacio B, Ng SC et al. Duration of intralipid's suppressive effect on NK cell's functional activity. *Am J Reprod Immunol* 2008;60:258–63.

32. Shreeve N, Sadek K. Intralipid therapy for recurrent implantation failure: New hope or false dawn? *J Reprod Immunol* 2012;93:38–40.

33. Clifford K, Rai R, Regan L. Future pregnancy outcome in unexplained recurrent first trimester miscarriage. *Hum Reprod* 1997;12:387–9.

34. Ober C, Karrison T, Odem RR et al. Mononuclear-cell immunisation in prevention of recurrent miscarriages: A randomised trial. *Lancet* 1999;354:365–9.

35. Porter TF, LaCoursiere Y, Scott JR. Immunotherapy for recurrent miscarriage. *Cochrane Database Syst Rev* 2006:CD000112.

36. Ata B, Tan SL, Shehata F et al. A systematic review of intravenous immunoglobulin for treatment of unexplained recurrent miscarriage. *Fertil Steril* 2011;95:1080–5.

37. Stephenson MD, Kutteh WH, Purkiss S et al. Intravenous immunoglobulin and idiopathic secondary recurrent miscarriage: A multicentered randomized placebo-controlled trial. *Hum Reprod* 2010;25:2203–9.

32

Autoimmunity and Recurrent Pregnancy Loss

Sonia Zatti, Andrea Lojacono, and Angela Tincani

Introduction

The aim of this chapter is to review the recent literature on the relationship between autoimmunity and pregnancy losses, whether in the first trimester, presenting as miscarriage, or second or third trimester intrauterine fetal death. Many autoantibodies are associated with reproductive failure but it is often unclear if the antibody is pathognomonic or not. In order to cause pregnancy loss, the autoantibody must react with a placental antigen. Some autoimmune diseases such as systemic lupus erythematosus (SLE), antiphospholipid syndrome (APS), diabetes mellitus, thyroid diseases, Crohn's disease, and other inflammatory bowel diseases have antibodies that are associated with pregnancy losses. In other cases, there may be autoantibodies against all stages of reproduction, but they are unrelated to autoimmune disease. Some of these antibodies have been associated with failure to conceive, such as anti-ovarian antibodies, anti-sperm antibodies, anti-endometrial antibodies, which are found in endometriosis, and anti-zona pellucida antibodies. Other antibodies may attack the trophoblast. Monoclonal antiphospholipid antibody reacts with human trophoblast, releasing apoptotic microparticles. Apoptosis of the cell membrane exteriorizes phospholipids such as phosphatidyl serine on the microparticles. Consequently, antiphospholipid antibodies (aPL) may be raised to phosphatidyl serine. Phosphatidyl ethanolamine is expressed by the trophoblast and may be an antigen for anti-phosphatidyl ethanolamine antibodies. If the trophoblast is the object of autoimmune activity, the fetus will later succumb, presenting as pregnancy loss. At later stages, IgG autoantibodies may cross the placenta and attack the embryo or fetus itself. Anti-Ro antibodies may act on the conducting system of the fetal heart leading to fetal heart block. Anti-laminin and anti-fibronectin antibodies may act against the cytoskeleton of the developing embryo. However, the association with pregnancy loss remains to be elucidated.

A combination of antibodies may be more relevant than one single antibody[1] and autoimmune conditions may be associated with a polyclonal pattern of antibodies rather than a monomorphic presentation.[2] Antiphospholipid antibodies (anticardiolipin, antiBeta2glycoprotein I, antiprothrombin, antiphosphatidylserine, and anytiphosphatidylethanolamine), which are strongly associated with pregnancy loss, are covered elsewhere in this book, and will not be discussed at length here. Many women with pregnancy loss carry several immunological disturbances related to[1] an increased predisposition to breakdown of immunological autotolerance and inflammatory responses and[2] dysregulation of the maternal immune response to specific fetal or trophoblast antigens.[3]

Autoimmune Mechanisms in Pregnancy

The adaptations of the immune responses to pregnancy are described in Chapter 27. Below is a brief outline, with emphasis on the changes occurring in autoimmunity.

Cytokine Balance

Cytokines play an important role in the maintenance of pregnancy by modulating the immune and endocrine systems. A full account of the immunobiology of pregnancy and pregnancy loss is given in

Chapter 27. Briefly, a correct balance between proinflammatory (Th-1) and antiinflammatory cytokines (Th-2) is thought to be essential for the continued development of pregnancy. The trophoblast when stimulated by progesterone produces interleukin (IL)-4 and IL-10 which induce Th0 cells to differentiate into TH2 cells in the decidua. The Th2-derived cytokines, IL-4 and IL-6, induce hCG release by the trophoblast. hCG stimulates the corpus luteum to secrete progesterone.[4] The balance between Th1/Th2 cytokines might be regulated by natural killer (NK) T cells in the decidua. The hormone hCG prevents apoptosis of the corpum luteum, thereby maintaining progesterone production and release of Th2 cytokines in a cytokine mediated cross-talk between the maternal endocrine system, decidua, immune system, and trophoblast.

Women with recurrent miscarriage are thought to produce higher concentrations of Th1 cytokines than parous women. This mechanism is thought to explain why approximately 70% of women with rheumatoid arthritis, which is a TH1 mediated disease, have a temporary remission of symptoms during pregnancy. SLE, however, which is a TH2 mediated disease, tends to relapse.

Natural Killer Cells

The number of endometrial granulated lymphocytes (EGLs) expressing some NK-markers, such as CD56, but not others such as CD16, CD57 increase in the late secretory stage, and account for 70–80% of decidual lymphocytes in the first trimester of pregnancy.[4] Decidual NK cells (uNK) are not cytolytic but produce interferon-γ (IFN-γ), which activates decidual macrophages. uNK cells may have critical functions in pregnancy by promoting appropriate vascularization of the implantation site and affecting placental size.[5] Th2 cytokines may influence uNK cells to prevent them from attacking the trophoblast. Th1 cytokines, however, such as IL-2 and IFN-γ, may induce NK killing activity. If activated, uNK may become cytotoxic and, as peripheral NK cells, attack the pregnancy, presenting as miscarriage.[6]

The preimplantation uNK cell density is higher in women with recurrent miscarriage. It has been reported[7] that IL-6 and IL-8 secretion from decidual uterine NK cells and macrophages, isolated from women with spontaneous miscarriage, is reduced compared to normal controls. IL-6 and IL-8 may play a role in spiral artery remodelling, failure of which may be associated with miscarriage. The proportions of immunosoppressive NK subset (NK3 and NKr1) are suppressed in miscarriages compared to normal pregnancy. Progesterone, prolactin, HCG, and soluble HLA-G1 could contribute to fetal tolerance by inducing the production of immunosoppressive NK subsets.[8]

Toll-Like Receptors (TLRs)

TLRs play a role in determining Th1/Th2 balance: their activation promotes a TH1 dominated immune response and inhibits TH2 cytokine production. Overexpression of TLR3 in the decidua can cause uNK activation and it might be correlated with pregnancy failure. A recent sutdy[9] demonstrated abnormally high TLR3 expression in patients with unexplained recurrent spontaneous miscarriage compared to a control group of healthy patients undergoing elective termination of pregnancy. Decidual NK cells promote immune tolerance and successful pregnancy by dampening inflammatory Th17 cells via IFN-γ secreted by the CD56 bright CD27+ NK subset. This response seems to be lost in patients with RM leading to a prominent Th17 response and extensive local inflammation.[10]

Autoantobodies and NK

A recent study[11] determined that women with reproductive failure who tested positive for autoantibodies (antiphospholipid and thyroid peroxidase antibodies) have the same uNK cells number that women who tested negative for these antibodies, hence the presence of autoantibodies does not to appear to affect the number of uNK cells in the endometrium around the time of implantation. However, increased numbers of NK cells are found in the peripheral blood in APS with pregnancy loss.[12]

Th1/Th2 and Cytokine Genotypes

Some studies suggest that the immunogenetic profile indicative of imbalance of Th2 cytokines is associated with pregnancy loss. Costeas et al.[13] have demonstrated that women with high abortion rates have distinct immunogenetic profiles, different to those in women with successful pregnancies. Additionally, IL-10 promoter gene polymorphisms are pivotal regarding pregnancy maintenance or loss.[7,14,15] Elevated concentration of IFN-γ have been observed in women with recurrent pregnancy loss (RPL), and consequently, the IFN-γ T/T genotype associated with higher IFN-γ production could be a risk factor for RPL.[15]

GM-CSF

Granulocyte-macrophage colony-stimulating factor (GM-CSF) plays an important role in Th1/Th2 balance as it stimulates the production of prostaglandins, tumor necrosis factor (TNF), IL-1, plasminogen activator and IL-6. Perricone et al.[16,17] found that women with RSA have significantly lower levels of GM-CSF.

Alloantibodies

At an early stage of pregnancy, alloantibodies are produced to paternal antigens in response to fetal antigens.[18] Their role in pregnancy maintenance is still unclear. On this basis, Beaman et al.[19] proposed a potential algorithm of assays to be performed to assess cause of recurrent miscarriage of immunological origin.

Autoantibodies

The presence of autoantibodies, such as anticardiolipin antibodies, antinuclear antibodies (ANA), and anti-double strand DNA antibodies, have often been reported in women with pregnancy loss even without overt autoimmune disease. However, these antibodies are also found in women with normal pregnancies.[3,20] In 2006, Shoenfeld et al.[21] published a study on the association between autoantibodies and reproductive failure. The authors assessed a number of autoantibodies in four groups of women: with autoimmune diseases, infertility, RPL, and controls. All patients were tested for the following antibodies: aPL, annexin-V, lactoferrin, thyroglobulin (TGG), thyroid peroxidase, prothrombin, ANA-Hep2, and anti-saccaromycetes cerevisiae (ASCA). The only antibodies found to be significantly higher in RPL patients than controls were ASCA, aPL, and anti-prothrombin antibodies. Anti-prothrombin antibodies and aPL were more prevalent in late pregnancy losses, ASCA antibodies had an equal prevalence in both early and late losses. Anti-prothrombin antibodies were associated with secondary aborter status, but not with primary aborter status. This might indicate that antibodies may be acquired after a first pregnancy, in which after embryonic death and apoptosis of the trophoblast membrane leads to externalization of phospholipids that can bind to prothrombin. ASCA was also associated with RPL in this study. ASCA antibodies can predict Crohn's disease development many years in advance.[22]

Antinuclear Antibodies

ANA positivity is a typical feature of many autoimmune diseases like SLE, but ANA can also be detected in healthy people. The possible role of ANA in reproductive disorders is largely undetermined,[23] and the relationship between ANA and RM remains controversial. However, ANA and antibodies against single- and double-stranded DNA (ssDNA, dsDNA) appear to be increased in about 35% of women with RSA, while their percentage is less than 10% in fertile women with no abortion history. However, Shoenfeld et al.[21] found a significantly increased frequency of ANA positivity only in RM women with autoimmune disease but not in RM women without autoimmune disease compared to controls. Antibodies against histones or non-DNA nuclear components (Sm, RNP, SSA, SSB, Scl70) are also found in some of these women.[24] The presence of ANA has been associated with increased inflammation around the placenta, inducing an environment that does not enhance the "acceptance" of the embryo. In these cases, anti-inflammatory prevention therapy with corticosteroids has been reported, but remains controversial.[25]

Anti-Ro/SSA and Anti-La/SSB

Patients positive for these antibodies have a 1–2% risk of congenital complete heart block (CHB) that can lead to fetal cardiac failure and intrauterine fetal death.[26–28] Some authors stated that this risk is as high as 55% when maternal hypothyroidism is associated to anti-Ro antibodies.[29,30] The Ig G isotype can cross the placenta from about 16 weeks of pregnancy and bind to cardiac cells. The antibodies seem to be responsible for impaired clearance of apoptotic cardiocytes. Once complete fetal heart block develops it is irreversible and leads to significant morbidity and potential mortality for the fetus. In pregnant patients with previous CHB, there is a 16% risk of recurrence. Therapy with fluorinated corticosteroids, such as dexamethasone or betamethasone, does not seem to be effective.[31,32] The recommended treatment for prophylaxis is low-dose intravenous immunoglobulin (IVIg),[33] which has been demonstrated not to be effective in reducing CHB and maternal antibody levels. Recent studies[34,35] have reported that hydroxycloroquine therapy may lower the incidence of cardiac complications in patient with antiRo antibodies.

Autoimmune Diseases

A Danish study published in 2008[36] reported that women with some immunological disorders (SLE, hyper and hypothyroidism, inflammatory bowel disease (IBD) and type 1 diabetes mellitus) have a higher risk of miscarriages. The risk of pregnancy loss increases after a diagnosis of autoimmune disease and this may be related to the breakdown of autotolerance and the predisposition to an increased inflammatory response. High plasma TNF-α levels have been reported to increase the risk of a subsequent miscarriage in women with previous pregnancy losses[37] and the plasma of women with euploid miscarriages have significantly higher levels of pro-inflammatory cytokines (TNF-γ, IFN-γ, and IL-6).[38]

In many autoimmune diseases, a deficiency of mannose binding lectin (MBL) correlates with more rapid progression due to an increased inflammatory response related to impaired clearance of apoptotic cells and immune complexes.[3]

Thyroid Disease: Antithyroid Antibodies

Thyroid autoimmunity (TAI) is the most common autoimmunity affecting 5–20% of normal pregnant women. Thyroid autoantibodies (ATA) have been suggested to be independent markers of "at-risk" pregnancy even with euthyroid status. Although the mechanism whereby ATA affects pregnancy is not known, TAI seems to be related to a Th1-cell-mediated autoimmune reaction. Anti-thyroid antibodies may reflect a predisposition for an underlying autoimmune disease, rather than overt thyroid hormone abnormalities, (as seen in Hashimoto's thyroiditis).[1] Recently, Twig et al.[22] have described that ATA exert their effect in both a thyroid stimulating hormone (TSH)-dependent and TSH-independent manner. The latter involves quantitative and qualitative changes in the profile of endometrial T-cells, which results in the reduced secretion of IL-4 and IL-10 together with the hypersecretion of IFN-γ. The suggestion is supported by the coexistence of ATA with nonorgan specific autoantibodies as well as with the increase and hyperactivity of cytotoxic NK cells in habitual aborters.[39] Hence, it has been suggested that ATA represent a generalized activation of the immune system (possibly a T-lymphocyte dysfunction), as they are found to coexist with activated T-cells in the uterus.[40] Additionally, thyroid autoimmunity frequently occurs concurrently with other autoimmune diseases such as SLE and Sjogren syndrome.[22]

Euthyroid women with TAI before pregnancy may develop overt hypothyroidism during pregnancy because of the increase in thyroid binding globulin (TBG), consequent decrease of FT4 and a compensatory TSH increase due to high estrogen and hCG levels.[17] TSH levels higher than 2.5 mIU/L in the first trimester double the risk of pregnancy loss, but not of preterm delivery, compared to women with lower TSH levels.[30,41] TSH has costimulatory activity for NK cells,[42] Consequently, the high rate of miscarriage may be related to a very mild thyroid "underfunction," in addition to autoimmune mechanisms, with the thyroid gland being less able to adapt to the increased requirements of pregnancy.

Some authors have reported a higher prevalence of anti-thyroid antibodies against either thyroglobulin (TG) or thyroid peroxidase (TPO) in women with miscarriages. Additionally the probability of abortion in women with ATA has been reported to be 10–32% versus 3–16% in controls.[40,43,44] However, other authors[21] have found no association between anti-thyroid antibodies and recurrent pregnancy losses. TGG antibodies also seemed to be more closely related to late pregnancy losses. In 2011, a meta-analysis[45] investigated the presence of anti-TPO and its relation to recurrent miscarriage and preterm birth. The meta-analysis included 30 articles with 31 studies (19 cohort and 12 case-control) involving 12,126 women. The presence of maternal thyroid autoantibodies was strongly associated with miscarriage and preterm delivery. Two randomized studies[44,46] evaluated the effect of treatment with levothyroxine on miscarriage. Both showed a fall in miscarriage rates, and meta-analysis showed a significant 52% relative risk reduction in miscarriages with levothyroxine supplementation (relative risk = 0.48, 0.25–0.92).

If thyroid autoimmunity is the explanation for pregnancy loss, treatment with IVIg, is expected, not only to neutralize the antibodies, but also to provide the required modulation of immune functioning. However, these women also seem to benefit from thyroid replacement therapy,[44] and the effect of thyroid replacement therapy in euthyroid women is greater than the overall effect of IVIg on the live birth rate.[44,45]

Diabetes

Type I diabetes is the result of an autoimmune process on the pancreas islet cells. Fluctuations in glucose levels can induce large variations in insulin levels, and lead to ketosis. Both insulin and ketone have an adverse effect in animal models and may affect human placenta, but the evidence for diabetes increasing the incidence of pregnancy loss is limited to uncontrolled type 1 diabetes in the presence of elevated glycosylated hemoglobin (HbA1C) levels.[47,48] Hence, before the introduction of insulin therapy in type 1 diabetes, successful pregnancy was achieved in only 2% of type 1 diabetic women. Well-controlled diabetes mellitus does not seem to be associated with recurrent pregnancy loss.[49] The goal of therapy in women of childbearing age should be a HbA1C level below 6,1%. Pregnancy planning and preconception tight control of blood sugar levels may reduce the risk of adverse pregnancy outcome.

Inflammatory Bowel Diseases

Inflammatory bowel diseases include Crohn's disease (CD) and ulcerative colitis (UC). Crohn's disease activity at time of conception has been reported to be associated with RPL.[21,50] However, this association has not been confirmed by other studies,[51,52] which identified IBD itself as a risk factor for an adverse pregnancy outcome. It is interesting that anti-saccharomycetes cerevisiae antibodies (ASCA) were found to be associated with recurrent pregnancy loss in Shoenfeld et al.'s[21] series (odds ratio for pregnancy loss 3.9, confidence interval 1.5–10.6). ASCA antibodies are associated with CD and other inflammatory bowel diseases, and can predict the development of CD many years in advance.[53] The clinical significance has not been determined, but it seems prudent that in cases of RPL with IBD, and ASCA antibodies, that the IBD should be in remission before another pregnancy is undertaken.

Other Autoantibodies and Immune Disturbances

Several "non classical" antibodies (directed to prothrombin or thromboplastin or mitochondrial antibodies of M5 type) have been observed in women with recurrent miscarriages, but their clinical significance remains unclear.[54] Another interesting finding in RPL with ANA or ATA is the increased presence of peripheral CD19+/CD5+ cells,[55] which are believed to produce polyvalent antibodies (mainly IgM) that are also directed against hormones (estradiol, progesterone, hCG) and neurotransmitters (endorphins, serotonin), and may be responsible for insufficient decidualization and decrease blood supply to the endometrium, respectively.

Potential Interventions

Many of the medications used for autoimmune diseases have been used to prevent pregnancy loss. Some of these medications are mentioned elsewhere in this book. Possible therapeutic approaches include low dose aspirin, low molecular weight heparin, glucocorticoid, immunoglobulin infusions (IVIg), and use of immunomodulatory drugs.

Aspirin and LMWH

Both aspirin and LMWH are used for patients with antiphospholipid syndrome and possibly unexplained adverse pregnancy outcomes; empirically this therapy was applied to women with unexplained RM.[56] Their role is discussed in APS in Chapter 21. The role of anticogulants in unexplained RPL is discussed in Chapter 25.

Glucocorticoids

Glucocorticosteroids can reduce inflammation and suppress the activity of several types of immune cells including T-cells[57] by inhibiting the transcription regulator NFkB (that promote proinflammatory cytokines as IL1β, IL 6, and TNFα). Prednisolone has been shown to reduce raised endometrial NK cells in women with RM.[58] Nakashima[59] treated patients with miscarriages and high NK cells activity: the patients with normalized NK cells activity after therapy had a lower number of pregnancy losses. In Bansal et al.'s[60] study, steroid therapy was started in the preconceptional period and restricted to early pregnancy in women with non-APS. The authors concluded that steroids may be helpful.[60] In pregnancy, only minute amounts of steroids cross the placenta, due to the expression of 11β-hydroxysteroid dehydrogenase in the placenta that inactivates cortisol.

In the case of autoimmune diseases, steroids may need to be used for the autoimmuine disease. In these cases, steroids are administered for maternal indications alone. However, steroid administration is associated with the same side effects as in nonpregnant women, Additionally, there is some evidence from case control studies, but not from prospective cohort studies, that high doses of steroids if taken in pregnancy, may increase the rate of cleft palate,[61] or of later effects such as reduced fetal growth.

Intravenous Immunoglobulin

IVIg treatment seems to reduce overexpressed Th1 activity and down regulates cytotoxic activity of NK cells[16,63,64] in the peripheral blood. This effect is seen immediately after infusion and it may be long acting for the entire pregnancy. IVIg reduces the cytotoxic activity of NK cells or may also increase circulating GM-CSF levels.[16] IVIg modulates macrophage activation[64] and B-cell function.[65] IVIg is used for numerous autoimmune conditions, such as agammaglobulinemia, immune thrombocytopenia purpura, chronic inflammatory demyelinating polyneuropathy, multiple sclerosis, Kawasaki disease, rheumatoid arthritis, and Guillain–Barré syndrome. If required in pregnancy, the medication can be used. There seem to be no real detrimental effects on the fetus. However, mild adverse events are reported in the mother in 1–15% of patients, these events can be fever, nausea, headache, mild tachycardia, blood pressure changes, etc. Severe adverse effects are rare, but include anaphylactic reactions, hemolytic anemia, viral infections, renal failure, and thrombotic events, but tend to occur in patients with IgA antibodies. The role of IVIg on unexplained pregnancy loss is controversial. Both sides of this controversy are presented in Chapters 28 and 31.

Anti-TNF-α Therapy

Anti-TNF-α therapy is widely used in autoimmune diseases (such as rheumatoid arthritis, SLE, Bechet's syndrome, and IBD). When used in conjunction with IVIg, etanercept or adalimumab have been found to be helpful in improving the live birth rate in women with RM compared with those receiving anticoagulation alone.[66] A recent study evaluated[67] etanercept therapy (four doses of 25 mg twice weekly before conception) for women with recurrent reproductive failure and increased NK-cell activity. NK-cell activity is significantly decreased after therapy, mainly in patients with subsequent pregnancy success but not in those with pregnancy failure.

However, the question of safety of anti-TNF-α in pregnancy has been only partially addressed. A prospective comparative observational study between 2002 and 2011 evaluated 83 anti-TNF-α exposed pregnant patients (35 infliximab, 25 etanercet, 23 adalimubab) versus 341 nonexposed patients. There was no difference in the incidence of congenital anomalies in two groups and no cases of VATER/ VACTERL association.[68] A retrospective multicenter study on IBD patients receiving TNF-α inhibitors reported no increased risk of complications during pregnancy and seemed to be safe for the newborn.[69] A recent meta-analysis including 462 exposed pregnant patients with IBD stated that the short-term risks of anti-TNF-α agents are low, even if the drug crosses the placenta from the end of the second trimester. However, intra uterine exposure may cause an increase in infections in infants and alterations in immune system development. For this reason, some authors suggest stopping anti-TNF-α agents in the second trimester. Certolizumab is derived from the Fab fragment of an anti-TNF monoclonal antibody and therefore can be continued throughout pregnancy. Anti-TNF agents are detected in breast milk, but in minimum doses.[70] However, current guidelines suggest that anti-TNF-α should be avoided in pregnancy until larger trials are conducted.[71,72]

Oral Hypoglycemic Agents

In most cases of diabetes, insulin is used, but recently oral hypoglycemic agents have been increasingly used in pregnancy. Metformin is an effective anti-hyperglycemic agent widely used in the treatment of type 2 diabetes. Metformin reduces hepatic glucose output, increases tissue insulin sensitivity and enhances peripheral glucose uptake; all these mechanisms decrease glucose levels but the risk of hypoglycemia is low because insulin production does not increase. Although metformin crosses the placenta, the umbilical cord concentration at delivery is usually half the level of the mother. The breast milk metformin concentration is low.

Metformin is considered a category B drug. The dose is 1500–2550 mg daily, but in pregnancy metformin clearance is enhanced and in late pregnancy metformin dose may need to be adjusted.

Generally, metformin is well-tolerated; common side effects are gastrointestinal symptoms (diarrhea, nausea, vomiting, adbominal discomfort); lactic acidosis is a very rare complication.

Metformin is also used in women with polycystic ovary syndrome (PCOS), which is characterized by insulin resistance. In PCOS, metformin restores the regularity of the menstrual cycle and enhances conception. A systematic review in 2013[73] reported that metformin is safe for the treatment of gestational diabetes and is more effective in overweight or obese women. In PCOS, metformin reduces the incidence of early pregnancy loss and preterm labor and protects against fetal growth restriction. Moreover, metformin may lead to a more favorable pattern of fat distribution in the newborn reducing long-term metabolic complications. Metformin reduces the incidence of neonatal hypoglycemia and weight gain in the mother.

The use of metformin is not associated with theratogenic effects, intrauterine deaths, or developmental delay, and appears to be safe in pregnancy. However, at present, there are no guidelines for the continuous use of metformin in pregnancy and so the duration of treatment has to be based on clinical experience.

Selenium

Selenium-dependent enzymes have some effects on thyroid function and the immune system.

Selenium deficiency is accompanied by loss of immune competence, affecting both B-cell-mediated immunity and B-cell function. In severe selenium deficiency, the lack of selenium dependent enzyme activity may contribute to oxidative damage of the thyroid cells leading to thyroid damage and fibrosis. Even in mild selenium deficiency, selenium supplementation has an impact on inflammatory activity in thyroid-specific autoimmune disease.[74] Recent studies suggest that selenium supplementation

(200 μg/day) reduces thyroid peroxidase antibody concentrations (TPO).[75] Increased concentrations of anti-thyroid peroxidase antibodies have been associated with RPL. TPO antibody was reduced by 4.3% at 3 months and 12.6% at 6 months in subclinical thyroiditis, and even more so in overt hypothyroidism (21.9% and 20.6% at 3 and 6 months, respectively), mainly in IgG1 and IgG3 subclasses.

Combination treatment with myo-inositol and selenomethionine has been shown to reduce TSH levels in patients with subclinical hypothyroidism due to autoimmune thyroiditis.[76] Myoinositol acts as a TSH second messenger. This reduction was more evident in the group supplemented with myo-inositol compared to the group treated with selenium alone. However, there is no direct evidence that selenium lowers the incidence of pregnancy loss in patients with thyroid autoimmunity.

Vitamin D3

Vitamin D3 has immunoregulatory effects and can downregulate TNFα and IFN γ.[77]

Patients with reduced Th1/Th2 balance have higher vitamin D3 levels; it is possible that vitamin D supplementation in RM women with deficiency might reduce adverse decidual inflammatory cytokines and Th17 cells.[78] Moreover, prevalence of vitamin D3 deficiency is 2.5-fold higher in patients with thyroid autoimmunity and correlates to the presence of thyroid antibodies.[78]

Conclusions

Further studies are required including randomized controlled trials and meta-analyses in order to determine the prevalence of each particular antibody in different type of pregnancy loss and the true incidence of pregnancy loss in the presence of different types or combinations of autoantibodies. Moreover, these studies should be corrected for confounding factors such as maternal age or other causes of miscarriages. The therapies used in autoimmune disease are also changing, constantly requiring new drugs to be assessed in terms of teratogenicity and other potentially harmful effects on mother and fetus.

REFERENCES

1. Marai I, Carp HJA, Shai S et al. Autoantibody panel screening in recurrent miscarriages. *Am J Reprod Immunol* 2004;51:235–40.
2. Gleicher N. Autoantibodies in normal and abnormal pregnancy. *Am J Reprod Immunol* 1992;28:269–73.
3. Christiansen OB. Reproductive immunology. *Mol Immunol* 2013;55:8–15.
4. Saito S. Cytokine network at the feto-maternal interface. *J Reprod Immunol* 2000;47:87–103.
5. Chen SJ, Yung-Liang L, Huey-Kang S. Immunologic regulation in pregnancy: From mechanism to therapeutic strategy for immunomodulation. *Clin Dev Immunol* 2012;2012:258391.
6. Nakamura O. Children's immunology, what can we learn from animal studies (1): Decidual cells induce specific immune system of feto-maternal interface. *J Toxicol Sci* 2009;34(Suppl 2):S331–9.
7. Pitman H, Innes BA, Robson SC et al. Altered expression of interleukin-6, interleukin-8 and their receptors in decidua of women with sporadic miscarriage. *Hum Reprod* 2013;28:2075–86.
8. Nakashima A Shima T, InadaK et al. The balance of the immune system between T cells and NK cells in miscarriages. *Am J Reprod Immunol* 2012;67:304–10.
9. Bao SH, Shuai W, Tong J et al. Increased expression of Toll-like receptor 3 in decidual natural killer cells of patients with unexplained recurrent spontaneous miscarriage. *Eur J Obstet Gynecol Reprod Biol* 2012;165:326–30.
10. Fu B, Li X, Sun R et al. Natural killer cells promote immune tolerance by regulating inflammatory TH17 cells at the human maternal-fetal interface. *Proc Natl Acad Sci U S A* 2012;27:E231–40.
11. Mariee NG, Tuckerman E, Laird S et al. The correlation of autoantibodies and uNK cells in women with reproductive failure. *J Reprod Immunol* 2012;95:59–66.
12. Perricone C, De Carolis C, Giacomelli R et al. High levels of NK cells in the peripheral blood of patients affected with anti-phospholipid syndrome and recurrent spontaneous abortion: A potential new hypothesis. *Rheumatology (Oxford)* 2007;46:1574–8.

13. Costeas PA, Koumouli A, Giantsiou-Kyriakou A et al. Th2/Th3 cytokine genotypes are associated with pregnancy loss. *Hum Immunol* 2004;65:135–41.

14. Prigoshin N, Tambutti M, Larriba J et al. Cytokine gene polymorphisms in recurrent pregnancy loss of unknown cause. *Am J Reprod Immunol* 2004;52:36–41.

15. Daher S, Shulzhenko N, Morgun A et al. Association between cytokine gene polymorphisms and recurrent pregnancy loss. *J Reprod Immunol* 2003;58:69–77.

16. Perricone R, De Carolis C, Giacomelli R et al. GM-CSF and pregnancy: Evidence of significantly reduced blood concentrations in unexplained recurrent abortion efficiently reversed by intravenous immunoglobulin treatment. *Am J Reprod Immunol* 2003;50:232–7.

17. Perricone C, De Carolis C, Perricone R. Pregnancy and autoimmunity: A common problem. *Best Pract Res Clin Rheumatol* 2012;26:47–60.

18. Orgad S, Loewenthal R, Gazit E et al. The prognostic value of anti-paternal antibodies and leukocyte immunizations on the proportion of live births in couples with consecutive recurrent miscarriages. *Hum Reprod* 1999;14:2974–9.

19. Beaman KD, Ntrivalas E, Mallers TM et al. Immune etiology of recurrent pregnancy loss and its diagnosis. *Am J Reprod Immunol* 2012;67:319–25.

20. Nielsen HS, Christiansen OB. Prognostic impact of anticardiolipin antibodies in women with recurrent miscarriage negative for lupus anticoagulant. *Hum Reprod* 2005;20:1720–8.

21. Shoenfeld Y, Carp HJA, Molina V et al. Autoantibodies and prediction of reproductive failure. *Am J Reprod Immunol* 2006;56:337–44.

22. Twig G, Shina A, Amital H et al. Pathogenesis of infertility and recurrent pregnancy loss in thyroid autoimmunity. *J Autoimmun* 2012;38:275–81.

23. Ticconi C, Rotondi F, Veglia M. Antinuclear autoantibodies in women with recurrent pregnancy loss. *Am J Reprod Immunol* 2010;64:384–92.

24. Kaider AS, Kaider BD, Janowicz PB et al. Immunodiagnostic evaluation in women with reproductive failure. *Am J Reprod Immunol* 1999;42:335–46.

25. Kwak JY, Gilman-Sachs A, Beaman KD et al. Reproductive outcome in women with recurrent spontaneous abortions of alloimmune and autoimmune causes: Preconception versus postconception treatment. *Am J Obstet Gynecol* 1992;166:1787–95.

26. Brucato A, Frassi M, Franceschini F et al. Risk of congenital complete heart block in newborns of mothers with anti-Ro/SSA antibodies detected by counterimmunoelectrophoresis: A prospective study of 100 women. *Arthritis Rheum* 2001;44:1832–5.

27. Buyon JP, Ben-Chetrit E, Karp S et al. Acquired congenital heart block: Pattern of maternal antibody response to biochemically defined antigens of the SSa/Ro-SSB/La system in neonatal lupus. *J Clin Invest* 1989;84:627–34.

28. Brucato A, Doria A, Frassi M et al. Pregnancy outcome in 100 women with autoimmune disease and anti-Ro/SSA antibodies: A prospective controlled study. *Lupus* 2002;11:716–21.

29. Vesel S, Mazic U, Blejec T et al. First-degree heart block in the fetus of an anti-SSA/Ro positive mother: Reversal after a short course of dexamethasone treatment. *Arthritis Rheum* 2004;50:2223–6.

30. Spence D, Hornberger L, Hamilton R et al. Increased risk of complete congenital heart block in infants born to women with hypothyroidism and anti-Ro and/or anti-La antibodies. *J Rheumatol* 2006;33:167–70.

31. Friedman DM, Rupel A, Buyon JP. Epidemiology etiology, detection and treatment of autoantibody-associated congenital heart block in neonatal lupus. *Curr Rheumatol Rep* 2007;9:101–8.

32. Breur JM, Visser GH, Kruize AA et al. Treatment of fetal heart block with maternal steroid therapy: Case report and review of the literature. *Ultrasound Obstet Gynecol* 2004;24:467–72.

33. Friedman DM, Llanos C, Izmirly PM et al. Evaluation of fetuses in a study of intravenous immunoglobulin s preventive therapy for congenital heart block: Results of a multi center, prospective,open-label clinical trial. *Arthritis Rheum* 2010;62:1138–46.

34. Izmirly PM, Kim MY, Llanos C et al. Evaluation of the risk of anti-SSA/Ro-SSB/La antibody-associated cardiac manifestations of neonatal lupus in fetuses of mothers with systemic lupus erythematosus exposed to hydroxychloroquine. *Ann Rheum Dis* 2010;69:1827–30.

35. Izmirly PM, Costedoat-Chalumeau N, Pisoni C et al. Maternal use of hydroxycloroquine is associated with a reduced risk of recurrent anti-SSA/Ro associated cardiac manifestations of neonatal lupus. *Circulation* 2012;126:76–82.

36. Christiansen OB, Steffensen R, Nielsen HS et al. Multifactorial etiology of recurrent miscarriage and its scientific and clinical implications. *Gynecol Obstet Invest* 2008;66:257–67.

37. Mueller-Eckhardt G, Mallman P, Neppert J et al. Immunogenetic and serological investigations in non-pregnant and in pregnant women with a history of recurrent spontaneous abortions. German RSA/IVIG Group. *J Reprod Immunol* 1994;27:95–109.

38. Calleja-Agius J, Jauniaux E, Pizzey AR et al. Investigation of systemic inflammatory response in first trimester pregnancy failure. *Hum Reprod* 2012;27:349–57.

39. Beer AE, Kwak JY, Ruiz JE. Immunophenotypic profiles of peripheral blood lymphocytes in women with recurrent pregnancy losses and in infertile women with multiple failed *in vitro* fertilization cycles. *Am J Reprod Immunol* 1996;35:376–82.

40. Stagnaro-Green A, Roman SH, Cobin RH et al. Detection of at-risk pregnancy by means of highly sensitive assays for thyroid autoantibodies. *JAMA* 1990;264:1422–5.

41. Negro R, Schwartz A, Gismondi R et al. Increased pregnancy loss rate in thyroid antibody negative women with TSH level between 2,5 and 5,0 in the first trimester of pregnancy. *J Clin Endoc Metab* 2010;95:E44–8.

42. Provinciali M, Di Stefano G, Fabris N. Improvement in the proliferative capacity and natural killer cell activity of murine spleen lymphocytes by thyrotropin. *Int J Immunopharmacol* 1992;14:865–70.

43. Pratt DE, Kaberlein G, Dudkiewicz A et al. The association of antithyroid antibodies in euthyroid nonpregnant women with recurrent first trimester abortions in the next pregnancy. *Fertil Steril* 1993;60:1001–5.

44. Vaquero E, Lazzarin N, De Carolis C et al. Mild thyroid abnormalities and recurrent spontaneous abortion: Diagnostic and therapeutical approach. *Am J Reprod Immunol* 2000;43:204–8.

45. Thangaratinam S, Tan A, Knox E et al. Association between thyroid antibodies and miscarriage and preterm birth: Meta-analysis of evidence. *Br Med J* 2011;342:2616.

46. Budenhofer BK, Ditsch N, Jerschke U et al. Thyroid (dys-)function in normal and disturbed pregnancy. *Arch Gynecol Obstet* 2013;287:1–7.

47. Carp HJA, Selmi C, Shoenfeld Y. The autoimmune bases of infertility and pregnancy loss. *J Autoimmun* 2012;38:266–74.

48. Gutaj P, Zawiejska A, Wender-Ozegowka E et al. Maternal factors predictive of first-trimester pregnancy loss in women with pregestational diabetes. *Pol Arch Med Wewn* 2013;123:21–7.

49. Clifford K, Rai R, Watson H et al. An informative protocol for the investigation of recurrent miscarriage: Preliminary experience of 500 consecutive cases. *Hum Reprod* 1994;9:1328–32.

50. Morales M, Berney T, Jenny A et al. Crohn's disease as a risk factor for the outcome of pregnancy. *Hepatogastroenterology* 2000;47:1595–98.

51. Naganuma M, Kunisaki R, Yoshimura N et al. Conception and pregnancy outcome in women with inflammatory bowel disease: A multicentre study from Japan. *J Crohns Colitis* 2011;5:317–23.

52. Mahadevan U, Sandborn WJ, Li D et al. Pregnancy outcomes in women with inflammatory bowel disease: A large community-based study from Northern Carolina. *Gastroenterology* 2007;133:1106–12.

53. Israeli E, Grotto I, Gilburd B et al, Anti-saccharomyces cerevisiae and antineutrophil cytoplasmic antibodies as predictors of inflammatory bowel disease. *Gut* 2005;54:1232–6.

54. Sherer Y, Tartakover-Matalon S, Blank M et al. Multiple autoantibodies associated with autoimmune reproductive failure. *J Assist Reprod Genet* 2003;20:53–7.

55. Beer AE, Kwak JYH, Gilman-Sacks A et al. New horizons in the evaluation and treatment of recurrent pregnancy loss. In: Hunt JS, ed. *Immunobiology of Reproduction*. New York: Serono Symposia USA, 1994. p. 316–34.

56. Branch DW, Gibson M, Silver R. Recurrent mmiscarriage. *New Engl J Med* 2010;363:1740–7.

57. Novac N, Baus D, Dostert A. Competition between glucocorticoid receptor and NFkappaB for control of the human FasL promoter. *FASEB J* 2006;20:1074–81.

58. Quenby S, Kalumbi C, Bates M et al. Prednisolone reduces preconceptual endometrial natural killer cells in women with recurent miscarriage. *Fertil Steril* 2005;84:980–4.

59. Nakashima A, Shima T, Inada K et al. The balance of the immune system between T cells and NK cells in miscarriage. *Am J Reprod Immunol* 2012;67:304–10.

60. Bansal AS, Bajardeen B, Thum MY. The basis and value of currently used immunomodulatory therapies in recurrent miscarriage. *J Reprod Immunol* 2012;93:41–51.

61. Gur C, Diav-Citrin O, Shechtman S et al. Pregnancy outcome after first trimester exposure to corticosteroids: A prospective controlled study. *Reprod Toxicol* 2004; 18:93–101.
62. Yamada H, Morikawa M, Furuta I et al. Intravenous immunoglobulin treatment in women with recurrent abortion: Increased cytokine levels and reduced Th1/Th2 lymphocyte ratio in peripheral blood. *Am J Reprod Immunol* 2003;49:84–9.
63. Kwak JY, Kwak FM, Gilman-Sach et al. Immunoglobulin G infusion treatment for women with recurrent spontaneous abortion and elevated CD56+ natural killer cells. *Early Pregnancy* 2000;4:154–64.
64. Ballow M. The IgG molecule as a biological immune response modifier: Mechanisms of action of intravenous immune serum globulin in autoimmune and inflammatory disorders. *J Allergy Clin Immunol* 2011;127:315–23.
65. Jordan SC, Toyoda M, Vo AA et al. Regulation of immunity and inflammation by intravenous immunoglobulin: Relevance to solid organ transplantation. *Exp Rev Clin Immunol* 2011;7:341–8.
66. Winger EE, Reed JL. Treatment with tumor necrosis factor inhibitors and intravenous immunoglobulin improve live birth rates in women with recurrent spontaneous abortion. *Am J Reprod Immunol* 2008;60:8–16.
67. Jerzak M, Ohams M, Gorski A et al. Etanercept immunotherapy in women with a history of recurrent reproductive failure. *Ginekol Pol* 2012;83:260–4.
68. Diav-Citrin O, Otcheretianski-Volodarsky A, Shechtman S et al. Pregnancy out come following gestational exposure to TNF-alpha-inhibitors. A prospective, comparative observational study. *Reprod Toxicol* 2013;24;43:C78–84.
69. Casanova MJ, Chaparro M, Domenech E et al. Safety of thiopurtines and anti TNFalpha drugs during pregnancy in patients with inflammatory bowel diseases. *Am J Gastroenterology* 2013;108:433–40.
70. Gisbert JP, Chaparro M. Safety of antiTNF agents during pregnancy and breastfeeding in women with inflammatory bowel disease. *Am J Gastroenterol* 2013;108:1426–38.
71. Roux CH, Brocq O, Breuil V et al. Pregnancies in rheumatic patients exposed to anti-tumor necrosis factor (TNF)-alpha therapy. *Rheumatology (Oxford)* 2007;46:695–8.
72. Verstappen SM, King Y, Watson KD et al. Anti-TNF therapies and pregnancy: Outcome of 130 pregnancies in the British Society for Rheumatology Biologics Register. *Ann Rheum Disease* 2011;70:823–26.
73. Lautatzis ME, Goulis DG, Vrontakis M. Efficacy and safety of metformin during pregnancy in women with gestational diabetes mellitus or polycystic ovary syndrome: A systematic review. *Metabolism* 2013;62:1522–34.
74. Gartner R, Gasnier BC, Dietrich JW et al. Selenium supplementation in patients with autoimmune-thyroiditis decreases thyroid peroxidase antibodies concentrations. *J Clin Endocrinol Metab* 2002; 87:1687–91.
75. Zhu L, Bai X, Teng WP et al. Effects of selenium supplementation on antibodies of autoimmune thyroiditis. *Zhounghua Yi Xue Za Zhi* 2012;92:2256–60. [In Chinese].
76. Nordio M, Pajalich R. Combined treatment with Myo-inositol and selenium ensures euthyroidism in subclinical hypothyroidism patients with autoimmune thyroiditis. *J Thyroid Res* 2013;2013:424163.
77. Bubanovic I. 1Alpha, 25-dihydroxy-vitamin-D3 as a new immunotherapy in treatment of recurrent spontaneous abortion. *Med Hypotheses* 2004;63:250–3.
78. Kivity S, Agmon-Levin N, Zisappi M et al. Vitamin D and autoimmune thyroid diseases. *Cell Mol Immunol* 2011;8:243–7.

33

Infections and Recurrent Pregnancy Loss

David Alan Viniker

Introduction

Any acute severe infection can be associated with occasional pregnancy loss. The role of infection in recurrent miscarriage is unclear.[1] In recent years there has been increasing interest in micro-organisms as possible causes of pathology in previously unexplained medical conditions.[2]

In this chapter, the relationship between infection and recurrent pregnancy loss is presented. Specific infections are reviewed, and the recent developments in molecular biology are discussed as they relate to future investigation.

Tuberculosis

Tuberculosis is a significant contributor to maternal mortality and is among the three leading causes of death among women aged 15–45 years in some poor and vulnerable areas. It may be associated with HIV infection. Diagnosis of tuberculosis in pregnancy may be challenging, as some symptoms may be ascribed to pregnancy with the normal weight gain in pregnancy temporarily masking the associated weight loss. Obstetric complications include occasional spontaneous abortion, placental insufficiency, preterm labor, and increased neonatal mortality.

Tuberculosis, is more commonly related to infertility than abortion, with only sporadic reports of pregnancy loss.[3,4] Saracoglu and colleagues[3] diagnosed 72 patients with pelvic tuberculosis from 1979 to 1989. The most common presentations were infertility (47.2%) pelvic or abdominal pain (32%), and abnormal bleeding (11%). There was one case of recurrent miscarriage. Physical examination was normal in 32% of the patients and chest X-ray was normal in 81%. The most common site of infection was the fallopian tubes with occlusion in 32 of the 34 patients having hysterosalpingography.

In a series of 25 cases of genital tuberculosis, 21 presented with infertility, three had postmenopausal bleeding and one was admitted with an acute abdomen.[4] Two women subsequently conceived but both aborted.

Listeria and other Intracellular Bacteria

Listeria is frequently found in processed and prepared foods and listeriosis is associated with high morbidity and death. Preventative measures are recommended, while monitoring and voluntary recall of contaminated items has effectively led to a 44% decrease in the prevalence of perinatal listeriosis in the USA.[5] Romana et al.[6] have put forward the case that latent listeriosis may cause recurrent miscarriage, as antilisteric antibodies have been detected by direct immunofluorescence studies. Romana et al.[6] investigated 309 women and found that 207 had a total of 334 miscarriages, 67 delivered prematurely, 75 had stillbirths, and 43 had malformed living or stillborn infants. Treatment resulted in the birth of 152 normal babies, all negative on immunofluorescence for antilisteric antibodies. Manganiello and Yearke[7] attempted to isolate *Listeria monocytogenes* from the cervix and endometrium of patients presenting with a history of two or more fetal losses. Endometrial tissue and endocervical swabs were cultured. During a 10-year study period, none of the patients with recurrent fetal loss were found to harbor the organism in their genital tract. Hence, *L. monocytogenes* could account for occasional fetal loss but not on a recurring basis. Manganiello and Yearke[7] concluded that routinely culturing for *L. monocytogenes* in patients with recurrent miscarriage is not warranted.

Pregnancy loss with *L. monocytogenes* may be related to interference with the immune tolerance to the fetus in pregnancy.[8]

Intracellular bacteria such as *L. monocytogenes*, *Brucella abortus* and various members of the order Chlamydiales, that grow either poorly or not at all on media used routinely to detect human pathogens could be the etiological agents of these obstetric conditions. There is growing evidence that *Chlamydia trachomatis*, *Chlamydia abortus*, and *Chlamydia pneumoniae* infections may also result in adverse pregnancy outcomes in humans. Moreover, newly discovered Chlamydia-like organisms are emerging as new pathogens in humans. For example, *Waddlia chondrophila*, a Chlamydia-related bacterium isolated from aborted bovine fetuses, has been implicated in human miscarriages. Future research should help us to better understand the pathophysiology of adverse pregnancy outcomes caused by intracellular bacteria and to determine the precise mode of transmission of newly identified bacteria, such as Waddlia and Parachlamydia. These emerging pathogens may represent the tip of the iceberg of a large number of as yet unknown intracellular pathogenic agents.[9] There relationship to recurrent pregnancy loss is unknown.

Torch Infections

There have been conflicting opinions on the role of cytomegalovirus (CMV) in recurrent miscarriage. Szkaradkiewicz and coworkers[10] found significantly elevated IgG in most of 11 women on the first day after a second consecutive trimester miscarriage. The control group were 15 women in the second trimester of a normal pregnancy. They concluded that in the majority of the studied women reactivation of chronic CMV infection occurred. Cook and colleagues[11] used the polymerase chain reaction (PCR) to detect CMV in gestational tissue of women with recurrent miscarriage. DNA was extracted from 25 samples of gestational tissue from 21 women with at least three unexplained spontaneous miscarriages. None of these specimens contained evidence of CMV DNA demonstrating that CMV is not a common direct cause of recurrent miscarriage.

In a prospective study of 280 women an analysis for IgG and IgM anti-toxoplasma was carried out. There was no evidence that toxoplasmosis has a role in recurrent abortion.[12]

Screening for TORCH infections (toxoplasmosis, rubella, cytomegalovirus, and herpes simplex virus) is unhelpful in the investigation of recurrent miscarriage. Whilst these infections can be associated with an individual pregnancy loss, they are illnesses generally contracted once, and therefore, should not result in recurrent pregnancy loss. The current recommendation is that TORCH screening in the investigation of recurrent miscarriage should be abandoned.[1]

Chlamydia

Mezinova et al.[13] have reported that chlamydia was found in 41.7% of 163 women with habitual miscarriage in their series. The miscarriage rate was 59.1% in the presence of chlamydia. However, all women treated for chlamydia infection went on to deliver at term. It was concluded that women with habitual miscarriage and chlamydia should receive appropriate therapy. Endometrial, endocervical, and urethral specimens have been obtained from 16 nonpregnant women with a history of recurrent miscarriage.[14] Chlamydia was isolated from the endometria of five women. No chlamydia were isolated from the cervix or urethra of two patients with proven endometrial involvement. This study demonstrated that eradicating intrauterine chlamydia infection before pregnancy improved pregnancy outcome in women with recurrent miscarriage. It was suggested that asymptomatic chlamydial infection might have an adverse effect on placentation.

An association between positive chlamydia serology and recurrent miscarriage has been reported by Kishore et al.[15] After excluding rhesus incompatibility, anatomical, endocrine, and chromosome abnormalities, serum anti-Chlamydia trachomatis IgM positivity was found in 46.5% of 47 patients with recurrent miscarriages compared to 13.8% of 29 age matched controls of normal pregnant women ($p < 0.001$). The prevalence of high titer IgG antibodies to *C. trachomatis* has been shown to be higher in recurrent miscarriage.[16] Seven (41%) of 17 women with three miscarriages and six (60%) of ten women with four miscarriages had chlamydial antibodies compared to 20 (14%) of 148 women with no miscarriages, six (13%) of 47 women with one miscarriage and four (12%) of 33 women with two miscarriages.[16] The incidence of three or more miscarriages was 31.8% for women with high titer IgG compared to 7.5% among women who were seronegative ($p < 0.001$). The association between high titer IgG to *C. trachomatis* and recurrent miscarriage may involve reactivation of latent chlamydia infection, endometrial damage from previous infection or an immune response to an epitope shared by chlamydial and fetal antigens.[16]

However, not all studies concur. Olliaro et al.[17] found no association between chlamydia and RPL in a study of 101 women with recurrent miscarriage.[7] Screening involved direct examination, culture and serological testing. The culture-positive and serology positive rates of 15% and 35% did not differ from other unselected populations. The time from last miscarriage or type of miscarriage was unrelated to *C. trachomatis* infection. The unselected population rates for chlamydia in this study were noticeably higher than generally expected. Others have also failed to find an association between IgG chlamydia antibodies and recurrent miscarriage.[18–20] Rae and colleagues[18] looked at IgG to chlamydia in 106 women with unexplained recurrent miscarriage and compared their findings with sera from a general antenatal population of 3890. Twenty-six (24.5%) women with recurrent miscarriage had positive serology compared with 788 (20.3%) controls. Chlamydial antibody seropositivity did not correlate with subsequent pregnancy outcome.

In a prospective study,[19] 70 patients with recurrent pregnancy loss attending a specialist recurrent miscarriage clinic were compared to 40 controls (40 normally pregnant women) and 94 asymptomatic sexually active women. There was no statistical difference in the frequencies of chlamydia IgG or IgA antibodies. In another study[20] of 504 patients with a history of two or more consecutive first trimester miscarriages, the presence of IgA and IgG antibodies to *C. trachomatis* did not influence subsequent pregnancy outcome.

There does not appear to be robust evidence to support serological investigations for chlamydia as part of the routine investigation of recurrent miscarriage but direct swab tests from the cervix may be taken and positive results treated appropriately.

Syphilis

In some parts of Africa, the incidence of syphilis seroreactivity in pregnant women is at least 10% and this is associated with spontaneous abortion, perinatal mortality, or a viable infant with congenital syphilis.[21] Screening for syphilis should be considered in at risk populations.

Bacterial Vaginosis

In women of reproductive age, lactobacilli are normally the predominant bacteria in the vagina. Lactobacilli are responsible for reducing the vaginal pH by metabolizing glycogen from squamous cells to lactic acid. The resulting acidic milieu provides protection against infection. Bacterial vaginosis (BV) has become the adopted nomenclature to describe a clinical condition characterized by an overgrowth of predominantly anaerobic bacteria within the vagina and a concomitant reduction or absence of lactobacilli. BV is recognized as the most common cause of vaginal discharge. Women may have symptoms of a characteristic vaginal discharge but are often asymptomatic. The discharge tends to be malodorous particularly after sexual intercourse. A remarkable feature of BV is the absence of a host reaction; thus, the suffix "osis" rather than "itis" as signs of inflammation are absent. In Gram-stained smears of the vaginal fluid, BV is diagnosed when three out of four of Amsel's criteria[22] are present, that is, the presence of clue cells—vaginal epithelial cells heavily coated with bacilli on wet preparation microscopy; vaginal pH greater than 4.5; a homogenous discharge; a strong fishy odor, which may be amplified on adding alkali to vaginal fluid. The organisms most often associated with BV are *Gardnerella vaginalis*, *Mycoplasma hominis*, *Ureaplasma urealyticum*, *Mobiluncus spp*, *Prevotella*, Porphyromonas, *Bacteroides* and *Peptostreptococcus spp.* It has been suggested that the clinical manifestations of BV depends on a synergistic interaction of a variety of micro-organisms. The Gram-negative organisms, including *Bacteroides*, are sensitive to metronidazole, whereas *Mycoplasma*, *Ureaplasma* and *Mobiluncus* are sensitive to macrolides such as erythromycin, and to the tetracyclines.

Seven hundred forty-nine consecutive women undergoing *in vitro* fertilization had a vaginal smear taken at the time of egg collection in a study comparing the prevalence of BV according to causation of infertility.[23] The smears were Gram-stained and graded as normal, intermediate or BV. The smears were normal in 63.6%, intermediate in 12.1% and BV in 24.3%. The rates of BV were 36.4% in tubal factor, 15.6% in male factor, 33.3% in anovulation, 12.5% in endometriosis, and 18.9% in unexplained infertility. Women with tubal infertility were three times more likely to have BV than women with male factor infertility, endometriosis, or unexplained infertility. Women with anovulation were also three times more likely to have BV compared to women with endometriosis or male factor infertility, which the authors suggested supports the theory that there is a hormonal influence on vaginal flora.

The lack of an animal model has made study of BV difficult and inhibited a full understanding of the etiology of the condition.[24] Recent research with murine rodents,[25,26] however, suggests that animal models can be used. In time, this may clarify our understanding of the relative contributions of several factors to the etiology of BV, which is central to the development of effective treatments and prophylaxis of this condition.

The detrimental effects on pregnancy, associated with BV, may be due to the bacteria ascending into the uterus.[27,28] One hypothesis suggests that micro-organisms, possibly those associated with BV, may surreptitiously inhabit the uterine cavity (bacteria endometrialis) where they are responsible for some common gynecological and obstetric enigmas.[28] Relatively little has been written about bacterial colonization of the endometrial cavity. The bacteriological investigation of the vagina and endometrial cavity are compared in Table 33.1. The healthy vagina is rich in micro-organisms, whereas the endometrial cavity is considered to be relatively sterile. Many micro-organisms colonize the vagina without necessarily being pathogenic. High vaginal swabs are frequently obtained in routine clinical practice, whereas the bacteriology of the endometrium has been studied almost entirely in research projects. The bacteriological diagnosis of BV is dependent on microscopic assessment of a wet preparation of the discharge or a Gram-stain rather than culture whereas investigation of the uterine cavity has depended on culture alone. The clinical significance of the varied patterns of bacteria found in the vagina remains controversial.

Our knowledge about intra-uterine micro-organisms is comparatively sparse and more difficult to interpret. Pathogenic micro-organisms can be found in the endometrial cavity without evidence of pelvic infection being visible at laparoscopy and with negative cervical cultures.[29] The bacteriology of the endometrial cavity has been investigated[30] immediately after a hysterectomy in 99 women. Nearly a quarter of all the patients in Moller et al.'s[30] study harbored one or more micro-organisms in the

TABLE 33.1

A Comparison of the Bacteriology of the Vagina and Uterine Cavity

Vagina	Uterine Cavity
Rich in micro-organisms	Relatively sterile
High vaginal swabs: routine clinical investigation	Sampling mainly confined to research centers
Bacterial vaginosis: diagnosis by microscopy of wet preparation or Gram-stain	Wet preparations and Gram-stain not studied
Culture unhelpful for bacterial vaginosis diagnosis	Cultures only. Specialist centers required for *Mycoplasma hominis* and *Ureaplasma urealyticum*
Possible marker for bacteria endometrialis	Micro-organisms can be present even with negative cervical cultures
Bacterial vaginosis: no clinical inflammation	Micro-organisms can occur with negative clinical examination

uterus, mostly *G. vaginalis*, *Enterobacter* or *Streptococcus agalactiae*. The samples were not tested for *Mycoplasmas* or *Mobiluncus*.

The brown rat and house mouse are two species of Muridae that are being increasingly used for medical research. Vaginal infection by a BV associated bacterium in an animal has been shown to parallel the human disease with regard to clinical diagnostic features.[26] Although *Gardnerella vaginalis* is frequently isolated in BV, there has been debate concerning the contribution of *G. vaginalis* to the etiology of BV, as it is also present in many healthy women. A new murine vaginal infection model with a clinical isolate of *G. vaginalis* has demonstrated that this model displays features used clinically to diagnose BV, including the presence of sialidase activity and exfoliated epithelial cells with adherent bacteria reminiscent of clue cells. *G. vaginalis* was capable of ascending uterine infection, which correlated with the degree of vaginal infection and level of vaginal sialidase activity. The results of this study suggest that *G. vaginalis* is sufficient to cause BV phenotypes and suggest that this organism may contribute to BV etiology and associated complications. The authors commented that this is the first time vaginal infection by a BV associated bacterium in an animal has been shown to parallel the human disease with regard to clinical diagnostic features. They predict that future studies with this model should facilitate investigation of important questions regarding BV etiology, pathogenesis, and associated complications.

The prevalence of BV in pregnancy varies from 9 to 23%.[31] Coitus during pregnancy is not related to BV or premature delivery. Pregnant women do not commonly develop BV after 16 weeks gestation. If present at 16 weeks, it spontaneously remits in approximately 30–50% of those reaching term.[32,33]

Premature Delivery

There is substantial evidence indicating that BV is associated with premature delivery.[31,34–40] The association with premature delivery may have implications for miscarriage, and raise the possibility that antibiotics may reduce the incidence of premature delivery. BV diagnosed in early pregnancy is particularly significant,[34] as the presence of BV in early pregnancy is associated with a two to threefold increased risk of preterm labor. Women who have abnormal vaginal flora that spontaneously returns to normal and who are not treated have as many abnormal outcomes as those treated with placebo, suggesting that the damage occurs in early pregnancy[35] or that the responsible micro-organisms have ascended into the uterine cavity.[28] In this context, it is disappointing that a study of interconceptional antibiotics to prevent preterm birth found that neither endometrial microbial colonization nor plasma cell endometritis were risk factors for adverse pregnancy outcome.[41]

In order to determine whether abnormal vaginal microflora is associated with premature labor, a study was conducted by McDonald et al.[36] in Australia. The assessment included cultures for aerobic and anaerobic bacteria, yeasts, genital mycoplasmas, and *G. vaginalis*. The results of 428 women in preterm labor were compared to 568 women in labor at term. Two distinct bacteriological groupings were associated with preterm labor, namely the BV group of organisms and a group of enteropharyngeal organisms. *G vaginalis* was found in 12% of women in preterm labor compared to 6% at term. The prevalence of *G. vaginalis* was even higher (17%) in women in preterm labor at less than 34 weeks of gestation. In an analysis of 12,937 women screened for BV, the odds ratio for preterm birth (<37 weeks of gestation) for asymptomatic BV-positive versus BV-negative women ranged from 1.1 to 1.6 and did not vary significantly with the gestational age at the time of screening.[37]

Vaginal fluid was collected for Gram-staining from 354 women in preterm labor with intact membranes between 24 and 34 weeks gestation in a prospective blinded study in Paris.[42] Normal flora was found in 254 of the 354 women tested (72.3%). Intermediate changes were found in 76 (21.7%) and BV in 24 (6.8%). Women with normal, intermediate and abnormal flora had 27 (10.6%), 14 (18.4%) and six (25.0%) births before 33 weeks, respectively. A history of spontaneous miscarriage after 14 weeks was the only risk factor associated with BV. Preterm delivery before 33 weeks was significantly associated with the flora grade ($p = 0.02$). It was concluded that the prevalence of BV and its association with preterm delivery are variable and should be interpreted differently for different populations. Although an association was found between BV and delivery before 33 weeks, the authors considered the predictive value of BV to be disappointing and the usefulness of testing for BV in women with premature labor was not demonstrated.

Unselected women with low-risk pregnancies attending the prenatal unit of a general hospital in Belgium were included in a study aimed to investigate the differential influences of abnormal vaginal flora, full and partial bacterial vaginosis, and aerobic vaginitis in the first trimester on preterm birth rate.[40] At the first prenatal visit, 1026 women were invited to undergo sampling of the vaginal fluid for wet mount microscopy and culture. Women without abnormalities of the vaginal flora in the first trimester had a 75% lower risk of delivery before 35 weeks compared with women with abnormal vaginal flora. In women with BV, partial BV had a detrimental effect on the risk of preterm birth for all gestational ages, but interestingly full BV did not. Preterm deliveries later than 24 + 6 weeks were more frequent when *M. hominis* was present. The authors commented that as metronidazole effectively treats full BV, but is ineffective against other forms of abnormal vaginal flora, their data may help to explain why its use to prevent preterm birth has not been successful in most studies.

Treatment and Premature Delivery

Effect of Antibiotics When BV Is an Incidental Finding

The effect of both metronidazole and clindamycin has been assessed on premature labor in randomized placebo studies and meta-analyses in low risk patients in whom BV was an incidental finding. McDonald et al.[43] reported a trial of metronidazole in women with a heavy growth of *G. vaginalis* or a Gram-stain indicative of BV at 19 weeks in 879 women. Metronidazole was administered at 24 weeks and at 29 weeks if *G. vaginalis* persisted. There was no difference in overall preterm births between metronidazole and placebo groups. In a subset of 46 women with a previous preterm birth metronidazole showed a significant reduction in spontaneous preterm birth 2/22 (9.1%) versus 10/24 (41.7%) in placebo treated patients. In this study antibiotics were most effective when there was a history of previous premature labor.

In Camargo et al.'s study of 785 low-risk Brazilian pregnant women,[44] 134 women with BV were treated with metronidazole, tinidazole, or secnidazole. Seventy-one women with BV received no treatment. Premature delivery occurred in 5.5% of the women without BV, 22.5% in women with untreated BV and 3.7% in treated women. Perinatal complications were significantly higher in those women with untreated BV. The risk ratios for premature rupture of the membranes was 7.5, preterm labor 3.4, preterm birth 6.0, and low birth weight 4.2.

Mothers with singleton pregnancies and no history of preterm delivery in whom BV was diagnosed by Gram-stain at 12 weeks gestation were randomized to receive vaginal clindamycin or placebo in Kurkinen-Raty et al.'s[45] study of 101 women with BV. Seventeen of 51 (33%) women were cured after clindamycin treatment compared to 17 out of 50 (34%) of the placebo treated group. The failure rate of clindamycin to cure BV was particularly high in this study. The preterm birth rate was 13.7% (7/51) in the clindamycin treated patients and 6.0% (3/50) in the placebo group. Premature delivery occurred in 20.7% (6/29) in those whom BV persisted compared to 0% (0/26) where BV was successfully treated. Hence, it is not sufficient to treat BV, but the bacteria must be eradicated.

Intravaginal clindamycin was also assessed by Rosenstein and colleagues.[35] Thirty-four women had normal vaginal flora at their first antenatal clinic visit, compared to 268 women who had abnormal vaginal flora. Follow up assessed for pregnancy outcome, vaginal flora and detection of *M. hominis* and *U. urealyticum* after treatment. There were no significantly different outcomes in pregnancy between treated and placebo groups. Women with grade III flora responded better to clindamycin than women with grade II flora by number of abnormal outcomes ($p = 0.03$) and return to normal vaginal flora. Women whose abnormal vaginal flora had spontaneously returned to normal and who were, therefore, not treated had as many abnormal outcomes as those receiving placebo, suggesting that damage by abnormal bacterial species occurred early in pregnancy.

The results of Lamont et al.'s[38] study do not concur with those of Kurkinen-Raty et al.[45] or Rosenstein et al.[35] In Lamont et al.'s[38] randomized, double blind study, 409 women, with abnormal genital tract flora on Gram-stain at 13–20 weeks of gestation, received clindamycin vaginal cream or placebo. Those who still had abnormal vaginal flora 3 weeks later received a subsequent course of the original treatment. There was a statistically significant reduction in the incidence of preterm birth in the clindamycin group (4%) compared with placebo (10%) ($p < 0.03$). It was concluded that clindamycin vaginal cream administered to women with abnormal vaginal flora before 20 weeks of gestation can decrease preterm birth by 60% and reduce the need for neonatal intensive care.

Antibiotics for treating bacterial vaginosis in pregnancy have been reviewed by Brocklehurst et al.[46] Randomized trials comparing antibiotic treatment with placebo or no treatment, or comparing two or more antibiotic regimens in pregnant women whether symptomatic or asymptomatic with bacterial vaginosis or intermediate vaginal flora and detected through screening. Twenty-one good quality trials were included involving 7847 women. Antibiotics were effective at eradicating bacterial vaginosis during pregnancy and reduced the risk of late miscarriage. Antibiotics did not reduce the risk of delivery before 37 weeks or the risk of preterm premature rupture of the membranes. In women with a previous preterm birth antibiotics did not alter the risk of another preterm birth. Treatment of women with abnormal vaginal flora may reduce the risk of delivery before 37 weeks. There were no useful differences between oral or vaginal delivery of antibiotics. The authors concluded that although bacterial vaginosis can be effectively treated with antibiotics, there was little evidence that treating all women with BV will prevent preterm birth.

Three meta-analyses have evaluated the potential benefit of treating BV in pregnancy. Brocklehurst et al.'s[46] meta-analysis, included 1504 women. Antibiotics were highly effective in eradicating infection. The effect of treating BV resulted in a trend to fewer births before 37 weeks of gestation, which was most marked in women with a previous preterm birth.

In Guise et al.'s[31] original meta-analysis, seven randomized controlled trials of BV treatment were included. BV treatment was found to be of no benefit for the average-risk woman. In women with previous preterm delivery, three of the studies showed a benefit of BV treatment for preterm delivery before 37 weeks. Two trials of high-risk women found an increase in preterm delivery less than 34 weeks in women who did not have BV but received BV treatment. Both meta-analyses concluded that there is no evidence in favor of screening all pregnant women for BV. For women with a history of previous preterm birth there is support for diagnosing and treating BV early in pregnancy to prevent a proportion of these women having a further preterm birth.

In an update to the study by Guise et al.,[24] Nygren et al.[47] performed a series of meta-analyses (using new and 2001 report data) to estimate the pooled effect of treatment on preterm delivery (<37 weeks, <34 weeks, or <32 weeks), on low birth weight (LBW), and on preterm premature rupture of membranes (PPROM). Seven new randomized controlled trials were found in the area of treatment of asymptomatic pregnant women with BV since the previous report was published in 2001. Meta-analysis of trials showed no treatment effects at any risk level for preterm delivery for preterm delivery. Two trials of high-risk women found an increase in preterm delivery less than 34 weeks in women who did not have BV but received BV treatment. Comparisons of patient populations, treatment regimens, and study designs did not explain the heterogeneity among studies.

In contrast, screening and treating BV in low risk pregnancies produced a statistically significant reduction in premature deliveries (R.R. 0.73) in Varma and Gupta's[48] meta-analysis, but there was no benefit in high-risk groups. It was hypothesized that premature delivery in high and low risk pregnant women are different entities and not linear extremes of the same syndrome. There are significant clinical and methodological differences between the above studies, which may account for the variation of the results and conclusions. Hay and colleagues[32] recommend that as BV is associated with second trimester miscarriage and preterm labor, treatment should be given no later than the beginning of the second trimester. Rosenstein and colleagues[35] concluded that earlier diagnosis and treatment may be more effective in preventing abnormal outcome and they suggested that screening and treating before pregnancy might be advantageous. Some have observed that treatment with topical vaginal antibiotics has proven to be less effective for the prevention of premature delivery than oral antibiotics.[49,50] This would indicate that the micro-organisms responsible for premature labor have ascended out of reach of topically administered antibiotics and the endometrial cavity would be the most likely place for them to initiate contractions. Some have found reduction of premature delivery only in those with a history of preterm birth.[31,43,51] Preterm delivery is the major cause of perinatal mortality and morbidity in the developed world. According to Lamont and Sawant[52] in up to 40% of cases, infection is a significant cause of spontaneous preterm labor. They recommend clindamycin as the antibiotic of choice.

Effect of Antibiotics on the Prevalence of BV

Antibiotics have been shown to affect the presence of BV. Clindamycin has been shown to be effective in eradicating the bacteria, whether used intravaginally,[53] or orally.[33] Abnormal flora were found after oral clindamycin in 10% of treated patients compared with 93% of placebo patients ($p < 0.001$) in Ugwumadu et al.'s[33] trial of 462 women (231 in the clindamycin and 231 in a placebo group). Normal flora was maintained in two thirds of women throughout pregnancy. The results of four weekly smears were compared in 135 women, 69 clindamycin treated and 66 placebo treated. For the clindamycin group, the prevalence of abnormal flora was 15% at 20 weeks and 17% at 36 weeks gestation compared with 69% at 20 weeks and 43% at 36 weeks in the placebo group. Borisov et al.[53] compared the effect of intravaginal clindamycin to the effect of metronidazole in 128 pregnant women with BV. BV was eradicated in 93% of the women using intravaginal clindamycin and in 87% of the group receiving the metronidazole. Both treatments were more effective than oral ampicillin for 7 days, which had a cure rate of 62%.

Ugwumadu et al.[33] concluded that as previous research had shown that spontaneous resolution of BV does not modify the risk of preterm birth, early screening and treatment should be advocated.

Effect of Antibiotics in Women with Previous Premature Labor

The effect of antibiotics has been assessed in women at high risk of premature labor with BV. The results of two studies indicate that antibiotics may reduce the incidence of premature labor. Both metronidazole and metronidazole together with erythromycin have been assessed in double blind placebo controlled trials. In Morales et al.'s[51] study, women with premature labour or premature rupture of the membranes in the preceding pregnancy were screened for BV between 13 and 20 weeks' gestation. Patients with a positive screen were randomized to receive metronidazole orally or placebo. Forty-four patients received metronidazole and 36 received placebo. The metronidazole group had fewer hospital admissions for preterm labor (27% vs. 78%), preterm births (18% vs. 39%), low birth weight infants (<2500 g) (14% vs. 33%), and premature rupture of the membranes (5% vs. 33%), respectively.

Hauth et al.[54] performed BV testing at 23 weeks in 624 pregnant women at risk of delivering prematurely. Patients were randomized on a 2:1 basis to receive treatment with erythromycin and metronidazole ($n = 426$) or placebo ($n = 190$). A second course of treatment was instituted for those women who still had BV at 28 weeks. In the antibiotic group 110 women delivered prematurely (26%) compared to 68 women in the placebo group (36%, $p = 0.01$). The association between treatment and lower rates of prematurity was observed only among the 258 women who had BV (31% with treatment vs. 49% with placebo; $p = 0.006$).

Miscarriage

Association between BV and Early Miscarriage

There have been a few studies linking BV with early first trimester miscarriage.[55–58] There is stronger evidence, however, that BV is related to late first trimester and second trimester loss[59,60] than early first trimester loss. The relationship between BV and early miscarriage has been assessed mainly in IVF patients, or threatened miscarriage, rather than recurrent miscarriage.

Miscarriage rates were assessed in 867 consecutive women undergoing IVF.[55] BV was found in 24.6% of the women before egg collection. There were no differences in the conception rates between those women with BV and those with normal vaginal flora. Twenty-two women (31.6%) with BV who conceived had a significantly increased risk of miscarriage in the first trimester compared with 27 women (18.5%) with normal vaginal flora. The increased rate of miscarriage remained significant after adjusting for factors known to increase the risk of miscarriage—maternal age, smoking, a history of recurrent miscarriage, no previous live birth, and polycystic ovary syndrome.

In a further study to investigate the effect of vaginal flora and vaginal inflammation on conception and early pregnancy loss, 91 women undergoing IVF were recruited.[56] At the time of embryo transfer, samples were taken for BV. The overall live birth rate was 30% and the rate of early pregnancy loss was 34%. Women with BV, intermediate flora and normal flora had early pregnancy loss rates of 33% (1/3), 42% (5/12), and 30% (3/10) ($p = 0.06$), respectively. It was concluded that IVF patients with BV may have increased rates of early pregnancy loss and that a larger prospective treatment trial to evaluate potential benefits of optimizing vaginal flora before IVF may be warranted; over the subsequent ten years no such study appears to have been reported.

The Nugent score and PCR were both used to assess the prevalence of BV in a study of 307 patients who were subsequently treated with IVF.[61] The primary outcome measure was the implantation rate. The secondary outcomes were clinical pregnancy rate, early and late miscarriage, premature rupture of membranes, preterm delivery, mode of delivery and birthweight. PCR revealed a prevalence of BV of 9.45%. Among women who performed vaginal douching, 22.2% were BV+ , whereas 7.9% of patients who did not douche were BV+ ($p = 0.028$). The embryo implantation rate was decreased between the BV– and BV+ groups (36.3% vs. 27.6%; $p = 0.418$), (not significant). There were no significant statistical differences between the groups in secondary obstetrical outcomes.

French et al.[62] reported that in a prospective analysis of 1100 pregnant women, 60% of women with first-trimester bleeding had one or more infections detected, such as BV (RR. 1.5), *T. vaginalis* (RR.2.3) and *C. trachomatis* (RR. 2.7). Each of these infections heightened the risk for preterm delivery in women with BV and first-trimester bleeding; BV (RR. 4.4), BV with *T. Vaginalis* (RR.3.0).

Association between BV and Late Miscarriage

The association with later pregnancy losses has been reported in a number of studies. Llahi-Camp et al.[59] found a history of one late miscarriage more than twice as commonly (27/130; 21%) compared to women who had only early miscarriages (31/370; 8%) ($p < 0.001$). In Llahi-Camp et al.'s[59] study, BV did not appear to be related to recurrent early miscarriage. Hay and coworkers[39] in a prospective study screened 783 women for BV at their first antenatal clinic visit. There were 12 late miscarriages (16–24 weeks of gestation), and a significant association with BV ($p < 0.001$). Oakeshott et al.[60] assessed 1,201 women presenting before 10 weeks of gestation prospectively. The relative risk of miscarriage associated with BV compared with women who were negative for BV before 16 weeks was 1.2. BV was associated with miscarriage at 13–15 weeks at a relative risk of 3.5. BV was therefore not strongly associated with early miscarriage but may be a factor for pregnancy loss after 13 weeks of gestation.

Donders et al.[63] assessed 228 women at 14 weeks of gestation, by culture for BV associated bacteria, in order to determine whether there is a relationship between BV and pregnancy loss up to 20 weeks. As screening was performed at 14 weeks, only second trimester losses could be assessed. The relative risk for pregnancy loss between 14 and 20 weeks was 5.4 in the presence of BV. *M. hominis* and *U. urealyticum* were also associated with an increased risk of late miscarriage.

Effect of Treatment of BV on Miscarriage

There is a general consensus in the literature that antibiotics reduce the incidence of late miscarriages and preterm labor in the presence of BV. In French et al.'s[62] study of 1100 pregnant women, systemic antibiotics reduced the rate of preterm birth for women with BV without first trimester bleeding (R.R. 0.37) and treatment of women with BV and first-trimester bleeding reduced preterm birth (R.R. 0.52). Clindamycin treatment was associated with a reduction in the number of late miscarriages and premature births in Berger and Kane's[64] study of women with asymptomatic BV between 12 and 22 weeks of gestation.

McGregor and colleagues[65] analyzed the effect of systemic treatment to reduce pregnancy loss (<22 weeks), preterm premature rupture of the membranes, and preterm delivery in a prospective controlled treatment trial. The overall presence of BV was 32.5%. BV was associated with pregnancy loss at <22 weeks (RR. 3.1). The relative risk of preterm premature rupture of the membranes was 3.5, and the relative risk of preterm birth was 1.9. In the treatment phase of the study women with BV received clindamycin orally. After treatment there were less preterm births ($RR = 0.5$) and preterm premature rupture of the membranes (R.R. 0.5).

Ugwumadu et al.[66] prospectively screened 6120 asymptomatic women at the first antenatal visit between 12 and 22 weeks of gestation. The 485 women with abnormal smears were randomly allocated to receive oral clindamycin or placebo. There were significantly fewer mid-trimester miscarriages or preterm deliveries in the clindamycin group (13/244) compared to the placebo group (38/241) ($p = 0.0003$).

In a multicenter, prospective randomized controlled trial,[67] 4429 low risk asymptomatic women were screened for BV at their first routine antenatal visit early in the second trimester. In the intervention group the women received standard antibiotic treatment and follow up for any detected infection; the number of preterm deliveries was significantly lower (3.0%) than in the control group (5.3%) ($p = 0.0001$). There were eight late miscarriages in the intervention group and 15 in the control group. It was concluded that introducing a simple infection screening program into routine antenatal care can significantly reduce late miscarriages and preterm births in a low risk group of pregnant women.

In Sweden, 9025 women were screened for BV in early pregnancy and 819 proved to be positive.[68] Only one of 11 women in the treatment group (vaginal clindamycin) compared to five of 12 women in the control group delivered before 33 completed weeks. Treatment was associated with 32 days longer gestation for the 23 participants who had late miscarriage or spontaneous preterm birth and significantly fewer infants had a birthweight below 2500. It was concluded that treatment was associated with significantly prolonged gestation and reduced cost of neonatal care. There was an overall saving of 27 euro per woman.

In a retrospective study, data from 2986 women in Vienna with singleton pregnancies presenting for routine antenatal care between 11 and 24 weeks was analyzed.[69] The women were screened for asymptomatic vaginal infection using Gram stain, differentiating between bacterial vaginosis, vaginal candidiasis, trichomoniasis, or combinations of any of the three. Women with infection received standard treatment and follow-up. Prenatal care was the same for women in the intervention and control groups, the only difference being the absence of screening and treating for vaginal infection in the control group. In the intervention group, the rate of preterm birth was significantly lower than in the control group (8.2% vs. 12.1%, $p < 0.0001$), as was the number of preterm infants with birth weights of 2500 g or below. A significant difference between groups was found for delivery before 33 weeks (1.9% vs. 5.4%, $p < 0.0001$). In this study, a simple screen-and-treatment program for common vaginal infections into routine antenatal care led to a significant reduction in preterm births in a general population of pregnant women.

Mycoplasmas

Di Bartolomeo and colleagues[70] established the prevalence of micro-organisms in 198 pregnant women with vaginal discharge. Endocervical and vaginal samples were assessed using direct methods, culture, immunodetection, and PCR looking for *C. trachomatis*, *Neisseria gonorrhoeae*, *Streptococcus agalactie*, *T. vaginalis*, *Candida*, *M. hominis*, *U. urealyticum*, and BV. In 51 cases (26%) one of the above were detected. BV was diagnosed in 30 cases (15%). *U. urealyticum* was found in 49%, *Candida* in 34%, *M. hominis* in 14.1%, *S. agalactie* in 5%, *T. vaginalis* in 4%, and *C. trachomatis* in 2.5%. *N. gonorrhoeae* was not detected. As the evidence suggested that vaginal colonization with genital mycoplasmas plays a role in complications of pregnancy, a study was set up to determine whether antibiotics would reduce spontaneous pregnancy loss.[71] The loss of a pregnancy included spontaneous miscarriage, stillbirths, premature infants who died or term infants who died from congenital pneumonia due to *U. urealyticum*. Women with spontaneous pregnancy wastage, and who were mycoplasma positive in the genital tract, were treated prospectively for 71 pregnancies. There was a significant reduction in pregnancy loss rate among those treated with doxycycline before pregnancy or erythromycin during pregnancy. The pregnancy loss rate in the untreated group was remarkably high with 22 of the 24 pregnancies being lost. There were 18 out of 37 pregnancies lost in the doxycycline only group, three lost out of 20 pregnancies in the erythromycin group and two of 12 treated pregnancies lost after doxycycline and erythromycin. The benefit was independent of maternal age, number of previous miscarriages or gestational age at miscarriage. It was concluded that antibiotics prescribed for women colonized with mycoplasmas could prevent recurrent spontaneous miscarriage.

The role of *U. urealyticum* in spontaneous and recurrent spontaneous miscarriage has been studied in 633 women.[72] Cervical colonization with *U. urealyticum* was found in 42.6% of 310 normal pregnant women, in 41.6% of 84 patients undergoing pregnancy termination, in 41.5% of normal fertile patients, in 53% of 122 patients with spontaneous miscarriage and in 64.5% of 76 women with recurrent miscarriage. The cervical colonization rate was significantly higher in patients with spontaneous miscarriage ($p < 0.05$) and recurrent spontaneous miscarriage ($p < 0.005$) compared to normal pregnant women. Endometrial colonization was more frequent in patients with recurrent miscarriage (27.6%) than in normal fertile women (9.7%) ($p < 0.05$). *U. urealyticum* was isolated in five of six women with intact membranes and uncontrollable preterm labor between 20 and 28 weeks of gestation. *U. urealyticum* was also isolated from the placenta in four patients and the amniotic fluid in two of four patients. It was concluded that *U. urealyticum* is a common commensal of the lower genital tract, but it may play a role in miscarriage and in uncontrollable preterm labor.

However, the role of *U. urealyticum* in adverse pregnancy outcomes is disputed. There was no difference in the incidence of premature rupture of the membranes, preterm labor or low-birth-weight infant between women carrying *U. urealyticum* and those women who were not carriers in Carey et al.'s[73] study. Carey et al.[73] assessed whether genital colonization with *U. urealyticum* was associated with adverse pregnancy outcome in 4934 women evaluated between 23 and 26 weeks of gestation. The prevalence of infection certainly seems to be higher when the abortus is cultured at mid trimester abortion or preterm labor. McDonald et al.[74] performed a prospective study of the changes in vaginal flora between midtrimester and labor in 560 women. Forty-five women delivered prematurely. *U. urealyticum* and *G. vaginalis* were both associated with preterm birth when present in the midtrimester.

Light and immunofluorescent microscopy were used to investigate 118 late miscarriages at 18–28 weeks of gestation.[75] Intrauterine infections were found in 86 cases with mycoplasmas being found in 44 (37%). One hundred and twenty-nine spontaneously delivered, nonmacerated midgestation placentae and fetuses, between 16 and 26 weeks of gestation, were examined and cultured for aerobic and anaerobic bacteria, genital mycoplasmas, and yeasts.[76] Micro-organisms were recovered in 85 (66%). Group B streptococcus was the most significant pathogen, being recovered in 21 cases. *Escherichia coli* (22 cases) and *U. urealyticum* (24 cases) were present mostly as mixed infections. Specimens from 51 spontaneous early miscarriages and 56 pregnancy terminations were investigated by culture for yeasts, Gram positive and Gram negative bacteria and genital mycoplasma.[77] Molecular diagnostic tests for DNA sequences were performed for *C. trachomatis*, herpes simplex viruses, adenovirus, and human papilloma virus. None of these were detected in normal pregnancies that were artificially terminated, whereas spontaneous miscarriage tissues were positive for at least one micro-organism in 31.5% of cases.

In the case of first trimester abortion, an association has not been found with mycoplasma or ureaplasma when placental specimens from aborted material were subjected to PCR for karyotyping and detection of bacterial and viral DNA.[78] There was no evidence of *M. hominis*, *U. urealyticum*, human cytomegalovirus or adeno-associated virus found. *C. trachomatis* DNA was detected once. However, Ye et al.[79] took endocervical swabs for mycoplasma in 58 women with spontaneous abortion and compared the outcome of pregnancy to a control group of 50 normal pregnant women. In the index cases, positive results for *U. urealyticum* and *M. hominis* were found in 74.1% (43/58) and 27.6% (16/58), respectively. These results were significantly different to those of the controls: the corresponding results being 48% (24/50) ($p < 0.01$) and 10% (5/50) ($p < 0.05$), respectively. It was concluded that mycoplasma infection could be one of the causes of early embryonic death.

A study from Albania[80] has found a high overall incidence of *M. hominis* (30.4%) and *U. urealyticum* (54.3%) in hospitalized women in the obstetric and gynecological department. The prevalence of these organisms was higher among women who had experienced miscarriage. Microbiological screening of vaginal flora and semen was performed 4 weeks before IVF for 951 couples.[81] Infections were found in 218 women (22.9%) and appropriate treatment was prescribed. There were 69 with *Candida albicans*, 49 with *U. urealyticum*, 43 with *G. vaginalis*, 24 with Streptococcus B or D and 22 with *E. coli*. The implantation rate was significantly reduced in patients with infection, 14.6% versus 19.3% ($p < 0.02$). Positive cultures from both vagina and semen was found in 77 couples with a spontaneous miscarriage rate of 46.7% compared to 17.6% with vaginal infection alone ($p < 0.01$). It was concluded that endocervical micro-organisms even when treated may affect implantation and this is enhanced when the semen has shown infection. The author has advocated testing for *M. hominis* and *U. urealyticum* following miscarriage but no evidence was put forward that this would lead to subsequent clinical improvement.

Antibiotics in Unexplained Pregnancy Losses

Antibiotics have been prescribed in some studies without bacteriological confirmation. The maternal and fetal outcomes of the next pregnancy were recorded in 254 couples attending an infertility clinic following one or more spontaneous miscarriages.[27] One hundred couples requested antibiotics—96 received doxycycline 100 mg twice daily for 4 weeks or tetracycline 500 mg four times daily for 4 weeks to cover *C. trachomatis* and mycoplasmas. In addition, 49 patients received erythromycin 500 mg four times daily for 2 weeks. Four patients received ampicillin or cephalexin. There was a significantly lower chance of miscarriage in the antibiotic treatment group (10%) compared to the untreated group (38%) ($p < 0.01$). Premature rupture of the membranes occurred in 4% of the treated group compared to 46% in the control group. The antibiotic group had a higher vaginal delivery rate (69% vs. 56%) ($p < 0.01$), lower incidence of fetal distress (6% vs. 26%), respiratory distress syndrome, neonatal infection, a higher birth weight and better Apgar scores. It was postulated that some spontaneous miscarriages may be caused by bacteria present in the genital tract at the time of conception and that these bacteria may have an adverse effect on the pregnancy.

Antibiotic therapy has been assessed for first-trimester threatened miscarriage in women with previous spontaneous miscarriage.[82] Only those at a gestational age of less than 9 weeks were included. Women with mild abdominal cramping received amoxicillin and erythromycin for 7 days. Severe abdominal pain was treated with amoxicillin and clindamycin for 7 days. Twenty-two of the 23 pregnancies were carried to term. It was concluded that antibiotics might prevent pregnancy loss in women with threatened miscarriage and that further clinical trials are warranted.

A randomized placebo-controlled trial was set up to determine whether metronidazole reduces early preterm labour in asymptomatic women with positive vaginal fetal fibronectin in the second trimester of pregnancy.[83] The women had at least one risk factor including mid-trimester loss or preterm delivery, uterine abnormality, cervical surgery or cervical cerclage. Nine hundred pregnancies were screened for fetal fibronectin at 24 and 27 weeks of gestation and the positive cases were randomized to receive a 7-day course of oral metronidazole or placebo. The primary outcome was delivery before 30 weeks of gestation and the secondary outcomes included delivery before 37 weeks. Fetal fibronectin was a good predictor of early preterm birth with positive predictive values at 24 weeks of gestation for delivery by 30 weeks of 26% and negative predictive value of 99%. The Trial Steering Committee stopped the study early; 21% (11/53) of the women receiving metronidazole delivered before 30 weeks compared with 11% (5/46) of those taking the placebo. Furthermore, there were significantly more preterm deliveries (<37 weeks) in women receiving the metronidazole 33/53 (62%) compared to placebo 18/46 (39%). Treatment was initiated relatively late and damage would have preceded the metronidazole as all the patients studied had positive fibronectin tests.

Patients with a history of previous recurrent second-trimester losses associated with failed cervical cerclage were prospectively included in a study of low-dose antibiotics until delivery.[84] Cerclage was performed at 14–24 weeks' gestation on the basis of transvaginal sonographic findings of cervical funneling. The outcome was evaluated by weeks of pregnancy gained in the current pregnancy as compared to the previous pregnancy. Ten patients were eligible for study and all ten achieved fetal viability. Pregnancy was prolonged by a mean of 13.4 ± 4.2 weeks beyond the previous pregnancy. This was highly statistically significant ($p < 0.001$). Continuous low-dose antibiotics prolonged pregnancy in patients with recurrent second-trimester pregnancy losses and prior failed cerclage. It was concluded that randomized clinical trials are needed to confirm the role of antibiotics in these high-risk pregnancies.

Future Developments

More than a century ago, Robert Koch devised a scientific standard for determining whether a disease is a result of a specific micro-organism. Koch's postulates stated that the pathogen should be isolated from the diseased host, grown in pure culture, and reproduce the disease when inoculated into a susceptible host. Interestingly, Koch accepted that his postulates were not always useful (cited by Fredricks and Relman[2]). In recent years, a previously unexpected infectious etiology has been demonstrated in a variety of clinical conditions. In gynecology, the role of the human papillomavirus in premalignant and malignant cervical disease has been confirmed, and in obstetrics, there appears to be a link between premature delivery and BV. In IVF, we are learning that micro-organisms in follicular fluid are associated with adverse pregnancy outcomes,[85] and the presence of periopathogenic micro-organisms or their products in human placentas may be related to the pathogenesis of pre-eclampsia.[86]

Helicobacter pylori has become established as the cause of peptic ulceration. Fredricks and Relman[2] have suggested that there are a number of chronic diseases, whose etiology remains obscure, but which have characteristics indicating a microbial involvement. These diseases include Crohn's disease, rheumatoid arthritis, systemic lupus erythematosis, atherosclerosis, multiple sclerosis, and diabetes mellitus. These authors suggest that traditional technology for detecting pathogens is not sufficiently sensitive to identify the micro-organisms responsible.

Whipple's disease illustrates the limitation of conventional bacteriology. Whipple described the disease that bears his name in 1907. The syndrome consists of polyarthritis, weight loss, diarrhea, malabsorption, and lymphadenopathy. Whipple observed rod-like bacillary structures in mesenteric lymph nodes raising the possibility of a bacterial etiology. Although the Whipple's bacillus could be seen by microscopy, it could not be grown in culture or in animal hosts and no successful serological test could be devised. It was not until the arrival of molecular biology that the bacillus could be characterized. Fredericks and Relman[2] concluded that failure to cultivate a micro-organism does not prove that a disease is not due to a pathogen. Bacteria may cause chronic systemic disease spanning decades. Furthermore, steroids may produce temporary improvement without proving that the disease is inflammatory or autoimmune rather than infectious. Finally, documented improvement or cure associated with antimicrobial agents in a chronic disease suggests a microbial origin.

Bacteria have a remarkable propensity to survive even in the most hostile environments, including sea ice and deep-sea hydrothermal vents with extreme temperatures and loaded with heavy metals.[87] The vast majority of micro-organisms are "unculturable" or "fastidious," which means that they cannot be identified by conventional culture techniques.[88] Over the last few years, the development and application of molecular diagnostic techniques has revolutionized diagnosis and monitoring of infectious diseases. Molecular biological techniques are increasingly being adopted into clinical laboratories. These molecular methods have made it possible to characterize mixed microflora in their entirety including those which cannot be grown in culture. Molecular studies of the vaginal flora have discovered many unculturable bacteria including bacteria in the Clostridiales order which are highly specific indicators of BV. A more complete understanding of vaginal microbial populations resulting from molecular biological techniques may lead to new strategies to maintain healthy vaginal floras and will provide opportunities to explore the role of novel bacteria in reproductive tract disease.[88]

Biofilms develop by bacteria aggregating in a hydrated polymeric matrix of their own synthesis on moist surfaces. They are inherently resistant to antimicrobial agents and are increasingly recognized to be at the root of many persistent and chronic bacterial infections.[89] Resistance of *H. pylori* infection to conventional therapies may be attributed to biofilm growing bacteria.[90] Fredricks and Relman[2] have observed that for more than a century bacteriologists have attempted to culture *Treponema pallidum* and *Mycobacterium leprae* without success but the pathogenicity of these organisms is not in doubt. These authors argue that just as we cannot cultivate known pathogens, we must accept the possibility that other pathogens may exist that resist cultivation. They have provided a set of guidelines to help prove microbial disease causation using molecular biological sequence-based evidence rather than culture.

Some have concluded that the best evidence suggests that infection is an occasional cause of sporadic spontaneous miscarriage and that recurrent miscarriage occurs with a much lower frequency. At the other extreme, mycoplasmas have been found in 74% of spontaneous miscarriages with embryonic death compared to 48% of the controls.[79]

Recently, attention has focused on the relationship between periodontal infection and adverse pregnancy outcomes, including late miscarriage.[91] Periodontal disease is one of the most common chronic infections with a prevalence of 10–60% depending on diagnostic criteria. So far there have been no reports on any association between first trimester miscarriage and periodontitis. An Indian study has shown a statistically significant relationship between maternal periodontitis and pregnancy duration.[91,92] The authors recommended that oral hygiene maintenance should become part of antenatal care. A larger study from Taiwan, however, did not confirm the relationship between periodontal health and premature delivery but found a relationship with low birth weight.[93]

The antiphospholipid syndrome has been linked to recurrent miscarriage and other pregnancy complications. It may respond to thromboprophylaxis improving the live birth rate.[94] Antiphospholipid antibodies may be associated with infection and one is left to contemplate the possibility that some cases of recurrent miscarriage could be related to underlying treatable infection. In this context it is of interest that antiphospholipid syndrome has been reported to disappear when *H. pylori* is eradicated.[95]

Whilst micro-organisms can be associated with miscarriage, the question will always arise as to whether they are pathogenic or opportunistic. Ultimately, from a clinical point of view, what really matters is whether treatment can reduce the occurrence of miscarriage. A few clinical studies so far have shown encouraging results and further research is warranted. It is recognized that screening for, and treatment of, BV in early pregnancy among high-risk women with a previous history of second-trimester miscarriage or spontaneous preterm labor may reduce the risk of recurrent late pregnancy loss and preterm birth. The fundamental question of efficacy of antibiotic treatment for BV before pregnancy in women with recurrent early miscarriage has yet to be addressed in clinical studies. Developments in serological tests and molecular biological techniques are enhancing our capability to detect evidence of infections in obstetrics and gynecology. Ultimately, there is the option of a trial of therapy with a presumptive diagnosis of genital infection being related to recurrent miscarriage without laboratory confirmation. The antibiotics of choice, metronidazole and the macrolides such as erythromycin, are relatively innocuous. Nevertheless, antibiotics should be used with caution as there is the potential risk of bacterial resistance.

REFERENCES

1. Royal College of Obstetricians and Gynaecologists. *The Investigation and Treatment of Couples with Recurrent Miscarriage. Guideline No. 17*. London: RCOG; 2011.
2. Fredricks DN, Relman DA. Infectious agents and the etiology of chronic idiopathic diseases. *Curr Clin Top Infect Dis* 1998;18:180–200.
3. Saracoglu OF, Mungan T, Tanzer F. Pelvic Tuberculosis. *Int J Gynaecol Obstet* 1992;37:115–20.
4. Figueroa-Damian R, Martinez-Velazco I, Villagrana-Zesati R et al. Tuberculosis of the female reproductive tract: Effect on function. *Int J Fertil Menopausal Stud* 1996;41:430–6.
5. Lamont RF, Sobel J, Mazaki-Tovi S et al. Listeriosis in human pregnancy: A systematic review. *J Perinat Med* 2011;39:227–36.
6. Romana C, Salleras L, Sage M. Latent listerosis may cause habitual abortion, intrauterine deaths, fetal malformations. When diagnosed and treated adequately normal children will be born. *Acta Microbiol Hung* 1989;36:171–2.
7. Manganiello PD, Yearke RR. A 10-year prospective study of women with a history of recurrent fetal losses fails to identify Listeria monocytogenes in the female genital tract. *Fertil Steril* 1991;56:781–2.
8. Rowe JH, Ertelt JM, Xin L et al. Listeria monocytogenes cytoplasmic entry induces fetal wastage by disrupting maternal Foxp3+ regulatory T cell-sustained fetal tolerance. *PLoS Pathog* 2012;8:e1002873.
9. Baud D, Greub G. Intracellular bacteria and adverse pregnancy outcomes. *Clin Microbiol Infect* 2011;17:1312–22.
10. Szkaradkiewicz A, Pieta P, Tulecka T et al. The diagnostic value of anti-CMV and anti-HPV-B19 antiviral antibodies in studies on causes of recurrent abortions. *Ginekol Pol* 1997;68:181–6.

11. Cook SM, Himebaugh KS, Frank TS. Absence of cytomegalovirus in gestational tissue in recurrent spontaneous abortion. *Diagn Mol Pathol* 1993;2:116–9.

12. Qublan HS, Jumaian N, Abu-Salem A et al. Toxoplasmosis and habitual abortion. *J Obstet Gynaecol* 2002;296–8.

13. Mezinova NN, Chuchupalov PD, Evdokimova NS et al. Effect of anti-chlamydial drugs on the effectiveness of the treatment of habitual abortion. *Akush Ginekol (Mosk)* 1991;7:30–2.

14. Mezinova NN, Chuchupalov PD. Endometrial Chlamydia infection in women with habitual abortion. *Akush Ginekol (Mosk)* 1992;2:25–6.

15. Kishore J, Agarwal J, Agarwal S et al. Seroanalysis of Chlamydia trachomatis and S-TORCH agents in women with recurrent spontaneous abortions. *Indian J Pathol Microbiol* 2003;46:684–7.

16. Witkin SS, Ledger WJ. Antibodies to Chlamydia trachomatis in sera of women with recurrent spontaneous abortions. *Am J Obstet Gynecol* 1992;167:135–9.

17. Olliaro P, Regazzetti A, Gorini G et al. Chlamydia trachomatis infection in sine causa recurrent abortion. *Boll Ist Sieroter Milan* 1991;70:467–70.

18. Rae R, Smith IW, Liston WA et al. Chlamydial serologic studies and recurrent spontaneous abortion. *Am J Obstet Gynecol* 1994;170;782–5.

19. Paukku M, Tulppala M, Puolakkainen M et al. Lack of association between serum antibodies to Chlamydia trachomatis and a history of recurrent pregnancy loss. *Fertil Steril* 1999;72:427–30.

20. Sugiura-Ogasawara M, Ozaki Y, Nakanishi T et al. Pregnancy outcome in recurrent aborters is not influenced by Chlamydia IGA and/or G. *Am J Reprod Immunol* 2005;53:50–3.

21. Schulz KF, Cates W Jr, O'mara PR. A synopsis of the problems in Africa in syphilis and gonorrhoea during pregnancy. *Afr J Sex Transmi Dis* 1986;2:56–7.

22. Amsel R, Totten PA, Spiegel CA et al. Nonspecific vaginitis. Diagnostic criteria and microbial and epidemiologic associations. *Am J Med* 1983;74:14–22.

23. Wilson JD, Ralph SG, Rutherford AJ. Rates of BV in women undergoing *in vitro* fertilisation for different types of infertility. *BJOG* 2002;109:714–7.

24. Turovskiy Y, Sutyak Noll K, Chikindas ML. The aetiology of bacterial vaginosis. *J Appl Microbiol* 2011;110:1105–28.

25. Teixeira GS, Carvalho FP, Arantes RM et al. Characteristics of Lactobacillus and Gardnerella vaginalis from women with or without bacterial vaginosis and their relationships in gnotobiotic mice. *J Med Microbiol* 2012; 61:1074–81.

26. Gilbert NM, Lewis WG, Lewis AL. Clinical features of bacterial vaginosis in a murine model of vaginal infection with Gardnerella vaginalis. *PLoS One* 2013;8:e59539.

27. Toth A, Lesser ML, Brooks-Toth CW et al. Outcome of subsequent pregnancies following antibiotic therapy after primary or multiple spontaneous abortions. *Surg Gynecol Obstet* 1986;163:243–50.

28. Viniker DA. Hypothesis on the role of sub-clinical bacteria of the endometrium (bacteria endometrialis) in gynaecological and obstetric enigmas. *Hum Reprod Update* 1999;5:373–85.

29. Lucisano A, Morandotti G, Marana R et al. Chlamydial genital infections and laparoscopic findings in infertile women. *Eur J Epidemiol* 1992;8:645–9.

30. Moller BR, Kristiansen FV, Thorsen P et al. Sterility of the uterine cavity. *Acta Obstet Gynecol Scand* 1995;74:216–9.

31. Guise JM, Mahon SM, Aickin M et al. Screening for bacterial vaginosis in pregnancy. *Am J Prev Med* 2001;20(Suppl. 3):62–72.

32. Hay PE, Morgan DJ, Ison CA et al. A longitudinal study of bacterial vaginosis during pregnancy. *Br J Obstet Gynaecol* 1994;101;1048–53.

33. Ugwumadu A, Reid F, Hay P et al. Natural history of bacterial vaginosis and intermediate flora in pregnancy and effect of oral clindamycin. *Obstet Gynecol* 2004;104:114–9.

34. Riduan JM, Hillier SL, Utomo B et al. Bacterial vaginosis and prematurity in Indonesia: Asociation in early and late pregnancy. *Am J Obstet Gynecol* 1993;169:175–8.

35. Rosenstein IJ, Morgan DJ, Lamont RF et al. Effect of intravaginal clindamycin cream on pregnancy outcome and on abnormal vaginal microbial flora of pregnant women. *Infect Dis Obstet Gynecol* 2000;8:158–65.

36. McDonald HM, O'Loughlin JA, Jolley P et al. Vaginal infection and preterm labour. *Br J Obstet Gynaecol* 1991;98:427–35.

37. Klebanoff MA, Hillier SL, Nugent RP et al. Is bacterial vaginosis a stronger risk factor for preterm birth when it is diagnosed earlier in gestation? *Am J Obstet Gynecol* 2005;192:470–7.

38. Lamont RF, Duncan SL, Mandal D et al. Intravaginal clindamycin to reduce preterm birth in women with abnormal genital tract flora. *Obstet Gynecol* 2003;101:516–22.

39. Hay PE, Lamont RF, Taylor-Robinson D et al. Abnormal bacterial colonisation of the genital tract and subsequent preterm delivery and late miscarriage. *BMJ* 1994:308:295–8.

40. Donders GG, Van Calsteren K, Bellen G et al. Predictive value for preterm birth of abnormal vaginal flora, bacterial vaginosis and aerobic vaginitis during the first trimester of pregnancy. *BJOG* 2009;116:1315–24.

41. Tita AT, Cliver SP, Goepfert AR et al. Clinical trial of interconceptional antibiotics to prevent preterm birth: Subgroup analyses and possible adverse antibiotic-microbial interaction. *Am J Obstet Gynecol* 2007;197:367.

42. Goffinet F, Maillard F, Mihoubi N et al. Bacterial vaginosis: Prevalence and predictive value for premature delivery and neonatal infection in women with preterm labour and intact membranes. *Eur J Obstet Gynecol Reprod Biol* 2003;108:146–51.

43. McDonald HM, O'Loughlin JA, Vigneswaran R et al. Impact of metronidazole therapy on preterm birth in women with bacterial vaginosis flora (Gardnerella vaginalis): A randomised, placebo controlled trial. *Br J Obstet Gynaecol* 1997;104:1391–7.

44. Camargo RP, Simoes JA, Cecatti JG et al. Impact of treatment for bacterial vaginosis on prematurity among Brazilian pregnant women: A retrospective cohort study. *Sao Paulo Med J* 2005;123:108–12.

45. Kurkinen-Raty M, Vuopala S, Koskela M et al. A randomised controlled trial of vaginal clindamycin for early pregnancy bacterial vaginosis. *BJOG* 2000;107:1427–32.

46. Brocklehurst P, Gordon A, Heatley E et al. Antibiotics for treating bacterial vaginosis in pregnancy. *Cochrane Database Syst Rev* 2013;CD000262.

47. Nygren P, Fu R, Freeman M, Bougatsos C et al. Screening and Treatment for Bacterial Vaginosis in Pregnancy: Systematic Review to Update the 2001 US Preventive Services Task Force Recommendation. Agency for Healthcare Research and Quality (US); Report Number 08–05106-EF-1; 2008.

48. Varma R, Gupta JK. Antibiotic treatment of bacterial vaginosis in pregnancy: Multiple meta-analyses and dilemmas in interpretation. *Eur J Obstet Gynecol Reprod Biol* 2006;124:10–4.

49. Majeroni BA. Bacterial vaginosis: An update. *Am Fam Physician* 1998;57:1285–9.

50. McGregor JA. Evidence based prevention of preterm birth/PROM: Infection and inflammation. Paper presented at The Problem with Prematurity II. St Thomas Hospital, London, September 7–9, 1998.

51. Morales WJ, Schorr S, Albritton J. Effect of metronidazole in patients with preterm birth in preceding pregnancy and bacterial vaginosis: A placebo-controlled, double-blind study. *Am J Obstet Gynecol* 1994;171:345–7.

52. Lamont RF, Sawant SR. Infection in the prediction and antibiotics in the prevention of spontaneous preterm labour and preterm birth. *Minerva Ginecol* 2005;57:423–33.

53. Borisov I, Dimitrova V, Mazneikova V et al. Therapeutic regimens for treating bacterial vaginosis in pregnant women, *Akush Ginekol (Sofiia)* 1999;38:14–6.

54. Hauth JC, Goldenberg RL, Andrews WW et al. Reduced incidence of preterm delivery with metronidazole and erythromycin in women with bacterial vaginosis. *N Engl J Med* 1995;333:1732–6.

55. Ralph SG, Rutherford AJ, Wilson JD. Influence of bacterial vaginosis on conception and miscarriage in the first trimester: Cohort study. *BMJ* 1999;319:220–3.

56. Eckert LO, Moore DE, Patton DL et al. Relationship of vaginal bacteria and inflammation with conception and early pregnancy loss following in-vitro fertilization. *Infect Dis Obstet Gynecol* 2003;11:11–7.

57. Ugwumadu AH. Bacterial Vaginosis in pregnancy. *Curr Opin Obstet Gynecol* 2002;14:115–8.

58. Leitich H, Bodner-Adler B, Brunbauer M et al. Bacterial vaginosis as a risk factor for preterm delivery: A meta-analysis. *Am J Obstet Gynecol* 2003;189:139–47.

59. Llahi-Camp JM, Rai R, Ison C et al. Association of bacterial vaginosis with a history of second trimester miscarriage. *Hum Reprod* 1996;11:1575–8.

60. Oakeshott P, Hay P, Hay S et al. Association between bacterial vaginosis or chlamydial infection and miscarriage before 16 weeks' gestation: Prospective community based cohort study. *BMJ* 2002;325:1334–7.

61. Mangot-Bertrand J, Fenollar F, Bretelle F et al. Molecular diagnosis of bacterial vaginosis: Impact on IVF outcome. *Eur J Clin Microbiol Infect Dis.* 2013;32:535–41.

62. French JI, McGregor JA, Draper D et al. Gestational bleeding, bacterial vaginosis and common reproductive tract infections: Risk for preterm birth and benefit of treatment. *Obstet Gynecol* 1999;93: 715–24.

63. Donders GG, Van Bulck B, Caudron J et al. Relationship of bacterial vaginosis and mycoplasmas to the risk of spontaneous abortion. *Am J Obstet Gynecol* 2000;183:431–7.

64. Berger A, Kane KY. Clindamycin for vaginosis reduces prematurity and late miscarriage. *J Fam Pract* 2003;52:603–4.

65. McGregor JA, French JI, Parker R et al. Prevention of premature birth by screening and treatment for common genital tract infections: Results of a prospective controlled evaluation. *Am J Obstet Gynecol* 1995;173:157–67.

66. Ugwumadu A, Manyonda I, Reid F et al. Effect of early oral clindamycin on late miscarriage and preterm delivery in asymptomatic women with abnormal vaginal flora and bacterial vaginosis: A randomised controlled trial. *Lancet* 2003;361:983–8.

67. Kiss H, Petricevic L, Husslein P. Prospective randomised controlled trial of an infection screening programme to reduce the rate of preterm delivery. *BMJ* 2004;329:371.

68. Larsson PG, Fåhraeus L, Carlsson B et al. Late miscarriage and preterm birth after treatment with clindamycin: A randomised consent design study according to Zelen. *BJOG* 2006;113:629–37.

69. Kiss H, Petricevic L, Martina S et al. Reducing the rate of preterm birth through a simple antenatal screen-and-treat programme: A retrospective cohort study. *Eur J Obstet Gynecol Reprod Biol* 2010;153:38–42.

70. Di Bartolomeo S, Rodriguez M, Sauka D et al. Microbiologic profile in symptomatic pregnant women's genital secretions in Gran Buenos Aires, Argentina. *Enferm Infecc Microbiol Clin* 2001;19:99–102.

71. Quinn PA, Shewchuk AB, Shuber J et al. Efficacy of antibiotic therapy in preventing spontaneous pregnancy loss among couples colonized with genital mycoplasmas. *Am J Obstet Gynecol* 1983;145:239–44.

72. Naessens A, Foulon W, Cammu H et al. Epidemiology and pathogenesis of U. urealyticum in spontaneous abortion and early preterm labor. *Acta Obstet Gynecol Scand* 1987;66:513–6.

73. Carey, JC, Blackwelder WC, Nugent RP et al. Antepartum cultures for Ureaplasma urealyticum are not useful in predicting pregnancy outcome. The Vaginal Infections and Prematurity Study Group. *Am J Obstet Gynecol* 1991;164:728–33.

74. McDonald HM, O'Loughlin JA, Jolley, PT et al. Changes in vaginal flora during pregnancy and association with preterm birth. *J Infect Dis* 1994;170:724–8.

75. Fedotova EP, Shastina GV. Intrauterine mycoplasmosis in late miscarriage. *Arkh Patol* 1994;56:61–5.

76. McDonald HM, Chambers HM. Intrauterine infection and spontaneous midgestation abortion: Is the spectrum of microorganisms similar to that in preterm labor? *Infect Dis Obstet Gynecol* 2000;8:220–7.

77. Penta M, Lukic A, Conte MP et al. Infectious agents in tissues from spontaneous abortions in the first trimester of pregnancy. *New Microbiol* 2003;26:329–37.

78. Matovina M, Husnjak K, Milutin N et al. Possible role of bacterial and viral infections in miscarriages. *Fertil Steril* 2004;81:662–9.

79. Ye LL, Zhang BY, Cao WL. Relationship between the endocervical mycoplasma infection and spontaneous abortion due to early embryonic death. *Zhonghua Fu Chan Ke Za Zhi* 2004;39:83–5.

80. Tavo V. Prevalence of Mycoplasma hominis and Ureaplazma urealyticum among women of reproductive age in Albania. *Med Arh* 2013;67:25–6.

81. Wittemer C, Bettahar-Lebugle K, Ohl J et al. Abnormal bacterial colonisation of the vagina and implantation during assisted reproduction. *Gynecol Obstet Fertil* 2004;32:135–9.

82. Ou MC, Pang CC, Chen FM et al. Antibiotic treatment for threatened abortion during the early first trimester in women with previous spontaneous abortion. *Acta Obstet Gynecol Scand* 2001;80:753–6.

83. Shennan A, Crawshaw S, Briley A. A randomised controlled trial of metronidazole for the prevention of preterm birth in women positive for cervicovaginal fetal fibronectin: The PREMET Study. *BJOG* 2006;113:65–74.

84. Shiffman RL. Continuous low-dose antibiotics and cerclage for recurrent second-trimester pregnancy loss. *J Reprod Med* 2000;45:323–6.

85. Pelzer ES, Allan JA, Waterhouse MA et al. Microorganisms within human follicular fluid: Effects on IVF. *PLoS One* 2013;8:e59062.

86. Barak S, Oettinger-Barak O, Machtei EE et al. Evidence of periopathogenic microorganisms in placentas of women with preeclampsia. *J Periodontol* 2007;78:670–6.

87. Nichols CA, Guezennec J, Bowman JP. Bacterial exopolysaccharides from extreme marine environments with special consideration of the southern ocean, sea ice, and deep-sea hydrothermal vents: A review. *Mar Biotechnol (NY)* 2005;7:253–71.

88. Fredricks DN, Marrazzo JM. Molecular methodology in determining vaginal flora in health and disease: Its time has come. *Curr Infect Dis Rep* 2005;7:463–70.

89. Costerton JW, Stewart PS, Greenberg EP. Bacterial Biofilms; A common cause of persistent infections. *Science* 1999;284:1318–22.

90. Cammarota G, Sanguinetti M, Gallo A et al. Review article: Biofilm formation by Helicobacter pylori as a target for eradication of resistant infection. *Aliment Pharmacol Ther* 2012;36222–30.

91. Farrell S, Ide M, Wilson RF. The relationship between maternal periodontitis, adverse pregnancy outcome and miscarriage in never smokers. *J Clin Periodontol* 2006;33:115–20.

92. Wang YL, Liou JD, Pan WL. Association between maternal periodontal disease and preterm delivery and low birth weight. *Taiwan J Obstet Gynecol* 2013;52:71–6.

93. Rai R, Regan L. Antiphospholipid syndrome and pregnancy loss. *Hosp Med* 1998;59:637–9.

94. Cicconi V, Carloni E, Franceschi F et al. Disappearance of antiphospholipid antibodies syndrome after Helicobacter pylori eradication. *Am J Med* 2001;111:163–4.

95. Mannem S, Chava VK. The relationship between maternal periodontitis and preterm low birth weight: A case-control study. *Contemp Clin Dent* 2011;2:88–93.

34

The Male Factor in Recurrent Pregnancy Loss and Embryo Implantation Failure

Richard Bronson

Only recently have we come to ask what role the male might play in pregnancy loss and embryo implantation failure, beyond contributing an abnormal set of paternal chromosomes at fertilization. Recent evidence suggests that these situations may be related to the transmission of previously unrecognized chromosomal microdeletions or via the epigenetic dysregulation of embryonic gene function by spermatozoal micro-RNAs. In addition, the composition of seminal plasma has been found to be highly complex, containing factors that play important roles in altering the uterine environment and the female immune system permissive of embryo implantation and trophoectoderm outgrowth leading to successful pregnancy. Much of the information presented in this chapter is quite new, suggesting tantalizing hints for clinical application through future translational research.

The Role of Spermatozoa in Pregnancy Loss

Chromosomes

Approximately 1% of sperm from normal ejaculates possess aneuploid sets of chromosomes, although this incidence rises with disordered spermatogenesis.[1] Diploidy is also rare in spermatozoa from men with normal semen quality. In contrast to observations in women, aneuploidy does not increase with male age, although the incidence of point mutation-related disease does. Exposure to chemotherapeutic agents and environmental pollutants have been shown to increase the incidence of sperm aneuploidy. The discovery in 1978 that human spermatozoa could penetrate zona-free hamster eggs allowed the first analysis of human sperm chromosomes;[2,3] however, the technique is difficult. Sperm fertilizing ability must be retained and the number of spermatozoa analyzed is low. Fluorescence *in situ* hybridization (FISH) analysis using chromosome-specific DNA probes was developed in the 1990s.[4] This technique allows sperm exhibiting abnormalities in motility or other aspects of fertilization to be assessed. Hundreds of sperm may be analyzed, but the number of chromosomes probed at any one time is limited.

Sperm Aneuploidy and Male Infertility and Following Laboratory-Assisted Reproduction

Infertile men have an increased risk for autosomal and sex chromosomal abnormalities in their sperm, which is roughly three times higher than in fertile controls.[1] In an earlier review,[5] no relationship was found between the frequency of aneuploidy and sperm morphology in the face of normal sperm concentration and motility. However, more recent studies have found increased aneuploidy rates in these cases.[6] The discrepancy may be due to the fact that teratospermia is only a descriptive rather than molecular diagnosis, and abnormal sperm shape may be caused by different etiologies.[7] Macrocephalic, multiflagellate sperm exhibit quite high frequencies of aneuploidy and polyploidy (50–100%), although their finding is uncommon. An increased incidence of sperm aneuploidy is observed in men with oligospermia, as the sperm concentration drops below 10 million/mL (Table 34.1).[5,6,8] Meiotic studies in men with nonobstructive azoospermia, using immunocytogenetic techniques, have demonstrated errors

TABLE 34.1

Comparison of Sperm Aneuploidy in Men with Mild, Moderate, and Severe Oligospermia

	Percent Aneuploid Sperm	**Percent Diploid Sperm**
Mild	0.72% (0.39–1.28)	1.13% (0.60–2.12)
Moderate	1.85% (0.39–4.24)	3.03% (0.53–4.01)
Severe	1.75% (0.79–3.32)	2.98% (0.98–7.69)

Source: Adapted from Martin RH. *Cytogenet Genome Res* 2005;111:245–9.
Note: Mild: oligospermia 10–20 million sperm/mL. Moderate: <10–1 million/mL. Severe: <1 million/mL. Ten men were studied in each group. Fluorescence *in situ* hybridization was performed for chromosomes 13,21,X,Y.

of chromosome synapsis and significantly reduced recombination. These men have an increased risk of aneuploidy in sperm that have been surgically removed from the testes.[9]

Sperm Aneuploidy and Cancer

Aneuploidy has been assessed by FISH for chromosomes 13, 21, X and Y before, and 6, 12 or 18–24 months after the initiation of chemotherapy in men with testicular cancer and Hodgkin's lymphoma and compared with age matched controls. At 6 months, all cancer patients showed significantly increased frequencies of XY disomy and nullisomy for chromosomes 13 and 21. Aneuploidy frequencies declined to pretreatment levels 18 months after treatment initiation, in general, but persisted in some chromosomes for up to 24 months. As noted by Tempest et al.,[10] it is important these men be made aware of the potentially increased risk of an aneuploid fetus from sperm cryopreserved prior to chemotherapy, and for conception to be avoided for up to 2 years after the initiation of treatment.

Chromosome Microdeletions and Duplications

Hysteroscopic observations of human embryos at the time of missed abortion prior to suction curettage have revealed that the majority of grossly abnormal embryos are aneuploid. However, a significant minority of these embryos were euploid, raising the possibility of the presence of lethal chromosomal micro-deletions or duplications that could not be detected by karyotyping.[11,12] Comparative genome hybridization (CGH) has the potential to allow simultaneous evaluation of all chromosomes at one time and has the resolution to identify submicroscopic copy number variations. Ivanka et al.[13] studied whole genome imbalances in immature germ cells found in ejaculates of six males with idiopathic azoospermia and normal karyotype, using microarray-based CGH. Copy number variations were found in sperm DNA of all analyzed patients. The most consistent were aberrations in Y-chromosome, which occurred in 5 out of 6 patients (83.3%). In addition to Y chromosomal micro-imbalance, several other affected loci were detected in autosomes. Stouffs et al.[14] used array-CGH to study a group of men with nonobstructive azoospermia, as documented on testis biopsy, in the absence of Y chromosome microdeletions and compared them with a group of normospermic males. Only genes documented by polymerase chain reaction (PCR) to be present in testicular tissue and not present in controls were considered significant. Ten regions of deletion or duplication were identified. The mechanisms whereby these genetic alterations lead to embryonic loss remains to be determined.

Effects of Environmental Toxicants on Chromosomes

A wide variety of environmental toxicants, such a pesticides, metals, and air pollutants have been shown to disrupt spermatogenesis.[15,16] For example, Marchetti et al.[17] investigated whether occupational exposures to benzene increase the incidence of sperm carrying structural chromosomal aberrations. FISH was used to measure frequencies of sperm carrying partial chromosomal duplications or deletions or breaks among 30 benzene-exposed and 11 unexposed workers in Tianjin, China. Exposed workers were categorized into low-, moderate-, and high-exposure groups based on urinary benzene. Chromosome breaks were significantly increased in the high-exposure group, raising concerns in exposed individuals for infertility, spontaneous abortions, as well as inherited defects in their children.

Epigenetics: The Role of Abnormal Sperm DNA Methylation in Early Pregnancy Loss

A growing body of evidence suggests the importance of the epigenetic structure of sperm DNA. During normal spermiogenesis, the majority of nuclear histones are replaced by protamines 1 and 2 (P1, P2), leading to a highly compacted nuclear structure containing P1 and P2 in approximately a 1:1 ratio. An abnormal P1/P2 ratio has been associated with reduced sperm concentration, abnormal sperm morphology, increased sperm DNA fragmentation, and reduced fertilization and implantation rates.[18]

The regulation of DNA methylation is essential to the normal function of gametes and embryo development.[19] Methylation is commonly found on cytosine residues of cytosine-phosphate-guanine dinucleotides (CpGs) that regulate gene transcription at specific sites of promoter regions. While hypomethylation facilitates gene activation due to increased accessibility of DNA by polymerase, hypermethylation blocks its access and inhibits gene expression. Although the oocyte has the capacity to correct some methylation defects in sperm, this most likely depends on the quality of the egg, as well as the degree to which methylation was abnormal.

Approximately 5% of sperm DNA remains bound to histones at developmental gene promoters, micro-RNA genes, and imprinted loci.[20] The deleterious effects of severe sperm DNA methylation defects on embryogenesis have been demonstrated in male mice and rats treated with the methylation inhibitor 5-aza-20-deoxycytidine. This resulted in a global decrease in sperm DNA methylation levels, reduced fertilization rates, and increased rates of preimplantation loss. On this basis, Aston et al.[21] hypothesized that abnormal embryo development in women, in the absence of known female causes, might be secondary to abnormal sperm epigenetic factors. They used an array-based DNA methylation assay to study the genome-wide methylation status of sperm DNA at more than 27,000 CpG sites in 13 men where abnormal embryo development after *in vitro* fertilization (IVF)/intracytoplasmic sperm injection (ICSI) was observed, in 15 men whose sperm displayed an abnormally high or low P1/P2 ratio, and 15 fertile normospermic controls. Altered methylation profiles were identified in three of 28 patients, but none of the controls.

The importance of environmental factors on genetic imprinting of the embryo, as mediated through the male, has been demonstrated by Adam Watkins et al. They reported at the 46th Annual Meeting of the Society for the Study of Reproduction, in 2013, that offspring in mice were heavier than normal, with impaired glucose tolerance, when males were fed a low-protein diet. Hypomethylation at calcium-signaling and apoptotic pathway loci in sperm was observed. The uteri of females mated to these animals also exhibited decreased expression of prostaglandin and lipoxygenese genes, and reductions in cytokine and glucose levels were observed as well. These findings suggest a uterine effect mediated directly by spermatozoa or by a component of seminal plasma.

Spermatozoal RNAs

Previously, RNAs detected in the spermatozoon were assumed to be either degraded leftovers following expulsion of the residual body during spermiogenesis, or contaminants from nongerm cells, as sperm were considered transcriptionally inert. Newer evidence, however, indicates that sperm retain specific coding and noncoding RNAs and a potential functional role after fertilization has been suggested. Sandler et al.[22] have recently reviewed the evidence that these sperm-derived RNAs are likely to play a role in early post-fertilization development. The population of sperm RNAs is complex, including rRNA, mRNA, and both large and small noncoding RNAs, such as miRNAs and piRNAs, which may possess functional potential. Of note, miR-34c is essential to early embryo development, being required for the first cellular division. Some noncoding RNAs may also act as epigenetic modifiers, inducing histone modifications and DNA methylation, perhaps playing a role in transgenerational epigenetic inherence.[23]

Evidence for this thesis is provided by Fullston et al.[24] who fed male mice a high fat diet, which caused a 21% increase in their adiposity. Both the male and female F1 offspring exhibited impaired glucose tolerance and insulin resistance. Although fed normal diets, these animals were also obese. Of interest, the F2 offspring were also affected, suggesting that environmental effects on fathers can affect subsequent generations. A global reduction in methylation of germ-cell DNA in male mice fed a high-fat diet was observed. In addition, altered content of micro-RNAs in the sperm of these mice was detected. Target genes of some these micro-RNA are known to be important for embryonic development and metabolic function. These studies provide support for the thesis that spermatozoa possess RNA subpopulations capable of altering the embryonic genome and that alterations in the pattern of epigenetic marking may lead to significant changes in offspring.

Reactive Oxygen Species, DNA Damage and Recurrent Implantation Failure

"Oxidative stress" results from exposure of spermatozoa to excess reactive oxygen species (ROS), such as hydrogen peroxide, superoxide anions, and hydroxyl radicals.[25] These can originate via generation of ROS by leukocytes, secondary to male genital tract infection, as a consequence of electron leakage from the spermatozoon mitochondria and by deficiency in the antioxidants present within the male reproductive tract.[26] The human sperm plasma membrane is especially vulnerable to oxidative stress because of its high content of polyunsaturated fatty acids such as docosahexaenoic acid, which plays a physiologic role in regulating sperm plasma membrane fluidity. It contains six double bonds per molecule and is the main substrate for lipid peroxidation in the presence of ROS, leading to loss of sperm motility and impaired gamete membrane fusion events occurring at fertilization. Sperm content of arachidonic acid and docosahexaenoic acid varies widely between individual men.[27] ROS also attack DNA bases (especially guanine) and phosphodiester backbones, inducing the formation of DNA base adducts. This process destabilizes the DNA structure resulting in DNA strand breaks. 8-hydroxy-20-deoxyguanosine (8OHdG) is the major oxidized base adduct formed in this process, and sperm of infertile men contain high levels of 8OHdG.

Spermatozoa are also particularly vulnerable to oxidative stress because of their deficiency in intracellular antioxidant enzymes due to limited cytoplasmic volume. Sperm then are especially dependent on antioxidants present in the male reproductive tract secretions. The epididymal fluid contains several antioxidants, including free radical scavengers such as vitamin C, uric acid, taurine, as well as the antioxidant enzyme superoxide dismutase and a unique form of glutathione peroxidase. Experimental deletion of this enzyme in male mice results in an increased incidence of miscarriage and birth defects in wild-type female mice mated to such males.

DNA in the sperm nucleus is more vulnerable to oxidative attack than the cellular mechanisms regulating sperm motility or sperm-oocyte fusion. Hence, there can be instances such as paternal smoking, where the DNA is oxidatively damaged but the spermatozoon remains capable of fertilizing the oocyte.[28] While the egg can survey the DNA damage present in the sperm chromatin and repair it following fertilization, this ability is likely to vary between oocytes and with maternal age.[29]

Hendricks and Hansen[30] have provided experimental evidence in cattle that oxidative damage to ejaculated sperm leads to formation of embryos with reduced competence for development. Treatment of bull sperm with menadione or *tert*-butyl hydroperoxide, to induce oxidative stress, reduced the proportions of oocytes that cleaved and those that developed to the blastocyst stage at day 8 after insemination. Burruel et al.[31] studied whether oxidative damage of rhesus macaque sperm induced by ROS *in vitro* would affect embryo development following ICSI of oocytes. Rhesus spermatozoa were treated with 1 mM xanthine and 0.1 U/mL xanthine oxidase, to promote oxidative damage and then assessed for motility, viability, and lipid peroxidation. Motile ROS-treated and control sperm were used for ICSI of MII oocytes. Embryo growth was evaluated for 3 days of culture to the 8-cell stage. ICSI of oocytes with motile sperm induced *similar* rates of fertilization and cleavage between treatments. However, development to 4- and 8-cell stage was significantly lower for embryos generated with ROS-treated sperm than for controls. Changes in transcript abundance resulting from sperm treatment with ROS were also observed in 2-cell embryos.

Clinical IVF experience in humans bears out these experiments. A systematic review of 28 studies evaluating sperm DNA damage and embryo development after IVF or ICSI revealed such an association

TABLE 34.2

Comparison of Sperm DFI and Outcome of *In Vitro* Fertilization
(IVF)/Intracytoplasmic Sperm Injection (ICSI)

DFI	≤ 9%	9–27%	≥ 27%
Percent eggs fertilized	80 ± 14%	78 ± 17%	80 ± 18%
Percent good embryo	52% (11/21)	52% (23/44)	48% (10/21)
Abortion rate (ICSI)	9% (1/11)	13% (3/23)	40% (4/10)
(IVF)	9% (2/23)	8% (3/36)	17% (2/12)

Source: Adapted from Lin MH et al. *Fertil Steril* 2008;90:352–9.
Note: DFI: DNA fragmentation index, reflecting the percent of spermatozoa with abnormal chromatin structure.

in half of the studies.[32,33] This heterogeneity may well be a reflection of the extent of DNA damage sustained by spermatozoa and the location of DNA adducts within the spermatozoon genome (Table 34.2). In addition, repair of sperm DNA by the oocyte after fertilization may vary between individuals, as previously noted.

Causes of Increased Reactive Oxygen Species

DNA damage has been linked to chemotherapy and radiotherapy, cigarette smoking, varicocele, hyperthermia, and aging.[34] Sperm motility and morphology have been shown to be impaired in smokers, correlating with serum cotinine levels, as a measure of nicotine intake.[35] As mentioned previously, seminal fluid contains several antioxidants that play a protective role against sperm oxidative damage. Unfortunately, these endogenous antioxidants are lowered in cigarette smokers. Seminal fluid vitamin C levels are lower in these men and in those with reduced oral intake of vitamin C, but they can be increased following increased dietary intake.[36,37] Increased levels of reactive oxygen species and sperm DNA damage can also be found in men with varicoceles[38] and after varicocele repair, sperm DNA fragmentation has been shown to decrease.[39] The presence of a varicocele in oligospermic men has also been associated with diminished seminal antioxidant capacity.

Anti-Oxidant Vitamins in the Treatment Oxidative Sperm DNA Damage

Two meta-analyses have been performed of studies regarding the use of antioxidant vitamins as treatment of DNA fragmentation secondary to oxidative stress. In one, 20 of the 65 published studies assessed were chosen for further analysis. Eleven were placebo-controlled. Overall, 19/20 studies showed a significant reduction of oxidative stress or DNA damage after oral antioxidant treatment. Sperm motility was improved in ten of 16 studies. There was no effect of antioxidants on sperm morphology and only three studies reported positive effects on sperm concentration. Ten studies reported fertilization or pregnancy rates, with six reporting a significant improvement.[40]

A second meta-analysis included 34 trials with 2876 couples in total.[41] Three of these trials reported live births. Men taking oral antioxidants had a statistically significant increase in live birth rate (pooled odds ratio [OR] 4.85, 95% confidence interval [CI] 1.92 to 12.24; $p = 0.0008$), when compared with those taking the control. This result, however, was based on only 20 live births from a total of 214 couples in three small studies. No studies reported harmful side effects of the antioxidant therapy used. It is clear that further well-designed, large randomized placebo controlled trials are needed to confirm these findings.

Effect of Paternal Age on Spermatozoa

While a slight paternal age-dependent increase in disomies of the sex chromosomes in spermatozoa have been reported,[42] age effects on autosomal aneuploidy are not detectable[7,42] (Table 34.3). In

TABLE 34.3

Is Age a Factor in Sperm Aneuploidy?

Age (n)	Aneuploidy[a]	Diploidy
20–29 (19)	65 ± 24	18 ± 18
30–39 (20)	58 ± 27	14 ± 10
40–49 (16)	50 ± 19	8 ± 5
50–59 (17)	47 ± 14	11 ± 5
60–80 (16)	58 ± 22	13 ± 12

Source: Adapted from Wyrobek AJ et al. *Proc Natl Acad Sci U S A* 2006;103:9601–6.

[a] 10,000 sperm were studied by fluorescence *in situ* hybridization for chromosomes 21, X, and Y in each man.

TABLE 34.4

Effect of Age of Men on Sperm DNA Damage

Age	Number	DFI (mean ± SD)
20–29	19	12.9 ± 7.7
30–39	20	16.3 ± 9.6
40–49	16	23.2 ± 14.9
50–59	17	35.4 ± 18.6
60–80	16	49.6 ± 17.3

Source: Adapted from Wyrobek AJ et al. *Proc Natl Acad Sci U S A* 2006;103:9601–6.

Note: DFI: DNA fragmentation index, as determined by flow cytometry, using the sperm chromatin structure assay. DFI: the ratio of red fluorescing sperm (exhibiting DNA damage) to the total [red + green] sperm, reflecting the percent spermatozoa with abnormal chromatin structure.

contrast, a significant increase in syndromes such as achondroplasia and Apert syndrome, due to single base mutations due to the continuous replication of male stem cells after puberty, have been found more frequently with increasing male age. Paternal age has been correlated with increased DNA damage in sperm donors and in men of infertile couples[43,44] (Table 34.4) and the resulting genetic mutations in the embryo might also lead to abortion. Slama et al.[45] performed a prospective study of 5121 women, who were interviewed when they were less than 13 weeks pregnant, then followed until birth. The risk of spontaneous abortion between weeks 6 and 20 of pregnancy was adjusted for maternal age. The adjusted hazard ratio of spontaneous abortion associated with paternal age of 35 years or more, compared with less than 35 years, was 1.27 (95% CI: 1.00–1.61). Among women aged less than 30 years, the hazard ratio of spontaneous abortion associated with paternal age of 35 years or more was 1.56 for first trimester spontaneous abortion and 0.87 for early second trimester spontaneous abortion.

Anti-Sperm Antibodies, Chlamydia, and Embryo Implantation Failure

An association has been found between the presence of antisperm antibodies in asymptomatic men and women with no history of *Chlamydia trachomatis* infection and immunity to the *C. trachomatis* 60-kDa heat shock protein (hsp60).[46] A soluble form of hsp60 has been detected in seminal fluid, and this finding correlates with the presence of anti-*chlamydial* antibodies in these individuals. These circulating antibodies appear to be reactive with a specific region of hsp60, which is a conserved epitope of the heat shock protein and shares 50% homology with an epitope on human spermatozoa. Witkin has proposed that as hsp60 is expressed on epithelial cells of human decidua, hsp-sensitized lymphocytes will be reactivated, leading to immune rejection of the embryo.[46]

Seminal Fluid as an Immune Modulator Promoting Early Pregnancy

Accumulating evidence has revealed the complexity of seminal fluid, beyond its role as a transport medium for sperm. These factors facilitate the implantation of embryos within the endometrium through perturbation of the female immune system, and in the regulation of trophectoderm outgrowth and early placental development. They include a high content of TGF-β[47] and PGE prostaglandins.[48] Semen contains 19-hydroxy PGE, which is not found in other secretions, and the concentration of PGE prostaglandins in human semen is many times higher than that found in other body fluids. Other factors in semen that may alter the female immune system include prostasomes,[49] polymines,[50] cytokines,[51] soluble Fc-gamma receptors,[52] pregnancy-associated plasma protein A (PAPP-A),[53] vascular endothelial growth factor (VEGF),[54] and HLA-G.[55]

Seminal prostasomes are small membranous vesicles produced by epithelial cells of the human prostate. Tarazona et al.[56] have shown by flow cytometric analysis that prostasomes express high levels of CD48, the ligand for the natural killer (NK) cell activating receptor CD244, and may modulate NK cell cytotoxicity, or lead to inhibition of cytokine secretion. Other ligands for NK receptors were not expressed in prostasomes. Addition of prostasomes from ejaculates of men with normal semen parameters to NK cell obtained from peripheral blood of healthy donors resulted in a decrease in CD244+ expression, in a dose-dependent manner.

Seminal fluid content of TGF-β is approximately five-fold that of serum and similar to that of colostrum.[57] The prostate has been identified as a major site of TGF-β in men, in contrast to rodents, where the seminal vesicle is its principal source. Robertson et al.[58] demonstrated that fetal loss and abnormalities are greater when preimplantation embryos are transferred to recipients after pseudo-pregnancy was induced in mice mated with seminal-vesicle-deficient males (without exposure to seminal fluid TGF-β), compared with seminal vesicle-intact intact males.

Gutsche et al.[59] studied the expression *in vitro* of cytokine mRNAs in human endometrial epithelial and stromal cells, demonstrating a concentration-dependent stimulation by seminal plasma of IL-1 beta, Il-6, and LIF mRNA. Semen exposure *in vivo* also induces neutrophil recruitment into the superficial epithelial layers of the cervix. Sharkey et al.[60] studied the changes in the leukocyte population and cytokines within the cervix following coitus. Matched cervical biopsies were obtained 48 hours apart in the periovulatory period and 12 hours following either unprotected sexual relations, vaginal intercourse using a condom, or in the absence of coitus. A significant increase in CD45+ cells consisting of CD14+ macrophages and CD1a+ dendritic cells expressing CD11a cells expressing MHC class II was observed *only* following semen exposure. mRNA expression of CSF2, IL-6, IL-1A, and IL-8 increased, as judged by quantitative reverse transcriptase polymerase chain reaction (RT-PCR) analysis of cDNA. When mRNA from cervical tissue biopsies was reverse transcribed into cDNA and hybridized to *Affymetrix* Human Gene 1.0ST arrays, 436 genes were found to be upregulated and 277 downregulated following semen exposure! Seminal TGF-β may play a role in mediating these events, though other cytokines and chemokines within semen, such as IL-8, CCL2 through CCL5, could also be important.

Effects of Seminal Fluid on Regulatory T Cell (T Reg) Lymphocytes

Successful pregnancy requires that the embryo be protected from damage by the maternal immune system, through a state of active immune tolerance. Robertson et al.[61] have recently reviewed emerging knowledge on how seminal fluid interacts with the female adaptive immune response in mice and humans, leading to the formation in the peri-implantation period of regulatory T cells (Treg) cells, which play a significant role in mediating this tolerance. Treg cells encounter antigens presented by a specific class of dendritic cells (DCs) that differentiate in the presence of TGF-β, IL10, granulocyte-macrophage colony-stimulating factor (GM-CSF), and IL-4. Prostaglandin E_2 appears to synergize with TGF-β in this role and enhances the inhibitory capacity of human CD4+ CD25+ Treg cells.[62]

Aluvihare et al.[63] showed, in mice, that CD4⁺CD25⁺ Treg cells increase in number within days after mating. Seminal fluid exposure activates and expands inducible regulatory T cell populations in lymph nodes draining the reproductive tract, which are then recruited to the uterus. In women, an estrogen-regulated increase in circulating CD4+CD25+FOXP3+ Treg cells has been observed during the late follicular phase of the menstrual cycle, followed by a decline in the luteal phase. Estrogen also causes elevated uterine expression of the chemokines CCL3, CCL4, and CCL5, which recruit Treg cells into the uterus. Seminal fluid components promote expansion of specific clones of paternal antigen-reactive Treg cells, acting in conjunction with their hormone-mediated peri-ovulatory expansion.[61]

Effects of Administration of Seminal Plasma on Establishing Pregnancy in Humans

Given the laboratory experiments in mice supporting a role of seminal fluid in promoting successful pregnancy, clinical studies have been performed, to determine whether seminal fluid exposure at the time of laboratory-assisted reproduction improved pregnancy rates. These studies have been inconsistent. Bellinge et al.[64] found that embryo implantation rates during *in vitro* fertilization and embryo transfer were higher in women exposed to semen at the time of follicular aspiration than in its absence. This effect was observed in a subpopulation of women with occluded fallopian tubes, eliminating the possibility of *in vivo* fertilization of oocytes that may not have been retrieved at follicular aspiration. Subsequently, Fishel et al.[65] failed to observe a difference in pregnancy rates when semen was deposited intra-vaginally, immediately after the time of oocyte recovery. Tremellen et al.[66] observed no difference in pregnancy rates following transfer of frozen embryos, in a group of women who had coitus at the time of embryo transfer versus a sexually abstinent group. However, the proportion of viable pregnancies at 6 weeks gestation was higher in the former group (OR 1.48, $p = 0.036$). In another study, when cryopreserved seminal plasma was placed intra-vaginally just after follicular aspiration, the clinical pregnancy rate was 37.3% in the SP group versus 25.7% in the saline control group, but this difference did not reach statistical significance.[67] Embryo implantation rates were not different in a third study in couples who had coitus at least once 12 hours after embryo transfer.[68] Friedler et al.[69] performed a double-blind, placebo-controlled study of 230 couples undergoing *in vitro* fertilization in which 500 µL of fresh seminal plasma was injected into the vaginal vault immediately after follicular aspiration. Number of ova recovered and number of cleaving embryos were comparable between groups. Although implantation rates were higher in the seminal fluid exposed group than in the controls (21.4% versus 16.9%), as were continuing pregnancy rates (32% versus 22.2%), these differences were not statistically significant. A study in which seminal fluid was placed intra-vaginally at the time of intra-uterine insemination (IUI) with spermatozoa washed out of semen also revealed no difference in pregnancy rate when compared with a saline control.[70] Unfortunately, all of these studies were of small size and often did not define their clinical populations well.

Clinical Studies of T Regulatory Cells in Women Experiencing Recurrent Pregnancy Loss

Jasper et al.[71] collected endometrial tissue during the mid-luteal phase from nulliparous women experiencing unexplained infertility of at least 2 years duration and who had failed to conceive despite transfer of ten or more good quality embryos following *in vitro* fertilization. Expression of mRNAs encoding T cell transcription factors, including Foxp3 (an enhancer gene that plays a role in Treg generation),[72] as well as TGF-β1-3, the major cytokines associated with Treg cell differentiation, the Th1 cytokines IFN-α and IL-12, and Th2 cytokines IL-4, IL-5, and IL-10 was determined. Women of proven fertility served as controls. All of the subjects abstained from coitus from the date of their last menses until endometrial sampling, or used condoms for contraception. A 43% reduction in endometrial mRNA encoding Foxp3 was found in the infertile group, but no difference in TGF-β1 and TGF-β2 between infertile and fertile women. Although TGF-β3 mRNA was reduced, this did not reach statistical significance. Th1 and Th2 cytokine expression was similar as well between groups. The diminished endometrial content of Foxp3 suggested that a possible decreased population of endometrial Treg cells of these women might play a role in compromised embryo implantation.

Sasaki et al.[73] enumerated using flow cytometry CD4+CD25^{bright} regulatory T cells in peripheral blood and decidua of women undergoing elective early pregnancy termination versus spontaneous abortion. The proportion of Treg cells was significantly lower in specimens from the latter group than those women undergoing induced abortions. Yang et al.[74] compared 34 healthy women who were undergoing elective pregnancy termination with 25 women with a mean number of 4.04 ± 1.24 successive spontaneous abortions in whom an etiology could not be found. Using flow cytometry to detect CD4+CD25^{bright} T cells, the population of these Treg cells was significantly lower in the decidua of recurrent aborters.

Schumacher et al.[75] have shown that tissue containing decidua and placenta from women undergoing spontaneous abortion had significantly decreased human chorionic gonadotropin (hCG) mRNA and protein levels associated with a decrease in Foxp3, neutropilin-1, IL-10 and TGF-β mRNA levels, when compared with normal pregnant women. They demonstrated, using *in vitro* migration assays, that Treg cells were attracted by hCG-producing trophoblasts and choriocarcinoma cells. Treg cells isolated from peripheral blood of pregnant women (30 weeks of gestation) as well as nonpregnant women after hCG exposure expressed the LH/hCG receptor on their surface. Given that abnormally low serum concentrations of human chorionic gonadotropin (hCG) are associated with pregnancies ending in spontaneous abortion, these finding raise the issue of whether the diminished number of Treg cells observed by Sasaki et al.[73] in women undergoing pregnancy loss are the cause or consequence of miscarriage.

Roberson[61] has cited data documenting a variation in the competence of seminal fluid from different men to induce cytokine responses in cervical cells, which appears to be correlated with its TGF-β content, as well as other signaling factors. A currently intriguing and unanswered question is whether the male sexual partners of those women who experience recurrent pregnancy loss associated with decreased numbers of Treg cells exhibit lower seminal fluid concentrations of TGF-β or E prostaglandins, which play roles in their generation.

Seminal Fluid HLA-G and Miscarriage

The nonclassical human leukocyte antigens, HLA-G, has been detected by Western blot analysis in human seminal plasma samples. HLA-G expression was shown by immunohistochemistry in normal testis and in epididymal tissue, but not in the seminal vesicle[55]. Soluble HLA-G in seminal plasma has been found to induce a tolerogenic phenotype in DCs[76] and can exert immune-modulatory effects in NK cells and promote Treg cell induction.[77]

REFERENCES

1. Martin RH. Cytogenetic determinants of male infertility. *Hum Reprod Update* 2008;14:379–90.
2. Rudak E, Jacobs P, Yanagimachi R. Direct analysis of the chromosome constitution of human spermatozoa. *Nature* 1978;274:911–3.
3. Martin RH, Balkan W, Burns K et al. The chromosome constitution of 1000 human spermatozoa. *Hum Genet* 1983;63:305–9.
4. Martin R, Spriggs E, Rudemaker A. Multicolor fluorescence *in situ* hybridization analysis of aneuploidy and diploidy frequencies in 225,846 sperm from 10 normal men. *Biol Reprod* 1996;54:394–8.
5. Sun F, Ko E, Martin RH. Is there a relationship between sperm chromatin abnormalities and sperm morphology? *Reprod Biol Endocrinol* 2006;4:1.
6. Templado C, Lroz L, Estop A. New insights on the origin and relevance of aneuploidy in human spermatozoa. *Mol Hum Reprod* 2013;16:634–43.
7. Bronson RA, Bronson SK, Oula LD. Ability of abnormally-shaped human spermatozoa to adhere to and penetrate zona-free hamster eggs: Correlation with sperm morphology and post-incubation motility. *J Androl* 2007;28:698–705.
8. Rademaker AW, Greene C et al. A comparison of the frequency of sperm chromosome abnormalities in men with mild, moderate, and severe oligozoospermia. *Biol Reprod* 2003;69:535–9.

9. Martin RH. Mechanisms of nondisjunction in human spermatogenesis. *Cytogenet Genome Res* 2005;111:245–9.

10. Tempest HG, Ko E, Chan P et al. Sperm aneuploidy frequencies analyzed before and after chemotherapy in testicular cancer and Hodgkin's lymphoma patients. *Hum Reprod* 2008;23:251–8.

11. Philipp T, Philipp K, Reiner A et al. Embryoscopic and cytogenetic analysis of 233 missed abortions: Factors involved in the pathogenesis of developmental defects of early failed pregnancies. *Hum Reprod* 2003;18:1724–32.

12. Rajcan-Separovic QY, Tyson C et al. Genomic changes detected by array CGH in human embryos with developmental defects. *Mol Hum Reprod* 2010;16:125–34.

13. Ivanka D, Vera D, Desislova N et al. Array comparative genomic hybridization (CGH) analysis of sperm DNA to detect copy number variations in infertile men with idiopathic azoospermia. *J Clin Med Res* 2010;2:42–8.

14. Stouffs K, Vandermaelen D, Massart A et al. Array comparative genomic hybridization in male infertility. *Hum Reprod* 2012;27:921–9.

15. Delbes G, Hales BF, Robaire B. Toxicants and human sperm chromatin integrity. *Mol Hum Reprod* 2009;16:14–22.

16. Rubes J, Selevan SG, Evenson DP et al. Episodic air pollution is associated with increased DNA fragmentation in human sperm without other changes in semen quality. *Hum Reprod* 2005;20:2776–83.

17. Marchetti E, Eskenazi B, Weldon RH et al. Occupational exposure to benzene and chromosome structure aberrations in the sperm of Chinese men. *Environ Health Perspect* 2012;120:229–34.

18. Balhorn R. The protamine family of sperm nuclear proteins. *Genome Res* 2007;8:227–35.

19. Jenkins TG, Carrell DT. The sperm epigenome and potential implications for the developing embryo. *Reproduction* 2012;143:727–34.

20. Hammoud SS, Nix DA, Zhang H et al. Distinctive chromatin in human sperm packages genes for embryo development. *Nature* 2009;460:473–8.

21. Aston KI, Punj V, Liu L et al. Sperm deoxyribonucleic acid methylation is altered in some men with abnormal chromatin packaging or poor *in vitro* fertilization embryogenesis. *Fertil Steril* 2012;97:285–92.

22. Sandler E, Johnson GD, Mao S et al. Stability, delivery and functions of human sperm RNAs at fertilization. *Nucleic Acid Res* 2013;41:4104–17.

23. Jodar M, Selvaraju S, Sendler E et al. The presence, role and clinical use of spermatozoal RNAs. *Hum Reprod Update* 2013;19:604–24.

24. Fullston T, Ohlsson Teague EM et al. Paternal obesity initiates metabolic disturbances in two generations of mice with incomplete penetrance to the F2 generation and alters the transcriptional profile of testis and sperm microRNA content. *FASEB J* 2013;27:4226–43.

25. Aitkin RJ, Bronson R, Smith TB et al. The source and significance of DNA damage in human spermatozoa: A commentary on diagnostic strategies and straw men fallacies. *Mol Hum Reprod* 2013;19:475–85.

26. Aitken RJ, De Iuliis. On the possible origins of DNA damage in human spermatozoa. *Mol Hum Reprod* 2010;16:3–13.

27. Ollero M, Powers RD, Alvarez JG. Variation of docosahexaenoic acid content in subsets of human spermatozoa at different stages of maturation: Implications for sperm lipoperoxidative damage. *Mol Reprod Develop* 2009;55:326–34.

28. Aitkin RJ, Gosdon E, Harkiss D et al. Relative impact of oxidative stress on the functional competence and genomic integrity of human spermatozoa. *Biol Reprod* 1998;59:1037–46.

29. Menezo Y, Dale B, Cohen M. DNA damage and repair in human oocytes and embryos: A review. *Zygote* 2010;18:357–65.

30. Hendricks KEM, Hansen PJ. Consequences for the bovine embryo of being derived from a spermatozoon subjected to oxidative stress. *Austral Veterinary J* 2010;88:307–10.

31. Burruel V, Klooster KL, Chitwood J et al. Oxidative damage to rhesus macaque spermatozoa results in mitotic arrest and transcript abundance changes in early embryos. *Biol Reprod* 2013;89:72.

32. Zini A, Jamal W, Cowan L, Al-Hathal N. Is sperm DNA damage associated with IVF embryo quality? A Systematic review. *J Assist Reprod Genet* 2011;28:391–7.

33. Lin MH, Kuo-Kuang LR, Li SH et al. Sperm chromatin structure parameters are not related to fertilization rates, embryo quality, and pregnancy rates in *in vitro* fertilization and intracytoplasmic sperm injection, but might be related to spontaneous abortion rates. *Fertil Steril* 2008;90:352–9.

34. Aitken RJ, Baker MA. Causes and consequences of apoptosis in spermatozoa; contributions to infertility and impacts on development. *Int J Dev Biol* 2013;57:265–72.
35. Zenzes MT. Smoking and reproduction: Gene damage to human gametes and embryos. *Hum Reprod Update* 2000;6:122–31.
36. Fraga CR, Motchnik PA, Shigenaga MK et al. Ascorbic acid protects against endogenous oxidative DNA damage in human sperm. *Proc Natl Acad Sci U S A* 1991;88:11003–6.
37. Fraga CG, Motchnik PA, Wyrobek AJ et al. Smoking and low antioxidant levels increase oxidative damage to sperm DNA. *Mutat Res* 1996;351:199–203.
38. Zini A, Dohie G. Are varicocoeles associated with increased deoxyribonucleic acid fragmentation? *Fertil Steril* 2011;96:1283–97.
39. Werthman P, Wixon R, Kasperson BS et al. Significant decrease in sperm deoxyribonucleic acid fragmentation after varicocelectomy. *Fertil Steril* 90;2008:1800–4.
40. Zini A, Al-Hathal N. Antioxidant therapy in male infertility: Fact or fiction? *Asian J Androl* 2011;13:371–84.
41. Showell MG, Brown J, Yazdani A et al. Antioxidants for male subfertility. *Cochrane Database Syst Rev* 2011;CD007411.
42. Sartorius GA, Nieschlag E. Paternal age and reproduction. *Hum Reprod Update* 2010;16:65–79.
43. Wyrobek AJ, Eskenazi B, Young S et al. Advancing age has differential effects on DNA damage, chromatin integrity, gene mutations, and aneuploides in sperm. *Proc Natl Acad Sci U S A* 2006;103:9601–6.
44. Dus M, Al-Hathal N, Sun-Gabriel M et al. High prevalence of isolated sperm DNA damage in infertile men with advanced paternal age. *J Assist Reprod Genet* 2013;30:843–8.
45. Slama R, Bouyer J, Windham G et al. Influence of paternal age on the risk of spontaneous abortion. *Am J Epidemiol* 2005;161:816–23.
46. Witkin SS, Askienazy-Elbhar M et al. Circulating antibodies to a conserved epitope of the Chlamydia trachomatis 60 kDa heat shock protein (hsp60) in infertile couples and its relationship to antibodies to C. trachomatis surface antigens and the Escherichia coli and human HSP60. *Hum Reprod* 1998;13:1175–9.
47. Robertson SA, Ingman WV, O'Leary S et al. Transforming growth factor beta—A mediator of immune deviation in seminal plasma. *J Reprod Immunol* 2002;57:109–28.
48. Kelly RW. Prostaglandins in primate semen: Biasing the immune system to benefit spermatozoa and virus? *Prostaglandins Leukot Essent Fatty Acids* 1997;57:113–8.
49. Burden HP, Holmes CBH, Persad R et al. Prostasomes: Their effects on human male reproduction and fertility. *Hum Reprod Update* 2006;12:283–92.
50. Shohat B, Maayan R, Singer M et al. Immunosuppressive activity and polyamine levels of seminal plasma in azo-ospermic, oligospermic, and normospermic men. *Arch Androl* 1990;24:41–50.
51. Maegawa M, Kanada M, Irahara M et al. A repertoire of cytokines in human seminal plasma. *J Reprod Immunol* 2002;54:33–42.
52. Thaler CJ, McConnache CR, McIntyre J. Inhibition of IgG-Fc-mediated cytotoxicity by seminal plasma IgG-Fc receptor antigens. *Fertil Steril* 1992;143:1937–42.
53. Bischof P, Martin-du-pan R, Lauber K et al. Human seminal plasma contains a protein that shares physicochemical, immunological and immunosuppressive properties with pregnancy-associated plasma protein-A. *J Clin Endocrin Metab* 1983;56:359–62.
54. Obermair A, Obruca A, Pohl M. Vascular endothelial growth factor and its receptors in male fertility. *Fertil Steril* 1999;72:269–75.
55. Larsen MH, Bzorek M, Pass MB et al. Human leukocyte antigen-G in the male reproductive system and in seminal plasma. *Mol Human Reprod* 2011;17:727–38.
56. Tarazona R, Delgado E, Guarnizo MC et al. Human prostasomes express CD48 and interfere with NK function. *Immunobiology* 2011;216:41–6.
57. Robertson SA. Seminal plasma and male factor signaling in the female reproductive tract. *Cell Tissue Res* 2005;322:43–52.
58. Robertson, SA, Guerin LR, Bromfeld JJ et al. Seminal fluid drives expansion of the CD4+CD25+ T regulatory cell pool and induces tolerance to paternal alloantigens in mice. *Biol Reprod* 2009;80:1036–45.
59. Gutsche S, von Wolff M, Strowitzki T et al. Seminal plasma induces mRNA expression of IL-10, IL-6, and LIF in endometrial epithelial cells in vitro. *Mol Hum Reprod* 2003;9:785–91.
60. Sharkey DJ, Tremellen KP, Jasper MJ et al. Seminal fluid induces leukocyte recruitment and cytokine and chemokine mRNA expression in the human cervix after coitus. *J Immunol* 2012;188:2445–54.

61. Robertson SA, Prins JR, Sharkey DJ et al. Seminal fluid and the generation of regulatory T cells for embryo implantation. *Am J Reprod Immunol* 2013;69:315–30.

62. Baratelli F, Liu Y, Zhu L et al. Prostaglandin E2 induces FOXP3 gene expression and T regulatory cell function in human CD4+ T cells. *J Immunol* 2005;175:1483–90.

63. Aluvihare VR, Kallikourdis M, Betz AG. Regulatory T cells mediate maternal tolerance to the fetus. *Nat Immunol* 2004;5:266–71.

64. Bellinge BS, Copelan CM, Thomas TD et al. The influence of patient insemination on the implantation rate in an *in vitro* fertilization and embryo transfer program. *Fertil Steril* 1986;46:252–6.

65. Fishel S, Webster J, Jackson P et al. Evaluation of high vaginal insemination at oocyte recovery in patients undergoing *in vitro* fertilization. *Fertil Steril* 1989;51:135–8.

66. Tremellen KP, Valbuenq D, Landaera J et al. The effect of intercourse on pregnancy rates during assisted reproduction. *Hum Reprod* 2000;15:2653–8.

67. Von Wolff M, Rosner S, Thone C. Intravaginal and intracervical application of seminal plasma in *in vitro* fertilization or intracytoplasmic sperm injection treatment cycles- a double-blind, placebo-controlled, randomized study. *Fertil Steril* 2009;91:167–72.

68. Afatoonian A, Ghandi S, Tabibnejad N. The effect of intercourse around embryo transfer on pregnancy rate in assisted reproductive technology cycles. *Int J Fertil Steril* 2009;2:169–72.

69. Friedler S, Ben-Ami L, Gidoni Y et al. Effect of seminal plasma application to the vaginal vault in *in vitro* fertilization or intracytoplasmic sperm injection treatment cycles—A double-blind, placebo-controlled, randomized study. *J Assist Reprod Genet* 2013;30:907–11.

70. Qasim SM, Trias A, Karacan M et al. Does the absence or presence of seminal fluid matter in patients undergoing ovulation induction with intrauterine insemination? *Hum Reprod* 1996;11:1008–10.

71. Jasper MJ, Tremellen KP, Robertson SA. Primary unexplained infertility is associated with reduced expression of the T-regulatory cell transcription factor Foxp3 in endometrial tissue. *Mol Hum Reprod* 2006;12:301–8.

72. Samstein RM, Josefowicz SZ, Arvey A et al. Extrathymic generation of regulatory T cells in placental mammals mitigates maternal-fetal conflict. *Cell* 2012;150:29–38.

73. Sasaki Y, Sakai M, Miyazaki S et al. Decidual and peripheral blood CD4 + CD25+ regulatory T cells in early pregnancy subjects and spontaneous abortion cases. *Mol Hum Reprod* 2004;10:347–53.

74. Yang H, Qiu L, Chen G et al. Proportional change of CD4+CD25+ regulatory T cells in decidua and peripheral blood in unexplained recurrent spontaneous abortion patients. *Fertil Steril* 2008;89:656–61.

75. Schumacher A, Brachwitz N, Sohr S et al. Human chorionic gonado tropin attracts regulatory T cells into the fetal-maternal interface during early human pregnancy. *J Immunol* 2009;182:5488–97.

76. Ristich V, Liang S, Zhang W et al. Tolerization of dendridic cells by HLA-G. *Eur J Immunol* 2005;35:1133–42.

77. Selman Z, Naji A, Zidi I et al. Human leukocyte antigen-G5 secretion in mesenchymal stem cells is required to suppress T lymphocyte and natural killer function and induce CD4 + CD25highFOXP3+ regulatory T cells. *Stem Cells* 2008;26:212–22.

35

Midtrimester Loss: The Role of Cerclage and Pessaries

Israel Hendler and Howard J. A. Carp

Introduction

Cervical insufficiency is defined as the inability of the uterine cervix to retain a pregnancy in the absence of contractions or labor. It is a clinical diagnosis characterized by recurrent painless cervical dilatation and spontaneous midtrimester loss of a viable fetus. Generally, in the absence of predisposing conditions, such as spontaneous rupture of the membranes, bleeding or infection, it may indicate a different origin for midtrimester loss rather than primary cervical malfunction or insufficiency.[1] Cervical insufficiency was first described in the English literature in 1678; however, even today the diagnosis is clinical and made in retrospect after a poor obstetric outcome. The diagnosis is difficult to make and is solely based upon careful history and review of the medical records, rather than accurate diagnostic imaging studies or other laboratory tools. True cervical insufficiency is probably uncommon; however, the lack of clear diagnostic criteria makes the incidence unknown.

Cervical cerclage was first introduced by Shirodkar in 1955; it is an appropriate and well-designed solution for true cervical insufficiency. However, due to lack of strict diagnostic criteria, the indication for cerclage are still far from clear as are the optimal methods and timing. This chapter focuses on the diagnosis of cervical insufficiency, the obstetric management of pregnant women at high risk for preterm delivery or midtrimester loss by ultrasonogarphic follow-up of cervical length, the particular problems of cerclage in recurrent pregnancy loss (RPL), the role of transcervical and transabdominal cervical cerclage, and the optimal timing and method of performing the procedure.

Pathophysiology

The pathophysiology of cervical insufficiency is poorly understood. The cervix develops from fusion and recanalization of the distal paramesonephric (Müllerian) ducts,[2] which is complete by approximately 20 weeks' gestation and is composed of both muscle and fibrous connective tissue. The fibrous component, which is responsible for the tensile strength of the cervix, increases in proportion from the external os towards the body of the uterus Cervical insufficiency is thought to be related to a defect in tensile strength at the cervicoisthmic junction.[3] Previous authors postulated a deficiency of cervical collagen, cervical elastin, or some other structural, mechanical component of cervical connective tissue that normally resists softening, effacement, and dilatation caused by the gravitational effect of the fetus and amniotic fluid. Although several theories of pathophysiology have been considered, the difficulty in obtaining biopsy samples from the human cervix before, during, and after term and preterm deliveries has hampered this understanding. In 1996, Iams et al.[4] challenged the traditional understanding of the cervix as being either "competent" or "incompetent." Transvaginal ultrasonography (TVU) of cervical length was performed in 2915 women at 23 weeks of gestation. Ultrasound revealed that the association between cervical length and the risk of preterm delivery is evident across the entire range of cervical lengths. Even among women whose cervical length was above the 10th percentile, the risk of preterm delivery increased as cervical length decreased. This suggests that the length of the cervix is an indirect indicator of its competence and it should be seen as a continuous rather than a dichotomous variable.

The length of the cervix is directly correlated with the duration of pregnancy: the shorter the cervix, the greater the likelihood of preterm delivery. However, the cervix is a dynamic structure in pregnancy, occasionally shortening with no apparent relationship to uterine contractions. Iams et al.[4] have proposed the model of a continuum of cervical compliance ("competence") similar to the natural biologic variation in the population in other physical traits, such as height and weight. In this model, cervical compliance and cervical length varies among women, and these qualities are just some of the components of uterine function that affect the timing of delivery. The length of the cervix during the second trimester in an obstetric population is distributed in a bell-shaped curve. The wide range in normal cervical length (the 10th and 90th percentiles are 25 and 45 mm, respectively) during this period is due, in part, to biologic variation, but may also result from premature cervical effacement. Although a short cervix is predictive of preterm birth, it is not diagnostic of cervical insufficiency and many women who have a congenitally short cervix deliver at term.[5–9]

Risk Factors for the Etiology of Cervical Insufficiency

Congenital Factors

A functional defect in the cervix can be caused by an anatomic abnormality (such as congenital Müllerian anomalies, including canalization defects (e.g., septate uterus), unification defects (e.g., bicornuate uterus), and even arcuate uterus, *in utero* diethylstilbestrol (DES) exposure, or collagen disorders (e.g., Ehlers–Danlos syndrome). Congenital defects may explain the familial tendency for cervical insufficiency. As an example, in one study, 34 of 125 (27%) women with cervical insufficiency had a first degree relative with the same diagnosis, but none of the 165 unaffected women had a family history of cervical insufficiency.

Acquired Factors

Obstetric Trauma

A cervical laceration may occur during labor or delivery, including spontaneous, forceps, vacuum, or cesarean births. Laceration might weaken the cervix, and contribute to cervical insufficiency.[10]

Mechanical Dilation

Mechanical dilation of the cervix during gynecologic procedures may weaken the cervix. Prior cervical mechanical dilatation is one of the most common associated risk factors. In a meta-analysis, an increasing number of voluntary pregnancy terminations was associated with an increasing risk of spontaneous preterm births.

Treatment of Cervical Intraepithelial Neoplasia

Cervical biopsy, laser ablation, loop electrosurgical excision procedures (LEEP), or cold knife conization may all weaken the cervix.[10,11] However, in most cases of presumed cervical insufficiency no known risk factor can be found.

Diagnosis of Cervical Insufficiency

Unfortunately, there are no reliable prepregnancy tests to confirm cervical insufficiency in "at-risk" women. In the past, clinicians have suggested a variety of tests including: assessment of the width of the cervical canal by hysterosalpingogram and/or by hysteroscopy, ease of insertion of cervical dilators of various diameters (Hegar test); the force required to withdraw a Foley catheter with its bulb inflated through the internal os; and different methods to measure force required to stretch the cervix using an intra-cervical balloon and vaginal examination on a weekly basis during the second trimester of pregnancy in high risk women with RPL to assess softening and shortening of the cervix. None of these has been validated in rigorous clinical studies. The obvious flaw with these techniques is the failure to account for the effects of pregnancy on the dynamic capabilities of the cervix.

With the advent of transvaginal ultrasonography and measurement of cervical length features such as shortening, effacement, and dilatation with the presence of funneling and prolapse of the membranes, have enabled clinicians to predict outcome long before symptoms occur; however, it is still unclear if cervical shortening is indicative of a primary cervical problem. Between 20 and 28 weeks, most women have a median cervical length of 35 mm that decreases gradually as pregnancy advances to about 30 mm at term. Without any reliable, objective method of distinguishing cervical insufficiency from other causes of premature cervical change, management is pragmatically based on combining features within the history (e.g., previous painless dilatation, cervical surgery) with ultrasound findings.

Cervical Cerclage

Transvaginal cerclage in pregnancy was first reported in 1955; the case was performed by Dr. V. Shirodkar, an Indian obstetrician. Shirodkar described 30 women who had 4–11 prior late miscarriages. Shirodkar emphasized that his work was confined to women in whom he could prove the existence of weakness of the internal os via repeated vaginal examinations. Many investigators have reported variations on the surgical technique of transvaginal cerclage, and the most common of these is the McDonald procedure. A variety of technical aspects of cervical cerclage have been investigated for their efficacy in prolonging gestation. Safety and effectiveness of technical aspects of cerclage may vary by the indications for this procedure. When first described cerclage was used for two indications: initially for prior second-trimester loss with painless cervical dilation in the current pregnancy (i.e., physical examination indicated) and soon after for recurrent second trimester loss, not attributable to other causes. Sixty years later cerclage is performed in 1:54–1:220 deliveries worldwide, although there is still confusion about the diagnostic criteria for cervical insufficiency and uncertainty regarding the benefits.

Techniques of Cerclage

McDonald's Cerclage

The McDonald's cerclage is performed using a permanent suture. It was originally described as follows: the bladder having been emptied, the cervix is exposed and grasped by Allis' or Babcock forceps. A purse string suture of No. 4 Mersilk on a Mayo needle is inserted around the exo-cervix as high as possible to approximate to the level of the internal os. This is at the junction of the vagina and smooth cervix. Five or six bites with the needle are made, with special attention to the stitches behind the cervix. These are difficult to insert and must be deep. The stitch is pulled tight enough to close the internal os, the knot being made in front of the cervix and the end left long enough to facilitate subsequent division. The ends are cut long to allow identification at term and facilitate removal.

Shirodkar Cerclage

Many modifications have been made, but in general, the Shirodkar technique involves dissection of the vaginal mucosa and retraction of the bladder and rectum to expose the cervix at the level of the internal os. The original technique was described as follows: (i) A strip of fascia lata 1/4 inch wide and 4 1/2 inches long, is removed from the outer side of the thigh, and each end of this strip is transfixed with a linen suture. (ii) The cervix is pulled down, a transverse incision is made above the cervix as in anterior colporrhaphy, and the bladder is pushed well up above the internal os. (iii) The cervix is then pulled forward, toward the symphysis pubis, and a vertical incision is made in the posterior vaginal wall, again at and above the internal os, going only through the vaginal wall. (iv) Through the right and left corner of the anterior incision, an aneurysm needle is passed between the cervix and the vaginal wall until its eye comes out of the posterior incision. (v) The linen attached to each end of the fascia is passed through the eye of the aneurysm needle, and the right end of the fascia is pulled retrovaginally forward into the anterior incision. The same thing is done from the left side. (vi) The two ends of the strip cross each other in front of the cervix and are tightened to close the internal os. The operator's left index finger in the internal os will indicate how much to pull on the strips. The assistant should be holding one end of the strip with an artery forceps. (vii) The two ends are stitched together by a number of stitches that take a bite of the muscle fibers of the lowest part of the lower uterine segment, using a small curved needle and fine linen. (viii) Extra portions of the fascia are cut out, and the anterior and posterior incisions are closed with chromic catgut No. 0.

Caspi et al.[12] described a modification using a single transverse incision in the anterior fornix. A monofilament suture is passed on each side, under the mucosa at the level of the internal os, from the anterior incision to exit through the mucosa of the posterior cervix, and is then tied. The modified procedure has been compared with the original technique of Shirodkar in a randomized trial in 90 subjects who lost their pregnancies despite having undergone McDonald's procedure or with cervical anatomy felt to be unfavorable for McDonald cerclage placement. Similar pregnancy outcomes were reported. The investigators believed that the modified Shirodkar technique has the advantages of simplicity, ease of removal, and lower incidence of severe vaginal discharge.

Evidence-Based Criteria for Cerclage Placement

History Indicated Cerclage

A minority of recurrent second trimester losses/births are primarily, and perhaps exclusively, caused by congenital or acquired structural weakness of the cervix, and can be treated effectively with support by a "history-indicated" cerclage. The largest randomized trial for history indicated cerclage was published in 1993 by the Medical Research Council/Royal College of Obstetrician and Gynecologists (MRC RCOG). One thousand two hundred and ninety-two pregnant women whose obstetricians were uncertain whether to recommend cervical cerclage, most of whom had a history of early delivery or cervical surgery were randomized to cervical cerclage or a policy of withholding the operation unless it was considered to be clearly indicated. The main outcomes were delivery before 33 or 37 completed weeks and the vital status of the infant after delivery. There were fewer deliveries before 33 weeks in the cerclage group (83 [13%] compared with 110 [17%], $p = 0.03$). There was a corresponding difference in very low birth weight deliveries (63 [10%] compared with 86 [13%], $p = 0.05$). The difference in the overall rate of miscarriage, stillbirth or neonatal death (55 [9%] compared with 68 [11%]) was less marked and was not statistically significant. The use of cervical cerclage was associated with increased medical intervention and a doubling of the risk of puerperal pyrexia. The authors concluded that the operation had an important beneficial effect in 1 in 25 cases in the trial. The authors recommended that, on balance, cervical cerclage should be offered to women with a history of three or more pregnancies ending before 37 weeks of gestation. It is now suggested to place history-indicated cerclage at 12 to 14 weeks for women who meet all of the following criteria: (i) two or more consecutive prior second trimester pregnancy losses or three or more early (<34 weeks) preterm births. (ii) Presence of risk factors for cervical insufficiency, including a history of cervical trauma and/or short labors or progressively earlier deliveries in successive pregnancies. (iii) Other causes of preterm birth (e.g., infection, placental bleeding, multiple gestation) have been excluded.

Ultrasound Indicated Cerclage

The majority of women with suspected cervical insufficiency do not meet the above criteria for history-indicated cerclage. In women with a history of spontaneous preterm birth, a systematic review of controlled studies showed that measurement of cervical length in the second trimester, especially before 24 weeks, predicted the risk of recurrent preterm birth. The use of a TVU cervical length <25 mm at <24 weeks to predict preterm birth at <35 weeks has a positive predictive value of 33.0%, and negative predictive value of 92.0%. Figure 35.1a shows the sonogram of a normal cervix on ultrasound. As shortening of cervical length seems to be a continuous process, ultrasound can detect dilatation of the internal os before the external os is affected. Figure 35.1b shows shortening of the cervical canal. The likelihood

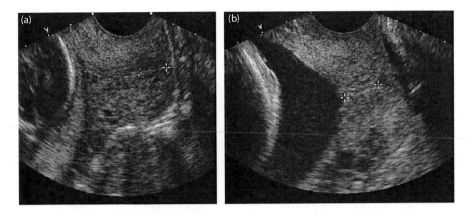

FIGURE 35.1 Ultrasound of cervical length. (a) Normal cervix of 35 mm length; (b) shortened cervix of 14 mm length. These sonograms shows normal cervices. The cervix in (a) is completely closed with a length of 35 mm as seen between the calipers. The cervix in (b) is 14 mm in length, but can still be competent.

ratio for spontaneous preterm birth <35 weeks is higher if the cervical length is shorter. Placement of cerclage upon identification of a short cervix ("ultrasound-indicated cerclage") is effective in reducing preterm births and results in pregnancy outcomes comparable to those with history-indicated cerclage, and avoids cerclage in about 60% of patients with a suggestive history. In a meta-analysis of randomized trials of women with singleton gestation, a prior spontaneous preterm birth and short cervical length <25 mm before 24 weeks, treatment with ultrasound-indicated cerclage significantly lowered the total neonatal morbidity and mortality (15.6 versus 24.8% without cerclage; relative risk [RR] 0.64, 95% confidence interval [CI] 0.45–0.91). The reduced morbidity was presumably a consequence of cerclage significantly reducing the frequency of preterm birth (delivery <35 weeks RR 0.70, 95% CI 0.55–0.89; 28.4% versus 41.3% in women without cerclage).[13,14]

In another meta-analysis of randomized trials of women with singleton gestations and prior preterm birth managed either by[1] cervical length screening with cerclage for short cervical length or[2] history-indicated cerclage, patients with ultrasound-indicated versus history-indicated cerclage had similar rates of preterm birth before 37 weeks (31% versus 32%, RR 0.97, 95% CI 0.73–1.29), preterm birth before 34 weeks (17% versus 23%, RR 0.76, 95% CI 0.48–1.20), and perinatal mortality (5% versus 3%, RR 1.77, 95% CI 0.58–5.35), and only 42% developed a short cervical length and received cerclage.[15]

Figure 35.2 shows funneling of the internal os and shortening of the cervical canal. However, trans-cervical ultrasonography has a number of drawbacks. Figure 35.3 shows an apparently normal looking cervix. Nevertheless, the application of light fundal pressure allows the insufficiency to become apparent, and grand multipara can have open cervices, without insufficiency. Hence, transcervical ultrasound is not always selective, as Figure 35.1b shows. In patients with recurrent first trimester losses, it is also not practical to screen all patients. Although the incidence of cervical incompetence,[16] midtrimester loss and preterm labor are higher after recurrent pregnancy loss[16,17] (see Figure 37.4 in Chapter 37), this higher incidence is probably not high enough to justify screening the entire population on a regular basis. In patients who are screened, it is advisable to start cervical length screening at 14 weeks, but screening may commence as early as 12 weeks in women with early second trimester losses, recurrent second trimester losses, or prior large cold knife conization. Ultrasound examination is generally repeated every 2 weeks until 24 weeks, as long as the cervical length is ≥30 mm, and increased to weekly if the cervical length is 25 to 29 mm, with the expectation that preterm cervical changes will precede overt preterm labor or membrane rupture symptoms by 3 to 6 weeks. Transvaginal ultrasound screening is usually discontinued at 24 weeks of gestation, as cerclage is not usually performed after this time.

Women with risk factors for cervical insufficiency, such as uterine anomalies, prior minor cervical surgery, or pregnancy termination, with no prior preterm delivery or late miscarriage and short cervical length have been reported to show a correlation between the risk of preterm birth and short cervical length,

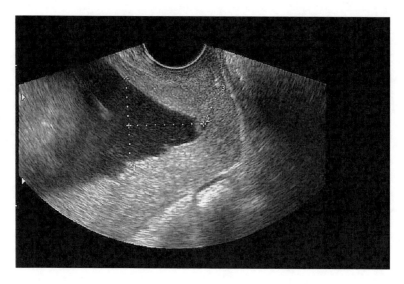

FIGURE 35.2 Sonogram of cervical incompetence. This figure shows funneling of the cervix with a dilation of the internal os. The remaining cervical canal from the funneling to the external os is extremely shortened.

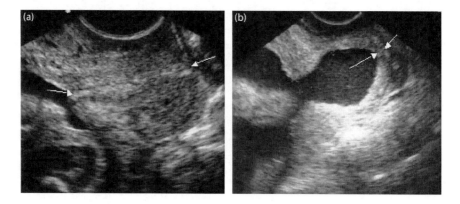

FIGURE 35.3 A dynamic cervix. (a) Cervix with no fundal pressure; (b) cervix with fundal pressure. The cervix was shortened from 28 to 0 mm during examination by light fundal pressure.

but data are limited. A wide range of recurrent preterm birth rates has been reported, depending on the cervical length threshold used and the gestational age at the time of measurement. Cerclage does not seem to benefit this population.

Progestogen administration has been reported to prevent preterm birth, either by 17 alpha hydroxy-progesterone caproate, vaginal micronized progesterone or dydrogesterone.[18–23] No randomized controlled trial has directly compared progestogen administration to cervical cerclage for the prevention of preterm birth in women with a sonographic short cervix in the midtrimester, singleton gestation, and previous preterm birth. An indirect comparison meta-analysis concluded that vaginal micronized progesterone and cerclage were equally efficacious in the prevention of preterm birth in this population[24] Based on evidence from the direct comparisons in the randomized trials discussed above, we treat women with prior preterm birth with intramuscular 17-alpha-hydroxyprogesterone caproate and then perform cerclage if the cervical length shortens to less than 25 mm. We perform a single TVU cervical length measurement at 18 to 24 weeks in women with risk factors for cervical insufficiency and no prior delivery, and treat those with a short cervix (≤20 mm) with vaginal micronized progesterone supplementation listed above. In a meta-analysis of five trials, administration of vaginal progesterone to women with a short cervix reduced the rate of spontaneous preterm birth and composite neonatal morbidity and mortality.

If the patient delivers preterm, or has another midtrimester loss, subsequent pregnancies are managed as described above. If the patient delivers at term, we again perform a single cervical length measurement at 18 to 24 weeks and administer vaginal micronized progesterone if the cervix is short.

Physical Examination Indicated Cerclage for Women Who Present with a Dilated, Effaced Cervix and Visible Membranes prior to 24 Weeks of Gestation

A patient may present before 24 weeks with minimal or no symptoms and physical examination reveals a dilated cervix. Occasionally, such findings may occur after diagnosis of a very short cervical length (e.g., <5 mm) on TVU. The management of these patients is governed primarily by whether the condition requires prompt delivery, for example, if there is overt infection, ruptured membranes, or significant hemorrhage. In the absence of indications for delivery, the gestational age and degree of cervical dilation are the next considerations. The goal of management is to both prolong the pregnancy and improve neonatal outcome in the likely event of preterm birth.[25-27]

Data from several studies suggest that a grossly dilated cervix with visible membranes may be an appropriate criterion for placement of a "physical examination indicated cerclage" in some cases (also called "heroic cerclage" or "emergency cerclage"). Placement of a physical examination indicated cerclage when a dilated cervix and visible membranes are detected on digital examination at <24 weeks appeared to prolong pregnancy and improve pregnancy outcome compared to expectant management in a small randomized trial, a prospective study, and retrospective cohort studies. Due to differences in patient populations, actual outcomes varied among these studies. Physical examination indicated cerclage in women with visible bulging membranes should only be considered in the absence of infection, labor, and vaginal bleeding (abruption).

In women without clinical signs of infection, amniocentesis should be considered in order to exclude subclinical infection.

Prior Successful Outcome after Cerclage

Prolongation of pregnancy after cerclage does not confirm the diagnosis of cervical insufficiency because many pregnancies with premature cervical effacement have good outcomes in the absence of surgical intervention. As discussed above, in randomized trials and controlled studies, about 60% of women with a history of early preterm birth or recurrent late miscarriage maintain cervical length above 25 mm and have low rates of recurrent preterm birth/loss without placement of a cerclage. Therefore, repeat cerclage in subsequent pregnancies is not mandatory.

In women who received a cerclage in a prior pregnancy without an appropriate indication, especially those who, after removal of cerclage at 36 to 37 weeks, did not go into labor in the subsequent 2 weeks, the risk of preterm birth in a subsequent pregnancy probably does not warrant a history-indicated cerclage; instead we suggest TVU cervical length screening.

Prior Unsuccessful Outcome after Cerclage

Transabdominal cerclage may be successful in women who deliver very preterm despite placement of a transvaginal cerclage.

Cervical Pessary

Another technique that has come into use for encircling the cervix is the cervical pessary. The Arabin pessary is the most commonly used such device. However, the idea of using a pessary is not new. In 1959, Cross described the use of a ring pessary in patients with cervical incompetence, lacerations or uterine malformations.[28] Since then, other devices have been used including the Hodge pessary and donut pessary. The pessary has been described to act by pressing the internal os closed from behind, and by changing the inclination of the cervical canal. This change of position may prevent direct pressure on the membranes at the internal os and on the cervix itself. The weight of the uterus may therefore be directed towards the lower anterior uterine segment rather than the cervix. The pessary has been reported to protect the cervical mucus plug by compressing the attachment of the remaining cervical tissue. The cervical mucus plug may protect the intrauterine cavity from ascending infection and subsequent miscarriage or preterm labor.[29,30]

The most commonly used pessary was designed by Arabin. It is a round cone-shaped flexible silicone pessary. The dome shape resembles the vaginal fornices, hence it attempts to encircle the cervix close to the internal os. It comes in different sizes and has perforations in the silicone to drain the vaginal discharge of the vaginal fornices.

Advantages of the Pessary

The pessary has a number of advantages over cerclage. The pessary can be fitted without anesthetic; it is not invasive, as cerclage. There is no foreign body inside the tissue of the cervix, which reduces the risk of infection. There is no fenestration from tearing of the cervical tissue, either by contractions, or pressure necrosis of the tissue under the suture. As with other pessaries, the Arabin pessary changes the uterocervical angle,[31,32] making the angle more acute, thus moving the weight of the uterus to the anterior segment. This change of angle is thought to prevent direct pressure on the membranes at the internal cervical os. The pessary also protects the cervical mucus plug by pushing the internal os closed. The cervical mucus plug may prevent ascending infection.[31,32] Cerclage, on the other hand introduces a foreign body close to the mucus plug and may enhance infection. If there is rupture of the membranes, suture cerclage should preferably be removed in order to prevent infection. The pessary can, however be left *in situ*, if the patient is managed conservatively.[33] In addition, removal is relatively easy. In some cases of cerclage, the suture may become embedded, making removal extremely difficult.

Correct Placement

If the Arabin pessary is used, the pessary should be lubricated, squeezed between thumb and fingers and introduced into the introitus. Inside the vagina, the pessary is unfolded, so that the smaller inner ring faces towards the cervix. The dome is pushed towards the fornices until the cervix is completely surrounded. Once in place, the pessary should not be felt by the patient. Subsequently, digital examination or ultrasound can be performed to confirm that the cervix protrudes through the inner ring. Arabin and Alfirevic[34] have published a table recommending different sizes to be used in different indications.

The pessary should be removed if delivery is imminent, or if contractions are effective. However, in normal circumstances, the pessary, as a suture, is removed at approximately 37 weeks. If there is cervical edema, removal may be painful. In any case, the cervix should be pushed back through the inner ring of the pessary dome.

Results

Unfortunately, there is insufficient evidence to make definite recommendations. In 1990, Quaas et al.[35] reported an observational study of the Arabin pessary in 107 patients. In 92 percent of patients, the pregnancy was maintained until 36 weeks with no reported complications. Arabin himself, published the results of a study on 46 women with a short cervical length <25 mm before 24 weeks.[36] Twenty-three had a pessary inserted, and the results compared to 23 women treated expectantly. The mean gestational age at delivery was 35+6 weeks in the pessary group and 33+2 weeks in the control group ($p = 0.02$).

There have been two randomized control trials of the pessary in patients with a short cervix (below 25 mm); however, the results are conflicting. In Goya et al.'s[33] trial, 385 women were selected on the basis of a short cervix on vaginal ultrasound between 18 and 22 weeks; 192 women were randomized to the pessary group. The use of the pessary was associated with a statistically significantly decrease in the incidence of preterm birth prior to 37 weeks compared with the 193 women in the expectant management group (22% versus 59%; respectively, RR = 0.36, 95% CI = 0.27–0.49). There were also fewer births before 34 weeks (6% versus 27%; RR = 0.24; 95% CI, 0.13–0.43), and before 28 weeks (2% versus 8%; RR, 0.25; CI, 0.09–0.73). Additionally, women in the pessary group required less tocolytics (RR 0.63; 95% CI 0.50–0.81) and corticosteroids (RR 0.66; 95% CI 0.54–0.81) than the expectant group. However, Hsui et al.[37] also assessed the pessary on 108 women with a singleton pregnancy who were selected for a short cervical length at routine second-trimester ultrasound. Fifty-three women were randomized to the pessary group, whereas 55 women formed the control group. The investigators attempted to make their control group placebo by simulating the insertion of a pessary. Pessary or sham treatment was blinded to the patients. The mean gestational age at delivery was 38.1 weeks in the pessary group compared with 37.8 weeks in the expectant management group. There was also no significant difference in the rates of delivery before 28, 34, or 37 weeks. However, in Hsui et al's[37] study, some of the women who would be expected to benefit were excluded, for example, women with a cerclage in a previous pregnancy, the presence of cervical dilatation, or a history of cervical incompetence were excluded.

In twin pregnancy, surgical cerclage is not generally thought to be helpful. However, the pessary has also been tested in twin pregnancy;[37,38] 403 women with twin pregnancy were treated with a pessary and the results compared with 410 women managed expectantly. Prophylactic use of the pessary did not reduce poor perinatal outcome. However, in the subgroup of women with a cervical length below 38 mm. at 20 weeks, the incidence of poor neonatal outcomes was 12% (9/78) for the pessary group and 29% (16/55) for the expectantly managed group. The major effect was due to significantly less deliveries before 32 weeks (14% versus 29%; RR, 0.49; 95% CI, 0.24–0.97).

Comparison of Treatment Modalities

There is only one publication comparing pessary treatment to cervical cerclage or progestogen treatment in patients with previous preterm births. Alfirevic et al.[39] compared three cohorts of women with previous preterm births and a short cervix; 142 women had a cerclage performed, 59 women received vaginal progesterone, and 42 were treated by pessary. There were no significant differences in terms of perinatal loss, neonatal morbidity, or preterm birth except for a higher rate of births before 34 weeks in the vaginal progesterone group compared to the pessary group.

REFERENCES

1. Dulay AT. Cervical insufficiency. *Merck Manual for Health Care Professionals*. Gynecology and Obstetrics: Abnormalities of Pregnancy. Available online from: http://www.merckmanuals.com/professional/gynecology_and_obstetrics/abnormalities_of_pregnancy/cervical_insufficiency.html.
2. Crosby WM, Hill EC. Embryology of the Mullerian duct system. Review of present-day theory. *Obstet Gynecol* 1962;20:507.
3. Danforth DN. The fibrous nature of the human cervix, and its relation to the isthmic segment in gravid and nongravid uteri. *Am J Obstet Gynecol* 1947;53:541–60.
4. Iams JD, Goldenberg RL, Meis PJ et al. The length of the cervix and the risk of spontaneous premature delivery. National institute of child health and human development maternal fetal medicine unit network. *N Engl J Med* 1996;334:567–72.
5. Berghella V, Owen J, MacPherson C et al. Natural history of cervical funneling in women at high risk for spontaneous preterm birth. *Obstet Gynecol* 2007;109:863–9.
6. Heath VC, Southall TR, Souka AP et al. Cervical length at 23 weeks of gestation: Prediction of spontaneous preterm delivery. *Ultrasound Obstet Gynecol* 1998;12:312–7.
7. Crane JM, Hutchens D. Transvaginal sonographic measurement of cervical length to predict preterm birth in asymptomatic women at increased risk: A systematic review. *Ultrasound Obstet Gynecol* 2008;31:579–87.
8. Committee opinion no. 522: Incidentally detected short cervical length. *Obstet Gynecol* 2012;119:879–82.
9. Tsoi E, Fuchs IB, Rane S et al. Sonographic measurement of cervical length in threatened preterm labor in singleton pregnancies with intact membranes. *Ultrasound Obstet Gynecol* 2005;25:353–6.

10. Harlap S, Shiono PH, Ramcharan S et al. A prospective study of spontaneous fetal losses after induced abortions. *N Engl J Med* 1979;301:677–81.

11. Sjøborg KD, Vistad I, Myhr SS et al. Pregnancy outcome after cervical cone excision: A case-control study. *Acta Obstet Gynecol Scand* 2007;86:423–8.

12. Caspi E, Schneider DF, Mor Z, Langer R, Weinraub Z, Bukovsky I. Cervical internal os cerclage: Description of a new technique and comparison with Shirodkar operation. *Am J Perinatol* 1990;7:347–9.

13. MRC/RCOG Working Party on Cervical Cerclage. Final report of the Medical Research Council/ Royal College of Obstetricians and Gynaecologists multicentre randomised trial of cervical cerclage *Br J Obstet Gynaecol* 1993;100:516–23.

14. Owen J, Hankins G, Iams JD et al. Multicenter randomized trial of cerclage for preterm birth prevention in high-risk women with shortened midtrimester cervical length. *Am J Obstet Gynecol* 2009;201:375. e1–8.

15. Berghella V, Odibo AO, To MS et al. Cerclage for short cervix on ultrasonography: Meta-analysis of trials using individual patient-level data. *Obstet Gynecol* 2005;106:181–9.

16. Sheiner E, Levy A, Katz M et al. Pregnancy outcome following recurrent spontaneous abortions. *Eur Jour Obst Gynecol Reprod Biol* 2005;118:61–5.

17. Hughes N, Hamilton EF, Tulandi T. Obstetric outcome in women after multiple spontaneous abortions. *J Reprod Med* 1991;36:165–6.

18. Spong CY, Meis PJ, Thom EA et al. Progesterone for prevention of recurrent preterm birth: Impact of gestational age at previous delivery. *Am J Obstet Gynecol* 2005;193:1127–31.

19. Meis PJ, Klebanoff M, Thom E et al. Prevention of recurrent preterm delivery by 17 alpha-hydroxyprogesterone caproate. *N Engl J Med* 2003;348:2379–85.

20. Da Fonseca EB, Bittar RE, Carvalho MH et al. Prophylactic administration of progesterone by vaginal suppository to reduce the incidence of spontaneous preterm birth in women at increased risk: A randomized placebo-controlled double-blind study. *Am J Obstet Gynecol* 2003;188:419–24.

21. Fonseca EB, Celik E, Parra M et al. Progesterone and the risk of preterm birth among women with a short cervix. *N Engl J Med* 2007;357:462–9.

22. Berghella V, Figueroa D, Szychowski JM et al. 17-alpha-hydroxyprogesterone caproate for the prevention of preterm birth in women with prior preterm birth and a short cervical length. *Am J Obstet Gynecol* 2010;202:351.

23. Hudic I, Szekeres-Bartho J, Fatušić Z et al. Dydrogesterone supplementation in women with threatened preterm delivery—The impact on cytokine profile, hormone profile, and progesterone-induced blocking factor. *J Reprod Immunol* 2011;92:103–7.

24. Conde-Agudelo A, Romero R, Nicolaides K et al. Vaginal progesterone vs. cervical cerclage for the prevention of preterm birth in women with a sonographic short cervix, previous preterm birth, and singleton gestation: A systematic review and indirect comparison metaanalysis. *Am J Obstet Gynecol* 2013;208:42.

25. Airoldi J, Pereira L, Cotter A et al. Amniocentesis prior to physical exam-indicated cerclage in women with midtrimester cervical dilation: Results from the expectant management compared to Physical Exam-indicated Cerclage international cohort study. *Am J Perinatol* 2009;26:63–8.

26. Pereira L, Cotter A, Gómez R et al. Expectant management compared with physical examination-indicated cerclage (EM-PEC) in selected women with a dilated cervix at 14(0/7)-25(6/7) weeks: Results from the EM-PEC international cohort study. *Am J Obstet Gynecol* 2007;197:483.

27. Berghella V, Ludmir J, Simonazzi G et al. Transvaginal cervical cerclage: Evidence for perioperative management strategies. *Am J Obstet Gynecol* 2013;209:181–92.

28. Cross R. Treatment of habitual abortion due to cervical incompetence. *Lancet* 1959;274:127.

29. Becher N, Adams Waldorf K, Hein M et al. The cervical mucus plug: Structured review of the literature. *Acta Obstet Gynecol Scand* 2009;88:502–13.

30. Lee DC, Hassan SS, Romero R et al. Protein profiling underscores immunological functions of uterine cervical mucus plug in human pregnancy. *J Proteomics* 2011;74:817–28.

31. Arabin B, Halbesma JR, Vork F et al. Is treatment with vaginal pessaries an option in patients with a sonographically detected short cervix. *J Perinat Med* 2003;31:122–33.

32. Goya M, Pratcorona L, Higueras T et al. Sonographic cervical length measurement in pregnant women with a cervical pessary. *Ultrasound Obstet Gynecol* 2011;38:205–9.

33. Goya M, Pratcorona L, Merced C et al. Cervical pessary in pregnant women with a short cervix (PECEP): An open-label randomised controlled trial. *Lancet* 2012;379:1800–6.
34. Arabin B, Alfirevic Z. Cervical pessaries for prevention of spontaneous preterm birth: Past, present and future. *Ultrasound Obstet Gynecol* 2013;42:390–9.
35. Quaas L, Hillemanns HG, du Bois A et al. The Arabin cerclage pessary-an alternative to surgical cerclage. *Geburtshilfe Frauenheilkd* 1990;50:429–33.
36. Arabin B, Halbesma JR, Vork F et al. Is treatment with vaginal pessaries an option in patients with a sonographically detected short cervix. *J Perinat Med* 2003;31:122–33.
37. Hui SY, Chor CM, Lau TK et al. Cerclage pessary for preventing preterm birth in women with a singleton pregnancy and a short cervix at 20 to 24 weeks: A randomized controlled trial. *Am J Perinatol* 2013;30:283–8.
38. Liem S, Schuit E, Hegeman M et al. Cervical pessaries for prevention of preterm birth in women with a multiple pregnancy (ProTWIN): A multicentre, open-label randomised controlled trial. *Lancet* 2013;382:1341–9.
39. Alfirevic Z, Owen J, Carreras Moratonas E et al. Vaginal progesterone, cerclage or cervical pessary for preventing preterm birth in asymptomatic singleton pregnant women with history of preterm birth and a sonographic short cervix. *Ultrasound Obstet Gynecol* 2013;41:146–51.

36

Midtrimester Loss and Viability

Flora Y. Wong and Victor Y. H. Yu

Introduction

Chapter 37 shows that women with recurrent miscarriage have a higher incidence of preterm labor. In addition, uterine anomalies and cervical incompetence are two causes of recurrent pregnancy loss that predispose to second trimester fetal loss. Women with recurrent second trimester fetal loss contribute disproportionately to the stillbirth rate, and second trimester delivery of live births contributes disproportionately to the neonatal mortality rate, thus, significantly increasing the overall perinatal mortality rate. However, a proactive policy of transfer *in utero* of high-risk pregnancies in danger of extremely preterm delivery in a tertiary perinatal center for management by maternal–fetal medicine specialists, together with competent resuscitation at birth and prompt initiation of neonatal intensive care by neonatologists, have been found to improve survival and quality-adjusted survival for extremely low birth weight (ELBW) infants born under 1000 g, including those born in the second trimester between 23 weeks and 26 weeks of gestation. However, morbidity remains high with the associated physical and social handicaps. Clinical protocols have been established for the management of those infants born alive at borderline viability, but continued advances made in the knowledge and technology in neonatal intensive care have resulted in revisions of medico-legal and ethical guidelines as the first edition of this book and will continue to do so. Principles behind decision-making on initiating and withdrawing intensive care will remain interpersonal and intimate, respectful to the infants' lives and their parents' autonomy, and sensitive to the emotional concerns of parents and staff.

Contribution of Extreme Prematurity to Perinatal Mortality

The State of Victoria in Australia has a population of about 6 million and a birth rate of about 14 per 1000. The legal requirements for birth registrations in the state are that a stillbirth must be registered if the gestation was 20 weeks' gestation and above or, if the period of gestation was not known, a birth weight of 400 g and over. Any infant, regardless of maturity or birth weight, who shows any sign of life after being born, must be registered as a live birth (and if death subsequently occurred within 28 days, as a neonatal death). Regional statewide perinatal mortality figures are generated from the information collected.[1] The scope of the perinatal death statistics includes all fetal deaths (at least 20 weeks' gestation or at least 400 g birth weight) and neonatal deaths (all live born babies who die within 28 completed days of birth, regardless of gestation or birth weight).

For the year 2009, there were a total of 73,241 births (of which 767 were stillbirths) in our state. The perinatal mortality rate (PMR), based on the above definitions, was 13.6 per 1000 births (the stillbirth rate was 10.5 per 1000 total births, and the neonatal death rate was 3.1 per 1000 live births). For the purpose of international comparison, the World Health Organization (WHO) recommended the publication of a standard mortality rate in which the numerator and denominator are restricted to heavier and more mature infants. A stillbirth is thus defined as a stillborn infant weighing at least 1000 g, or if the weight is not known, born after at least 28 weeks' gestation. A neonatal death is defined as a death occurring within 7 days of birth in an infant whose birth weight is at least 1000 g or, if the weight is not known, an infant born after at least 28 weeks. Our perinatal mortality rate, in accordance with

TABLE 36.1

Contribution of Low Birth Weight and Preterm Births to Perinatal
Deaths in the State of Victoria (Year 2009)

		Births (%)	Perinatal Deaths (%)
Birth weight			
	<2500g	6.4	82.4
	<1500g	1.2	70.1
	<1000g	0.6	63.6
Birth weight			
	<37 weeks	7.6	83.3
	<32 weeks	1.3	70.6
	<28 weeks	0.5	60.7

these WHO definitions, was 3.9 per 1000 births (stillbirth rate 2.8 per 1000, neonatal death rate 1.1 per 1000). Table 36.1 shows that ELBW infants have a major impact on perinatal mortality statistics that is disproportional to their numbers.

Changing Viability in Extremely Preterm Infants

Population-based studies from a designated geographical region, rather than from a single institution, are essential for the assessment of the true impact of maternal–fetal and neonatal intensive care practices on the survival and long-term neurodevelpmental outcome of extremely preterm live births. Significant numbers of preterm infants born outside perinatal centers might not be transferred by a neonatal emergency transport service (NETS) to institutions with a neonatal intensive care unit (NICU), and they would die at their hospital of birth. Our research group, the Victorian Infant Collaborative Study (VICS) has been reporting on the long-term outcome of a population-based ELBW cohort born in the State of Victoria since 1979–80 and up to 14 years of age from the original report in 1983[2] up to 2013.[3] Within the state, there are three level III perinatal centers, each with its NICU and a fourth stand-alone NICU in a children's hospital. There are 39 level II special-care units and 150 level I maternity units with small neonatal nurseries attached.

Place of Birth and Outcome

The three perinatal centers deliver only about one-quarter of the State of Victoria's births. However, 70% of ELBW births were being delivered in the three hospitals even during the early years, indicating that there was already an effective effort being made to identify women with high-risk pregnancies who might deliver an ELBW infant, and they were being referred *in utero* by midwives and obstetricians in the community for consultation by maternal–fetal medicine specialists within our perinatal centers. For the remaining 30% ELBW infants who were born outside the perinatal centers, less than half (42%) were transferred for neonatal intensive care after birth; those not referred, with very few exceptions, died. The perinatal mortality rate of ELBW infants was significantly lower in those born in the perinatal centers compared with those born elsewhere (72% vs. 93%) as were the stillbirth rate (36% vs. 59%), and neonatal death rate (56% vs. 82%).[4,5]

By the late 1990s, more than 90% of ELBW were delivered in perinatal centers in Victoria. The survival rate of ELBW infants was significantly higher in those born in the perinatal centers compared with those born elsewhere. The difference in survival rates between inborn and outborn infants widened progressively over time: the survival advantages for inborn infants over outborn infants were 12.0% in 1979–1980, 30.1% in 1985–1987, 36.5% in 1991–1992, and 43.6% in 1997.[6]

The VICS study defined long-term disability as severe if the child had cerebral palsy and was unable to walk, low IQ defined as a psychological test score of more than two standard deviations below the mean, or bilateral blindness. Not only did our inborn ELBW infants have a significantly higher survival rate compared with those who were outborn, the inborn survivors had also a significantly lower severe disability rate. Quality-adjusted survival rate, estimated according to proportion of survivors with various severity of disability, was found to be significantly higher in inborn infants across the eras between the 1970s and the 1990s.[6] The high disability rate of outborn infants was attributable to suboptimal perinatal care, secondary to a failure or a delay in initiating intensive care among these outborn infants. The progressively decreasing proportion of outborn ELBW infants over time reflects predominantly obstetric decision-making. It is important that the message of the advantages of *in utero* referral for ELBW infants reaches all those involved in obstetric decision-making—not only obstetricians, but also other health personnel such as general practitioners and nurses, as well as the parents of infants concerned.

Transfer *In Utero* Improves Outcome

The benefits of a more proactive transfer-*in-utero* policy to level III perinatal centers for management were established when the early VICS regional cohort was compared with later VICS regional cohorts born in 1997 and 2005. Not only was there a significant improvement in ELBW survival rate over the 3 decades from 25.6% in 1979–1980 to 66.9% in 2005,[7] but there was a significant increase in quality-adjusted survival (based on level of disability) among ELBW survivors at our 2-year assessment: from 19.4% in 1979–1980 to 57.1% in 2005[7] (Table 36.2). Severe disability was defined as cerebral palsy in children unlikely ever to walk, Bayley-III Scales or Cognitive Scale and Language Composite Scale scores of less than −3 standard deviations (SD) (compared with the mean and SD for the controls comprising of randomly selected normal birth-weight and term infants) or blindness; moderate disability as cerebral palsy in nonambulant children who were likely to walk or sensorineural deafness requiring amplification or developmental scores from −3 SD to less than −2 SD; and mild disability as cerebral palsy in ambulant children or developmental scores from −2 SD to less than −1 SD. "Utilities" for survivors were assigned according to the severity of the disability: 0.4 for severe, 0.6 for moderate, 0.8 for mild, and 1 for no disability. Utilities were multiplied for children with multiple disabilities, and therefore, the lowest utility possible for survivors was 0.064. Infants who died had a utility of 0. Infants who survived but were not assessed were assigned a utility of 1. Quality-adjusted survival rates were calculated by summing the utilities and dividing by the number of live births.

The VICS study identified that the primary factor in the improved outcome was the significant increase in the proportion of the state's ELBW infants was born within the three perinatal centers (from 70% to >90%). A secondary factor was a greater number of outborn ELBW live births who received resuscitation and prompt intensive care even at the level II hospitals prior to the arrival of NETS.[8] Comparing cohorts of ELBW infants born in 1979–1980 with those born in 1997, at 8 years of age,

TABLE 36.2

Improving Survival and Quality-Adjusted (QA) Survival in a Population-Based Study of Extremely Low Birth Weight (ELBW) Infants

Birth Weight (g)	Percentage of ELBW Infants in the Time Period				
	1979–1980 (*n* = 348)	1985–1987 (*n* = 560)	1991–1992 (*n* = 423)	1997 (*n* = 226)	2005 (*n* = 257)
500–749					
Survival	6	9	33	63	45
QA survival	4	8	26	47	36
750–999					
Survival	37	57	72	86	90
QA survival	28	48	62	73	79
Total					
Survival	26	38	57	75	67
QA survival	19	32	48	61	57

severe intellectual impairment was reduced from 10.3% to 4%, blindness from 7% to 1.8%, deafness from 4.6% to 2.4%, while the cerebral palsy rate showed a trend of small nonsignificant increase from 6.6% to 9.7%.[9] Notably, these figures show a large number of disabilities compared to normal birth-weight controls.[9] On the other hand, in spite of an increase in the consumption of hospital resources that inevitably results from a proactive treatment policy, economic evaluation of efficiency in terms of cost-effectiveness and cost–utility has remained unchanged.[10]

Risk of Recurrent Pregnancy Loss and Prematurity

Women with a history of pregnancy loss, when compared with those who have delivered a live birth, are known to have a higher risk of pregnancy loss in previous and subsequent pregnancies. In our study of women who had delivered an ELBW infant, the frequency of pregnancy loss in previous pregnancies was 41%. In subsequent pregnancies it was 31%.[11] These rates are higher than that of 10–20% reported for our general population. The perinatal mortality rate is also known to increase more than three-fold among women with one prior preterm birth and at least one prior pregnancy loss. In our study of women who had delivered an ELBW infant, the perinatal mortality rate of their subsequent pregnancies was 51.7 per 1000 births. This was four times higher than that reported for our general population in the same time period (12.8 per 1000 births of at least 20 weeks' gestation and 400 g birth weight). We also know that significantly more infants are born preterm when there is a previous history of perinatal loss or prematurity. In our study of women who had delivered an ELBW infant, the prematurity rate was 28% and the low birth weight rate was 34% in subsequent pregnancies, which was about six times higher than that of the general population. Those women who had a diagnosis of cervical incompetence were at the highest risk of a subsequent preterm birth. The low birth weight rates among live births subsequent to the birth of an ELBW infant in our study was 36% less than 2500 g, 11% less than 1500 g, and 5% less than 1000 g.

Outcome According to Gestational Age

The use of birth weight as a framework for the reporting of outcome data is a convenient system for neonatologists who have an accurate measurement on which to base the study. However, gestational age, not birth weight, is the parameter used by obstetricians as a guide to critical decisions on the management of the mother and fetus. A proactive attitude among physicians in recent years has improved the survival prospects, even among extremely preterm births of less than 26 weeks' gestation.[12] There is a tendency to underestimate birth weight in preterm infants before birth, and the perinatal mortality of those with clinical underestimation of birth weight is known to be higher than those with correctly estimated birth weight. Therefore, studies with gestation as an independent variable in determining outcome are required to assist obstetricians, neonatologists and parents in their decision-making process especially prior to an extreme preterm birth.[13,14]

The first VICS regional cohort based on gestational age cohort consisted of 316 infants consecutively born in the three years, 1985–87, at 24–26 weeks of gestation.[15] Gestational age was calculated from dates obtained by menstrual history, usually confirmed by ultrasound before 20 weeks of gestation. Of the 95 5-year-old survivors, one was untraced but who was assessed at 2 years to be free of disability. Overall survival rate to 5 years was 30% and the severe disability rate among survivors was 11% (Table 36.3). There was no trend in increasing disability with lower gestational age. Cerebral palsy was diagnosed in 13%, bilateral blindness in 5%, deafness requiring hearing aids in 2%, and IQ more than two SD below the mean in 7%. These outcome data were mostly favorable and better than that reported in other contemporaneous regional cohorts born in other parts of the world.

Postnatal surfactant replacement therapy was introduced for routine clinical use in 1991 in the State of Victoria. It has been proven to reduce mortality in randomized controlled trials within NICUs, but regional data are vital to assess the impact of such a therapeutic innovation on a whole population. Therefore, in our post-surfactant era (1991–92), VICS studied 401 infants consecutively born at 23–27 weeks of gestation in the State of Victoria.[16] Of the 225 two-year extremely preterm survivors, 219 (97%) were assessed, in addition to 242 contemporaneous normal birth weight controls in which 2%

TABLE 36.3

Extremely Preterm Infants: Survival and Disability Rates among Survivors in the Three Eras

	1985–1987	**1991–1992**	**1997**	**2005**
Survival rate	(*n* = 316)	(*n* = 428)	(*n* = 217)	(*n* = 270)
23 weeks	0%	10%	45%	22%
24 weeks	12%	33%	41%	51%
25 weeks	28%	58%	77%	67%
26 weeks	45%	72%	88%	82%
27 weeks	–	77%	88%	89%
Degree of disability	(*n* = 95)	(*n* = 219)	(*n* = 148)	(*n* = 172)
Severe	11%	8%	16%	4%
Moderate	7%	13%	12%	17%
Mild	25%	25%	24%	29%
None	61%	54%	49%	51%

were found to have severe disability. Compared with our regional 1985–1987 cohort from the presurfactant era, survival rate had improved significantly (Table 36.3) with no significant change in their severe disability rate (20% at 23 weeks, 14% at 24 weeks, 6% at 25 weeks, 9% at 26 weeks, and 1% at 27 weeks). The rate of blindness was, however, significantly lower in 1991–1992 (from 5% to 2%).

When parents are counseled at different time periods before and after the birth of their extremely preterm infant, they wish to know not only whether their child would survive but also whether their child would survive with or without disability. The 1991–1992 VICS regional cohort of infants born at 23–27 weeks of gestation was assessed again at 5 years of age to allow a more certain estimate of disability, and to determine how the prognosis offered to parents changed with increasing postnatal age and when different perinatal variables were taken into account.[17] Sixty-seven of the 401 extremely preterm infants (17%) were born outside level III perinatal centers. Their place of birth was a significant factor for survival: 62% for inborn infants and 28% for outborn infants. The attitude of the attending physician determined whether intensive care was offered. Overall, 16% of live births at 23–27 weeks were not offered intensive care and died on the first day: 69% at 23 weeks, 35% at 24 weeks, 6% at 25 weeks, 2% at 26 weeks, and 1% at 27 weeks. Nine percent of inborn infants were not offered intensive care compared with 54% of outborn infants. Variables that were associated positively with survival on day one were increasing maturity, antenatal corticosteroid therapy, multiple births, female sex, and not being small for gestational age, and on day seven, grade three or four cerebroventricular hemorrhage. Outcome data were available for 221 (98%) survivors (and 245 contemporaneous normal birth weight controls): nonambulatory cerebral palsy was diagnosed in 7%, bilateral blindness in 2%, deafness requiring hearing aids in 1%, and IQ score more than two SD below the mean for the normal birth weight controls in 15%. Variables that were associated positively with survival free of major disability on day one were postnatal surfactant therapy and the other factors associated with survival *per se*. On day 28 and at hospital discharge, variables significantly associated with a lower rate of survival free of major disability were grade three or four cerebroventricular hemorrhage, cystic periventricular leukomalacia, postnatal dexamethasone therapy, and surgery. Almost half the extremely preterm survivors had none of these adverse prognostic variables (47%), and their major disability rate was 7%, not significantly different from the rate of 3% for normal birth weight children. The risks of major disability increased to 17% with one adverse variable, 47% with two variables, and 67% with three variables.

The subsequent VICS regional cohort based on gestational age consisted of 208 consecutive live births at 23–27 weeks' gestation and 188 contemporaneous normal birth weight controls born in the State of Victoria during 1997.[18] Compared with our regional 1991–1992 cohort, the survival rate to 2 years of age had improved at each week of gestation with no significant changes in the disability rate (Table 36.3). As the gain from a significant increase in survival was greater than the loss from a marginal increase in disability among survivors, the rate of survival free of disability was higher in 1997 compared with 1991–1992 both overall and in all gestational age subgroups. There was no gestational age below which most survivors were disabled.

The most recent VICS regional cohort studied 270 livebirths at 22–27 weeks' gestational age, born consecutively in Victoria during 2005,[19] of which 172 (63.7%) survived to 2 years, not significantly different from the survival rate of 69.6% for those born in 1997. Rates of severe developmental delay and severe disability were significantly lower than in the very preterm survivors born in 1997. Quality-adjusted survival rates in the extremely preterm cohorts rose from 42.1% in 1991–92 to 55.1% in 1997, but did not increase in 2005 (53.4%).[19] The rate of cerebral palsy in our 2005 cohort is lower than that in those born in Victoria in the 1990s (9.8% in 2005 versus 12% in 1997). One possible explanation for this might be that most survivors would have received caffeine (which is known to reduce cerebral palsy in very preterm infants[20]) in 2005 but not in the 1990s. Another possible explanation is that the use of postnatal corticosteroids, also known to cause cerebral palsy, decreased substantially after the early 2000s compared with the 1990s.[21]

Comparison with Other Regional Studies

In a review of survival rates for extremely preterm infants born in North America, none of the studies had regional or population-based cohorts that could be directly compared with our VICS study.[22] Two regional cohorts reported from the United Kingdom had survival rates at individual weeks of gestation lower than that in our study. In the Trent region of England, with an annual birth rate similar to that Victoria (60,000), the survival rates to discharge home in a cohort from 1994 to 1997 were 14% at 23 weeks, 26% at 24 weeks, 41% at 25 weeks, 61% at 25 weeks, 75% at 27 weeks, and 85% at 28 weeks.[23] For the same time period, survival rates from our VICS cohort were 25% at 23 weeks, 46% at 24 weeks, 79% at 25 weeks, 85% at 26 weeks, 82% at 27 weeks, and 91% at 28 weeks. The EPICure study reported the outcome at 2.5 years of 23–25 weeks of gestation live births born in the United Kingdom in 1995.[24] Comparative data from the VICS study of cohorts born both prior to the EPICure cohort (1991–1992) and after the EPICure cohort (1997) are shown in Table 36.4. The 1991–1992 Australian cohort, which was 3 years before the 1995 UK cohort, already had better survival, and the survival rate of the infants born at 23–25 weeks' gestation in the 1997 Australian cohort was more than double that of the UK cohort (69% versus 29%) (Table 36.4). Hospital survival rates reported from a regional cohort from the Netherlands relating to infants born in 1995 were extremely poor. The majority of deaths in that study at 23 and 24 weeks occurred before admission to the NICU: 2% at 23 weeks, 3% at 24 weeks, 29% at 25 weeks, and 54% at 26 weeks.[25] Survival without disability rate was 23% in the EPICure study,[24] compared to 48% in the VICS study in 1997.[19] For the VICS cohort in 2005, survival rates to 2 years of age have plateaued for ELBW infants in the late 1990s. The survivors in 2005 had lower rates of severe developmental delay and severe disability compared with the late 1990s, but overall survival without disability rate remained similar to the 1990s. The one significant trend over a longer period of time, from the late 1970s to 2005, in ELBW survivors has been the fall in the rate of blindness (from 6% in 1979–1980 to 0% in 2005).[7] The EPICure2 study in the United Kingdom reporting on livebirths at 23–26 weeks of gestation in 2006[26,27] showed both survival and survival without disability have increased from the 1995 cohort, but still lower than that reported in the VICS study in 2005 (Table 36.4).

Others have also reported long-term outcomes by birth weight from cohorts born in the 2000s. Wilson-Costello et al.[28] reported the results of a large, single-center, uncontrolled study of the outcomes

TABLE 36.4

Comparison between the Population-Based Victorian Infant Collaborative Study (VICS) and EPICure Data for Infants Born at 23–25 Weeks' Gestation

	VICS 1991–1992	EPICure 1995	VICS 1997	VICS 2005	EPICure 2006
Survival rate	38%	29%	69%	64%	51%
23 weeks	10%	10%	41%	22%	19%
24 weeks	33%	26%	41%	51%	40%
25 weeks	58%	43%	73%	67%	66%
Survival without disability	54%	23%	48%	51%	34%

of ELBW infants born in 2000–2005 compared with cohorts from the 1980s and 1990s. Of their cohort of 223, the survival rate of 71% at 20 months was similar to the VICS cohort in 2005; the rate had also plateaued since the 1990s. Tommiska et al.[29] compared data from the Finnish national register for ELBW infants born in 1996–1997 with those born in 1999–2000. Survival, the rates of cerebral palsy, and blindness did not change significantly over time; no control data were available.[29] In contrast to the results in the VICS study, a population based Swiss study has shown an increase in survival for extremely preterm infants at the limit of viability (22–25 completed weeks' gestation) between 2000–2001 and 2003–2004. Survival rose from 31% to 40%, with most of the increase due at 25 weeks' gestation; there were no controls and no long-term outcome data.[30]

Ethical Dilemmas Following Extreme Preterm Birth

Ethical problems of selective nontreatment arise in caring for extremely preterm infants when clinical decisions have to be made after the birth of a live born infant to either withhold or withdraw intensive care.[31] Studies have shown great variability in doctors' attitudes and their management policies for extreme prematurity. There is a tendency for both obstetricians and neonatologists to underestimate the potential for survival and overestimate the risks of disability for extremely preterm infants.[32–34] This problem becomes especially acute for parents who have lost a number of pregnancies, and the ELBW infant may be the only live infant that they will have. Many neonatologists continue to selectively resuscitate extremely preterm infants at birth, which means that live born infants are left to die through withholding of intensive care. If doctors believe that the infant has little prospect for survival or survival without disability, it is probable that their clinical management would be delayed or less than optimal and may in fact be creating a self-fulfilling prophecy.[35] An Australian survey in the 1980s had shown at that time a great number of neonatologists selectively resuscitate extremely preterm infants at birth, suggesting that many of these live births were left to die through withholding of neonatal intensive care.[32] More recent national surveys conducted in 2000 showed a more proactive resuscitation policy among Australian obstetricians and neonatologist (Table 36.5).[33,34]

Decision to Withhold Intensive Care

In the majority of level III perinatal centers within developed countries, all infants with a birth weight of more than 500 g or a gestation of 24 weeks or more are offered intensive care. At Monash Medical Centre (MMC) in Australia, we have reported that 10% of 442 extremely preterm live births born at 23–28 weeks of gestation over a 10-year period, 1977–1986, were not offered intensive care, 4% had obvious major malformations, and 6% were considered "nonviable," for which resuscitation at birth was not offered or was not successful.[36] The proportion of live births in which treatment was withheld at the time of delivery was 37% at 23 weeks, 17% at 24 weeks, 8% at 25 weeks, 1% at 26 weeks, 1% at 27 weeks, and 0% at 28 weeks. This approach to offering intensive care was considered ahead of its times even in developed countries 20–30 years ago.[37] During an identical period, 1977–1986, in another level III perinatal center within a few kilometers of MMC, 42% of similar live births born at 24–26 weeks of gestation were not offered intensive care, all of whom died.[36] This accounted for a lower survival rate among their infants born at 23–28 weeks of gestation compared with those in MMC (29% versus 44%), as the survival rate among those who were offered intensive care was

TABLE 36.5

Percentage of Australian Doctors Who Would Recommend to Parents that Their Extremely Preterm Infants Be Resuscitated at the Time of Birth

	22 weeks	23 weeks	24 weeks	25 weeks
Obstetricians	9%	33%	59%	79%
Neonatologists	13%	48%	92%	100%

similar. Our practice during the 1990s was consistent with what the Royal College of Paediatrics and Child Health in the United Kingdom had published in 1997, which stated that it would not be unreasonable to consider withholding treatment in an infant born at 23 weeks weighing little more than 500 g.[38] There is a general consensus in developed countries even to this day that parents of a 22-week infant should be discouraged from seeking active treatment and offered palliative care, those of a 23-week infant should be supported for noninitiation of treatment, those of a 24-week infant should be advised of commencement of resuscitation with noninitiation of intensive care treatment if parents and clinicians felt this was indicated, whereas those of a 25–26 week infant should be encouraged to consent to intensive care.[39–41]

Decision to Withdraw Intensive Care

However, a proactive policy to initiate intensive care must take into consideration that a decision to withdraw intensive care might have to be made in selective infants at a later stage in the course of the infant's treatment. In the event that the infant's subsequent clinical course indicates that further curative efforts are futile or lack compensating benefit, intensive care should be discontinued and palliative care, which provides symptomatic relief and comfort, should be introduced. This approach, termed "individualized prognostic strategy" has been advocated as an acceptable and preferred mode of operation in the NICU, one that has been endorsed by the Canadian Pediatric Society and the American Academy of Pediatrics.[42,43] The attending neonatologist has the primary role as an advocate for the infant and medical advisor to the parents, whereas the parents act as surrogates for their infant. The shift in emphasis from curative to palliative treatment requires consensus among all those involved in the care of the infant, both medical and nursing staff, as well as consent from the parents who should be closely involved in this widely shared decision-making process. At MMC, over an 8-year period 1981–1987, intensive care was withdrawn prior to death in 65% of 316 deaths.[44] Among these infants, death was considered to be inevitable in the short term even with the continuation of neonatal intensive care in 70% of the cases. In the remainder, the risk of severe brain damage was considered to be so great that death was considered preferable to a life with major disability. Therefore, in our NICU, full treatment until death is uncommon and occurred in only one-third of cases. This experience was not unique as studies from other developed countries showed that 30–80% of deaths in their NICU follow a deliberate withdrawal of life sustaining treatment.[45–47] Some centers have reported that the primary mode of death in a NICU was withdrawal of life-sustaining support.[48]

There are three clinical situations in which selective withdrawal of intensive care is appropriate. First, there are few who would disagree that withdrawal of intensive care is morally and ethically acceptable when death is considered to be inevitable and the infant is in the process of dying whatever treatment is provided. Intensive care would be considered in these cases a futile exercise and not in the best interest of the infant. Examples in this category include those infants with severe respiratory failure or fulminating sepsis who have persistent or worsening hypoxemia, acidosis, and hypotension unresponsive to ventilatory and inotropic support. There is no obligation to provide futile medical care in such cases, as no infant with progressive multiple organ failure survives even without withholding cardiopulmonary resuscitation. Second, it is appropriate to consider withdrawal of intensive care even when death is not inevitable with continued treatment, but there is a significantly high risk of severe physical and mental disability should the infant survive. Such a decision should not raise too many moral and ethical problems if the infant's development of self-awareness and intentional action is believed to be virtually impossible or there is no prospect of the infant ever being able to act on his or her own behalf. One scenario is that of an extremely preterm infant with large, bilateral parenchymal hemorrhages, infarcts, and/or leukomalacia in the brain. Third, which is more controversial as an issue, is when survival with moderate disability is possible with treatment, but the infant is likely to suffer persistent pain, require recurrent hospitalization and invasive treatment throughout life, and to experience early death in childhood or early adulthood. This situation may arise with a preterm infant with severe chronic lung disease nonresponsive to dexamethasone and with no prospect of being weaned from mechanical ventilation, but for whom lung transplant is still considered an experimental option.

The one principle with which all the guidelines proposed in the United Kingdom, Canada, USA, and Australia agree, is that if continued life for the infant with treatment is a worse outcome than death, then the principle of *primum non nocere* imposes a professional, moral, and humanitarian duty upon neonatologists to withhold or withdraw life sustaining treatment. Infants cannot benefit from such treatment and death is not the worst outcome for them if they cannot be rescued from irreversible medical deterioration and death, cannot have life prolonged without major sensorineural sequelae, and cannot be relieved of ongoing pain and suffering. When the process of dying is being artificially prolonged, most would agree that the harm of continued treatment exceeds any potential benefit. However, decisions based on quality of life considerations are more difficult as there is inevitably imprecision in predicting the risk of intolerable disability or suffering.

Medico-Legal Perspective

Very few cases of selective nontreatment have reached the courts. It is considered appropriate for these difficult decisions to be made within the context of the infant/neonatologist/parent relationship and experience has shown that there is no excessive abuse in such private decision-making processes. The legal position appears to recognize the importance of respecting parental decisions but emphasizes that the law court has the right to intervene and overrule a decision if that is necessary to protect the best interests of the infant. The British legal system, for example, had upheld selective nontreatment in the three categories of neonatal conditions referred to previously. First, selective nontreatment was ruled to be legally acceptable when death was inevitable in the case of a hydrocephalic preterm infant on the verge of death. Second, legal precedence for selective nontreatment for an infant with severe brain damage, who was neither dying nor in severe pain, was found in a case presenting to court with a high risk of multiple sensorineural disabilities. Third, selective nontreatment was considered lawful in an infant where the benefits of life with treatment failed to outweigh the burdens of a "demonstrably awful life" of pain and suffering.

The Decision-Making Process

The importance of less medical paternalism and more informed parental involvement in the decision-making process of selective nontreatment must be emphasized. The neonatologist should never make unilateral decisions regarding the right to die. Adequate and consistent parental communication carried out by medical and nursing staff must begin with the admission of all infants into the NICU so that trust can be developed between the parents and staff irrespective of outcome.[49] An open-visiting policy for families is essential to promote such parental contact.[50] A realistic assessment of the infant's clinical condition should be given by the neonatologist to the parents as soon as possible. The medical facts should be presented with an honest, sympathetic, and caring attitude. Often the information has to be repeated and reinforced by the entire staff. Otherwise, misunderstandings and unrealistic expectations can lead to confusion, suspicions, bitterness, and frank hostility. As with most medical decisions made by neonatologists that require parental informed consent, much of the discussion on selective nontreatment depends on trust in the knowledge, judgment, and integrity of the doctor. When a consensus has been reached by the NICU staff that selective nontreatment is an appropriate option to raise with the parents, one or more intense and intimate meetings would be required so that the crucial set of discussions could take place and in which a decision could be reached on the matter. These meetings usually involve both of the parents, the attending neonatologist, a nurse representative, and a nonmedical staff member who can act as the parents' advocate, such as a medical social worker. Ways of minimizing the chances of unresolved disagreements and of maximizing the chances of a just and ethical conclusion have recently been reviewed.[51]

The principles underlying clinical practice and the decision-making process should be the same for developed and developing countries, but there must be less medical paternalism and more informed parental involvement in developing countries. Compared to developed countries, communications between the medical and nursing staff and the parents are less adequate in developing countries. In most developed countries, intensive care being routinely offered to all who have reached 24 weeks of gestation. Limited resources in developing countries, however, necessitate a different intervention point, which may be 26 weeks or even 28 weeks.[52] In recurrent pregnancy loss, additional factors need to be taken into consideration, as the parents may have undergone numerous losses before reaching this stage. They may be subject to further early losses, and may not reach this stage again.

Palliative Care

The neonatologist's duty does not end with the decision for selective nontreatment. The principles and guidelines for palliative care demand that basic nursing care should continue with the emphasis to provide comfort to the infant. Electronic monitoring of physiological parameters, diagnostic investigations (such as x-rays and blood tests), medications (including oxygen and antibiotics), and therapeutic procedures (including resuscitation, all forms of assisted ventilation and intravenous infusion), which might prolong the dying process, should be discontinued. Prolonged terminal weaning, defined as a stepwise or gradual decreasing of ventilator support over a period of hours, is considered inappropriate. Dragging out the withdrawal serves only to prolong the dying process and any attendant suffering. The argument that the sudden withdrawal of ventilator support resembles an intentional killing does not hold merit, as in both cases, a treatment on which the infant depends for life is being discontinued and death is the expected outcome. The infant should be nursed in a normal cot and warmth provided by light clothing. If the infant has apparent distress, symptomatic relief should be provided, such as suctioning to remove oropharyngeal secretions and sedation with normal therapeutic doses of morphine, on a p.r.n. basis, even if the pain relief measures may inadvertently shorten the dying process.

A controversial issue involves the withdrawal of enteral nutrition and hydration during palliative care. Preterm or sick infants require gavage feeding, although it has been advocated that this feeding method is part of medical treatment and should therefore be discontinued during palliative care, others consider it as basic nursing care which must not be withheld under any circumstances.[53] A number of court decisions have supported the withdrawal of nutrition, thus equating the administration of artificial nutrition with other medical procedures.[54] Precedence has been set in a British court on the legality of withholding gavage feeding. Nevertheless, most neonatologists would be reluctant not to provide gavage feeding, even when it might be lawful and appears to be in the infant's best interest. There is an obvious perception of a moral difference between withdrawing ventilatory support and withholding fluids or nutrition with selective nontreatment. The underlying principle is that naturally or artificially administered hydration and nutrition may be given or withheld, depending on the infant's comfort.

Parents need a quiet place to be with their infant during the dying process. They may wish that other family members and religious advisors be present. Hospice concepts have been applied to neonatal care by providing a family room that is private yet close to the NICU and by training NICU staff in more supportive approaches towards the families.[55,56] Such a program allows the staff to cope better with the dying infants offered selective nontreatment and facilitates the grieving process in the parents. In certain circumstances, withdrawal of intensive care may be arranged to take place in the home, so that death can occur in a more comforting environment for the family.

Conclusions

A proactive policy of resuscitation at birth and prompt initiation of intensive care has been shown to be associated with an improvement in the survival of extremely preterm infants, including those born in the second trimester, in regional population-based studies within the State of Victoria in Australia. As a greater percentage of live births were offered intensive care in our series of studies that spanned over 20 years, the survival rate rose progressively in all birth weight and gestation subgroups among extremely low birth weight infants, including those who were born at borderline viability down to 23 weeks of gestation. Their quality-adjusted survival rate also rose progressively, as the large gains in survival over time had not been offset by significant increases in survival with disability. Cost-effectiveness and cost–utility ratios remained stable overall, with efficiency gains in the smaller infants over time, as more such infants were being transferred *in utero* and were born in level III perinatal centers with the regionalization of perinatal–neonatal healthcare programs. Multicentered collaboration to conduct long-term studies of geographically defined cohorts provides unique information not available from institution-based studies. Such data are vital for answering questions such as "how low should we go?" Quality outcomes depend more on the comprehensive organization of an effective system of networking perinatal–neonatal services within a geographically determined region, than on the introduction of expensive high-technology therapies within individual neonatal intensive care units.

Among the many neonatal ethical problems, the one that neonatologists are faced with on a regular basis involves the issue of selective nontreatment, that is, clinical decisions made after the birth of a live born infant to either withhold or withdraw treatment in certain clinical situations. If medical doctors believe that the infant has little prospect for intact survival, their management would be suboptimal and they create a self-fulfilling prophecy. A policy establishing criteria for initiating life-sustaining treatment must be developed with proper consideration of the cultural, social, and economic factors operating in the developed or developing country. There are infants whose subsequent clinical course after initiation of neonatal intensive care will indicate that further curative efforts are futile or lack compensating benefit. A policy establishing criteria for withdrawing life-sustaining treatment must also be developed, to allow the appropriate use of palliative care in these instances. The clinical situations in which selective nontreatment is taking place in the neonatal intensive care unit are: (i) when death is considered to be inevitable whatever treatment is provided; (ii) even when death is not inevitable, there is a significantly high risk of severe physical and mental disability should the infant survive; and (iii) when survival with moderate disability is possible, but the infant is likely to experience ongoing pain and suffering, repeated hospitalization and invasive treatment, and early death in childhood.

REFERENCES

1. Consultative Council on Obstetric and Paediatric Mortality and Morbidity. *Annual Report for the Year 2009*. Melbourne: Health Department of Victoria; 2009.
2. Kitchen WH, Campbell N, Drew JH et al. Provision of perinatal services and survival of extremely low birth weight infants in Victoria. *Med J Aust* 1983;2:314–8.
3. Roberts G, Burnett AC, Lee KJ et al. Quality of life at age 18 years after extremely preterm birth in the post-surfactant era. *J Pediatr* 2013;163:1008–13.
4. Lumley J, Kitchen WH, Roy RND et al. The survival of extremely low birth weight infants in Victoria: 1982–85. *Med J Aust* 1988;149:242–6.
5. Lumley J, Kitchen WH, Roy RND et al. Method of delivery and resuscitation of very low birth weight infants in Victoria: 1982–85. *Med J Aust* 1990;152:143–6.
6. Doyle LW. Changing availability of neonatal intensive care for extremely low birthweight infants in Victoria over two decades. *Med J Aust* 2004;181:136–9.
7. Doyle LW, Roberts G, Anderson PJ. Changing long-term outcomes for infants 500–999 g birth weight in Victoria, 1979–2005. *Arch Dis Child Fetal Neonatal* 2011;96:443–7.
8. Victorian Infant Collaborative Study Group. Improving the quality of survival for infants of birth weight <1000 g born in non-Level III centres in Victoria. *Med J Aust* 1993;158:24–7.
9. Roberts G, Anderson PJ, Doyle LW. Neurosensory disabilities at school age in geographic cohorts of extremely low birth weight children born between the 1970s and the 1990s. *J Pediatr* 2009;154:829–34.
10. Victorian Infant Collaborative Study Group. Evaluation of neonatal intensive care for extremely low birth weight infants in Victoria over two decades: II. Efficiency. *Pediatrics* 2004;113:510–4.
11. Yu VYH, Davis NG, Mercado MF et al. Subsequent pregnancy following the birth of an extremely low birth-weight infant. *Aust NZ J Obstet Gynaecol* 1986;26:115–9.
12. Yu VYH, Doyle LW. Survival and disabilities in extremely tiny babies. *Sem Neonatol* 1996;1:257–65.
13. Yu VYH, Carse EA, Charlton MP. Outcome of infants born at less than 26 weeks gestation. In: McIntosh N, Hansen T, eds. *Current Topics in Neonatal Care*. Philadelphia: Saunders, 1996. p. 67–84.
14. Yu VYH. *The Extremely Tiny Baby*. London: Saunders, 1996.
15. Victorian Infant Collaborative Study Group. Outcome to five years of age of children 24–26 weeks' gestational age born in the State of Victoria. *Med J Aust* 1995;163:11–4.

16. Victorian Infant Collaborative Study Group. Outcome at 2 years of children 23–27 weeks' gestation born in Victoria in 1991–92. *J Paediatr Child Health* 1997;33:161–5.

17. Victorian Infant Collaborative Study Group. Outcome at 5 years of age of children 23–27 weeks' gestation: Refining the prognosis. *Pediatrics* 2001;108:134–41.

18. ictorian Infant Collaborative Study Group. Neonatal intensive care at borderline viability—Is it worth it? *Early Hum Dev* 2004;80:103–13.

19. Doyle LW, Roberts G, Anderson PJ. Outcomes at age 2 years of infants <28 weeks' gestational age born in Victoria in 2005. *J Pediatr* 2010;156:49–53.

20. Schmidt B, Roberts RS, Davis P et al. Long-term effects of caffeine therapy for apnea of prematurity. *N Engl J Med* 2007;357:1893–1902.

21. Doyle LW, Halliday HL, Ehrenkranz RA et al. Impact of postnatal systemic corticosteroids on mortality and cerebral palsy in preterm infants: Effect modification by risk for chronic lung disease. *Pediatrics* 2005;115:655–61.

22. Lorenz JM. The outcome of extreme prematurity. *Sem Perinatol* 2001;25:348–59.

23. Draper ES, Manktelow B, Field DJ et al. Prediction of survival for preterm births by weight and gestational age: Retrospective population based study. *Br Med J* 1999;319:1093–7.

24. Wood NS, Marlow N, Costeloe K et al. Neurologic and developmental disability after extremely preterm birth. EPICure Study Group. *N Engl J Med* 2000;343:378–84.

25. den Ouden AL, van Baar AL, Dorrepaal CA et al. Overlevingskans van zeer immature pasgeborenen in Nederland. *Tijdschr Kindergeneeskd* 2000;142:241–6.

26. Costeloe KL, Hennessy EM, Haider S et al. Short term outcomes after extreme preterm birth in England: Comparison of two birth cohorts in 1995 and 2006 (the EPICure studies). *BMJ* 2012;345:e7976.

27. Moore T, Hennessy EM, Myles J et al. Neurological and developmental outcome in extremely preterm children born in England in 1995 and 2006: The EPICure studies. *BMJ* 2012;345:e7961.

28. Wilson-Costello D, Friedman H, Minich N et al. Improved neurodevelopmental outcomes for extremely low birth weight infants in 2000–2002. *Pediatrics* 2007;119:37–45.

29. Tommiska V, Heinonen K, Lehtonen L et al. No improvement in outcome of nationwide extremely low birth weight infant populations between 1996–1997 and 1999–2000. *Pediatrics* 2007;119:29–36.

30. Fischer N, Steurer MA, Adams M et al. Survival rates of extremely preterm infants (gestational age <26 weeks) in Switzerland: Impact of the Swiss guidelines for the care of infants born at the limit of viability. *Arch Dis Child Fetal Neonatal* 2009;94:407–413.

31. Yu VYH. The extremely low birth weight infant: An ethical approach to treatment. *Aust Paediatr J* 1987;23:97–103.

32. de Garis C, Kuhse H, Singer P et al. Attitudes of Australian neonatal paediatricians to the treatment of extremely preterm infants. *Aust Paediatr J* 1987;23:223–6.

33. Mulvey S, Partridge JC, Martinez AM et al. The management of extremely premature infants and the perceptions of viability and parental counselling practices of Australian paediatricians. *Aust N Z J Obstet Gynaecol* 2001;41:269–73.

34. Munro M, Yu VYH, Partridge JC et al. Antenatal counselling, resuscitation practices and attitudes among Australian neonatologists towards life support in extreme prematurity. *Aust N Z J Obstet Gynaecol* 2001;44:275–80.

35. Martinez AM, Partridge JC, Yu VYH et al. Physician counseling practices and decision-making for extremely low birth weight infants in the Pacific Rim. *J Paediatr Child Health* 2005;41:209–14.

36. Yu VYH, Gomez JM, Shah V et al. Survival prospects of extremely preterm infants: A 10-year experience in a single perinatal centre. *Am J Perinatol* 1992;9:164–9.

37. Yu VYH. Selective non-treatment of newborn infants. *Med J Aust* 1994;161:627–9.

38. RCPCH Ethic Advisory Committee. *Withholding or Withdrawing Life Saving Treatment in Children. A Framework for Practice.* London: Royal College of Paediatrics and Child Health; 1997.

39. Rennie JM. Perinatal management at the lower margin of viability. *Arch Dis Child* 1996;74:F214–8.

40. Lui K, Bajuk B, Foster K et al. Perinatal care at the borderlines of viability: A consensus statement based on a NSW and ACT consensus workshop. *Med J Aust* 2006;185:495–500.

41. Wilkinson AR, Ahluwalia J, Cole A et al. Management of babies born extremely preterm at less than 26 weeks of gestation: A framework for clinical practice at the time of birth. *Arch Dis Child Fetal Neonatal* 2009;94:2–5.

42. Fetus and Newborn Committee, Canadian Pediatric Society; Maternal-Fetal Medicine Committee, Society of Obstetricians and Gynecologists of Canada. Management of the woman with threatened birth of an infant of extremely low gestational age. *Can Med Assoc J* 1994;151:547–53.

43. AAP Committee on Bioethics. Ethics and the care of critically ill infants and children. *Pediatrics* 1996;98:149–52.

44. Carse EA, Yu VYH. Deaths following withdrawal of treatment in a neonatal intensive care unit. In: Wiknjosastro GK, ed. *Proceedings of the 5th Congress of the Federation of Asia-Oceania Perinatal Societies*. Denpasar: Perinatal Society of Indonesia; 1988. p. 55.

45. Whitelaw A. Death as an option in neonatal intensive care. *Lancet* 1986;2:328–31.

46. Kelly NP, Rowley SR, Harding JE. Death in neonatal intensive care. *J Paediatr Child Health* 1994;30:419–22.

47. Eventov-Friedman S, Kanevsky H, Bar-Oz B. Neonatal end-of-life care: A single-center NICU experience in Israel over a decade. *Pediatrics* 2013;131:e1889–96.

48. Weiner J, Sharma J, Lantos J et al. How infants die in the neonatal intensive care unit: Trends from 1999 through 2008. *Arch Pediatr Adolesc Med* 2011;165:630–4.

49. Yu VYH. Caring for parents of high-risk infants. *Med J Aust* 1977;2:534–7.

50. Yu VYH, Jamieson J, Astbury J. Parents' reactions to unrestricted parental contact with infants in the intensive care nursery. *Med J Aust* 1981;1:294–6.

51. Tripp J, McGregor D. Withholding and withdrawing of life sustaining treatment in the newborn. *Arch Dis Child* 2006;91:F67–71.

52. Partridge JC, Martinez AM, Nishida H et al. International comparison of care for very low birth weight infants: Parents' perception of counseling and decision-making. *Pediatrics* 2005;116:263–71.

53. Doyal L, Wilsher D. Towards guidelines for withholding and withdrawal of life prolonging treatment in neonatal medicine. *Arch Dis Child* 1994;70:F66–70.

54. Mirale ED, Mahowald MB. Withholding nutrition from seriously ill newborn infants: A parent's perspective. *J Pediatr* 1988;113:262–5.

55. Yu VYH. Death as an option in the neonatal intensive care unit. The ethics of withdrawal of life-support. In: Burrows GD, Petrucco OM, Llewellyn-Jones D, eds. *Psychosomatic Aspects of Reproductive Medicine and Family Planning*. Melbourne: York Press; 1987. p. 112–9.

56. Whitfield JM, Siegel RE, Glicken AD et al. The application of hospice concepts to neonatal care. *Am J Dis Child* 1982;136:421–4.

37

Obstetric Outcomes after Recurrent Miscarriage

Howard J. A. Carp

Introduction

Most work on recurrent miscarriage has concentrated on the causes, prognosis, treatment, and subsequent live birth rate. However, this group of patients is also at a higher risk for obstetric complications such as bleeding, fetal anomalies, pre-eclampsia, intrauterine growth restriction (IUGR), preterm labor, and perinatal mortality. Consequently, prenatal care should be modified to seek these complications. It is unclear whether these late obstetric complications are associated with specific conditions such as antiphospholipid syndrome or hereditary thrombophilias or are associated with recurrent pregnancy loss *per se*. Various interventions have also been reported to affect the incidence of later obstetric complications. These interventions include paternal leucocyte immunization and intravenous immunoglobulin for unexplained recurrent pregnancy loss, anticoagulants and aspirin or intravenous immunoglobulin for antiphospholipid syndrome, and anticoagulants for hereditary thrombophilias. This chapter assesses some of the obstetric complications associated with different forms of recurrent pregnancy loss and the treatment modalities that have been used.

Method of Study

Publications describing the obstetric complications in recurrent miscarriage were sought by a thorough literature search, including online databases, Medline, and Embase. The original database of the "Recurrent Miscarriage Trialists group" is held by the author as one of the data contributors to that database. Figures were also obtained from one of the author's own database that contains information on 3000 patients attending the recurrent miscarriage clinic of the Sheba Medical Center, Tel Hashomer, Israel. The figures were entered into a computerized database and the figures analyzed.

Statistical Analysis

Odds ratios with 95% confidence intervals (CI) were calculated for for developing obstetric complications, such as vaginal bleeding, anomalies, pre-eclampsia, IUGR, perinatal mortality, placental abruption, and placenta praevia. When true incidences were available from cohort studies the relative risk were calculated. These figures were also compared in subgroups of patients and after various treatment interventions.

Incidence of Obstetric Complications after Recurrent Miscarriage

Most of the literature on obstetric complications comes from an era after antiphospholipid syndrome had been defined, but before hereditary thrombophilias had been defined. Reginald et al.[1] in a retrospective observational cohort study assessed the results of 175 pregnancies in 97 recurrently miscarrying women whose subsequent pregnancy progressed beyond 28 weeks. However, the underlying causes of recurrent miscarriage of this group of women were not documented. The results were not compared with a control group attending the same hospital, but with standard figures from Scotland between 1973 and 1979. A significantly higher incidence of preterm deliveries, perinatal deaths, and intrauterine growth restriction was found. In contrast, Hughes et al.[2] examined the obstetric outcome in 88 women with a past history of three or more consecutive pregnancy losses and compared the results to a control group drawn from their local obstetric population. The incidence of small-for-gestational-age infants (3.4%), preterm delivery (12.5%), and perinatal mortality (0%) were no different to the control group. As in Reginald et al.'s[1] study, there was no mention of antiphospholipid syndrome. However, an increased incidence of gestational diabetes and pregnancy induced hypertension was found. Tulppala et al.[3] conducted a prospective study of 32 deliveries in 63 women with recurrent miscarriage and presented the results of a detailed investigative protocol, including antiphospholipid syndrome. The incidence of growth retardation (20%), preterm delivery (9.7%), and impaired glucose tolerance (22.8%) appeared to be increased. Unfortunately, the results were not compared to any control population. Jivraj et al.[4] studied a cohort of 162 women with recurrent miscarriage compared to local controls, and found an increased incidence of the same complications as Reginald et al.,[1] but also an increaded incidence of cesarean sections, which were performed for the above obstetric conditions. Although that study did define the causes of pregnancy loss in the control group, the figures were too small to allow comparisons to be drawn between different groups of patient. Thom et al.[5] examined Washington State birth certificate records for 1984 to 1987 to examine the association between spontaneous abortion, recurrent miscarriage (RM) and adverse outcomes in the subsequent live birth. The results of 638 women with three or more miscarriages were compared to those of women with no prior spontaneous abortions ($n = 3099$). Women with RM had a higher risk of delivery at less than 37 weeks' gestation, placenta previa, premature rupture of membranes, breech presentation, and congenital malformations. The most recent series is a population-based study, reported by Sheiner et al.[6] in which all singleton pregnancies were assessed in women with and without two or more consecutive recurrent abortions; 154,294 singleton deliveries occurred between 1988 and 2002 and 7503 of these deliveries occurred in patients with recurrent miscarriage. The following complications were found to be associated with recurrent miscarriage: advanced maternal age, cervical incompetence, diabetes mellitus, hypertensive disorders, placenta previa and abruptio placenta, mal-presentations, and premature ruputre of membranes. A higher rate of cesarean section was also found in patients with previous recurrent miscarriages compared to controls (15.9% and 10.9%, respectively [odds ratio = 1.6; 95% CI, 1.5–1.7]). More recently, a literature review by van Oppenraaij et al.[7] for the ESHRE Special Interest Group for Early Pregnancy (SIGEP) reported that recurrent miscarriage is associated with an increased risk for pre-eclampsia, placental abruption, placenta praevia, premature rupture of membranes, preterm delivery, intrauterine growth retardation, preterm delivery, low birth weight, and congenital anomalies.

An attempt was made to determine the common odds ratio for various late complications of pregnancy after recurrent miscarriage compared to controls. Reginald et al.'s[1] series could not be included as there was no relevant control group. Tulppala et al.'s[3] series could not be included as there was no control group. The other four publications were combined in a meta-analysis.

Vaginal Bleeding

The incidence of bleeding was only described in Reginald et al.'s series, quoted by Beard.[8] Hence no common odds ratio (OR) could be calculated. Vaginal bleeding seems to be increased in pregnancies that develop. Vaginal bleeding is a common complication occurring in 50 of 162 women in Reginald's series[7] and 50 of 102 patients in the author's series.[9] The reason for this bleeding remains unclear; 75% of habitual abortions are blighted ova.[9] However, when the pregnancy succeeds and there is a live embryo within the uterus, bleeding still occurs in 40–50% of patients.

Anomalies

There is little information available on anomalies. Sheiner et al.'s[6] study reports two anomalies in 29 patients. Although a very small series, the figures are higher than expected. Analysis of the figures in the RMITG trial[10] showed an anomaly rate of 4%. In the author's series, there were three anomalies in 99 developing pregnancies in nontreated patients. However, in the RMITG and author's series, no control group is available. In Thom et al.'s report,[5] women with a history of recurrent miscarriage were

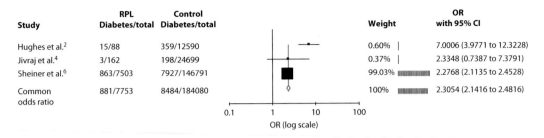

FIGURE 37.1   Odds ratio for gestational diabetes in recurrent pregnancy loss.

found to have a higher risk of delivering a child with congenital malformations (relative risk [RR] 1.8, 95% CI 1.1–3.0) than normal controls. However, many embryos with severe anomalies will be lost as miscarriages (see Chapter 11), and routine ultrasound systems scans will pick up a number of additional fetuses with anomalies. As many patients with malformations in the fetus elect to terminate the pregnancy, the incidence of anomalies at birth may not be higher today than in the general population.

Diabetes

Three papers describe the prevalence of diabetes. Hughes et al.,[2] Jivraj et al.,[4] and Sheiner et al.[6] as a control group was available, their common OR could be determined for 7753 patients with recurrent miscarriage and 172,490 control patients. The prevalence of diabetes was 11.75% and 4.95% in recurrently miscarrying and control patients, respectively. The odds ratios are summarized in Figure 37.1. As can be seen, there was a common OR of 2.30 for gestational diabetes in recurrent pregnancy loss. This figure was statistically significant (95% CI 2.14–2.49). Tulppala et al.[3] also found a prevalence of 22.6% (7/31 patients tested).

Pregnancy Induced Hypertension

Hughes et al.,[2] Jivraj et al.,[4] Thom et al.,[5] and Sheiner et al.[6] quoted the incidence of pregnancy induced hypertension (PIH). The figures are summarized in Figure 37.2. In order to obtain significant numbers, the figures for pre-eclampsia and other forms of pregnancy induced hypertension were analyzed as a whole. The common OR was 1.13 (CI 1.01–1.25), which was statistically significant. Neither Reginald et al.[1] nor Tulppala et al.[3] quote figures for pregnancy induced hypertension.

Intrauterine Growth Restriction

The same four papers as above give figures for IUGR. Thom et al.[5] quoted a relative risk of RR 2.0, 95% CI 1.4–2.8. Reginald et al.[1] reported a 33% incidence in 344 pregnancies prospectively followed up, and reported that this showed a relative risk of 3 compared to the standard Scottish population.

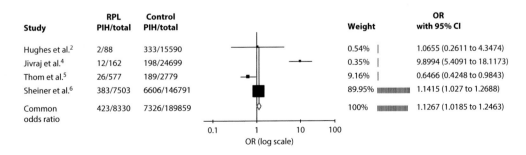

FIGURE 37.2   Odds ratio for pregnancy induced hypertension in recurrent pregnancy loss.

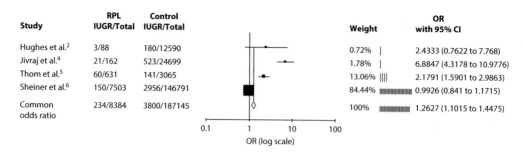

FIGURE 37.3 Odds ratio for intrauterine growth restriction in recurrent pregnancy loss.

Tulppala et al.[3] also reported a 20% incidence (6/30 pregnancies). However, when the four papers with control groups are taken together, the common OR for developing IUGR is 1.26 (CI 1.10–1.44) (Figure 37.3). The relationship between two or more miscarriages and IUGR (OR 1.4, 95% CI 1.2–1.6) has been found in a large population-based Danish study.[11]

Placental Abruption

Only Thom et al.[5] and Sheiner et al.[6] have reported a higher risk of placental abruption after two or more miscarriages. None of the other publications mentioned reported on placental abruption specifically. The results are summarised in Figure 37.4. There was a common OR of 5.8 (CI 5.1–6.6).

Placenta Previa

RM has been associated with an increased risk of placenta praevia (RR 6.0, 95% CI 1.6–22.2) in subsequent ongoing pregnancies in Thom et al.'s[5] study. None of the other publications mentioned above reported on placenta previa specifically. The results are summarized in Figure 37.3.

Preterm Labor

Comparative figures are available for preterm labor from Hughes et al.'s[2] and Jivraj et al.'s[4] and Thom et al.'s[5] series. Figure 37.5 summarizes the results. Again, there was a statistically significant association between preterm labor and recurrent pregnancy loss. The common OR was 1.74 (CI 1.38 – 2.19). In Reginald et al.'s[1] series, there was a 28% incidence of preterm labor. The relative risk was 3.3 when compared to the Scottish data for the equivalent period. Tulppala et al.[3] quoted a 9.7% incidence in their series.

Perinatal Mortality

Again, there was an increased tendency for mortality after recurrent pregnancy loss with a common OR of 1.22 (CI 1.02–1.46). This is summarised in Figure 37.6. However, the perinatal mortality may be artificially low due to obstetric intervention for other complications in pregnancy. Reginald et al.[1]

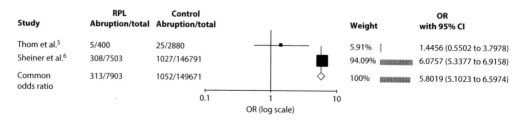

FIGURE 37.4 Odds ratio for placental abruption.

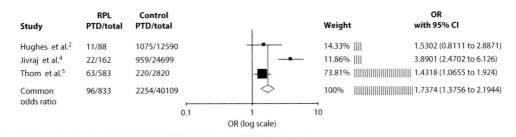

Study	RPL PTD/total	Control PTD/total		Weight		OR with 95% CI
Hughes et al.[2]	11/88	1075/12590		14.33%	||||	1.5302 (0.8111 to 2.8871)
Jivraj et al.[4]	22/162	959/24699		11.86%	||||	3.8901 (2.4702 to 6.126)
Thom et al.[5]	63/583	220/2820		73.81%	|||||||||||||||||||	1.4318 (1.0655 to 1.924)
Common odds ratio	96/833	2254/40109		100%	||||||||||||||||||||	1.7374 (1.3756 to 2.1944)

FIGURE 37.5 Odds ratio for preterm labor in recurrent pregnancy loss.

Study	RPL Mortality/total	Control Mortality/total		Weight		Association measure with 95% CI
Hughes et al.[2]	0/88	4.6/1000		0.37%	|	1.1032 (0.0599 to 20.3054)
Jivraj et al.[4]	2/162	247/24699		1.59%	|	1.2374 (0.3051 to 5.0189)
Sheiner et al.[6]	128/7503	2055/146791		98.04%	▨▨▨	1.2224 (1.021 to 1.4636)
Common odds ratio	130/7753	2306.6/172490		100%	▨▨▨	1.2227 (1.023 to 1.4612)

FIGURE 37.6 Odds ratio for perinatal mortality in recurrent pregnancy loss.

reported considerably higher than the standard figures for England and Wales in the same period of time with 19 perinatal deaths in 118 infants (16.1%) when the perinatal mortality was 10.1/1000. Tulppala et al.[3] does not quote perinatal mortality.

It seems, therefore, that the currently available literature on the obstetric and neonatal outcome of pregnancies from women with a history of recurrent miscarriage shows a consistently worse prognosis. However, it is unclear whether the worse prognosis is only found in patients with predisposing causes, such as antiphospholipid syndrome and hereditary thrombophilias, or is also present in patients with unexplained pregnancy losses.

Antiphospholipid Syndrome

In the author's series,[12] the outcome of 24 pregnancies in patients with lupus anticoagulant and five or more first trimester abortions was compared to 22 pregnancies in women with no antiphospholipid antibodies and five or more miscarriages. The subsequent number of first trimester miscarriages, and the live birth rate was similar in both groups of patients. However, the incidence of second or third trimester fetal deaths, intrauterine growth restriction, and need for premature induction of labor or preterm cesarean section was significantly higher in the antiphospholipid syndrome (APS) patients. The similar live birth rate was only obtained by early obstetric intervention to prevent intra-uterine fetal deaths. A number of other publications have attested that the risk of obstetric complications is high in antiphospholipid syndrome.[13,14] The incidence of pre-eclampsia is particularly high in APS.[14,15] IUGR has been reported with a frequency ranging from 30% to 12% in different series. Some series show a significant increase in the incidence of IUGR,[16,17] whereas other studies have not confirmed the increased incidence.[18,19] The incidence of preterm labor is also increased in APS patients.[16] Recently, Bouvier et al.[20] have reported the results of 513 women with APS and 791 women negative for antiphospholipid antibodies who served as controls. Among women with a history of recurrent miscarriage, APS women were at a higher risk than other women of pre-eclampsia, placenta-mediated complications, and neonatal mortality.

The currently accepted optimal treatment regimen for APS is heparin or low molecular weight heparin (LMWH) with the addition of low dose aspirin. However, anticoagulants do not seem lower the incidence of obstetric complications associated with this syndrome.[21–23] Intravenous immunoglobulin (IVIg) may have a beneficial effect in APS, as the action and production of aPL are inhibited by IVIg.

The F(ab') fragment of IVIg inhibits binding of anticardiolipin antibody to cardiolipin in dose dependent manner.[24] The F(ab') fragment of IVIg inhibits lupus anticoagulant activity.[25] IVIg lowers levels of ACA after each infusion.[26] IVIg may contain antiidiotypic antibodies to aPL, or inactivate B cell clones leading to decreased autoantibody production.[27] IVIg seems to have no apparent benefit over anticoagulants in terms of live births. However, when the obstetric complications are considered, a different clinical picture emerges. Vaquero et al.[28] compared IVIg to prednisone and aspirin. The prevalence of IUGR and preterm labor was similar in both groups, but the prevalence of pregnancy induced hypertension and gestational diabetes was significantly lower ($p < 0.05$) after IVIg (5% of 41 patients and 14% of 22 patients, respectively) for each condition. Branch et al.[29] compared IVIg to placebo; there were fewer cases of IUGR after IVIg (14% of seven patients compared to 33% of nine patients, respectively), and fewer admissions to the neonatal intensive care unit (14% of seven patients after IVIg compared to 44% of nine, respectively). Harris and Pierangelli[30] reported that pre-eclampsia, IUGR, and prematurity were reduced when IVIg was compared to prednisone and aspirin or heparin and aspirin.

Hereditary Thrombophilias

There have recently been numerous publications associating genetic predispositions (hereditary thrombophilias) to thrombosis with pregnancy loss. Hereditary thrombophilias include proteins C, S or antithrombin III deficiencies, activated protein C resistance (APCR), factor V Leiden mutation, the prothrombin gene mutation (G20210A), and excessive factor VIII. The features of hereditary thrombophilias and the effects on obstetric complications are discussed in the chapter on clotting disorders. Kuperminc et al.[31] have reported an association between thrombophilias and severe pre-eclampsia, placental abruption, IUGR, and stillbirth. However, these findings have been disputed by Infante-Rivard et al.[32] who also performed a case control study, and recently by Rodger et al., in a comparative cohort study.[33] Sheiner et al.[6] have drawn attention to the fact that the other publications on obstetric complications in recurrent pregnancy loss were written at a time when the hereditary thrombophilias had not yet been recognized. In their series, higher rates of IUGR, CS, low Apgar scores, and perinatal mortality were found among the 22 patients with known thrombophilia as compared to the controls, although the differences did not reach statistical significance. In the author's series of 21 pregnancies with factor V Leiden that were followed up prospectively, there was one case of HELLP syndrome, but no other obstetric complications, and no deep vein thrombosis or pulmonary embolus (author's series).

There are isolated reports[34–36] of using anticoagulants in the presence of thrombophilias to lower the late obstetric complications. However, there is, as yet, insufficient evidence that anticoagulants actually reduce the incidence of late obstetric complications. Further trials need to be performed in order to determine whether anticoagulants do indeed reduce the incidence of obstetric complications.

Obstetric Complications after Alloimmunization

Two methods of alloimmunization have been used in the past in order to improve the subsequent live birth rate in recurrently aborting women: active immunization with paternal leucocytes and passive immunization using IVIg. In order to summarize the obstetric complications either with or without immunotherapy, the various series in the literature were pooled in order to obtain a sufficient number of patients available for meaningful comparison. The databases of Beard,[8] the RMITG meta-analysis,[10] and the author's series were combined in order to compare the obstetric complications after paternal leucocyte immunization. As paternal leucocyte immunization (PLI) has now gone out of favor, there are no new series. Nine hundred and seventy-nine immunized patients were available for analysis compared to 483 nonimmunized patients. The prevalence of IUGR, perinatal mortality, and the incidence of anomalies were assessed. These figures are summarized in Table 37.1. As can be seen there was a significantly lower incidence of preterm labor, perinatal mortality, and intrauterine growth restriction after paternal leucocyte immunization than in controls. The incidence of fetal anomalies was not significantly different in both groups of patients. As the RMITG meta-analysis[10] did not assess bleeding

TABLE 37.1

Preterm Labor, Intrauterine Growth Restriction, Perinatal Mortality and Anomalies with Paternal Leucocyte Immunization Compared to Controls

	Immunized (979)		Controls (483)		Relative Risk
Preterm labor	39	(3.9%)	52	(10.8%)	0.63 CI (0.49–0.79)
Growth retardation	17	(1.7%)	59	(12.2%)	0.32 CI (0.21–0.49)
Prenatal mortality	9	(0.9%)	21	(4.3%)	0.44 CI (0.26–0.47)
Anomalies	25	(2.6%)	19	(3.9%)	0.84 CI (0.65–1.10)

Note: The incidences of the various obstetric complications are shown in parentheses. Figures include 92 immunized and 175 nonimmunized patients from Beard's[8] series, 759 immunized patients and 279 nonimmunized patients from the RMITG register,[9] and 128 immunized patients and 29 nonimmunized patients in the author's series. CI: confidence interval.

TABLE 37.2

Bleeding and Preeclampsia with Paternal Leucocyte Immunization Compared to Controls

	Immunized (216)		Controls (191)		Relative Risk
Bleeding	83	(38%)	64	(34%)	1.10 CI (0.92–1.33)
Preeclampsia	27	(13%)	57	(30%)	0.55 CI (0.40–0.76)

Note: The incidences of the various obstetric complications are shown in parentheses. Figures include 88 immunized and 162 nonimmunized patients from Beard's[8] series and 128 immunized patients and 29 nonimmunized patients in the author's series. CI: confidence interval.

and pre-eclampsia, data could only be obtained from Beard[8] series and the author's series. Two hundred and sixteen immunized patients and 191 control patients were available for analysis. These figures are summarized in Table 37.2. As can be seen the incidence of pre-eclampsia was lower in immunized women. However, there was no significant difference in the incidence of vaginal bleeding, which remained high in 38% and 34% in immunized and control women, respectively.

Table 37.3 shows the obstetric complications after IVIg in the 136 women in the author's series. There is no relevant control group, as some of the patients were administered IVIg after failure of paternal leucocyte immunization. The figures were compared to nonimmunized patients in the registers above and those in control patients in other series on IVIg in the literature. The incidences of growth retardation, perinatal mortality, bleeding and pre-eclampsia, were all lower after IVIg, but the incidence of preterm labor and anomalies did not seem to be affected. However, these results should be interpreted with caution due to the nature of the control group.

TABLE 37.3

Obstetric Complications after Intravenous Immunoglobulin (IVIg) Compared to Controls

	IVIg		Controls		Relative Risk
Preterm labor	15/136	(11%)	52/483	(10.8%)	1.02 CI (0.53–1.96)
Growth retardation	6/136	(4%)	59/483	(12.2%)	0.39 CI (0.18–0.86)
Pernatal mortality	2/136	(1.5%)	21/483	(4.3%)	0.39 CI (0.10–0.47)
Bleeding	5/136	(3.7%)	64/191	(34%)	0.14 CI (0.06–0.33)
Preeclampsia	4/136	(2.9%)	57/191	(30%)	0.13 CI (0.05–0.34)
Anomalies	1/136	(0.7%)	19/483	(3.9%)	0.22 CI (0.03–1.51)

Note: The figures show the incidence of anomalies as a function of the total number of patients in the sample. The incidences of the various obstetric complications are shown in parentheses. IVIg figures are from the author's series, the control figures are pooled data from the literature. CI: confidence interval.

Cytokines as Mediators of Pregnancy Loss and Obstetric Complications

Cytokines are low molecular weight peptides or glycopeptides, which are produced by lymphocytes, monocytes/macrophages, mast cells, eosinophils, and blood vessel endothelial cells. Cytokines seem to influence all stages of pregnancy. A full account of their actions is given in Chapter 27. An inappropriate cytokine balance has been reported to act in early pregnancy causing natural killer cell activation,[37] placental apoptosis,[38] teratogenesis,[39] and excessive coagulation. Hence, cytokine imbalance is one of the mechanisms which have been proposed to underlie recurrent miscarriage. The effect of cytokine imbalance on coagulation may explain some of the effects of hereditary thrombophilias.

Late obstetric complications have also been shown to be associated with altered cytokine levels. Pre-eclampsia is associated with reduced interleukin (IL)-10 and higher IL-2 production from peripheral blood mononuclear cells,[40,41] high serum IL-8, and tumor necrosis factor (TNF)-α.[42] In preterm births, cytokine involvement has been reported,[43] particularly increased amniotic IL-6, IL-8, and TNF-α have been reported.[44–47] Progesterone is often used to prevent preterm labor. Hudic et al.[48] prospectively compared serum concentrations of the anti-inflammatory cytokine, IL-10 and the pro-inflammatory cytokines IL-6, TNF-α, and interferon (IFN)-γ in women with threatened preterm delivery who were given the synthetic progestogen dydrogesterone to women with threatened preterm delivery who were not given progesterone supplementation. Progestogen treatment was associated with a significantly longer gestation than women who were given progesterone. Additionally, women treated by dydrogesterone had significantly higher serum levels of IL-10 than controls and lower concentrations of IFN-γ. In intrauterine growth restriction, the TGF-β in cord blood and the mRNA for IL-10 are significantly reduced, whereas IL-8 mRNA is significantly higher[49,50] and placental TNF-α secretion is enhanced.[50]

The various interventions used for improving the live birth rate in recurrent miscarriage, may have their effects by modulating cytokine balance, and modulation of cytokine balance may also influence the incidence of later obstetric complications. As stated in the chapter on coagulation disorders, it is possible that heparin or enoxaparin may work by anti-inflammatory mechanisms rather than anticoagulation. Heparin increases serum TNF binding protein, hence protecting against systemic harmful manifestations.[51] Low molecular weight heparins inhibit TNF-α production.[52] Thrombosis results in an inflammatory response of the vein wall. Both heparin and LMWH limit the anti-inflammatory response, but in Downing et al.'s[53] series, LMWH was more effective than heparin in limiting neutrophil extravasation and was the only intervention to decrease vein wall permeability.

The mode of action of PLI is unclear. PLI may also alter the balance between Th-1 and Th-2 cytokines. PLI has been reported to reduce IFN-γ, and increase the secretion of IL-10, and TGF-β[54] and has also been shown to modulate the serum IL-6 and soluble IL-6 receptor levels to the values observed in normal pregnancy.[55] IVIg has numerous actions. The actions of IVIg in pregnancy, including the effects on APS, have been summarized elsewhere.[56] In addition to various other mechanisms, IVIg, as PLI, depresses natural killer cell function[57] and enhances the action of Th-2 cytokines.[58]

Conclusions

Patients with recurrent miscarriage seem to form a high-risk group for later obstetric complications. Late obstetric complications have been described in APS and hereditary thrombophilias. However, there is insufficient evidence at present to determine whether the late obstetric complications occur exclusively in these two conditions, or whether they are associated with recurrent miscarriage *per se*. Immunomodulation seems to reduce the incidence of some of these complications. The role of anticoagulants in reducing obstetric complications is more doubtful. However, careful surveillance is required in pregnancies following recurrent miscarriage in order to detect obstetric complications. Further prospective cohort studies are necessary in order more accurately define the patient at risk and the effect of treatment modalities.

REFERENCES

1. Reginald PW, Beard RW, Chapple J et al. Outcome of pregnancies progressing beyond 28 weeks gestation in women with a history of recurrent miscarriage. *Brit J Obstet Gynaecol* 1987;94:643–8.
2. Hughes N, Hamilton EF, Tulandi T. Obstetric outcome in women after multiple spontaneous abortions. *J Reprod Med* 1991;36:165–6.
3. Tulppala M., Palosuo T., Ramsay T et al. A prospective study of 63 couples with a history or recurrent spontaneous abortion: Contributing factors and outcome of subsequent pregnancies. *Hum Reprod* 1993;8:764–70.
4. Jivraj S, Anstie B, Cheong YC et al. Obstetric and neonatal outcome in women with a history of recurrent miscarriage: A cohort study. *Hum Reprod* 2001;16:102–6.
5. Thom DH, Nelson LM, Vaughan TL. Spontaneous miscarriage and subsequent adverse birth outcomes. *Am J Obstet Gynecol* 1992;166:111–6.
6. Sheiner E, Levy A, Katz M et al. Pregnancy outcome following recurrent spontaneous abortions. *Eur Jour Obst Gynecol Reprod Biol* 2005;118:61–5.
7. van Oppenraaij RH, Jauniaux E, Christiansen OB et al. Predicting adverse obstetric outcome after early pregnancy events and complications: A review. *Hum Reprod Update* 2009;15:409–21.
8. Beard RW. Clinical associations of recurrent miscarriage. In: Beard RW. Sharp F, eds. *Early Pregnancy Loss: Mechanisms and Treatment.* London: RCOG; 1988. p. 3–8.
9. Carp HJA, Toder V, Mashiach S et al. Recurrent miscarriage: A review of current concepts, immune mechanisms, and results of treatment. *Obst Gynecol Surv* 1990;45:657–69.
10. Worldwide collaborative observational study and meta-analysis on allogenic leucocyte immunotherapy for recurrent spontaneous abortion. Recurrent Miscarriage Immunotherapy Trialists Group. *Am J Reprod Immunol* 1994;32:55–72.
11. Basso O, Olsen J, Christensen K. Risk of preterm delivery, low birthweight and growth retardation following spontaneous abortion: A registry-based study in Denmark. *Int J Epidemiol* 1998;27:642–6.
12. Carp HJA, Menashe Y, Frenkel Y et al. Lupus anticoagulant: Significance in first trimester habitual abortion. *J Reprod Med* 1993;38:549–52.
13. Tincani A, Balestrieri G, Danieli E et al. Pregnancy complications of the antiphospholipid syndrome. *Autoimmunity* 2003;36:27–32.
14. de Jesús GR, Rodrigues G, de Jesús NR et al. Pregnancy morbidity in antiphospholipid syndrome: What is the impact of treatment? *Curr Rheumatol Rep* 2014;16:403.
15. Lima F, Khamashta MA, Buchanan NM et al. A study of sixty pregnancies in patients with the antiphospholipid syndrome. *Clin Exp Rheumatol* 1996;14:1316.
16. Branch DW, Silver RM, Blackwell JL et al. Outcome of treated pregnancies in women with antiphospholipid syndrome: An update of the Utah experience. *Obstet Gynecol* 1992;80:614–20.
17. Kutteh WH, Ermel LD. A clinical trial for the treatment of antiphospholipid antibody-associated recurrent pregnancy loss with lower dose heparin and aspirin. *Am J Reprod Immunol* 1996;35:4027.
18. Pattison NS, Chamley LW, McKay EJ. et al. Antiphospholipid antibodies in pregnancy: Prevalence and clinical associations. *Br J Obstet Gynaecol* 1993;100:909–13.
19. Lynch A, Marlar R, Murphy J et al. Antiphospholipid antibodies in predicting adverse pregnancy outcome. A prospective study. *Ann Intern Med* 1994;120:470–5.
20. Bouvier S, Cochery-Nouvellon E, Lavigne-Lissalde G et al. Comparative incidence of pregnancy outcomes in treated obstetric antiphospholipid syndrome: The NOH-APS observational study. *Blood* 2014;123:404–13.
21. Shehata HA, Nelson-Piercy C, Khamashta MA. Management of pregnancy in antiphospholipid syndrome. *Rheum Dis Clin North Am.* 2001;27:643–59.
22. Backos M, Rai R, Baxter N et al. Pregnancy complications in women with recurrent miscarriage associated with antiphospholipid antibodies treated with low dose aspirin and heparin. *Br J ObstetGynaecol* 1999;106:102–7.
23. Branch DW, Silver RM, Blackwell JL et al. Outcome of treated pregnancies in women with antiphospholipid syndrome: An update of the Utah experience. *Obstet Gynecol* 1992;80:614–20.
24. Caccavo D, Vaccaro F, Ferri GM et al. Anti-idiotypes against antiphospholipid antibodies are present in normal polyspecific immunoglobulinsfor therapeutic use. *J Autoimmun* 1994;7:537–48.

25. Galli M, Cortelazzo S, Barbui T. *In vivo* efficacy of intravenous gammaglobulins in patients with lupus anticoagulant is not mediated by anti-idiotypic mechanisms. *Am J Hematol* 1991;38:184–8.

26. Kwak JY, Quilty EA, Gilman-Sachs A et al. Intravenous immunoglobulin infusion therapy in women with recurrent spontaneous abortions of immune etiologies. *J Reprod Immunol* 1995;28:175–88.

27. Wegmann TG. The cytokine basis for cross-talk between the maternal immune and reproductive systems. *Curr Opin Immunol* 1990;2:765–9.

28. Vaquero E, Lazzarin N, Valensie H et al. Pregnancy outcome in recurrent spontaneous abortion associated with antiphospholipid antibodies: A comparative study of intravenous immunoglobulin versus prednisone plus low-dose aspirin. *Am J Reprod Immunol* 2001;45:174–9.

29. Branch DW, Peaceman AM, Druzin M et al. A multicenter, placebo-controlled pilot study of intravenous immune globulin treatment of antiphospholipid syndrome during pregnancy. The pregnancy loss study group. *Am J Obstet Gynecol* 2000;182:122–7.

30. Harris EN, Pierangeli SS. Utilization of intravenous immunoglobulin therapy to treat recurrent pregnancy loss in the antiphospholipid syndrome: A review. *Scand J Rheumatol Suppl* 1998;107:97–102.

31. Kupferminc MJ, Eldor A, Steinman N et al. Increased frequency of genetic thrombophilia in women with complications of pregnancy. *N Engl J Med* 1999;340:9–13.

32. Infante-Rivard C, Rivard GE, Yotov WV et al. Absence of association of thrombophilia polymorphisms with intrauterine growth restriction. *N Engl J Med* 2002;347:19–25.

33. Rodger MA, Walker MC, Smith GN et al. Is thrombophilia associated with placenta-mediated pregnancy complications? A prospective cohort study. *J Thromb Haemost* 2014;12:469–78.

34. Younis JS, Ohel G, Brenner B et al. Familial thrombophilia—The scientific rationale for thrombophylaxis in recurrent pregnancy loss. *Hum Reprod* 1997;12:1389–90.

35. Brenner B, Hoffman R, Blumenfeld Z et al. Gestational outcome in thrombophilic women with recurrent pregnancy loss treated by enoxaparin. *Thromb Hemost* 2000;83:693–7.

36. Riyazi N, Leeda M, de Vries JI et al. Low-molecular-weight heparin combined with aspirin in pregnant women with thrombophilia and a history of preeclampsia or fetal growth restriction: A preliminary study. *Eur J Obstet Gynecol Reprod Biol* 1998;80:49–54.

37. King A, Jokhi PP, Burrows TD et al. Functions of human decidual NK cells. *Am J Reprod Immunol* 1996;35:258–60.

38. Baines MG, Duglos AJ, de Fougerolles AR et al. Immunological prevention of spontaneous early embryo resorption is mediated by non specific immunostimulation. *Am J Reprod Immunol* 1996;35:34–42.

39. Savion S, Brengauz-Breitmann M, Torchinsky A et al. A possible role for granulocyte macrophage-colony stimulating factor in modulating teratogen-induced effects. *Teratog Carcinog Mutagen* 1999;19:171–82.

40. Darmochwal-Kolarz D, Rolinski J, Leszczynska-Goarzelak B et al. The expressions of intracellular cytokines in the lymphocytes of preeclamptic patients. *Am J Reprod Immunol* 2002;48:381–6.

41. Orange S, Horvath J, Hennessy A. Preeclampsia is associated with a reduced interleukin-10 production from peripheral blood mononuclear cells. *Hypertens Pregnancy* 2003;22:1–8.

42. Velzing-Aarts FV, Muskiet FA, Van der Dijs FP et al. High serum interleukin-8 levels in afro-caribbean women with pre-eclampsia. Relations with tumor necrosis factor-alpha, duffy negative phenotype and von Willebrand factor. *Am J Reprod Immunol* 2002;48:319–22.

43. Park JS, Park CW, Lockwood CJ et al. Role of cytokines in preterm labor and birth. *Minerva Ginecol* 2005;57:349–66.

44. Fortunato SJ, Menon R, Lombardi SJ. Role of tumor necrosis factor-alpha in the premature rupture of membranes and preterm labor pathways. *Am J Obstet Gynecol* 2002;187:1159–62.

45. Jacobsson B, Mattsby-Baltzer I, Andersch B et al. Microbial invasion and cytokine response in amniotic fluid in a Swedish population of women in preterm labor. *Acta Obstet Gynecol Scand* 2003;82:120–8.

46. Maymon E, Ghezzi F, Edwin SS et al. The tumor necrosis factor alpha and its soluble receptor profile in term and preterm parturition. *Am J Obstet Gynecol* 1999;181:1142–8.

47. Ognjanovic S, Bryant-Greenwood GD. Pre-B-cell colony-enhancing factor, a novel cytokine of human fetal membranes. *Am J Obstet Gynecol* 2002;187:1051–8.

48. Hudic I, Szekeres-Bartho, J, Zlatan F et al. Dydrogesterone supplementation in women with threatened preterm delivery—The impact on cytokine profile, hormone profile, and progesterone-induced blocking factor. *J Reprod Immunol* 2010;92:103–7.

49. Hahn-Zoric M, Hagberg H, Kjellmer I et al. Aberrations in placental cytokine mRNA related to intrauterine growth retardation. *Pediatr Res* 2002;51:201–6.

50. Holcberg G, Huleihel M, Sapir O et al. Increased production of tumor necrosis factor-alpha TNF-alpha by IUGR human placentae. *Eur J Obstet Gynecol Reprod Biol* 2001;94:69–72.

51. Lantz M, Thysell H, Nilsson E et al. On the binding of tumor necrosis factor (TNF) to heparin and the release *in vivo* of the TNF-binding protein I by heparin. *J Clin Invest* 1991;88:2026–31.

52. Baram D, Rashkovsky M, Hershkoviz R et al. Inhibitory effects of low molecular weight heparin on mediator release by mast cells: Preferential inhibition of cytokine production and mast cell-dependent cutaneous inflammation. *Clin Exp Immunol* 1997;110:485–91.

53. Downing LJ, Strieter RM, Kadell AM et al. Low-dose low-molecular-weight heparin is anti-inflammatory during venous thrombosis. *J Vasc Surg* 1998;28:848–54.

54. Gafter U, Sredni B, Segal J et al. Suppressed cell-mediated immunity and monocyte and natural killer cell activity following allogeneic immunization of women with spontaneous recurrent abortion. *J Clin Immunol* 1997;17:408–19.

55. Zenclussen AC, Kortebani G, Mazzolli A et al. Interleukin-6 and soluble interleukin-6 receptor serum levels in recurrent spontaneous abortion women immunized with paternal white cells. *Am J Reprod Immunol* 2000;44:22–9.

56. Carp HJA, Sapir T, Shoenfeld Y. Intravenous immunoglobulin and recurrent pregnancy loss. *Clin Rev Allergy Immunol* 2005;29:327–32.

57. Ruiz JE, Kwak JY, Baum L et al. Effect of intravenous immunoglobulin G on natural killer cell cytotoxicity *in vitro* in women with recurrent spontaneous abortion. *J Reprod Immunol* 1996;31:125–41.

58. Graphou O, Chioti A, Pantazi A et al. Effect of intravenous immunoglobulin treatment on the Th1/Th2 balance in women with recurrent spontaneous abortions. *Am J Reprod Immunol* 2003;49:21–9.

38

Coping with Repeated Pregnancy Loss: Psychological Mechanisms

Keren Shakhar

Recurrent miscarriage (RM) is clearly a stressful experience, but very little is known about what sets its emotional experience apart from isolated spontaneous miscarriages and about other forms of infertility. This chapter aims to describe how RM affects the daily life, self-esteem, marital and social relations of couples experiencing RM and how they cope with this experience. The degree of emotional anguish couples experience largely depends on the significance they ascribe to RM. This meaning is influenced not only by the couples' views, but also by the perception of infertility and the view of prenatal life in their specific society.

Psychological Reactions to Recurrent Miscarriage

RM is a type of infertility that confronts couples with repeated cycles of hope and despair. Many couples view parenthood as an indispensable component of their marriage and many cases of RM occur before they have had a child. Young couples often take their ability to conceive for granted and are only concerned with the question when to have a child. RM shatters their basic expectations about family life. What is expected to be a fulfilling experience is instead an experience of loss and disappointment. These miscarriages usually occur at a very sensitive phase in the couple's development: becoming parents is a transitional stage that requires reconstruction of identities and preparation for new roles.

Only few studies have specifically addressed the psychological difficulties of couples suffering from more than one miscarriage, focusing, as a rule, on the women. It is estimated that around 30% of women with RM are depressed and that even a higher proportion have high levels of state and trait anxiety.[1,2] These studies suggest that the second miscarriage has a harsher emotional impact than the first.[3–5] Surprisingly, no differences in psychological distress were found between women who have had a child prior to the miscarriages and those who have not.[1–3] Some mothers report feeling guilty for failing to provide a sibling for their child and fear that their child feels lonely.

When women with RM conceive again they exhibit high levels of anxiety and have difficulty getting through each day.[6] This anxiety is manifested as general tension, despondence, and premonitions of miscarriage and may be exhibited by weeping, fear of detecting bleeding, extreme anxiety over any abdominal pain, constant checking for signs of pregnancy, avoidance of other pregnant women, and reluctance to discuss the pregnancy with anyone, including husbands.[6,7] Some women show less emotional attachment to their subsequent pregnancies, and avoid thinking about their future child.[6,8] Although this type of reaction may alleviate the constant anxiety and protect women emotionally if they eventually miscarry, it also diminishes the pleasure women can derive from being pregnant and may prevent grief from being processed. It is unclear how deep into pregnancy women are less attached to their embryo and whether it complicates the transition to motherhood.

As the psychological literature on RM is limited, and as women with RM must cope with both miscarriages and potential infertility, what is known about these two entities will be examined next.

Coping with a Miscarriage

The reaction to a sudden loss of pregnancy varies greatly among different couples: some exhibit little or no reaction, whereas others demonstrate a significant decline in their coping ability[9,10] and may feel emptiness and guilt, increased anxiety and depressive symptoms.[10,11] These depressive symptoms can include staying in bed and doing nothing, difficulty in performing daily tasks, and a feeling of a physical illness. One month after miscarriage approximately half of the women are still depressed[3] and for many depression may persist up to half a year after the miscarriage.[11]

Many couples experiencing a miscarriage undergo a process of grieving[9] (to be described later). They mourn the lost child, their failed hopes for the child, and their unaccomplished parenthood. Unlike the grief over the death of a relative, these couples generally do not receive social support, and may face insensitive attitudes. Sometimes the miscarriage occurs before the couple had shared the news of the pregnancy with anyone, leaving them lonely in the grieving process. It is crucial to understand that even if the embryo was lost at a very early gestational week, many couples already regard their embryo as a baby, name or nickname him, talk to him, ascribe him with a specific personality, and imagine his future.

Unfortunately, family members and friends may not know how to respond to the bereaved couple, and may not grasp what the pregnancy meant to them.[12] A break in communications sometimes occurs due to lack of response or because the couples consider the response inappropriate.[13] Typical attempts at consolation include "at least you can get pregnant," "maybe it's good you miscarried, the baby was probably abnormal," "how can you grieve so much, you were barely pregnant," and "you can always conceive again." While these perspectives may help some couples, many others do not want to forget their miscarried child at this time, and resist the possibility that someday they would feel as if the loss has never happened.[6] Friends and family may feel guilty of their pregnancies and may sometimes try to hide their pregnancy or talk less about their children, resulting in the couple feeling distanced from their friends, which can result in social withdrawal.[12] In addition, the couple may feel that family and friends expect them to conceive again to quickly replace their loss.

Apart from being emotionally disturbing, miscarriage can be physically traumatic; it may involve sudden pain, loss of blood, rapid hospitalization, and curettage.[13] Some women identify the physical process of miscarriage as the most stressful aspect of RM.

There has been considerable research on variables that moderate the influence of miscarriage on well-being, some of which may vary with time since the loss. Some of these mediators are uncontrollable: young age is associated with lower well-being;[5] a later gestational week of miscarriage has harsher psychological consequences. However, other factors that are related to adverse well-being can be controlled: attributing high personal significance to miscarriage, low investment and satisfaction in domains of life other than parenthood, lack of social support, and use of passive coping strategies.[9,14] Placing greater value in the relationship with spouses was also associated with higher scores on well-being.

It is noteworthy that the nature of the experience of an isolated miscarriage may be different to that of RM. First, unlike an isolated miscarriage, which has little prognostic value, in RM, each additional miscarriage reduces the prospects of having children. The prognostic meaning that couples associate with the miscarriage can further damage their sense of well-being. In addition, the repeated losses may exacerbate the experience or teach couples to cope with it.

Coping with Infertility

Coping with infertility has been extensively explored over the last 50 years. Many researchers describe infertility as a psychological crisis that includes loss of self-esteem, increased anxiety, sexual problems, anger, depression, and self-blame.[15–17] The uncertainty of having biological children evokes a sense that life is unpredictable and that significant events in life are not under control. Couples may also feel socially isolated as they avoid social gatherings to evade interactions with pregnant women or children. Some couples cannot bear being expected to hold someone else's child or to listen to stories about the pleasures and difficulties others are experiencing when raising children. These often remind them of their loss.

The Unique Experience of Recurrent Miscarriage

Loss of self-esteem, guilt and self-blame may be even more evident in women suffering from RM. Unlike many fertility problems, where the cause is either unknown or is attributed to both partners, in RM, women often feel that they are to blame because it was their body that could not support the pregnancy. This feeling is reinforced by the medical examinations the couples undergo: most clinical examinations evaluate possible etiologies in the women.

Levels of stress and anxiety in women with RM are especially high during pregnancy and may peak around the gestational week when previous miscarriages occurred.[6] This is unlike most other fertility problems where conception is the aim itself, and once achieved, the mission has largely been accomplished. The decision to conceive again is often very complex as women often consider whether they can bear another miscarriage.

The Grieving Process

Couples experiencing RM will often grieve for their lost children, their lost parenthood, their biological failure, the loss of control over their life, and for the possibility that they would not have biological children.[11,16] Unlike losing a child, the couples do not have memories of the baby and their loss is often not acknowledged by society.[9] There are no rituals associated with mourning a miscarriage. Couples may feel reluctant to share the experience with others, often cannot take days off from work, and may lack the time they would like to grieve for the loss. Couples may also be torn between their hopes for a successful pregnancy and their grief. This grief process is often characterized by intense fluctuations in emotions ranging from crying to laughing to being angry. This grief process may last for months and even years and often extends into the subsequent pregnancies that serve as reminders for previous losses and can trigger intense emotions. Many couples may be very surprised by their mood swings and the intensity of the emotions they experience. They may not be aware that this is a normal reaction to their loss.

Although there is no single right way to grieve, several stages of grief are commonly experienced. Not everyone passes through each of these stages and couples differ in the amount of time they spend at each stage. The following list of stages is mostly based on Mennings' experience in his work as a counselor with infertile couples.[18]

Denial, Shock, and Numbness[9,19]

This stage often begins with the shock that another miscarriage has occurred and it is characterized by the feeling that "this can't be happening to me." Couples sometimes do not even admit to themselves that something may be wrong. This reaction serves as a defense mechanism and it will usually diminish as couples begin to acknowledge their loss, usually within hours to days. This emotional numbness and denial should not be confused with "lack of caring."

Anger[8,19]

During this stage, couples are preoccupied with the miscarriages they have had and a feeling of unfairness surrounds their thoughts. The couple also experiences an intense yearning for the lost child, for the lost parenthood, pregnancy, and dreams. The anger associated with the unfairness of the entire experience can focus on the pain and inconvenience associated with miscarriage, with the tests and treatments, with the social pressure they encounter from family and friends, and with comments regarding their miscarriages and childlessness. The anger may also include broader targets such as abortion rights advocates, people who easily carry to term, and the medical team. Social support and respect can help abate this anger.

Isolation[19]

As described in the previous section, many couples exhibit social withdrawal. Couples often feel that their experience is unique and that others whose experience of being pregnant is joyous cannot comprehend what they are going through.

Guilt[8,19]

Women sometimes feel that the recurrent miscarriages are a punishment for something they did. They may regret actions they took or failed to take prior to the miscarriages.

Depression[1,8]

At this stage, there is full penetration of the loss. Thoughts such as "my life is over, I can't go on," "I don't care anymore" are very frequent. Some women may feel a sense of great loss, mood fluctuations, and loneliness.

Rebuilding and Healing

There is disagreement whether complete healing can occur. Still, at this stage the couple starts dealing with the reality of the situation. They restructure the event, organize their activities and plan to move forward in life.

What Domains of Life Are Affected

Self-Esteem[16,17]

Most people view the ability to conceive and have children as central to their personal identity, many women view motherhood as an integral part of their self-worth and femininity.[20] This may also be reinforced by religious percepts for example, "reproduce and fill the earth."

Loss of Control[6,12,16]

For many women RM is the first experience of a major loss of control over their life, their body, and their ability to plan the future.

Relationship with Peers[12,16]

As previously discussed, couples may feel excluded from friends whose interests focuses on children and may seek new reference groups to belong to.

Marital Stress[1,12,21]

While the experience of infertility can improve marital adjustment for some couples, it may damage the relationships of others and increase marital stress.[21] This diversity may occur because couples may differ from each other in their attitude toward the losses, in their grief response and in their motivation to have children. In addition, women may feel guilty for failing their spouse's expectations and feel responsible for his pain. Many women fear that their partner would leave them to find someone else with whom to have children.

Sexual Life[21,22]

RM, like other fertility problems, may increase sexual discontent. Couples may feel a pressure to quickly conceive again, and with it an increased demand to have sex at certain times. Not being in the mood, or being absent due to various reasons, such as business trips, may increase the tension.

Financial Costs

RM frequently taxes couples with financial costs: visits to a specialist, tests, treatment, and absence from work.

The Male Partner

Spouses are often very lonely in their experience of RM. The woman is usually considered as the patient—women experience the physical miscarriage, their reproductive system is assumed to hold the cause, and they are subject to most of the diagnostic tests. The idea that the spouse may also experience intense grief is often forgotten. Compared to women, the grief of male partners is less active and is expressed for a shorter duration.[23] Men are often ready to carry on with their lives earlier than women and are less interested in repeatedly discussing the miscarriage.[10,17]

Spouses frequently find themselves in a very delicate position: while they themselves endure crisis, grieve, and need support, they feel that they ought to be strong to emotionally support their partners. As a result, spouses suppress their feelings of loss and do not share it with their partners. They may struggle to say the right words and fear that what they say would make their partners feel worse. Many of them fail to realize that their female partner wants to know they also grieve the loss. Also, although the spouses may have the best intentions of providing support, there are gender differences in coping strategies with life stressors,[24] and men tend to give instrumental rather than social support, leaving women feeling unsupported and the male partners feeling guilty and unappreciated.

The Physician

Although the physician and the couple share the desire for pregnancy to succeed, the cooperation between them is complex and may be very vulnerable. The challenge facing the physician when first seeing couples with RM is almost impossible; there is often very limited time and the components of a medical consultation are very consuming. This is usually a time when the couple's anxiety and stress are very intense and they are very attentive and sensitive to every word and gesture. Their first visit to the specialist can itself evoke many emotions: frustration, anger, stress, and inadequacy. This visit reminds them of past miscarriages, confronts them with their lack of control, clarifies that they should prepare for more miscarriages, and confirms that they have a medical condition that might leave them childless. Physicians are often unaware that the high stress the couple experiences interferes with their ability to process the information received at the visit. Thus, a very common experience for many patients undergoing diagnosis is that they often cannot recall what the physician said and tend to misinterpret what has been told to them.

The Value of Psychological Support in Couples with RM

Clearly, the experience of RM increases levels of distress, depressive symptoms, and anxiety. RM can affect almost every aspect of life, and its emotional burden usually becomes heavier during pregnancy. To lower levels of distress, couples often withdraw from friends and do not receive the social support they need. Obviously, these couples could benefit from psychological support. Although various psychological therapies exist and should be offered to the couple suffering from RM, most couples desire to receive some of the support from the medical team. Thus, before describing various psychological supports that can be offered, there are several issues that should be taken into consideration as part of the "tender loving care." Even if such elements cannot be incorporated into medical care, awareness to the needs of the couples can itself help them feel understood.

Couples wish to be treated and followed up by the same physician. They want their physician to inquire about their psychological well-being and offer them help if needed. Even if they choose to not seek psychological support, such inquiry makes them feel that they are being understood. Women often report that they would like their partner to be more involved. This can be partly achieved by adding his name to medical files and addressing him with questions. Once pregnancy is achieved, the couple would like to meet their physician to discuss their life styles and schedule examinations that can assure them that pregnancy is proceeding as expected (e.g., βhCG, ultrasound every 2 weeks). If miscarriage occurs, couples wish to inform their physician and discuss the situation. They want to be assured they have not done anything to harm pregnancy.[25] If women are hospitalized, they should not be roomed with pregnant women.

What Kind of Psychological Supports Can Be Offered?

Support Groups

One way to compensate for the lack of social support from family and friends is to seek couples who share similar experiences. Meeting other couples with RM can decrease the sense of loneliness and reassure couples that their reactions and feelings are normal.[26] Unfortunately, women suffering from RM usually do not know other women in their situation and internet forums that are specific for RM hardly exist. Organizing support groups consisting of couples with RM can definitely meet this need.

Teaching Couples about the Grieving Process

As most couples are unaware that the intense emotional turbulence they experience is a normal and a common reaction to the loss, they become upset by their reaction. Teaching them about the common grief process can help them accept their grief, and proceed with it in their own way and pace.

Activities for Reducing Anxiety

Physical activity, art, meditation, relaxation, and yoga can reduce general anxiety in a nonspecific manner.

Cognitive Restructuring[27]

The individual interpretation of RM influences the emotions evoked by this experience. Some of the negative thoughts are automatic and erroneous. Challenging these thoughts and restructuring them into more truthful and positive thinking can improve well-being. Such techniques were shown to diminish stress, anxiety, depression, and self-blame, and to increase enjoyments in everyday life, in having each other, in work, etc. An example of a common automatic thought in women with RM may be "I'll never have any children." This thought is definitely not true and should be challenged. Some examples may be "This process is very painful for me but there is a chance that I will eventually have children." In addition, the significance attributed to having biological children can be reframed as well.

Sometimes spouses fail to recognize what their partners are going through; this may create a cycle of disrupted communication that decreases couples' enjoyment in doing things together and increases their martial stress. A fruitful dialogue can be achieved by learning to listen more to each other, by acknowledging each other's feelings, by being aware of the different coping strategies, and by recognizing each other's needs.

Learning of Other Parenting Options

Although not all couples feel ready to explore other means to achieve parenthood, many could benefit from meeting couples who have chosen to adopt or use the aid of a surrogate mother. This not only informs them of the procedures and the emotions associated with choosing other paths, but it also confronts them with "their worst nightmare." Although they may not decide to follow these paths, couples often realize this is not a bad option as they have imagined and some of the fear that is associated with infertility may be relieved.

Discussing Legitimacy

Many women with RM report that they feel it is illegitimate to quit trying or to seek alternative means for parenthood. Discussing their legitimacy to decide that they want a break or to stop trying to conceive again may relieve some of the pressure some women experience.

As emotional anxiety tends to peak during pregnancy, some psychological therapy should also be offered during this period. Clearly some of strategies listed can only be offered between pregnancies but they can relieve the psychological burden in subsequent pregnancies.

Can Stress Contribute to Recurrent Miscarriage?

A common question that bothers couples with RM is whether excessive stress can adversely affect pregnancy and lead to miscarriage. This question is difficult to examine in humans as a relationship between psychological factors and miscarriage cannot be interpreted as a causal relationship.

The best support for the potential contribution of psychological factors to RM comes from studies evaluating the effect of psychological support on miscarriage rates in women suffering from RM.[28–30] Interventions ranged from basic "tender loving care" to relaxation workshops and audiocassettes, weekly ultrasound examinations, and other psychological interventions that assure couples that their pregnancy is proceeding as expected. Remarkably, in all studies, women who received psychological support had two to four-fold lower miscarriage rates than those who did not. Although these studies suffer from methodological problems, it is doubtful whether these flaws can account for such a marked reduction in miscarriage rates (on average from 72% to 23%).

One possible pathway that can mediate the effects of stress on miscarriage is through the effect of stress on natural killer (NK) cells. Studies in mice have shown that stress more than tripled the resorption rates in miscarriage-prone mice and that depletion of NK cells prevented this effect.[31] In humans, we have recently shown that the number and activity of peripheral NK cells in RM, which have previously been shown to predict the outcome of subsequent pregnancy, is a transient response to the blood withdrawal.[32] A cannula was inserted into the veins of women with RM and controls, and blood was drawn immediately and 20 minutes later. NK activity and cell number were increased in RM patients in the first blood withdrawal, but declined to a level similar to that of the control in the second blood withdrawal. These levels remained almost unchanged in the control groups. This may suggest that the increased NK activity and numbers often observed in women with RM reflects hypersensitivity to the stress of blood withdrawal rather than the immunological steady state. It remains to be determined whether such hypersensitivity is also predictive of pregnancy outcome.

If stress indeed contributes to miscarriage in women with RM, it could lead couples into a vicious circle. The first miscarriage could be due to some biological cause such as an abnormal karyotype. Such a miscarriage can increase stress levels during the subsequent pregnancy and consequently boosts the risk of another miscarriage. If another miscarriage occurs it increases stress levels again, and consequently, the chances of another miscarriage.

Summary

More than any other fertility problem, RM submits patients to repeated cycles of hope and despair. Although management of emotions is not considered part of the physician role, adopting an inclusive psychosocial perspective would greatly improve the treatment of couples with RM. The anxiety, depression, anger, and frustration these couples experience are critically influenced by the significance they bestow on their miscarriages, by the pressure they perceive from family and friends, and by how much emotion and social support they receive. A supportive and empathic approach by the medical team can ease this suffering, and psychological interventions can be used to improve the couples' coping and enhance their well-being. Such intervention may not only relieve the emotional burden of RM but also lower the risk of another miscarriage. Although some clinicians may doubt such effects, the evidence for such a possibility exceeds the support for several medical interventions already employed in RM. Larger randomized studies should examine this possibility more carefully. Until proven, the psychosocial hypothesis should be raised with caution as it can lead women to blame themselves for the miscarriage.

REFERENCES

1. Klock SC, Chang G, Hiley A et al. Psychological distress among women with recurrent spontaneous abortion. *Psychosomatics* 1997;38:503–7.
2. Craig M, Tata P, Regan L. Psychiatric morbidity among patients with recurrent miscarriage. *J Psychosom Obstet Gynaecol* 2002;23:157–64.
3. Friedman T, Gath D. The psychiatric consequences of spontaneous abortion. *Br J Psychiatry* 1989;155:810–3.
4. Aoki K, Furukawa T, Ogasawara M et al. Psychosocial factors in recurrent miscarriages. *Acta Obstet Gynecol Scand* 1998;77:572–3.
5. Neugebauer R. Depressive symptoms at two months after miscarriage: Interpreting study findings from an epidemiological versus clinical perspective. *Depress Anxiety* 2003;17:152–61.
6. Cote-Arsenault D, Bidlack D, Humm A. Women's emotions and concerns during pregnancy following perinatal loss. *MCN Am J Matern Child Nurs* 2001;26:128–34.
7. Liddell HS, Pattison NS, Zanderigo A. Recurrent miscarriage—Outcome after supportive care in early pregnancy. *Aust N Z J Obstet Gynaecol* 1991;31:320–2.
8. Madden ME. The variety of emotional reactions to miscarriage. *Women Health* 1994;21:85–104.
9. Lee C, Slade P. Miscarriage as a traumatic event: A review of the literature and new implications for intervention. *J Psychosom Res* 1996;40:235–44.
10. Athey J, Spielvogel AM. Risk factors and interventions for psychological sequelae in women after miscarriage. *Prim Care Update Ob Gyns* 2000;7:64–9.
11. Nikcevic AV, Tunkel SA, Nicolaides KH. Psychological outcomes following missed abortions and provision of follow-up care. *Ultrasound Obstet Gynecol* 1998;11:123–8.
12. Imeson M, McMurray A. Couples' experiences of infertility: A phenomenological study. *J Adv Nurs* 1996;24:1014–22.
13. Bansen SS, Stevens HA. Women's experiences of miscarriage in early pregnancy. *J Nurse Midwifery* 1992;37:84–90.
14. Brier N. Understanding and managing the emotional reactions to a miscarriage. *Obstet Gynecol* 1999;93:151–5.
15. Greil AL, Slauson-Blevins K, McQuillan J. The experience of infertility: A review of recent literature. *Sociol Health Illn* 2010;32:140–62.
16. Gonzalez LO. Infertility as a transformational process: A framework for psychotherapeutic support of infertile women. *Issues Ment Health Nurs* 2000;21:619–33.
17. Pasch LA, Dunkel-Schetter C, Christensen A. Differences between husbands' and wives' approach to infertility affect marital communication and adjustment. *Fertil Steril* 2002;77:1241–7.
18. Menning BE. The emotional needs of infertile couples. *Fertil Steril* 1980;34:313–9.
19. Matthews AM, Matthews R. Beyond the mechanics of infertility—Perspectives on the social-psychology of infertility and involuntary childlessness. *Fam Relat* 1986;35:479–87.
20. Becker G, Nachtigall RD. "Born to be a mother": The cultural construction of risk in infertility treatment in the U.S. *Soc Sci Med* 1994;39:507–18.
21. Monga M, Alexandrescu B, Katz SE et al. Impact of infertility on quality of life, marital adjustment, and sexual function. *Urology* 2004;63:126–30.
22. Seibel MM, Taymor ML. Emotional aspects of infertility. *Fertil Steril* 1982;37:137–45.
23. Beutel M, Willner H, Deckardt R et al. Similarities and differences in couples' grief reactions following a miscarriage: Results from a longitudinal study. *J Psychosom Res* 1996;40:245–53.

24. Jordan C, Revenson TA. Gender differences in coping with infertility: A meta-analysis. *J Behav Med* 1999;22:341–58.

25. Musters AM, Koot YE, van den Boogaard NM et al. Supportive care for women with recurrent miscarriage: A survey to quantify women's preferences. *Hum Reprod* 2013;28:398–405.

26. Musters AM, Taminiau-Bloem EF et al. Supportive care for women with unexplained recurrent miscarriage: Patients' perspectives. *Hum Reprod* 2011;26:873–7.

27. Beck JS. *Cognitive Therapy: Basic and Beyond*. New York: The Guilford Press; 1995.

28. Tupper C, Weil RJ. The problem of spontaneous abortion. *Am J Obstet Gynecol* 1962;83:421–4.

29. Stray-Pedersen B, Stray-Pedersen S. Etiologic factors and subsequent reproductive performance in 195 couples with a prior history of habitual abortion. *Am J Obstet Gynecol* 1984;148:140–6.

30. Rai R, Clifford K, Regan L. The modern preventative treatment of recurrent miscarriage. *Br J Obstet Gynaecol* 1996;103:106–10.

31. Arck PC, Merali FS, Stanisz AM et al. Stress-induced murine abortion associated with substance P-dependent alteration in cytokines in maternal uterine decidua. *Biol Reprod* 1995;53:814–9.

32. Shakhar K, Rosenne E, Loewenthal R et al. High NK cell activity in recurrent miscarriage: What are we really measuring? *Hum Reprod* 2006;21:2421–5.

39

Methodological Issues in Evidence-Based Evaluation of Treatment for Recurrent Miscarriage

Salim Daya

Introduction

The philosophy of employing evidence from valid and current studies to assist in making clinical decisions is now widely acknowledged as desirable for improving the quality of care provided to patients. The principles of this evidence-based approach to health care management involve searching the literature for studies and critically appraising them to answer clearly defined and focused questions generated from encounters with patients presenting with their clinical problems. This approach is necessary to guide management in obstetrics and gynecology, including the subspecialty of infertility dealing with the problem of recurrent miscarriage.

Miscarriage is the most common complication of pregnancy, occurring in 10–15% of pregnancies. It is defined in North America as any loss occurring before 20 weeks of gestation; in Europe, the definition includes any pregnancy loss before 24 weeks of gestation. Although accurate prevalence figures are not available, it has been estimated that 2–5% of women have three or more miscarriages.[1,2] Consequently, the burden of illness requiring health care assessment and intervention is not insignificant and calls for accurate diagnostic testing and provision of efficacious therapies. Over the years, increased attention has focused on the evaluation and management of recurrent miscarriage. These efforts have led to the development of protocols for diagnostic evaluation in couples with this disorder so that a plan of care can be outlined based on the findings. However, to date, there is no consensus on the optimal evaluation and management strategy to effectively address the problem of recurrent miscarriage. The problem is made more challenging by the fact that the published literature is generally of poor quality and often has contradictory findings, in part, due to sampling variability, but largely due to studies of low validity. The approach of systematically gathering the evidence and pooling outcome data with meta-analyses is an attempt to bring some order to this field, but it too has its pitfalls leading in some instances to erroneous inferences and misleading recommendations for clinical care.

Several years ago, the Special Interest Group for Early Pregnancy under the auspices of the European Society for Human Reproduction and Embryology updated their guidelines for the investigation and medical treatment of recurrent miscarriage.[3] Unfortunately, the paucity of good quality evidence led to the conclusion that many of the proposed investigations require further evaluation within research programs. In addition, tender loving care and health advice were the only interventions that did not require further study; most of the other proposed therapies either require more investigation of their efficacy with randomized trials or are associated with more harm than benefit.[3] More recently, the Practice Committee for the American Society for Reproductive Medicine issued an opinion on the evaluation and treatment of recurrent pregnancy loss.[4] They indicated that evaluation could begin after two pregnancy losses, but in 50% of these women, no defined etiology can be identified.

Reliable inferences regarding therapeutic interventions can only be drawn from trials that have addressed all the important elements necessary for internal validity. Some of these requirements will be discussed in this chapter by highlighting the common pitfalls that are encountered and illustrating them with examples. In addition, by addressing these issues, it is hoped the reader will become more versed in reviewing the literature on recurrent miscarriage management so that the judicious and explicit use of the best current evidence can be made to guide clinical management.

Methodological Issues in the Assessment of Evidence from Therapeutic Trials in Recurrent Miscarriage

Definition of Recurrent Miscarriage (Defining the Population)

The term miscarriage is used to describe a pregnancy that fails to progress resulting in death and expulsion of the embryo or fetus. The generally accepted definition stipulates that the fetus or embryo should weigh 500 g or less,[1] a stage that corresponds to a gestational age of up to 20 weeks. Unfortunately, this definition is not used consistently, and pregnancy losses at higher gestational ages are also classified as miscarriage in some countries. Additionally, the literature is replete with studies on women with pregnancy loss, a term that includes miscarriage and pregnancies that have ended in stillbirth or preterm neonatal death. Thus, from a definition perspective, it is important to characterize the population being studied so that comparisons across therapeutic trials can be made more appropriately and reliably. Unfortunately, the ASRM Practice Committee has further complicated the issue by referring to the term "recurrent pregnancy loss" that includes women with two or more failed clinical pregnancies (gestational age not specified).[4] Furthermore, although the committee recognizes the importance of identifying a threshold of three or more losses for epidemiological studies, it endorses the evaluation of women who have had two first trimester miscarriages. Consensus on this issue is urgently required so that the data gathering and evaluation process is consistent and will yield more reliable and externally valid conclusions.

Recurrent miscarriage defines a clinical condition in which a woman has had at least three miscarriages. However, because the pregnancy history in women with recurrent miscarriage may include pregnancies that have ended in live birth, three different groups can be identified. The groups should be assessed separately because the risk of subsequent miscarriage within each group varies.[1]

Primary Recurrent Miscarriage Group

This group consists of women with three or more consecutive miscarriages with no pregnancy progressing beyond 20 weeks' gestation.

Secondary Recurrent Miscarriage Group

This group consists of women who have had three or more miscarriages after a pregnancy that, having gone beyond 20 weeks' gestation, may have ended in live birth, stillbirth or neonatal death.

Tertiary Recurrent Miscarriage Group

This is a group that has not been well characterized or studied and consists of women who have had at least three miscarriages that are not consecutive but are interspersed with pregnancies that have progressed beyond 20 weeks' gestation (and may have ended in live birth, stillbirth, or neonatal death.)

These three groups are mutually exclusive and distinct and should be evaluated separately because the group being selected will undoubtedly influence the prognosis for a successful outcome. The current approach of combing all three groups together does not allow the effect of the experimental intervention to be detected easily because the prognosis is determined by the relative contribution of subjects from each of the three groups.

Exclusion of Implantation Failures (Avoiding Clinical Heterogeneity)

The widespread availability of treatment with assisted reproduction has created a challenge for the management of women who repeatedly fail to conceive despite undergoing uterine transfer of good quality embryos. Repeated implantation failure (RIF) is now a recognized entity defined as failure to achieve a pregnancy after at least three cycles of *in vitro* fertilisation[5] in which at least ten high-grade embryos were transferred into the uterus. It has been suggested that RIF and recurrent miscarriage represent different ends of the same disorder.[6] This position is difficult to accept because the former is a preimplantation failure that results in no pregnancy, whereas the latter is a post-implantation failure that results in no live birth. Although there may be some overlap in the two conditions from the diagnostic protocol perspective, it is evident from the results of these tests that the two entities are distinct and should not be combined. For example, studies of cytokine expression in the endometrium have produced conflicting and sometimes contradictory findings in these two conditions.[7] Similarly, there is no evidence that measuring serum levels of antiphospholipids is of benefit in RIF in contrast to measurement in women with recurrent miscarriage.[8]

Evidence from such studies indicates that RIF and recurrent miscarriage are two distinct entities that should not be lumped together as if they represent different aspects of a spectrum of reproductive failure. By investigating them separately, and by conducting efficacy trials in each group separately, the problem of clinical heterogeneity is avoided and the benefit (or lack thereof) of interventions can be evaluated more accurately.

Baseline Risk of Miscarriage (Establishing the Control Event Rate)

Initial estimates of the likelihood of a successful pregnancy in women with previous miscarriages were based on the assumption that the overall miscarriage rate consists of the sum of two independent rates, one resulting from a random factor and the other from a recurrent factor in miscarriage sequences. Such mathematical calculations demonstrated a higher risk of miscarriage in a subsequent pregnancy as the number of previous miscarriages increased; the chance of a fourth pregnancy going to term in women with three previous miscarriages is considerably lower than that of a third pregnancy going to term with two previous miscarriages.[1] For many years, these mathematical estimates of miscarriage rate were used as control rates against which the efficacy of therapeutic regimens for recurrent miscarriage was assessed. The reliability of these rates was challenged after evidence from a number of clinical studies suggested that the miscarriage rate after three consecutive miscarriages was substantially lower than had been predicted by the earlier mathematical models.[1]

Despite the varied methods of ascertainment, the results of the studies showed remarkable consistency in finding a positive correlation between risk of miscarriage and the number of previous miscarriages. This effect of prior losses on subsequent probability of live birth was confirmed using the data from the placebo arm of studies in unexplained recurrent miscarriage and provided a quantitative estimate of the risk.[9] It is clear from this evidence that the number of previous miscarriages is an important covariate, which has to be taken into account when planning therapeutic trials. Women with a higher number of previous miscarriages constitute a group with a more severe form of recurrent miscarriage than those with relatively lower numbers of previous miscarriages. Consequently, the magnitude of the treatment effect is expected to be much larger in these more severe forms of the disorder (because the control event rate is so much lower) and is likely to be more easily detected if the subjects are grouped by severity.[10] Thus, the ideal trial should have stratification for the number of previous miscarriages, with randomization of subjects to control or experimental interventions being performed within each stratum.

To date, such a study with a priori stratification has not been undertaken. Instead, the general (and incorrect) approach has been to select the study sample from the population of women having three or more miscarriages, and ignore stratification for number of previous miscarriages. The consequence is a sample that is likely to consist of a higher proportion of women with lower numbers of previous miscarriages thereby reducing the probability of detecting a significant treatment effect.

Controlling for Female Age (Reducing Selection Bias)

The risk of miscarriage resulting from chromosomal anomalies in the fetus increases with maternal age, especially after the age of 35. Additionally, women who have recurrent miscarriages tend to have more pregnancies and have their pregnancies at a later age than those who have successful outcomes. The relationship of gravidity with female age and the relationship of chromosomal anomalies and female age suggest that the increased risk of miscarriage with gravidity, in part, can be ascribed to the effect of maternal age. Thus, clinical trials of treatment efficacy must take female age into consideration during the design phase by using stratification for this covariate. This approach will avoid the possibility of bias that may show the treatment to be less favorable if the experimental group has a higher proportion of older women than the control group.

Controlling for Male Partner (Reducing Selection Bias)

An important determinant of fertilization and embryo development is the integrity of sperm DNA. Although sperm with DNA damage can fertilize oocytes, the risk of miscarriage is increased. A systematic review and meta-analysis of 16 cohort studies comprising 2969 couples demonstrated a significant relationship between a high proportion of sperm with DNA damage and miscarriage.[11] Although the magnitude of the effect varied among the studies, the association was seen consistently across most of these studies.

DNA damage can be induced by a variety of mechanisms during spermatogenesis and spermiogenesis. However, a higher level of DNA damage was observed in ejaculated sperm compared with testicular sperm suggesting that most sperm DNA damage is acquired at the post-testicular level.[12] Post-testicular DNA fragmentation can be induced by oxygen free radicals affecting sperm during transit through the male reproductive tract and by radiation, chemotherapy, and environmental factors such as smoking and air pollution.[13]

Although sporadic miscarriages are associated with high rates of aneuploidy in the products of conception, in women with recurrent miscarriage the frequency of embryonic aneuploidy in such tissue was found to decrease significantly as the number of previous miscarriages increased.[14] This observation suggests that in this population factors such as sperm DNA fragmentation may be responsible for the miscarriage.

The importance of the male partner in contributing to the risk of miscarriage is relevant because it has been observed that women who have recurrent miscarriages with one male partner may have successful pregnancies with another male partner. This issue of partner specificity is an important consideration in avoiding selection bias when evaluating treatment efficacy. To ensure homogeneity of the sample and maximize the probability of detecting a true treatment effect, couples should be chosen for a trial on treatment efficacy only if the consecutive miscarriages experienced by the subject have occurred with the same male partner.

Clearly Defined Objective (Articulating the Research Question)

Before commencing a trial, it is important to articulate the objective clearly and concisely so that the inferences that are drawn from the results can be communicated without ambiguity. To do so requires formulating the research question that is relevant to the problem at hand and is structured in four parts; the population being evaluated, the experimental intervention being tested, the control intervention used as the comparator, and the outcome that has clinical importance. A lack of clarity in the objective formulation becomes evident when the findings are discussed, because often several different outcomes have been considered and attempts have been made to develop an explanation for the findings that has strayed from the original idea for which the study was commissioned.

Randomization (Ensuring Similarity among Intervention Groups)

The randomized controlled trial (RCT) has become the gold standard in evaluating treatment efficacy. Randomization of subjects to receive either experimental or control intervention generates two groups that are generally similar in all respects except for the single factor (the intervention) being studied. This approach ensures that any significant difference in the outcome between the two groups is likely due only to this single factor. In addition, by ensuring their equal distribution in the two groups, it guards against differences in factors not known to be important to the outcome of interest.

There are many methods of randomization, including simple coin tossing, drawing straws, and the use of computer-generated random number tables. The use of block randomization is an additional maneuver that produces equal numbers of subjects in each group, a result not usually obtained with the other simpler methods of randomization. Another approach that is not infrequently used is that of quasi-randomization, wherein subjects are allocated using either the subject's clinical chart number (even number for the experimental group and odd number for the control group), or the subject's date of birth (first half of the year for the experimental group and second half of the year for the control group), or the day of the week when the subject is seen in the clinic (Monday, Wednesday, and Friday for the experimental group and Tuesday, Thursday, and Saturday for the control group). Additionally, alternation is often used to create two intervention groups by alternating the assignment between experimental and control interventions for each successive subject enrolled in the trial (i.e., first subject allocated to the experimental group, the second subject to the control group, the third subject to the experimental group, and so on). When carried out properly, both quasi-randomization and alternation are fairly simple and effective methods for generating experimental and control groups. However, both methods have several pitfalls, including the openness of the process and, in the case of quasi-randomization, the allocation of unequal numbers of subjects to each group.

To improve validity of the trial and to minimize post-randomization withdrawals of subjects (for reasons such as change of mind, relocation to another city, and so on), it is important to perform randomization as late as possible, preferably just prior to the intervention being administered.

Concealment of Group Allocation (Avoiding Selection bias)

Selection bias is encountered when potentially eligible subjects are selectively excluded from the trial because of prior knowledge of the group to which they would have been allocated had they participated in the trial. Although randomization is generally effective in creating equally balanced groups, it does not guard against selection bias, because the investigator may have a notion of the efficacy (or lack thereof) of the experimental intervention and may consciously or unknowingly steer subjects towards or away from this intervention. An effective strategy to avoid selection bias is to ensure information regarding the group allocation is concealed from the investigators and care providers until the subject is irreversibly committed to the trial. In the absence of concealment, it has been shown that the effect of an experimental intervention may be overestimated by as much as 40%.[15,16]

There are several methods to conceal group allocation including: (i) covering each consecutive assignment on the random list with opaque tape that is removed to reveal the group only when the next eligible subject is enrolled; (ii) the use of consecutively numbered opaque envelopes containing the group assignment; and (iii) the use of an individual not directly involved with the trial. Although the first two methods are simple and pragmatic, they are not tamper-proof and need to be policed to prevent investigators from looking ahead of time under the tape or in the envelope to determine where their preferred intervention is located in the random sequence of assignments. The use of a third party, such as a telephone operator located at a site distant from the study center and who can be contacted at the time of enrolment, or a pharmacist who is responsible for dispensing the treatments, provides the highest level of security because it ensures the randomization list is kept away from the investigators.

The openness of the quasi-randomization and alternation methods makes them less reliable to prevent selection bias unless all eligible subjects are enrolled sequentially. From a methodological perspective, the debate over the validity of using these methods in efficacy trials is still ongoing.

Blinding or Masking (Avoiding Ascertainment Bias)

The response to an intervention may not be due entirely to the active chemical compound administered or the surgical procedure performed, but may be influenced by other factors, such as the subject's expectations, the enthusiasm and reputation of the health care provider, and the nature of the intervention. Consequently, the outcome of a trial may be biased (ascertainment bias) if the subject, the investigator, or the outcomes assessor has knowledge of the intervention the subject is receiving. Blinding (or masking), is a strategy whereby those involved in the trial are kept unaware of the identity of the intervention and is used to prevent ascertainment bias because it eliminates the influence (either positive or negative) knowledge of the intervention being administered may have on the estimation of the treatment effect.

Blinding is not the same as allocation concealment; the role of blinding is in safeguarding the randomization sequence after allocation has been performed. For subjects enrolled in the trial, blinding enhances their compliance with the treatment protocol and encourages them to complete the trial. A subject who perceives the experimental intervention to be better than the control intervention may be less willing to remain in the trial, comply with the treatment protocol, or adhere to the follow-up procedures if she is aware that she has not received the experimental intervention. Additionally, in the absence of blinding, the treatment effect is overestimated leading to incorrect inferences about the value of the experimental intervention.[16] The magnitude of the overestimation is much larger in infertility trials with pregnancy as the outcome measure.[17]

The testing of subjects under conditions of intentional ignorance may include the use of dummy interventions, such as placebo and sham surgery. These methods ensure that none of the subjects and, where possible, the trial personnel, is able to recognize whether the intervention administered is active or inert until the code is broken at the conclusion of the trial. A placebo is designed to be indistinguishable in physical properties from the active intervention. However, when a standard treatment exists, it should be used as the comparator for the new intervention, and every effort should be taken to make the interventions indistinguishable from each other by the trial participant. To do so often requires the use of a double-dummy approach (i.e., two placebos), especially if the routes of administration of the two interventions are different, for example, oral versus intravenous, so that the subject receives both oral and intravenous agents, one of which will be a placebo in the experimental group and vice versa for the control group.

The magnitude of the placebo effect (the response observed in the placebo group) is difficult to quantify, unless the placebo is compared with no treatment. Estimates of the benefit have ranged from none to between 35% and 75% of trial participants showing improved outcome.[18] The observation that the use of "tender loving care" was more efficacious than when it was not used in women with recurrent miscarriage undergoing another pregnancy[19] suggests that in recurrent miscarriage research, the placebo effect is likely to be of significant magnitude for which appropriate measures should be taken when designing an efficacy trial.

In trials evaluating surgical procedures, the use of placebo poses a unique challenge.[20] Placebo surgery (also known as a sham operation) requires the subject to undergo all preparations (including anesthesia and surgical incision) essential to the true operation except the surgical procedure itself. The beneficial effect of the sham operation has been attributed to the placebo effect, with estimates that the placebo response in surgery may be of the same magnitude (about 35%) as that observed in medical trials.[21] The placebo effect in surgery may be defined as the difference between the overall effect of surgery and that attributable to the procedure itself.[22] This realization has prompted researchers to reintroduce the sham operation to evaluate surgical interventions so that the high standard required in efficacy studies can be maintained. The risks to subjects undergoing a sham operation are not trivial and it is important to balance these risks against the potential benefits to society-at-large if the surgical procedure is proven effective. It is also important that future patients be spared from the risks and cost of an ineffective surgical procedure. However, if there is no proven alternative therapy available, then the sham operation for surgical therapy trials is a desirable and valid approach to evaluate the efficacy of the intervention, provided an appropriate risk assessment has been undertaken.[23]

In recurrent miscarriage management, there are very few instances when surgical treatment can be considered. Hence, the use of the sham procedure has not yet been explored. Examples that come to mind are cerclage for cervical incompetence and hysteroscopic resection of a uterine septum. For the latter, despite the fact that hysteroscopic resection is now considered by many to be the standard of care for the treatment of women who have a uterine septum and subfertility, the evidence for its efficacy compared to no treatment is lacking.[24]

Co-Intervention (Avoiding Treatment Bias)

The appeal of a randomized trial is the assurance that random allocation of the subjects to experimental or control groups results in the subjects in these groups having similar characteristics at baseline, so that the efficacy of the experimental intervention can be tested cleanly and quantified reliably without interference from any extraneous factors. In this context, it is important to ensure that, except for the interventions being compared, the management protocol is held the same for both groups. Co-intervention occurs when one group is provided with additional care (such as supplementary treatment, more monitoring, easier access to health care personnel, and so on) that is not offered to the other group. The efficacy of the experimental intervention will be biased by co-intervention leading to incorrect estimation of the size of the treatment effect. Also, with co-intervention, the research question changes from the original question, "is the experimental intervention more efficacious than the control interventions?" to the new question, "is experimental treatment in addition to the co-intervening care more efficacious than control intervention?"

Sample Size Estimation (Ensuring the Ability to Detect a Difference in Outcome)

In an efficacy trial with comparable groups, any difference observed in the primary outcome event is due either to chance or to the effect of the experimental intervention. The possibility of finding a treatment effect of the magnitude observed in such a trial is expressed by a probability value (*p*-value) that indicates how likely an ineffective treatment would have been expected to produce the result observed. The lower the *p*-value, the less likely is the effect due to chance and the more likely is it due to the experimental intervention being evaluated. By convention, the threshold of this likelihood is taken to be a probability value of 0.05, such that when the *p*-value is less than 0.05, the observed data are inconsistent with the experimental intervention being ineffective (i.e., the experimental intervention is more efficacious than the control intervention).

In clinical trials, it is important to be able to detect, with a high level of confidence, a clinically meaningful difference between experimental and control interventions. To do so requires conducting a trial with sufficient numbers of subjects to avoid a chance finding (type I error) and to avoid missing the detection of a true difference if one exists (type II error). The ideal situation is to conduct the trial with a sample size just large enough to test the null hypothesis. The goal is to increase the signal-to-noise ratio by recognizing that statistical "noise" (i.e., variability) is inversely proportional to the square root of the sample size (i.e., noise decreases as the sample size increases). When the variation within groups gets larger (the louder the noise) or when the difference in outcomes between the groups gets smaller (the fainter the signal), the larger is the sample size needed to detect the signal.

The size of the sample needed to adequately test the hypothesis of treatment efficacy can be calculated using a standard formula or with the use of readily available software programs. The size of the treatment effect (the "signal") is the difference in magnitude between the outcomes in the experimental and control groups, and is selected by the investigators because it has clinical relevance and importance. The clinically important difference that is chosen is the smallest difference below which the experimental treatment would not be expected to alter current clinical management. In addition, an indication of the variability (the "noise") is obtained from the standard deviation for outcomes that are continuous variables; for proportions, the difference in event rates is all that is needed. It is also necessary to select appropriate values for the probability of making errors of hypothesis testing (typically, 0.05 for type I and 0.2 for type II errors). Finally, it should be established whether the statistical test used to compare the difference in outcomes is to be based on a one-tailed (difference in outcomes in one direction, i.e., benefit with experimental intervention) or two-tailed (difference in outcomes in either direction, i.e., benefit or harm with the experimental intervention).

In recurrent miscarriage research, the outcome events of most clinical relevance are clinical pregnancy or live birth, the rates of which are generally high. The sample size required to test the efficacy of most interventions purported to improve pregnancy rates is often small enough to permit the trial to be undertaken. For example, the control event rate (i.e., success rate with placebo or no treatment) after three miscarriages is expected to be 65%, and any experimental intervention that can improve the outcome to that expected in the normal population (i.e., 85%) would produce an absolute treatment effect of 20%, a difference that is clinically important, implying that for every five women with recurrent miscarriage treated with the experimental intervention, one additional successful outcome would be obtained compared to the control intervention.

To detect this magnitude of difference in clinical pregnancy rates would require a sample size of 162 (81 in each group) using a two-tailed hypothesis test with probabilities for types I and II errors set at 0.05 and 0.2, respectively. Accruing this number of subjects is not difficult in centers specializing in the evaluation and management of recurrent miscarriage, but may require several years to complete a trial in institutions with an average volume of clinical activity. Consequently, in everyday practice, smaller trials are usually conducted because they are easier to complete in a shorter period of time. Unfortunately, because they are insufficiently powered to test the null hypothesis, the results obtained often lead to erroneous inferences being drawn unless the results from these trials can be pooled with meta-analysis to generate more precise estimates of the treatment effect.

Reviewing the literature on recurrent miscarriage demonstrates an urgent need for trials with adequate power to be carried out so that conclusions about treatment efficacy can be made more reliably. For example, a systematic review of immunotherapy for recurrent miscarriage included 12 trials with an average sample size of 53 (range 22–131).[25] Only one of the 12 trials had a sufficiently large sample size with 131 subjects. Similarly, a systematic review of treatment for recurrent miscarriage in women with antiphospholipid antibody or lupus anticoagulant included 13 trials with an average sample size of 66 (range 16–202).[26] This review contained only one trial with a sufficiently large sample size of 202 subjects. Thus, if progress is to be made in recurrent miscarriage research, larger trials are necessary to test the efficacy of new (and existing) interventions.

Avoiding Historical Controls (Avoiding Overestimation of the Effect of Treatment)

Despite the acknowledgement that the randomized trial is the ideal study design in evaluating therapeutic efficacy, clinical decisions are often made from evidence derived from non-randomized, observational studies, such as cohort, case-control, and historical-control. When randomized trials were compared with observational studies to answer the same clinical question, between-study heterogeneity was observed more frequently among observational studies.[27] Some of this variability was reduced after historical-control studies were excluded from the analyses.

A historical-control study is one in which the outcome of an intervention is compared to the outcome observed prior to the administration of the experimental intervention. In recurrent miscarriage research, this design is used fairly frequently to support claims of improved efficacy of new interventions. As an example, a historical-control study was performed to determine whether metformin administered to women with polycystic ovary syndrome to achieve pregnancy and then continued throughout the pregnancy would reduce the likelihood of first trimester miscarriage.[28] Among the ten women evaluated in the study, their collective history of 22 previous pregnancies without metformin included 16 (73%) miscarriages. In contrast, the current pregnancy on metformin therapy ended in miscarriage in only one woman (10%). The authors statistically (and incorrectly) compared the two rates of miscarriage and concluded that there was a significant benefit with metformin use. This approach is invalid from both design (inappropriate controls) and analytical (lack of independence) perspectives.

There is also evidence that demonstrates historical-control studies are associated with an overestimation of the effect of treatment.[27] Thus, historical-control studies should be avoided in recurrent miscarriage research because treatment estimates derived from them are less reliable than those from prospectively undertaken controlled studies.[29]

Intention-to-Treat Analysis (Avoiding Post-Randomization Exclusion of Data)

In trials of treatment efficacy, the purpose of randomization is to avoid bias in the selection of subjects so that comparable experimental and control groups can be studied to provide a reliable estimate of the size of the treatment effect. Once a subject has been randomized into the trial, she needs to be included in the analyses, even if she never began the treatment or stopped taking the treatment part way through the trial. After randomization, any changes in the composition of the groups, such as withdrawing from treatment, being excluded from the analysis for failing to follow protocol, crossing over to the alternative intervention group, and so on, will disturb the balance between them and may affect their comparability. Therefore, it is important to ensure that subjects not only remain in the groups to which they were allocated, but also complete the study.

Unfortunately, despite diligent attention to detail and monitoring of trial progress, the ideal goal of achieving perfect compliance is often not reached. The usual approach to dealing with such post-randomization withdrawals is to analyze the data from only those who completed the assigned treatment (i.e., per-protocol analysis) and ignore those who deviated from the protocol. Although this approach seems sensible, it is not correct from a methodological perspective because the power of the study to detect a clinically meaningful treatment effect is reduced. Also, by confining the analysis only to those who are compliant with the protocol will produce an estimate of the treatment effect that is biased because non-compliance is not a random occurrence and may be associated with a poorer (or better) outcome. The correct approach is to perform the analysis according to the original random assignment using an *intention-to-treat* method whereby all subjects allocated to one group at the time of randomization are analyzed together as representing the intervention originally assigned to that group.

In most clinical trials, because it is expected that there will be some degree of non-compliance, the intention-to-treat analysis will tend to underestimate the effect of the experimental intervention. Maintaining group similarity and preserving the balance among prognostic factors in the study groups produce a cautious method for evaluation and minimizes the likelihood of making a type I error in hypothesis testing.

A good strategy to reduce the numbers of post-randomization withdrawals is to perform the random allocation as late as possible, preferably just prior to the administration of the intervention.

Lack of Superiority, Equivalence and Non-Inferiority (Ensuring Appropriate Testing of the Null Hypothesis)

The placebo-controlled trial is the optimal design for evaluating the efficacy of new treatments. However, once efficacy of a treatment has been established, newer treatments should be compared against these standard active treatments because the use of placebo for such subsequent evaluation is considered unethical.

In general, efficacy trials of active treatments are designed to determine whether a new (experimental) intervention is superior to the standard (control) intervention. The objective of such superiority trials is to rule out equality of the interventions by rejecting the null hypothesis that there is no difference between the two treatments. Ideally, such trials are undertaken with the expectation that the new intervention will fare better and the objective is to demonstrate this fact unequivocally. More commonly, though, the new intervention is only expected to demonstrate similar efficacy to the standard intervention so that health care providers can offer their patients a choice of treatment options. The objective in such a trial is to demonstrate equivalent efficacy (equivalence) of the two interventions.

A common mistake, when a superiority trial fails to reject the null hypothesis of no difference, is to conclude that the two interventions are equivalent. For example, consider a trial with a sample size of 50 women with recurrent miscarriage in which the standard intervention produced a live birth rate of 65%, and the experimental treatment intervention produced a live birth rate of 85%. This difference in pregnancy rates of 20% is not statistically significant and may lead one to conclude that the two interventions are the same (i.e., equivalent). This is an incorrect interpretation as a lack of proof of superiority may be consistent with equivalence, it is not proof that equivalence is present. If the same result were observed in a sample of 200 women, the observed treatment effect would be statistically significant. The current practice of conducting small comparative trials that fail to show superiority of the new intervention should be avoided when trying to evaluate equivalence, because the "lack of evidence of a difference" is not synonymous with "evidence of a lack of difference."

The goal in an equivalence trial is to rule out differences of clinical importance in the primary outcome between two interventions. To calculate a sample size for an equivalence trial requires defining a priori a clinically important difference, starting with the assumption that there is a zero difference in the outcome event rates between the two interventions. The null hypothesis (in contrast to that in a superiority trial) is stated differently as a minimum difference that is acceptable that would render the two interventions interchangeable.[30] By rejecting this null hypothesis in favor of the alternative hypothesis that the difference in outcomes between the two interventions is zero, one can conclude that the interventions are equivalent.

It should be recognized that the outcome event rate with the experimental intervention might be slightly larger or slightly smaller than that with the control intervention. Thus, a range of possible outcome event rates can be generated. By starting with a 0% difference in outcome event rates, a confidence interval around this value is chosen to represent the clinically important range within which any differences in outcome rates can lie for interventions that are considered equivalent. Equivalence can be claimed when the trial is completed, if the observed difference in outcome event rates lies entirely within the range selected for clinical importance. The smaller the selected range, the larger the sample size required. Thus, the execution of an equivalence trial is challenging because it requires a much larger sample size than that of a superiority trial.

An alternative strategy that avoids the need for a very large sample size is to conduct a "non-inferiority" trial. The objective of the active-controlled, non-inferiority trial is not to demonstrate superiority, but to establish that the effect of the experimental intervention, when compared to the control intervention, is not below some prestated non-inferiority margin. In other words, given that it is impossible to prove the null hypothesis of no difference, an operational definition must be considered that allows the experimental intervention to be inferior to the standard (control) intervention by a clinically tolerable amount (i.e., the experimental intervention is "not much inferior" to the control intervention). Clinicians have to decide on the amount of non-inferiority they are willing to accept as medically insignificant or tolerable as a basis for non-inferiority claims. Such an approach is often used for newer drugs that may have lower side effects, better tolerance, or lower cost than the standard intervention. For a non-inferiority evaluation, the null hypothesis states that the control intervention is superior to the experimental intervention. The alternative hypothesis is that the experimental intervention is not inferior to the control intervention.

The design of a non-inferiority trial requires specifying the non-inferiority margin that is the extent to which the outcome with the control intervention can exceed that with the experimental intervention and still render the experimental intervention non-inferior to the control intervention. The null hypothesis states that the outcome with the control intervention is at least as large as or exceeds this margin; if the null hypothesis cannot be rejected then the control intervention is more efficacious than the experimental intervention. Rejection of the null hypothesis is required to establish non-inferiority of the control intervention. It should be noted that according to the alternative hypothesis, the experimental intervention might perform better than the control intervention, but not to an extent greater than the inferiority margin that has been established.

Because the direction of effect being assessed is one-sided (i.e., the experimental intervention is not inferior to the control intervention), a one-sided hypothesis test is performed. Thus, by not requiring a two-sided hypothesis test, the sample size required will be much lower. However, if the experimental treatment performs better than the control intervention (and the outcome event rate exceeds the non-inferiority margin), one cannot conclude that it is superior, because the trial design was not set up to test this hypothesis.

Before a non-inferiority trial can be undertaken, it is necessary to confirm that the control intervention has been shown to be better than placebo. Furthermore, it is important to select a non-inferiority margin that is small enough to not exceed that which has clinical relevance; choosing a large inferiority margin will risk the generalization of the study findings, because it can be argued that such a large difference is clinically meaningful suggesting that the control intervention is superior to the experimental intervention. Finally, it has to be assumed that the control intervention is superior to placebo (had such a comparison taken place). To do so requires the inferiority margin to be smaller than the smallest effect size the experimental intervention would be expected to produce had it been compared to placebo. In this context, for the experimental intervention to be designated as being "at least as good as" the control intervention, it has to retain at least 50% of the superiority of the control intervention over placebo.[31,32]

Onset of Treatment (Maximizing the Magnitude of the Effect of Treatment)

A major problem in the management of recurrent miscarriage is the assumption that diagnostic tests carried out in the nonpregnant state are used to identify potential causes of the miscarriages that have already occurred. Treatment is then offered to prevent miscarriage in a subsequent pregnancy. Unfortunately, there is no standardization in many of the treatment protocols regarding the onset of treatment. For example, intravenous immunoglobulin has been administered before conception in some studies, and only after confirmation of the pregnancy in other studies.[33] Sometimes treatment is instituted only after fetal cardiac activity has been demonstrated as seen with the use of heparin in women with elevated antiphospholipid levels.[26] In this situation, the likelihood of a successful outcome without treatment once fetal cardiac activity has been demonstrated is relatively high and it will result in efficacy studies failing to accurately quantify the magnitude of the treatment effect with the experimental intervention.

The optimal time of onset of therapy will vary depending on the cause of the recurrent miscarriages, but it makes sense to commence treatment before conception for most causes that can be identified using the current diagnostic protocol. Clearly, consensus on this issue is urgently required so that treatment benefit can be maximized.

Censoring Subjects Who Fail to Conceive (Avoiding Treatment Bias)

Another methodological concern in efficacy trials is the restriction of the number of cycles of preconceptional treatment patients may undergo. If these women do not conceive then they are withdrawn from the study and replaced by other women who take their place in the trial. This strategy violates the principle of randomization and introduces treatment bias by enrolling women with high fecundity rates. It becomes difficult to generalize the results of such trials to the population of women with recurrent miscarriage.

Women with recurrent miscarriage compared to those with sporadic miscarriage have a longer interpregnancy conception interval (i.e., length of time taken for conception to occur after a previous miscarriage increases with the number of miscarriages).[34,35] The pathologic mechanism for this observation is not clear. One possible hypothesis is that fear of miscarriage in a subsequent pregnancy induces significant stress that may adversely influence the hypothalamus and result in subtle ovulatory dysfunction.[1] Thus, it is clear that for treatments commenced before conception, a sufficient length of time will be required before pregnancy can be achieved. For this reason and for the methodological reasons discussed, women enrolled into randomized trials of treatment for recurrent miscarriage should not be withdrawn just because pregnancy has not occurred in a short period of time.

Karyotypic Analysis of the Products of Conception in Treatment Failures (Improving Accuracy of Treatment Effect Estimation)

The risk of having aneuploidy arising *de novo* is present in all pregnancies. Consequently, it is possible that women receiving experimental or control interventions may experience another miscarriage for this reason, which has nothing to do with the intervention itself. Hence, it is prudent to submit all products of conception in efficacy trials to karyotypic analysis to exclude the presence of aneuploidy. Without this information, it is impossible to ascertain whether the miscarriage is the result of a failure of the intervention administered or a *de novo* chromosomal anomaly. The magnitude of the size of the treatment effect will be affected without adjusting for the miscarriages that were inevitable because of aneuploidy.

Improvement in ultrasonographic technology has resulted in images of early pregnancy having higher resolution to permit earlier diagnosis of pregnancy failure, a process that is assisted with serial measurement of serum levels of progesterone and human chorionic gonadotropin. Thus, it is possible to collect fetal and trophoblast tissue early and in a non-contaminated state so that karyotypic analyses can be carried out successfully without any jeopardy to the cell culture, which had been a problem when tissue was collected in a non-sterile manner. Furthermore, improved techniques in cytogenetics have permitted more accurate and reliable assessments of the products of conception to be made. Given these improvements in our diagnostic ability, it is even more important that every effort be taken to study the products of conception in every case of miscarriage in therapeutic trials, so that a more valid assessment of the efficacy of the experimental treatment can be performed.

Systematic Reviews (Improving the Precision of the Treatment Effect)

Although single randomized controlled trials are useful in evaluating efficacy and estimating the treatment effect, there is growing recognition that the use of systematic reviews to pool knowledge from a complete body of work is a better strategy to gather the best evidence to make decisions about therapeutic interventions. Systematic reviews are very reliable because their approach is structured, consisting of clearly stated objectives, predefined eligibility criteria in searching for relevant studies, collation of findings from studies that have been evaluated for validity, and statistical pooling of the data with meta-analysis. This approach generates estimates of treatment effect that are more precise than can be obtained from individual primary studies.

The Cochrane Collaboration was established in 1993 and it is focused on preparing and publishing systematic reviews of highest quality studies. There are currently 54 Cochrane Review Groups, each covering a specific area of health care. Seven of these groups deal directly with the field of obstetrics and gynecology and women's health. Among these groups, the Menstrual Disorders and Subfertility group is focused on RCTs of treatment for subfertility. There are now over 5000 published RCTs on subfertility and 170 full Cochrane reviews (until June 2013).[36] However, when searching the database of reviews, there are, to date, only 11 reviews on recurrent miscarriage. Clearly, much work remains to be done in this area to increase the numbers of systematic reviews evaluating treatments for recurrent miscarriage. In doing so, the field can be advanced by providing more reliable and precise estimates of the effect of treatment.

Adherence to Guidelines (Enhancing External Validity)

Evidence from clinical research should be evaluated for validity before it is applied to clinical practice. Subsequently, evidence of high quality should be incorporated into clinical guidelines to direct physicians on improving the level of care they provide to their patients. These guidelines will evolve as newer and valid evidence is gathered. Although such a process of integrating evidence into clinical practice is logical and sensible, the true state of affairs in the area of recurrent miscarriage leaves a lot to be desired. For example, although guidelines for recurrent miscarriage have incorporated knowledge from diagnostic tests and efficacy of therapy, the adherence to these guidelines by practitioners has been shown to be very poor.[37]

A recent study assessed the quality of care in couples with recurrent miscarriage according to a set of guideline-based quality indicators and analyzed whether variation in this care was related to determinants at the level of the patient, the professional, or the hospital.[38] Adherence to these indicators was found to be low, with wide variation among hospitals, resulting in appropriate care being administered to less than 50% of the couples. Thus, despite being evidence-based, the new guidelines were not being readily adopted in clinical practice. Furthermore, when professionals were asked about their adherence to guidelines, it was observed that there was a 30–40% over-estimation compared to their actual adherence.[39]

The importance of adherence to guidelines for recurrent miscarriage becomes clear when assessing external validity of trials of therapeutic efficacy. The sample selected for study is chosen from the population of women with recurrent miscarriage that satisfies inclusion criteria based on currently accepted standards. However, if the standards being applied in clinical practice are at variance to guidelines because of non-adherence by practitioners, then extrapolation of the evidence from efficacy trials to the general population becomes less reliable and may result in the treatment effect being minimized, thereby reducing the effectiveness of the interventions.

Summary

Therapeutic decision-making relies on the availability of good quality evidence generated from studies of high quality, high internal validity, and without bias. In the area of efficacy evaluation of therapy for recurrent miscarriage, the randomized trial is the gold standard and should be designed and executed with attention to methodological details outlined in this chapter. The starting point requires defining the research objective that is clearly articulated as a research question describing the patient population, experimental and control interventions, and outcome of interest. The population should be clearly defined and women with repeated implantation failure should be excluded. The subjects selected for the trial should be randomly allocated to the experimental or control interventions to ensure similarity in the composition of the group. The allocation sequence should be concealed from all investigators and health care personnel involved with the trial so that bias in selecting participants can be avoided.

Whenever possible, attempts should be made to blind subjects, investigators, health care personnel providing care, and outcomes assessors so that ascertainment bias can be avoided. Further bias of treatment assessment can be avoided by ensuring that co-intervention does not occur and historical controls are avoided.

Testing the null hypothesis of no difference in outcomes between the experimental and control intervention requires enrolling sufficiently large numbers of participants so that a clinically important treatment effect can be detected. Smaller sample sizes will usually lead to erroneous inferences about treatment efficacy. Wherever possible, stratification should be performed for the number of previous miscarriages. In addition, stratification, or subgrouping, by female age should be considered. Treatment should be commenced prior to pregnancy and should be continued for a sufficient length of time to permit pregnancy to occur; post-randomization withdrawals of subjects who fail to conceive after a short period of time should be avoided.

All analyses should be undertaken using an intention-to-treat approach so that post-randomization exclusion of data does not occur. The approach of the study from the perspectives of superiority, equivalence, or non-inferiority should be established before the trial begins so that the required numbers of participants can be accrued and the hypothesis testing can be directed appropriately. The products of conception should be submitted for karyotypic analysis for all intervention failures so that more accurate estimates of the effect of treatment can be generated.

The reporting of the results should follow the guidelines established by the Consolidated Standards of Reporting Trials (CONSORT).[40] This statement consists of a checklist and flow diagram for reporting the results from randomized controlled trials and prompts investigators to ensure that important elements in clinical trial design have been addressed. The issues raised in this chapter are important for creating the basis for using an evidence-based approach to inform therapeutic decisions in clinical practice.

Finally, systematic reviews of randomized controlled trials should be undertaken to improve the precision of the treatment effect of interventions for recurrent miscarriage and the practice of therapeutics in this field should adhere to established guidelines that are developed from such high quality and valid evidence.

REFERENCES

1. Daya S. Habitual abortion. In: Copeland LJ, Jarrell JF, eds. *Textbook of Gynecology*. 2nd ed. Philadelphia: WB Saunders; 2000. p. 227–71.
2. Mills JL, Simpson JH, Driscoll SG et al. Incidence of spontaneous abortion among normal women and insulin-dependent women whose pregnancies were identified within 21 days of conception. *N Engl J Med* 1988;319:1617–23.
3. Jauniaux E, Farquharson RG, Christiansen OB et al. Evidence-based guidelines for the investigation and medical treatment of recurrent miscarriage. *Hum Reprod* 2006;21:2216–22.
4. The Practice Committee of the American Society for Reproductive Medicine. Evaluation and treatment of recurrent pregnancy loss: A committee opinion. *Fertil Steril* 2012;98:1103–11.
5. Tan BK, Vandekerckhove P, Kennedy R et al. Investigation and current management of recurrent IVF treatment failure in the UK. *BJOG* 2005;112:773–80.
6. Nardo LG, Li TC, Edwards RG. Introduction: Human embryo implantation failure and recurrent miscarriage: Basic science and clinical practice. *Reprod Biomed Online* 2006;13:11–2.
7. Laird S, Tuckerman EM, Li TC. Cytokine expression in the endometrium of women with implantation failure and recurrent miscarriage. *Reprod Biomed Online* 2006;13:13–23.
8. Stern C, Chamley L. Antiphospholipid antibodies and coagulation defects in women with implantation failure after IVF and recurrent miscarriage. *Reprod Biomed Online* 2006;13:29–37.
9. Daya S. Immunotherapy for unexplained recurrent spontaneous abortion. *Infertil Reprod Med Clin N Am* 1997;8:65–77.
10 Carp HJ, Toder V, Torchinsky A et al. Allogenic leukocyte immunization after five or more miscarriages. Recurrent Miscarriage Immunotherapy Trialists Group. *Hum Reprod* 1997;12:250–5.
11. Robinson L, Gallos ID, Conner SJ et al. The effect of sperm DNA fragmentation on miscarriage rates: A systematic review and meta-analysis. *Hum Reprod* 2012;27:2908–17.

12. Greco E, Scarselli F, Iacobelli M et al. Efficient treatment of infertility due to sperm DNA damage by ICSI with testicular spermatozoa. *Hum Reprod* 2005;20:226–30.

13. Sakkas D, Alvarez JG. Sperm DNA fragmentation: Mechanisms of origin, impact on reproductive outcome, and analysis. *Fertil Steril* 2010;93:1027–36.

14. Ogaswara M, Aoki K, Okada S et al. Embryonic karyotype of abortuses in relation to the number of previous miscarriages. *Fertil Steril* 2000;73:300–4.

15. Chalmers TC, Celano P, Sacks HS et al. Bias in treatment assignment in controlled clinical trials. *N Engl J Med* 1983;309:1359–61.

16. Schultz KF, Chalmers I, Hayes RJ et al. Empirical evidence of bias: Dimensions of methodological quality associated with estimates of treatment effects in controlled trials. *JAMA* 1995;273:408–12.

17. Khan KS, Daya S, Collins JA et al. Empirical evidence of bias in infertility research: Overestimation of treatment effect in crossover trials using pregnancy as the outcome measure. *Fertil Steril* 1996;65:939–45.

18 Daya S. The placebo effect. *Evid Based Obstet Gynecol* 2000;2:1.

19. Stray-Pedersen B, Stray-Pedersen S. Etiological factors and subsequent obstetric performance in 195 couples with a prior history of habitual abortion. *Am J Obstet Gynecol* 1983;148:140–6.

20. Daya S. Issues in surgical therapy evaluation: The sham operation. *Evid Based Obstet Gynecol* 2000;2:31–2.

21. Beecher HK. Surgery as placebo. A quantitative study of bias. *JAMA* 1961;176:1102–7.

22. Johnson AG. Surgery as a placebo. *Lancet* 1994;344:1140–2.

23. American Medical Association. Report of the AMA House of Delegates, 2000 Annual Meeting, Recommendation #5. Available online from www.ama-assn.org.

24. Bosteels J, Kasius J, Weyers S et al. Hysteroscopy for treating subfertility associated with suspected major uterine cavity abnormalities. *Cochrane Database Sys Rev* 2013;CD009461.

25. Porter TF, LaCoursiere Y, Scott JR. Immunotherapy for recurrent miscarriage. *Cochrane Database Sys Rev* 2006;CD000112.

26. Empson M, Lassere M, Craig J et al. Prevention of recurrent miscarriage for women with antiphospholipid antibody or lupus anticoagulant. *Cochrane Database Sys Rev* 2005;CD002859.

27. Ioannidis JPA, Haidich A-B, Pappa M et al. Comparison of evidence of treatment effects in randomized and nonrandomized studies. *JAMA* 2001;286:821–30.

28. Glueck CJ, Phillips H, Cameron D et al. Continuing metformin throughout pregnancy in women with polycystic ovary syndrome appears to safely reduce first-trimester spontaneous abortion: A pilot study. *Fertil Steril* 2001;75:46–52.

29. Daya S. Evaluation of treatment efficacy—Randomization or observation? *Evid Based Obstet Gynecol* 2001;3:111–3.

30 Daya S. Issues in assessing therapeutic equivalence. *Evid Based Obstet Gynecol* 2001;3:167–8.

31. D'Agostino Sr RB, Massaro JM, Sullivan JM. Non-inferiority trials: Design concepts and issues—The encounters of academic consultants in statistics. *Statist Med* 2003;22:169–86.

32. Jones B, Jarvis P, Lewis JA et al. Trials to assess equivalence: The importance of rigorous methods. *BMJ* 1996:313:36–9.

33. Daya S, Gunby J. Porter E et al. Critical analysis of intravenous immunoglobulin therapy for recurrent miscarriage. *Hum Reprod Update* 1999;5:475–82.

34. Strobino BR, Kline J, Shrout P et al. Recurrent spontaneous abortion: Definition of a syndrome. In: Porter IH, Hook EB, eds. *Human Embryonic and Fetal Death*. New York: Academic Press; 1980. p. 315.

35. Fitzsimmons J, Jackson D, Wapner R et al. Subsequent reproductive outcome in couples with repeated pregnancy loss. *Am J Med Genet* 1983;16:583.

36. Farquhar C, Moore V, Bhattacharya S et al. Twenty years of Cochrane reviews in menstrual disorders and subfertility. *Hum Reprod* 2013;28:2883–92.

37. Franssen MT, Korevaar JC, van der Veen F et al. Management of recurrent miscarriage: Evaluating the impact of a guideline. *Hum Reprod* 2007;22:1298–303.

38. van den Boogaard E, Hermens RPMG, Franssen AMHW et al. Recurrent miscarriage: Do professionals adhere to their guidelines. *Hum Reprod* 2013;28:2898–904.

39. Hrisos S, Eccles MP, Francis JJ et al. Are there valid proxy measures of clinical behaviour? A systematic review. *Implement Sci* 2009;4:37.

40. Moher D, Schulz KF, Altman D. The CONSORT statement: Revised recommendations for improving the quality of reports of parallel-group randomized trials. *Lancet* 2001;357:1191–4.

40

Investigation Protocol for Recurrent Pregnancy Loss

Howard J. A. Carp

Introduction

In the first edition of this book, three guidelines for management of recurrent pregnancy loss (RPL) were compared and contrasted, they were the protocol of the Royal College of Obstetricians (RCOG),[1] the American College of Obstetricians and Gynecologists (ACOG)[2] and the European Society of Human Reproduction and Embryology (ESHRE).[3] The chapter in the first edition showed that each of the guidelines were different with widely differing recommendations. The RCOG guideline has been updated, with the latest edition published in 2011.[4] The ESHRE protocol has not been updated, and the ACOG guideline was replaced by the American Society of Reproductive Medicine (ASRM) guideline in 2012.[5] In addition, there are Dutch and Danish guidelines available. In the 7 years since the first edition of this book, it was hoped that the various guidelines would have developed a unified approach. Alas, this has not happened, and the guidelines are still very different in their approach to RPL.

Although the purpose of an investigation protocol is to assist physicians as to which investigations are worthwhile in order to reach a diagnosis, the various protocols may confuse the physician. The physician may comply with the guideline of his own national or regional organization, but there is a real problem when the leading professional organizations do not concur. Virtually all the protocols classify RPL as one homogeneous condition, and try to suggest a group of investigations or treatment either centered on an evidence based approach or the experience of the particular authors. However, treating RPL as one homogenous condition takes no account of individual circumstances in different patients. The prognosis is different in different patients. The author classifies patients into those with a good, medium or poor prognosis. Stravelos and Li[6] classify patients as type I, in which RPL occurs by chance, there is no underlying pathology and a good prognosis; and type II unexplained RPL, which occurs due to an underlying pathology that is currently not yet identified by routine clinical investigations and a poorer prognosis. Good or bad prognosis is dependent on certain factors: primary and secondary aborters,[7] those losing late or early pregnancy losses, as late losses have a worse prognosis,[8] and recently those losing karyotypically abnormal from those losing karyotypically normal embryos, as euploid abortions are associated with a worse prognosis than aneuploid abortions.[9] Additionally, treatment is often controversial, as demonstrated by the various debates in this book. We are of the opinion that there may not be one approach to treatment. For example, in antiphospholipid syndrome (APS), low molecular weight heparins (LMWH), and aspirin may be the standard treatment, but a different approach is indicated in the patient who continues losing pregnancies despite treatment. In this chapter, some of the standard protocols will be discussed, and some other approaches discussed that might be appropriate in particular patients.

Inclusion Criteria

The standard protocols listed above differ about who should be investigated and the criteria for investigation. The ASRM protocol,[5] recommends investigation after two or more pregnancy losses, whereas the RCOG[4] and ESHRE[3] protocols only recommend assessment after three or more losses. However, no protocol defines pregnancy loss. A problem arises with preclinical or biochemical pregnancy losses. In these cases, no pregnancy sac can be visualized on ultrasound. The incidence of biochemical losses is so high that the relevance of biochemical pregnancy losses is questionable. All biochemical pregnancies are by definition, pregnancies of unknown location, therefore some biochemical pregnancies will be ectopic gestations. Hence, the recent revised definitions of the American Society for Reproductive Medicine,[10] where clinicians are advised not to consider biochemical pregnancy losses as miscarriages when assessing RPL. However, none of the investigation protocol says whether these "biochemical pregnancies" should be considered pregnancy losses. A positive hCG level may be due to "phantom," endometrial or pituitary hCG. This problem has become especially common since the wide use of *in vitro* fertilization, where hCG testing is often performed 12 days after exogenous hCG administration. Although hCG should be cleared from the circulation by 12 days, some may still be present in certain patients leading to a false positive result. The author[11] has previously defined a biochemical pregnancy as three or more spontaneous pregnancies with a βhCG level between 10 and 1000 IU/L in a cycle in which no hCG was administered, no pregnancy sac was demonstrated on ultrasound, and menstruation delayed by no more than 1 week. This definition has since been accepted by ESHRE.[12] However, the author has tended to become more restrictive, and now only accepts a biochemical pregnancy as such if there are two readings that show a rising level. Patient No. 6 below presented with a problem of recurrent biochemical pregnancies. If biochemical pregnancies recur three times, the author considers these events as early pregnancy losses.

Similar confusion surrounds the upper level of pregnancy loss. Traditionally any pregnancy that has been lost prior to viability was considered as abortion. The more recent North American definition includes pregnancy losses up to 20 weeks as a miscarriage. However, there are many exceptions to this rule. Preston et al.,[13] in a leading paper on hereditary thrombophilias, assessed "miscarriages" as up to 27 weeks. Ober et al. (Ober, personal communication) in the paper most often quoted to show that paternal leucocyte immunization is ineffective,[14] included nonconsecutive abortions and pregnancies up to 29 weeks. Laskin[15] in a leading article usually quoted to show that steroids have no place in antiphospholipid syndrome included patients with pregnancy losses up to 31 weeks. It is difficult to believe that that research on patients with two losses at 27, 29, or 31 weeks have relevance to patients with five or more losses of blighted ova. We tend to agree with the conclusions laid out by Farquharson et al.,[12] that recurrent pregnancy loss needs to be much better defined before any relevant investigation or treatment protocols can be determined.

Standard Protocols

The RCOG protocol[1] was originally published in 1997, updated in 2003, and most recently updated in 2012.[4] The protocol attempts to be evidence based as far as possible. Evidence is classified as in Table 40.1. The recommendations are made for and against various causes of miscarriage and methods of treatment are graded according to the level of evidence available. Areas lacking evidence are called "good practice points," based on the clinical experience of the guideline development group. The evidence is mainly taken from the Cochrane Register of Controlled Trials. The guideline recommends fetal karyotyping, three dimensional ultrasound, hydrosonography or hysteroscopy for uterine anomalies, APS testing and interpretation according to the updated "Sapporo" criteria,[16] and treatment with heparin and aspirin. Interestingly, parental karyotyping, which was recommended in the previous versions of the guideline, are no longer recommended except when an unbalanced chromosome abnormality is identified in the products of conception. The protocol claims that there is insufficient evidence to

TABLE 40.1

Levels of Evidence

Ia	Evidence obtained from meta-analysis of randomized controlled trials
Ib	Evidence obtained from at least one randomized controlled trial
IIa	Evidence obtained from at least one well-designed controlled study without randomization
IIb	Evidence obtained from at least one other type of well-designed quasi-experimental study
III	Evidence obtained from well-designed nonexperimental descriptive studies, such as comparative studies, correlation studies, and case studies
IV	Evidence obtained from expert committee reports or opinions and/or clinical experience of respected authorities

assess progesterone and hCG supplementation, and bacterial vaginosis. Assessment of thyroid function, antithyroid antibodies, alloimmune testing and immunotherapy, and assessment of TORCH and other infective agents are not recommended. The protocol reserves judgment on factor V Leiden or the other hereditary thrombophilias, claiming that there may be an association with second trimester miscarriage, but not first trimester miscarriage. The RCOG protocol[4] is the generally accepted norm within the UK. The guideline states that a significant proportion of cases of recurrent miscarriage remain unexplained, despite detailed investigation, and that the prognosis for a successful future pregnancy with supportive care alone is in the region of 75%. However, the most recent version of the guideline states that the prognosis worsens with increasing maternal age and the number of previous miscarriages.

The RCOG guideline takes no account of specific types of pregnancy loss, and does not distinguish between different types of patient. There are no suggestions regarding patients who subsequently miscarry despite the reassurance of a 75% prognosis for a live birth. The fact that the guideline states "the use of empirical treatment in women with unexplained recurrent miscarriage is unnecessary and should be resisted," has denied many British patients with large numbers of miscarriages, treatment which may be effective in certain subgroups of patient.

The ASRM guideline[5] is much less dogmatic than the RCOG guideline. Two pregnancy losses are recognized as warranting investigation. The ASRM guideline does not base its recommendations on a strictly evidence based approach, and states that new and controversial etiologies should not be investigated or treated. Various suspected causes of RPL are either recommended or not recommended, or claimed to be of doubtful value. As the RCOG guideline, the ASRM guideline does not take account of different types of patient, or different prognoses; it does state clearly that it should not be construed as dictating an exclusive course of treatment or procedure. The guideline also states that variations in practice may be warranted based on the needs of the individual patient, resources, and limitations unique to the institution or type of practice. Unlike the RCOG guideline,[4] the ASRM guideline recommends parental karyotyping, and suggests that the couple should be offered prenatal diagnosis if one parent has a chromosomal aberration. Karyotyping of the abortus is recommended. The guideline states that assessment of the uterine cavity is advised and it supports resection of a septum. Although the contribution of uterine septa to first trimester loss is claimed to be controversial, the resection of intra-uterine adhesions and polyps is also said to be controversial without good evidence of effect. Screening is recommended for antiphospholipid antibodies and recommended treatment is with aspirin and unfractionated heparin rather than low molecular weight heparins. Progesterone support is said to be ineffective, but may have a place in some patients. The ASRM guideline does not recommend screening for antithyroid antibodies, or infections such as chlamydia, mycoplasma, or bacterial vaginosis. Alloimmune testing, paternal leucocyte immunization nor intravenous immunoglobulin G (IVIg) are also not recommended; hCG supplementation is not mentioned.

The ESHRE guideline[3] was published in 2006, and 8 years later, requires updating. However, ESHRE, as with RCOG, restricts the definition of recurrent miscarriage to three or more consecutive miscarriages. It takes account of different types of patient as the introduction states: "The number of previous miscarriages and maternal age are the most important covariates and they have to be taken into account when planning therapeutic trials. The ideal trial should have stratification for the number of previous miscarriages and maternal age, with randomization between control and experimental treatments within each stratum." The protocol discusses investigations of cause and treatment interventions separately, and unlike the RCOG guidelines, does not quote the level of evidence for its recommendations. The protocol does recommend testing blood sugar levels and thyroid function tests, antiphospholipid antibodies (LAC and aCL), parental karyotyping, and assessment of the uterine cavity by pelvic ultrasound or hysterosalpingography. Hysteroscopy and laparoscopy are reserved as "advanced investigations" but the protocol does not make clear which patients warrant "advanced investigations." There is a new category of investigations, known as investigations that should be used in the framework of a clinical trial. These include fetal karyotyping, testing of NK cells, luteal phase endometrial biopsy, and homocysteine levels. Treatment is classified separately from investigation in this protocol. Both tender loving care and health advice, such as diet, abstention, or reduction of coffee intake, smoking, and alcohol are described as established treatments. However, no evidence, results, or references are quoted to justify calling these treatment modalities established treatment. The following are said to require more RCTs before definite recommendations can be made: aspirin and low molecular weight heparins,

TABLE 40.2

Comparison of Three Protocols for the Investigation and Treatment of Recurrent Pregnancy Loss

Investigation or Treatment	RCOG Protocol	ASRM Protocol	ESHRE Protocol
Parental karyotyping	Not recommended	Recommended	Recommended
Fetal karyotyping	Recommended	Recommended	Trial required
Uterine cavity assessment	Recommended	Insufficient evidence	Recommended
Resection of uterine septum	Insufficient evidence	Should be considered	–
APS assessment (ACA and LA)	Recommended	Recommended	Recommended
Treatment of APS with heparin and aspirin	Recommended	Recommended	Insufficient evidence
Luteal Phase investigation	–	Not recommended	Insufficient evidence trials required
Progesterone supplementation	Insufficient evidence	Insufficient evidence	Insufficient evidence. More RCTs required
hCG supplementation	Insufficient evidence	–	–
Bacterial vaginosis	Insufficient evidence	Not recommended	–
Hereditary thrombophilias	Recommended for second trimester losses	Not recommended	Recommended as advanced investigation
Anticoagulants for hereditary thrombophilia	Insufficient evidence	–	Insufficient evidence
Thyroid function	–	Recommended	Recommended
Glucose challenge test	–	–	Recommended
Prolactin estimation	–	Recommended	–
TORCH Testing	Not recommended	Not recommended	Not recommended
Alloimmune testing	Not recommended	Not recommended	Insufficient evidence
Immunotherapy	Not recommended	Not recommended	Insufficient evidence. RCT required for IVIg and third party leucocytes, PLI no proven effect.
Tender loving care	Insufficient evidence	Recommenderd	Recommended
Diet, smoking, alcohol	–	–	Recommended
Folic acid for hyperhomocysteinemia	–	–	Insufficient evidence
Vitamin supplementation	–	–	Not recommended
Steroids	Not recommended	Not recommended	Not recommended

Note: RCOG: Royal College of Obstetricians; ASRM: American Society of Reproductive Medicine; ESHRE: European Society of Human Reproduction and Embryology; APS: antiphospholipid syndrome; RCT: randomized controlled trial; IVIg: intravenous immunoglobulin G.

or unfractionated heparin for APS, anticoagulants for inherited thrombophilia, progesterone supplementation, intravenous immunoglobulin, folic acid in women with hyperhomocysteinemia, and immunization with third-party donor leucocytes. However, immunization with paternal leucocytes is said to be of no proven benefit as is multivitamin supplementation. Steroids are said to be associated with more harm than benefit during the first half of pregnancy. Again, no evidence or references are provided.

Table 40.2 contrasts the recommendations for various investigations and treatment modalities in the three protocols. Reliance on these guidelines will leave the physician in a quandary as to which investigations to perform and which treatment to offer.

Factors Affecting Subsequent Prognosis

The chance of a third pregnancy loss after two miscarriages is usually quoted to be approximately 20%, and the chance of a fourth miscarriage after three previous miscarriages is usually quoted to be approximately 40%. However, some studies have failed to find a difference in the subsequent live birth rate between two and three previous losses.[17] In certain forms of recurrent pregnancy loss,

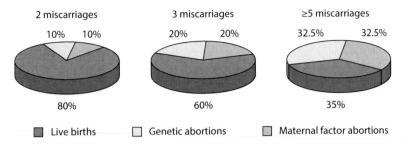

FIGURE 40.1 Number of previous abortions and effect of treatment for maternal factors. Patients with two miscarriages have an 80% chance of a live birth if untreated. If 50% of subsequent miscarriages are chromosomally abnormal, any treatment aimed at correcting a maternal cause of miscarriage, can only raise the live birth rate from 80% to 90%. In order to show a statistical significance between 80% and 90%, will require a mega-trial. Hence most treatment regimens used on patients with two miscarriages will be ineffective. Treating patients with three miscarriages, can only raise the live birth rate by 20%. However, if treatment is used on patients with a poor prognosis, the live birth rate can be raised by 32%, making it relatively easy to show a statistically significant effect of treatment.

the recurrence rate is unknown, for example, in recurrent biochemical pregnancies, after *in vitro* fertilization, antiphospholipid syndrome, or in the older woman. However, there are certain factors that help to predict the prognosis. These are: (i) number of previous pregnancy losses. As the number of previous losses increases, the chance of a live birth decreases.[18] (ii) Primary, secondary or tertiary aborter status, the secondary aborter has a better prognosis than the primary aborter.[7] (iii) Karyotype of previous miscarriage. The patient with an aneuploid abortion has a better chance of a live birth.[9,19] Figure 4.1 in Chapter 4 shows the prognosis according to fetal karyotype. (iv) Concurrent infertility.[20,21] (v) Maternal age.[18,21] (vi) Antipaternal complement dependent antibodies (APCA) have also been reported to be predictive of a successful pregnancy outcome.[20,22] (vii) Natural killer (NK) cells.[23,24] (viii) Early or late pregnancy losses, as the patient with late losses tends to have a worse prognosis.[8] The most important predictive factor is the number of previous miscarriages. Figure 1.1 in Chapter 1 shows the decreasing live birth rate with the increasing number of miscarriages. Carp et al.[7] have previously published figures for their series. After three miscarriages, there was a 55% live birth rate in untreated patients with unexplained recurrent pregnancy loss (33 of 85 patients). The incidence of live births was 45% after four miscarriages (17 of 38 patients, 41% after five miscarriages (10 of 24 patients), 13% of patients with six miscarriages (2 of 15 patients), and 23% after 7–12 miscarriages (4 of 17 patients).

Figure 40.1 shows the effect of assessing treatment on patients with two miscarriages. If there is a subsequent 80% live birth rate, and 50% of subsequent miscarriages are chromosomally abnormal, any treatment aimed at correcting a maternal cause of miscarriage can only raise the live birth rate from 80% to 90%. In order to show a statistical significance between 80% and 90%, a mega-trial will be required. Hence, any trial that includes patients with two miscarriages will show any treatment to be ineffective. Even the ASRM guideline,[5] which recognizes two or more miscarriages as the basis for investigation and treatment, suggests that research trials should be limited to patients with three or more pregnancy losses. Table 40.3 shows a rough scale of the prognosis according to the various prognostic factors, and should give physicians and patients a rough idea as to the relative prognosis.

Good Prognosis Patients

These patients include young patients with two or possibly three first trimester miscarriages. "Good prognosis" patients probably require very little investigation. However, they do require reassurance of their prognosis and "tender loving care." Ultrasound scans on a regular basis can reassure the patient and their partner that the pregnancy is progressing normally. The early pregnancy centers in the UK are invaluable in this approach, especially if they allow the patient access on a "walk in" basis. The patient

TABLE 40.3

Relative Prognoses According to Clinical Features

	Good Prognosis	Medium Prognosis	Poor Prognosis
Number of miscarriages	2	4	5
	3		6
			7
			8
			9
Age	20s	30s	40s
Karyotype of abortus	Aberrant	Normal	Normal
1° or 2° aborter	2°	1° or 3°	1° or 3°
Early or late losses	Early	Early	Late
Infertility	Normal fertility		Infertility
Antipaternal complement dependent antibodies	Positive	Negative	Negative
Natural killer cells	Normal		High

should be reassured that in the event of another miscarriage, further investigations will be carried out, including karyotyping of the abortus, and possibly embryoscopy. It is doubtful whether "good prognosis" patients need pharmacological support on an empirical basis. A question arises regarding patients who have undergone partial investigations. For example, if a patient with two blighted ova is found to have a septum, it is questionable whether the septum is the cause, or whether it should be resected. A septum has been described to cause abortions of live fetuses in the second or third trimester's after a "mini labour."[25] Therefore, should the septum be left *in situ*? As there is no evidence that it is the cause, or should it be resected, as it may cause late abortions and pre-term labor? These questions should be discussed with the patient and partner. It is important to remember that the patient's views are as valid as those laid down in official guidelines. In any recurrent miscarriage clinic, the majority of patients will have a good prognosis. Their good prognosis should not influence the management of patients with a poor prognosis. Chapter 41 shows a treatment protocol for treating good or medium prognosis patients, which differentiates between pregnancy loss due to embryonic aneuploidy and treating losses due to maternal factors.

Medium Prognosis Patients

This group of patients will include women with three and possibly four miscarriages. The prognosis for a live birth is approximately 60% after three miscarriages (40% after four miscarriages) (Figure 40.1). If these patients are included in a trial, Figure 40.1 shows that treatment of maternal factors can raise the live birth rate by approximately 25%. Again, a trial of treatment for maternal factors would need large numbers to achieve the power to show a statistically significant benefit of treatment. For example, paternal leucocyte immunization was shown to have a statistically significant benefit in the RMITG trial of 419 patients,[20] but not in Ober et al.'s[14] trial of 200 patients. We believe that these patients should be investigated, and the standard protocols assessed above give an indication of the criteria for investigation. In this group of patients, investigation may vary depending on the clinical presentation. Various clinical presentations and their likely causes are described below. In "medium prognosis" patients, treatment should be directed at the cause as far as possible. However, despite extensive investigations, the cause is often not apparent. In these cases, there may be a place for empirical hormone support with progesterone or hCG, as there is evidence,[26–29] although debatable, that these hormones may improve the prognosis by approximately 25%. This treatment is empiric, as there is no investigation in the interval between pregnancies that can diagnose a hormonal deficiency. A problem may arise when the clinical presentation is at variance with the laboratory investigations. For example, should a patient with antiphospholipid antibodies and a chromosomally abnormal abortus in a previous pregnancy be treated by anticoagulants? As with "good prognosis" patients, skill and experience may be necessary to interpret the results.

If there is a presumptive diagnosis, treatment should be prescribed accordingly. Some examples are given below

1. Parental chromosomal aberrations. Opinions are divided as to whether these patients have a worse prognosis.[30–33] Additionally, they seem to lose eukaryotypic abortuses.[34] Only few abortuses inherit the aberration in an unbalanced form (five of 39 abortuses in Carp et al.'s[34] series). However, if the fetus does inherit the chromosomal aberration in an unbalanced form, preimplantation genetic diagnosis (PGD) may be appropriate treatment.

2. Fetal karyotypic aberrations. When aberrations are present, there is usually a good prognosis. However, there are a few patients with repeat aneuploidy. This was found in 19% of patients in Carp et al.'s[34] series, and 10% of patients in Sullivan et al.'s[35] series. PGD is appropriate in cases of repeat aneuploidy.

3. Antiphospholipid antibodies are generally accepted as a cause of pregnancy loss. At present, treatment seems to be indicated. However, the "Sapporo" criteria of two readings at least 12 weeks apart, should be observed before a definitive diagnosis.[16] It may be that the strict "Sapporo" criteria should be relaxed in RPL as suggested in Chapter 20, but there is no placebo control trial on anticoagulant and aspirin treatment in APS or reproductive auto-immune failure syndrome (RAFS). In a questionaire[36] which was sent to 16 experts in obstetrics, rheumatology, immunology and internal medicine in the USA, UK, France, Spain, Netherlands, Italy, Israel, Argentina, and Brazil, the general opinion was to treat with LMWH and low dose aspirin from the moment that pregnancy was diagnosed. However, until now, there has been no evidence that aspirin has a therapeutic effect. On the contrary, a meta-analysis of three trials of aspirin has failed to find any therapeutic effect.[37]

4. Hereditary thrombophilias are controversial as to their role in pregnancy loss. They seem to be associated with late losses rather than early losses.[13] However, the literature is divided on this issue. Hereditary thrombophilias, protein C, and antithrombin activities are measured by chromogenic assays, and free protein S antigen is measured by ELISA. Patients were diagnosed having protein C, protein S, or antithrombin deficiency if the value of the corresponding protein is below 2 standard deviations of the mean level. Protein C resistance is assessed by clotting techniques. Factor V Leiden, the C677T substitution in the MTHFR gene, and the G20210A substitution in the factor II gene is detected by polymerase chain reaction amplification. However, the testing is costly. Serum fasting homocysteine levels are possibly better indicators than MTHFR. At present, we treat patients with hereditary thrombophilias with anticoagulants, usually the low molecular weight heparin enoxaparin. We have found this medication to raise the live birth rate by 25% in a comparative cohort, but nonrandomized study.[38] Randomized trials are sorely needed in order to determine if this approach is justified.

5. There is also a dearth of trials to determine the place of uterine malformations. Classically, hysterosalpingography was used to make the diagnosis of uterine anomalies, however, x-ray is uncomfortable for the patient and can only diagnose the uterine cavity. Hysterosalpingography cannot distinguish between a septate and bicornuate uterus. Recently, hysteroscopy has tended to replace x-ray. Hysteroscopy is associated with much less discomfort, but also cannot distinguish between a septate and bicornuate uterus. However, it is the best procedure for diagnosing other intrauterine pathology such as polyps, fibroids, etc. Three-dimensional (3D) ultrasound is probably the best procedure for distinguishing between a septate and bicornuate uterus. This distinction is essential if hysteroscopic setotomy is considered. However, 3D ultrasound requires specialized equipment and highly trained staff.

Poor Prognosis Patients

The author defines these patients as those with five or more consecutive miscarriages. Stravelos and Li[17] classify these patients as type 2 RPL. They have been poorly described in the literature and they have formed the subjects of few trials. These patients constitute approximately 20% of the patients in the Recurrent Miscarriage Immunotherapy Trialists Group register, and 30% of the patients in our service.[39] However, the proportion will be fewer in patients in centers using the ASRM definition of RPL as two or more miscarriages. The feature that distinguishes these patients is that they have usually had all the investigations and empirical treatments available. Hormone supplements, anticoagulants, hysteroscopic surgery, and often *in vitro* fertilization have been tried. Additionally, there may be APS patients who have failed treatment, patients who continue miscarrying after surgery for uterine anomalies, and in our service, patients who have been treated with anticoagulants for hereditary thrombophilias without success. However, most of these patients have not had fetal karyotyping performed. After five or more miscarriages, the chance of fetal chromosomal aberrations is less than after three miscarriages. Ogasawara et al.[9] have shown clearly that the incidence of chromosomal aberrations decreases with the number of miscarriages. Our approach in these patients is to perform controversial testing and treatment. These patients cannot be assured of a good prognosis as described in the various guidelines. A cytotoxic cross match between maternal serum and paternal cells to detect APCA may be helpful. The absence of these antibodies indicates a poorer prognosis,[20] and the presence of these antibodies indicates a better prognosis.[22] The numbers and activity of NK cells can also be helpful. Increased numbers of NK cells have been found in the peripheral blood in RPL,[40] particularly in primary aborters.[41] Increased numbers and activity of NK cells have also been associated with a poorer prognosis in the subsequent pregnancy.[42,43]

In poor prognosis patients in whom other forms of treatment have failed, immunotherapy seems to confer a greater benefit that after two or three miscarriages.[39,44–46] The randomized trials and meta-analyses of paternal leucocyte immunization are not appropriate for judging the effect on "poor prognosis" patients, as the results have been obscured by the good and medium prognosis patients. IVIg has also not been found to be effective when all patients are judged as a homogeneous group.[40] However, when "poor prognosis" patients are selected, IVIg has been found to improve the live birth rate.[45,46] Immunotherapy is probably more appropriate in patients losing karyotypically normal embryos.[47]

As with the "medium prognosis" patients, we attempt to karyotype the embryo. If immunotherapy fails, and the embryo is karyotypically normal, surrogacy may offer the only possibility of a live birth. If however, the pregnancy is karyotypically abnormal, a second pregnancy can be attempted with immunotherapy, as immunotherapy cannot prevent chgromosomal aberrations. If, however, the patient loses two karyotypically abnormal embryos, PGD should be offered.

The Resistant Patient

The patient with three miscarriages has an approximately 60–70% chance of a subsequent live birth and a 30–40% chance of a fourth miscarriage. The patient with four miscarriages has a 50–60% chance of a subsequent miscarriage. Therefore, after three miscarriages 15–24% of patients will have two subsequent miscarriages (see Figure 1.1). None of the guidelines listed above provide any guidance for the resistant patient, only for the initial pregnancy. The following is the authors approach. If a subsequent miscarriage occurs in the first trimester, the embryo should be karyotyped. If conventional karyotyping fails due to culture failure etc., it is possible to obtain DNA from the abortus, and perform CGH. Alternatively, embryoscopy can be performed to exclude anomalies, if embryoscopy is available. If the embryo is aneuploid or otherwise abnormal, the aneuploidy may be an isolated event and the prognosis is better for the next pregnancy (see Chapter 4). If treatment had been administered for a maternal cause of pregnancy loss, the fetal abnormality may be a confounding factor, and it is fully justified to repeat the same treatment. However, in cases of repeat aneuploidy, preimplantation genetic screening (PGS) should be performed.

If the embryo is normal on genetic testing, other forms of therapy should be considered. For example, if progesterone support had been given, hCG or immunotherapy might need to be considered.

If a subsequent loss occurs in the second or third trimesters, hysteroscopy may need to be performed (if not previously performed) or repeated in order to exclude uterine anomalies. If anticoagulants had been used for APS, an increased dose may be indicated. In the very resistant cases with five or more miscarriages, unconventional or non-evidence based treatment may be indicated, such as intravenous immunoglobulin, or surrogacy.

Specific Forms of Pregnancy Loss

The majority of recurrent pregnancy losses are losses of blighted ova, in which no fetal heartbeat or even a fetal shadow was ever detected on ultrasound. We tend to assess these patients based on their prognosis, as listed above, and to treat them according to karyotypic findings.

Recurrent Second Trimester Fetal Death

This group of patients has a poorer prognosis than after first trimester losses.[8] It is therefore justified to investigate and treat after two losses. The chance of a second trimester loss being due to chromosomal aberrations is less than in first trimester miscarriages. However, there may be fetal structural anomalies. Hence, detailed ultrasound may assist the diagnosis. Another possibility for diagnosing fetal structural anomalies is embryo-fetoscopy. Diabetes should be excluded as diabetes predisposes to fetal anomalies.

Thrombotic mechanisms, either due to APS or hereditary thrombophilias, are more likely to cause fetal demise than first trimester miscarriages.[13,48] If either of these is found, in the presence of recurrent second trimester fetal deaths, treatment by anticoagulants is warranted. New thrombophilias are constantly being identified. Microparticles and protein Z deficiency are two such examples. These thrombophilias are not usually excluded in any investigation protocol. However, there is insufficient evidence of effect to use anticoagulants on an empirical basis in the absence of APS or hereditary thrombophilia. To date, no trial has assessed anticoagulants in unexplained recurrent second trimester losses.

Drakeley et al.[49] have summarized a database analysis of 636 patients attending a UK miscarriage clinic. Second trimester miscarriages accounted for 25% of miscarriages in their series; 33% tested positive for aPL, there was a 4% prevalence of uterine anomaly, 3% could be explained by infections and 2% of patients were hypothyroid. In 50% of patients, no diagnosis was apparent. However, hereditary thrombophilias were not investigated in that series.

Losses of Live Embryos

Live embryos may be lost in the first or second trimesters. The distinguishing feature of these losses is that the uterus starts to contract, and vaginal bleeding precedes fetal demise. There may be placental separation and retroplacental hematoma formation. These forms of pregnancy loss are relatively rare, comprising approximately 11% of recurrent pregnancy losses.[50] These pregnancy losses are less likely to be due to an embryonic or fetal factor, and more likely to be due to a uterine or other maternal factor. However, patients with this clinical presentation have not been investigated as a separate group. Hence, there is no evidence to support any conclusions about this group. In the first trimester, there is a typical history. Embryonic development is normal. The uterus suddenly starts to contract and abortion can ensue. Abortion may be fast, within half an hour,[50] or may take longer. In this type of miscarriage, we recommend testing for uterine anomalies and infections. In patients who are pregnant, and present with a hematoma, empirical prophylactic antibiotics may have a place in preventing the hematoma from becoming infected. In the case of an infection, uterine contractions rapidly follow with expulsion of the uterine contents. Pelinescu-Onciul[51] has reported that the orally active progestogen dydrogesterone is effective in preventing retroplacental hematoma progressing to miscarriage.

In the case of second trimester losses of live fetuses, uterine anomalies, infections and possibly diabetes (which predisposes to infections), should be investigated. In the presence of contractions in the second trimester, tocolytic agents may be appropriate, and progestogens indicated to prevent contractions, although progestogens are not usually effective after contractions have started. Again, the appropriate trials to determine an optimal course of management have not been carried out.

Unfortunately, many patients do not know the character of the miscarriage. They will only know the character of the miscarriage if ultrasound has previously been performed in order to detect a fetal heartbeat.

Mixed Pattern of Pregnancy Losses

In many cases, each pregnancy loss may have a different clinical presentation. For example, there may be a blighted ova followed by an abortion of a live fetus in the second trimester, followed by a missed abortion. These mixed patterns of pregnancy loss are relatively frequent in patients with three losses, but rare in the patients with five or more losses. In the patients with a mixed pattern of pregnancy loss, the cause is more likely to be due to chance, and the prognosis is good. Inclusion of these patients in a trial of treatment may well confound the results, and raise the live birth rate of a control group of patients. In the author's opinion, they probably do not require active treatment. If included in any research protocol, they should be considered as a separate group of patients.

Case Presentations

The following section illustrates certain difficult cases in order to show their different presentations and the likely causes and methods of management.

Patient No. 1

The patient age 22, para 0, presented after six miscarriages between 8 and 9 weeks. No fetal heart had ever been detected, except in the fourth pregnancy when a fetal heart was said to be present at 6 weeks. However, the pregnancy showed no fetal shadow from 7 weeks onwards until curettage was performed for a blighted ovum at 9 weeks. The fourth pregnancy was found to have a normal 46XX karyotype. The following features had been investigated and found to be normal: parental karyotypes 46XX and 46XY. Lupus anticoagulant, anticardiolipin antibodies, and hereditary thrombophilias were normal. The hormone levels LH, FSH, and prolactin were normal. Mid luteal progesterone levels were 18 ng/mL. Thyroid function was normal. There was no diabetes. Hysteroscopy showed a normal cavity. Anti-paternal complement dependent antibodies were negative. The third pregnancy was treated with progesterone supplements. The fourth and fifth pregnancies were treated with enoxaparin and aspirin on an empirical basis. The sixth pregnancy was untreated. The patient was treated by paternal leucocyte immunization between the sixth and seventh pregnancies. Immunizations were boosted until seroconversion occurred with the development of anti-paternal complement dependent antibodies directed towards paternal HLA antigens. The seventh pregnancy was uneventful. No additional medications were administered. The seventh pregnancy terminated in the delivery of a female infant, 3580 g at 40 weeks. The eighth pregnancy was also a normal delivery. Paternal leucocyte immunization is not often used at present due to a widespread conviction that it is ineffective. It is not recognized as a standard treatment by the FDA in the U.S. until another trial is performed in the U.S. to show efficacy.

Patient No. 2

The patient, age 24, Para 0, presented after three miscarriages between 12 and 16 weeks. From the history, it was apparent that these were abortions of live fetuses. Hysteroscopy showed a large and thick septum that divided the uterus. The external contour of the uterus was shown to be normal on laparoscopy. The septum was resected hysteroscopically until the fundus of the uterus. The fourth pregnancy terminated as a blighted ovum at 8 weeks. Although a fourth miscarriage may sound like a failure of treatment, this was not so, as the blighted ovum was found to be triploid. The fifth pregnancy terminated as induced labor at 42 weeks, and the sixth pregnancy in spontaneous labor at 40 weeks.

Patient No. 3

The patient age 30, Para 1, a secondary aborter presented after three mid-trimester losses. The first pregnancy terminated as an uncomplicated delivery of a female infant 4050 g. The second pregnancy terminated as a fetal death at 17 weeks, and the third pregnancy as a fetal death at 19 weeks. Parental karyotyping was normal. Glucose challenge tests and thyroid function were normal. Hysteroscopy showed a normal uterine cavity. Thrombophilia testing showed the patient to be homozygous for the MTHFR mutation.[52,53] However, homocysteine levels were normal. The fourth and fifth pregnancies were treated with enoxaparin 40 mg from detection of the fetal heartbeat. However, these pregnancies terminated at 18 and 16 weeks, respectively, with intra-uterine fetal deaths. The sixth pregnancy was treated with enoxaparin 80 mg daily. The pregnancy terminated as a cesarean section at 39 weeks. A live male infant of 3240 g was delivered. Although the dose of 40 mg has been compared to 80 mg in a large cohort of patients,[54] both doses have been found to be equally effective. There may be individual patients in whom the larger doses are required.

Patient No. 4

This patient, aged 38, was a secondary aborter with two live births followed by six miscarriages, most of which were missed abortions in which a previous fetal heart was lost between 10 and 12 weeks. Investigation showed APCA to be positive. There was no APS, thrombophilia, or other cause apparent for the miscarriages. The parental karyotype was 46XX and 46XY with a balanced translocation: t(14:13)(p11:q12). The subsequent pregnancy was a missed abortion at 10 weeks. Again, a previously detected fetal heartbeat was lost. This pregnancy was found to be 46XY, -4, tder (4:13), that is, monosomy 4. Instead of the second chromosome 4, there was a chromosome with a small section of chromosome 4 and the translocated section of chromosome 13 and 14. In other words, there was partial 4 monosomy, partial 13, and partial 14 trisomies. The patient has been advised to have PGD or PGS if she desires another child. Meantime, the patient has decided to complete her family with two children.

Patient No. 5

The patient aged 40, para 0 presented after four pregnancy losses. There had been ruptured membranes at 20 weeks, two intra-uterine fetal deaths at 20 weeks, accompanied by hypertension and gestational diabetes. The fourth pregnancy was a missed abortion at 14 weeks. These four pregnancies were achieved from four cycles of zygote intra-fallopian transfer (ZIFT). There were no apparent explanations for the pregnancy losses. There was no aPL or hereditary thrombophilia. Hysteroscopy was normal. The parental karyotype was 46XX/46XY. The fifth pregnancy was achieved by the eighth cycle of *in vitro* fertilization following 22 months of infertility. The fifth pregnancy was treated with aspirin 100 mg. however; the pregnancy was terminated artificially at 22 weeks for severe pre-eclampsia with HELLP syndrome.

The patient was advised surrogacy. However, she conceived spontaneously while arranging for surrogacy. She was treated empirically with enoxaparin 40 mg daily and aspirin 100 mg. At 12 weeks, nuchal translucency screening was normal. A Shirodkar suture was inserted at 13 weeks, due to the previous ruptured membranes at 20 weeks. However, pre-eclampsia and gestational diabetes developed at 18 weeks, followed by fetal demise. The patient has undergone surrogacy. The surrogate gestational carrier has delivered a healthy male infant.

Patient No. 6

A patient, aged 33, presented with the following history: first pregnancy, "biochemical pregnancy" βhCG level unknown. The second pregnancy was twins. One twin died at 18 weeks with a sacrococcygeal tumor, the second was delivered at 32 weeks with microcephalus. The third pregnancy was a missed abortion at 10 weeks. A fetal heartbeat was previously present but was lost at 10 weeks.

Fourth pregnancy: cesarean section. Male infant 3045 g. Fifth pregnancy: biochemical, βhCG = 600; sixth pregnancy: biochemical pregnancy, βhCG = 1200; seventh pregnancy: biochemical pregnancy, βhCG = 800; eighth pregnancy: biochemical pregnancy, βhCG = 866. This clinical picture may be outside the ASRM definition of recurrent pregnancy loss. However, she requires investigation and treatment. Investigation showed no aPL, thrombophilia, uterine anomaly, hormonal imbalance, or parental chromosomal aberrations.

Conclusions

Recurrent pregnancy loss is not one homogeneous condition. Hence, there is no one protocol that is applicable. The aim of the standard protocols is entirely laudable, to advise physicians with little experience of RPL as to the optimal methods of diagnosis and treatment. Hence, the standard protocols try to guarantee that the patient receives effective treatment, and that ineffective treatment is not used. However, the standard protocols listed above might have done more harm than good, as they treat recurrent pregnancy loss as one homogeneous group. Hence, their recommendations preclude the treatment of subgroups of patients. The development of an optimal investigation protocol depends on reaching an accurate diagnosis of cause and directing treatment to that diagnosis. Fetal karyotyping and embryoscopy hold out the possibility of more accurately diagnosing embryonic or fetal causes of pregnancy loss. Treatments that have not been shown to be effective when tried on a large cohort of patients may be found to be highly effective when only used on a subgroup of patients with an accurate diagnosis.

REFERENCES

1. Royal College of Obstetricians and Gynaecologists. *The Management of Recurrent Miscarriage. Guideline No. 17*. London: RCOG; 2003.
2. American College of Obstetricians and Gynecologists. Management of recurrent early pregnancy loss, ACOG practice bulletin number 24, February 2001. *Int J Gynecol Obstet* 2002;78:179–90.
3. Jauniaux E, Farquharson RG, Christiansen OB et al. Evidence-based guidelines for the investigation and medical treatment of recurrent miscarriage. *Hum Reprod* 2006;21:2216–22.
4. Royal College of Obstetricians and Gynaecologists. *The Investigation and Treatment of Couples with Recurrent Miscarriage. Guideline No. 17*. London: RCOG; 2011.
5. Practice Committee of American Society for Reproductive Medicine. Evaluation and treatment of recurrent pregnancy loss: A committee opinion. *Fertil Steril* 2012;98:1103–11.
6. Saravelos SH, Li TC. Unexplained recurrent miscarriage: How can we explain it? *Hum Reprod* 2012;27:1882–6.
7. Carp HJA. Update on Recurrent Pregnancy Loss. In: Ratnam SS, Ng SC, Arulkumaran S, eds. *Contributions to Obstetrics and Gynaecology*. Singapore: Oxford University Press; 2000, pp. 75–107.
8. Goldenberg RL, Mayberry SK, Copper RL et al. Pregnancy outcome following a second-trimester loss. *Obstet Gynecol* 1993;81:444–6.
9. Ogasawara M, Aoki K, Okada S et al. Embryonic karyotype of abortuses in relation to the number of previous miscarriages. *Fertil Steril* 2000;73:300–4.
10. American Society for Reproductive Medicine. Definitions of infertility and recurrent pregnancy loss. *Fertil Steril* 2008;90:S60.
11. Carp HJA, Toder V, Mashiach S et al. The effect of paternal leucocyte immunization on implantation after recurrent biochemical pregnancies and repeated failure of embryo transfer. *Am J Reprod Immunol* 1994;31:112–5.
12. Farquharson RG, Jauniaux E, Exalto N. ESHRE Special Interest Group for Early Pregnancy (SIGEP). Updated and revised nomenclature for description of early pregnancy events. *Hum Reprod* 2005;20:3008–11.
13. Preston FE, Rosendaal FR, Walker ID et al. Increased fetal loss in women with heritable thrombophilia. *Lancet* 1996;348:913–6.
14. Ober C, Karrison T, Odem RR et al. Mononuclear-cell immunisation in prevention of recurrent miscarriages: A randomised trial. *Lancet* 1999;354:365–9.

15. Laskin CA, Bombardier C, Hannah ME et al. Prednisone and aspirin in women with autoantibodies and unexplained recurrent fetal loss. *N Engl J Med* 1997;337:148–53.

16. Miyakis S, Lockshin MD, Atsumi T et al. International consensus statement on an update of the classification criteria for definite antiphospholipid syndrome (APS). *J Thromb Haemost* 2006;4:295–306.

17. Jaslow CR, Carney JL, Kutteh WH. Diagnostic factors identified in 1020 women with two versus three or more recurrent pregnancy losses. *Fertil Steril* 2010;93:1234–43.

18. Lund M, Kamper-Jørgensen M, Nielsen HS et al. Prognosis for live birth in women with recurrent miscarriage: What is the best measure of success? *Obstet Gynecol* 2012;119:37–43.

19. Carp H, Toder V, Aviram A et al. Karyotype of the abortus in recurrent miscarriage. *Fertil Steril* 2001;75:678–82.

20. Recurrent Miscarriage Immunotherapy Trialists Group. Worldwide collaborative observational study and metaanalysis on allogenic leucocyte immunotherapy for recurrent spontaneous abortion. *Am J Reprod Immunol* 1994;32:55–72.

21. Cauchi MN, Pepperell R, Kloss M et al. Predictors of pregnancy success in repeated miscarriages. *Am J Reprod Immunol* 1991;26:72–5.

22. Orgad S, Gazit E, Lowenthal R. et al. The prognostic value of Antipaternal Antibodies and leukocyte immunizations on the proportion of live births in couples with consecutive recurrent miscarriages. *Hum Reprod* 1999;14:2974–9.

23. Aoki K, Kajiura S, Matsumoto Y et al. Preconceptional natural-killer-cell activity as a predictor of miscarriage. *Lancet* 1995;345:1340–2.

24. Shakhar K, Ben-Eliyahu S, Rosen E. et al. Primary versus secondary recurrent miscarriage: Differences in number and activity of peripheral NK cells. *Fertil Steril* 2003;80:368–75.

25. Rock JA, Jones HW. The clinical management of the double uterus. *Fertil Steril* 1977;28:798–806.

26. Daya S. Efficacy of progesterone support for pregnancy in women with recurrent miscarriage: A metaanalysis of controlled trials. *Br J Obstet Gynaecol* 1989;96:275–80

27. Oates-Whitehead RM, Haas DM, Carrier JA. Progestogen for preventing miscarriage. *Cochrane Database Syst Rev* 2003;CD003511.

28. Morley LC, Simpson N, Tang T. Human chorionic gonadotrophin (hCG) for preventing miscarriage. *Cochrane Database Syst Rev* 2013;CD008611.

29. Carp HJA. Recurrent miscarriage and hCG supplementation: A review and metaanalysis. *Gynecol Endocrinol* 2010;26:712–6.

30. Carp HJA, Feldman B, Oelsner G et al. Parental karyotype and subsequent live births in recurrent miscarriage. *Fertil Steril* 2004;81:1296–301.

31. Franssen MT, Korevaar JC, van der Veen F et al. Reproductive outcome after chromosome analysis in couples with two or more miscarriages: Index [corrected]-control study. *BMJ* 2006;332:759–63.

32. Barber JC, Cockwell AE, Grant E et al. Is karyotyping couples experiencing recurrent miscarriage worth the cost? *BJOG* 2010;117:885–8.

33. Sugiura-Ogasawara M, Ozaki Y, Sato T et al. Poor prognosis of recurrent aborters with either maternal or paternal reciprocal translocations. *Fertil Steril* 2004;81:367–73.

34. Carp HJA, Guetta E, Dorf H et al. Embryonic karyotype in recurrent miscarriage with parental karyotypic aberrations. *Fertil Steril* 2006;85:446–50.

35. Sullivan AE, Silver RM, LaCoursiere DY et al. Recurrent fetal aneuploidy and recurrent miscarriage. *Obstet Gynecol* 2004;104:784–8.

36. Tincani A, Branch DW, Levy RA et al. Treatment of pregnant patients with antiphospholipid syndrome. *Lupus* 2003;12:524–9.

37. Empson M, Lassere M, Craig JC et al. Recurrent pregnancy loss with antiphospholipid antibody: A systematic review of therapeutic trials. *Obstet Gynecol* 2002;99:135–44.

38. Carp HJA, Dolitzky M, Inbal A. Thromboprophylaxis improves the live birth rate in women with consecutive recurrent miscarriages and hereditary thrombophilia. *J Thromb Hemost* 2003;1:433–8.

39. Carp HJA, Toder V, Torchinsky A et al. Allogeneic leucocyte immunization in women with five or more recurrent abortions. *Hum Reprod* 1997;12:250–5.

40. Seshadri S, Sunkara SK. Natural killer cells in female infertility and recurrent miscarriage: A systematic review and meta-analysis. *Hum Reprod Update* 2014;20:429–38.

41. Shakhar K, Ben-Eliyahu S, Loewenthal R et al. Differences in number and activity of peripheral natural killer cells in primary versus secondary recurrent miscarriage. *Fertil Steril* 2003;80:368–75.

42. Aoki K, Kajiura S, Matsumoto Y et al. Preconceptional natural-killer-cell activity as a predictor of miscarriage. *Lancet* 1995;345:1340–2.

43. Coulam CB, Beaman KD. Reciprocal alteration in circulating TJ6+ CD19+ and TJ6+ CD56+ leukocytes in early pregnancy predicts success or miscarriage. *Am J Reprod Immunol* 1995;34:219–24.

44. Daya S, Gunby J. The effectiveness of allogeneic leucocyte immunization in unexplained primary recurrent spontaneous abortion. *Am J Reprod Immunol* 1994;32:294–302.

45. Carp HJA, Toder V, Gazit E. Further experience with intravenous immunoglobulin in women with recurrent miscarriage and a poor prognosis. *Am J Reprod Immunol* 2001;46:268–73.

46. Yamada H, Kishida T, Kobayashi N et al. Massive Immunoglobulin Treatment in women with four or more recurrent spontaneous primary abortions of unexplained aetiology. *Hum Reprod* 1998;13:2620–3.

47. Clark DA, Daya S, Coulam CB et al. Implications of abnormal human trophoblast karyotype of the evidence-based approach to the understanding, investigation, and treatment of recurrent spontaneous abortion. *Am J Reprod. Immunol* 1996;35:495–8.

48. Grandone E, Margaglione M, Colaizzo D et al. Factor V Leiden is associated with repeated and recurrent unexplained fetal losses. *Thromb Haemost* 1997;77:822–4.

49. Drakeley AJ, Quenby S, Farquharson RG. Mid-trimester loss—Appraisal of a screening protocol. *Hum Reprod* 1998;13:1975–80.

50. Carp HJA, Toder V, Mashiach S et al. Reccurrent miscarriage: A review of current concepts, immune mechanisms, and results of treatment. *Obst Gyn Surv* 1990;45:657–69.

51. Pelinescu-Onciul D. Subchorionic hemorrhage treatment with dydrogesterone. *Gynecol Endocrinol* 2007;23(Suppl 1):77–81.

52. Arruda VR, Von zuben PM, Chiapurini LC et al. The mutation Ala677-Val in the methylene tetrahydrofolate reductase gene: A risk factor for arterial disease and venous thrombosis. *Thromb Haem* 1997;77:818–21.

53. Nelen WL, Blom HJ, Thomas CM et al. Methylenetetrahydrofolate reductase polymorphism affects the change in homocysteine and folate concentrations resulting from low dose folic acid supplementation in women with unexplained recurrent miscarriages. *J Nutr* 1998;128;1336–41.

54. Brenner B, Hoffman R, Carp H, Dulitsky M, Younis J, LIVE-ENOX Investigators. Efficacy and safety of two doses of enoxaparin in women with thrombophilia and recurrent pregnancy loss: The LIVE-ENOX study. *J Thromb Haemost* 2005;3:227–9.

41

A New Algorithm for Evaluation and Treatment of Recurrent Pregnancy Loss

William H. Kutteh, Raymond W. Ke, and Paul R. Brezina

Introduction

Recurrent early pregnancy loss is a profound personal tragedy to couples seeking parenthood and a formidable clinical challenge to their physician. Great strides have been made in characterizing the incidence and diversity of this heterogeneous disorder. However, when to evaluate a couple and what constitutes a complete evaluation is, at the time of the writing of this chapter, in a state of flux. The American Society for Reproductive Medicine (ASRM) has recently released a committee opinion on the evaluation and treatment of RPL.[1] Although the traditional definition of recurrent pregnancy loss (RPL) included those couples with three or more spontaneous, consecutive pregnancy losses, the ASRM now defines RPL as "two or more failed clinical pregnancies."[1] Clinical pregnancy is defined as a "pregnancy documented by ultrasonography or histopathological examination." The definition has been changed as several studies have indicated that the risk of recurrent miscarriage after two successive losses is only slightly lower (24–29%) than that of women with three or more spontaneous abortions (31–33%).[2] Thus, evaluation and treatment can reasonably be started after two consecutive miscarriages,[1,3] especially when the woman is older than 35 years of age, or when the couple has had difficulty conceiving.[4] Using this definition, RPL can be found in about 1–2% of reproductive aged women[5] and a definite cause of pregnancy loss can be established in over half of couples after a thorough evaluation[3,6] and successful outcomes will occur in over two-thirds of all couples.[3,7]

We outline here a new proposed algorithm for the evaluation and treatment of RPL (Figure 41.1). Under this new schema, no diagnostic/therapeutic action is recommended following one miscarriage, as a single loss is usually a sporadic event. The overall risk of loss of a clinically recognized pregnancy loss is 15%,[2,8] but studies that evaluated the frequency of pregnancy loss, based on highly sensitive tests for quantitative hCG, indicated that the total clinical and preclinical losses in women aged 20–30 is approximately 25%, while the loss rate in women aged 40 or more is at least double that figure.[2,8] ASRM currently only recommends including clinical pregnancies, and makes no recommendations on the nonclinical losses.

An evaluation of an RPL patient should always include a complete history, including documentation of prior pregnancies, any pathologic tests that were performed on prior miscarriages, any evidence of chronic or acute infections or diseases, any recent physical or emotional trauma, history of cramping or bleeding with a previous miscarriage, any family history of pregnancy loss, and any previous gynecologic surgery or complicating factor. A summary of the diagnosis and management of recurrent pregnancy loss includes an investigation of genetic, endocrinologic, anatomic, immunologic, and iatrogenic, causes (Table 41.1).

Chapter 40 outlines different types of RPL, and the management of couples with a high order of miscarriages and a poor prognosis. However, the majority of couples have two or three missed miscarriages in the first trimester, and this algorithm refers to that majority of patients. In women with a high number of miscarriages, recurrent aneuploidy or those who continue miscarrying despite treatment, modifications to this algorithm may be necessary. It is interesting that the ASRM has lowered the number of miscarriages in the definition of RPL in order to provide guidance for the great majority of patients, whereas the editor of this book tries to concentrate on the much fewer number of patients with five or more miscarriages.

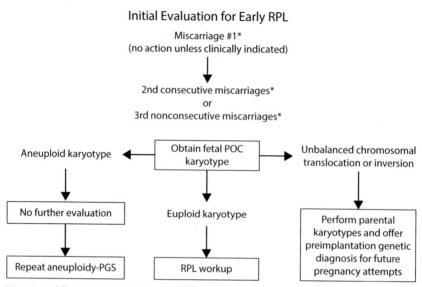

FIGURE 41.1   Initial evaluation for early recurrent pregnancy loss (RPL). This figure outlines an algorithm for the initial evaluation of early RPL. Arrows are provided that guide the reader through various outcomes possible during the RPL evaluation and appropriate "next steps" in diagnostic management.

TABLE 41.1

Diagnosis and Management of Recurrent Pregnancy Loss

Etiology	Diagnostic Evaluation	Therapy
Genetic	Karyotype partners	Genetic counseling
	Karyotype POC	Donor gametes, PGD
Anatomic	Hysterosalpingogram	Septum transection
	Hysteroscopy	Myomectomy
	Sonohysterography	Lysis of adhesions
	Transvaginal 3D US	
Endocrinologic	Midluteal progesterone	Progesterone
	TSH	Levothyroxine
	Prolactin	Bromocriptine, Dostinex
	HgbA1c	Metformin
Immunologic	Lupus anticoagulant	Heparin + aspirin
	Antiphospholipid antibodies	Heparin + aspirin
	Anti β2 glycoprotein	Heparin + aspirin
Psychologic	Interview	Support groups
Iatrogenic	Tobacco, alcohol use, obesity	Eliminate consumption
	Exposure to toxins, chemicals	Eliminate exposure

Note: POC: products of conception; PGD: preimplantation genetic diagnosis; 3D US: three-dimensional ultrasound: TSH: thyroid stimulating hormone.

Algorithm of Management

In our proposed algorithm for the evaluation and treatment of RPL, shown in Figure 41.1. Fetal karyotype is recommended after either the second consecutive or third nonconsecutive miscarriage. Products of conception (POC) obtained from early nonviable pregnancies may be sent for traditional karyotype

Workup for Early RPL

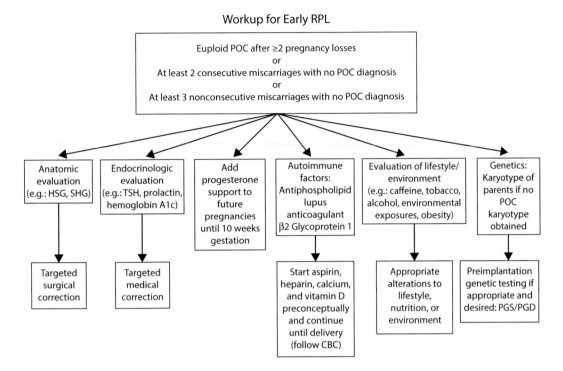

Not included in this decision tree are more controversial types of testing and therapies such as those dealing with microbiologic factors, thrombophilic factors, immunotherapy, and other evaluations though these may be appropriate in certain clinical situations.

FIGURE 41.2 Workup for early recurrent pregnancy loss (RPL). This figure outlines an algorithm for the full workup of early RPL. Arrows are provided that guide the reader through various outcomes possible during the RPL evaluation and appropriate "next steps" in diagnostic and therapeutic management. HSG: hysterosalpingogram; SHG: sonohysterogram; TSH: thyroid stimulating hormone; aPL: antiphospholipid antibodies; LAC: lupus anticoagulant; β2GP1: β2 glycoprotein 1; POC: products of conception; ASA: aspirin; PGS: preimplantation genetic screening; PGD: preimplantation genetic screening.

or, as we recommend, be sent for 23 chromosome pair microarray evaluation. POC obtained from early nonviable pregnancies are sent for 23 chromosome pair microarray evaluation. The results of this POC karyotype guide further evaluation (Figure 41.1). If the POC are found to be aneuploid, no further evaluation or treatment is recommended at that juncture because the cause for the loss is known; however, all future early miscarriages should also be subject to karyotypic evaluation. Chromosomal testing of the products of conception from a second miscarriage may confer a cost savings measure,[9,10] as chromosomal testing may save the patient the expense, time, and effort of a full work up for maternal causes of RPL. If repeat aneuploidy is found, preimplantation genetic screening (PGS) should be considered. If an unbalanced chromosomal translocation or inversion is identified in the fetal POC, then the workup would focus on performing parental karyotypes and offering appropriate therapeutic options such as PGD. If the fetal POC are found to be chromosomally normal, then a full RPL workup for maternal factors should be performed. If the fetal POC karyotypes have not been performed previously, then we recommend a full RPL workup after at least two consecutive miscarriages (Figure 41.2).

Full Workup for Maternal Factors

All the maternal factors are fully discussed in other chapters of this book. The following shows what we believe to be an appropriate workup for the patient with two or more early euploid miscarriages and the literature to support their investigation. Although there may not be grade one evidence for all of the following features, and some may not have been recommended by ASRM or the other guidelines summarized in the previous chapter, none has been assessed in euploid pregnancy loss, with the aneuploid losses excluded.

Anatomic Causes of RPL

The relevance of congenital and acquired uterine anomalies is summarized in Chapter 26.

The most common congenital abnormality associated with pregnancy loss is the septate uterus. The spontaneous abortion rate is high, averaging about 65% of pregnancies in some studies.[11] A septum was found significantly more frequently in women with primary RPL than women with secondary RPL in our recent study.[12] Uncontrolled studies suggest that resection of the uterine septum results in higher delivery rates than in women without treatment. Other congenital abnormalities, such as uterine didelphys, bicornuate, and unicornuate uterus are more frequently associated with later trimester losses or preterm delivery.

Intrauterine cavity abnormalities, such as submucosal leiomyomas and polyps, can contribute to pregnancy loss. Until recently, it was felt that only submucous leiomyomas should be surgically removed prior to subsequent attempts at pregnancy. However, several recent studies investigating the implantation rate in women undergoing *in vitro* fertilization (IVF) have clearly demonstrated decreased implantation with intramural leiomyomas in the range of 30 mm.[13] When smaller leiomyomas are identified, it is unclear if myomectomy is beneficial.[14]

At present, there is no prospective study evaluating the efficacy of uterine surgery. However, Sugiura-Ogasawara[11] has reported a case control study of 1570 patients, with two or more miscarriages, where uterine anomalies impacted on the progression of normal (euploid) pregnancies.

Cervical incompetence commonly causes pregnancy loss in the second, rather than first, trimester. It may be associated with congenital uterine abnormalities such as septate or bicornuate uterus. Rarely, it may be congenital following *in utero* exposure to diethylstilbestrol.[15] It is postulated that most cases occur as a result of surgical trauma to the cervix from conization, loop electrosurgical excision procedures, overdilaton of the cervix during pregnancy termination, or obstetric lacerations.[16]

Endocrinologic Causes of RPL

Endocrine factors may contribute to 8–12% of recurrent pregnancy loss. They are fully summarized in Chapter 13. An endocrinologic evaluation is a critical component of the RPL workup.

Luteal Phase Deficiency

Luteal phase deficiency (LPD) is defined as an inability of the corpus luteum to secrete progesterone in high enough amounts or for too short a duration. The preponderance of evidence suggests that LPD is a preovulatory event most likely linked to an alteration in the preovulatory estrogen stimulation, which may indicate poor oocyte quality and a poorly functioning corpus luteum.[17,18] However, progesterone levels are subject to large fluctuations because of pulsatile release of the LH hormone. Moreover, there is a lack of correlation between serum levels of progesterone and endometrial histology.[19] Additionally, low levels of progesterone may reflect a pregnancy that is failing due to aneuploidy, or other embryonic factors. Hence, the role of progesterone supplementation is debated in Chapters 14, 15 and 16 in this book. However, a recent Cochrane review evaluating 15 trials concluded that there was a benefit to the routine administration of progesterone to all women with a history of RPL.[20]

Untreated Hypothyroidism

We investigate thyroid function as hypothyroidism may increase the risk of miscarriage. A study of over 700 patients with recurrent pregnancy loss identified 7.6% with hypothyroidism.[21] It has also been suggested that thyroid antibodies are elevated in women with recurrent pregnancy loss. A retrospective study of 700 patients with recurrent pregnancy loss demonstrated that 158 women had antithyroid antibodies but only 23 of those women had clinical hypothyroidism on the basis of an abnormal thyroid stimulating hormone (TSH) value.[22] The presence of antithyroid antibodies may imply abnormal T-cell function, and therefore, more of an immune dysfunction rather than an endocrine disorder may be responsible for the pregnancy losses. The Endocrine Society recommends that patients with RPL be treated to keep a TSH level of between 1.0 and 2.5 uIU/mL in the first trimester.[23] For TSH levels found to be between 2.5 and 10 mIU/mL, a starting levothyroxine dose of at least 50 µg/d is recommended.[23] The role of thyroid autoimmunity and dysfunction are described in the chapters on endocrinology and autoimmunity.

Abnormal Glucose Metabolism

Patients with poorly controlled diabetes are known to have an increased risk of spontaneous miscarriage, which is reduced to normal spontaneous loss rates when women are euglycemic preconceptually.[24] Testing for fasting insulin and glucose is simple and treatment with insulin-sensitizing agents can reduce the risk of recurrent miscarriage.[25] More recently, determining the average load of blood glucose through testing of hemoglobin A1C has become an increasingly utilized modality to evaluate insulin resistance.[1] Because there is strong evidence that obesity and/or insulin resistance are associated with an increased risk of miscarriage, weight reduction in obese women is a first step in the treatment. Metformin seems to improve pregnancy outcome, but the evidence for this treatment is limited to a few cohort studies. Metformin is a category B medication in the first trimester of pregnancy and appears to be safe. Other endocrine abnormalities, such as thyroid disorders and diabetes, should be corrected prior to conception.

Hyperprolactinemia

Normal circulating levels of prolactin may play an important role in maintaining early pregnancy. Data from animal studies suggest that elevated prolactin levels may adversely affect corpus luteal function; however, this concept has not been proven in humans.[26] A recent study of 64 hyperprolactinemic women showed that bromocriptine therapy was associated with a higher rate of successful pregnancy and that prolactin levels were significantly higher in women who miscarried.[27]

Diminished Ovarian Reserve

Follicle stimulating hormone (FSH) is thought to be a marker of the number of follicles available for recruitment on any given menstrual cycle. Therefore, elevated levels of FSH in the early follicular phase of the menstrual cycle are representative of diminished ovarian reserve. More recently, other markers, such as decreased anti-Müllerian hormone, have been introduced to identify diminished ovarian reserve. Although the frequency of elevated day 3 FSH levels in women with recurrent miscarriage is similar to the frequency in the infertile population, the prognosis of recurrent miscarriages is worsened with increased day 3 FSH levels.[28] Although no treatment is available, testing may be helpful in women over the age of 35 with recurrent pregnancy loss, and appropriate counseling should follow.

Immune Factors as the Cause of RPL

In some instances, there is a failure in normal control mechanisms that prevent an immune reaction against self, resulting in an autoimmune response.[29] Autoantibodies to phospholipids, thyroid antigens, nuclear antigens and others have been investigated as possible causes for pregnancy loss.[21]

Antiphospholipid Antibody Syndrome (APS)

APS and antiphospholipid (aPL) antibodies have been fully described in previous chapters. There is still controversy concerning testing for phospholipids other than lupus anticoagulant, anti-beta 2 glycoprotein I antibodies, and anticardiolipin antibodies. However, an increasing number of studies suggest that antibodies to phosphatidyl serine are also associated with pregnancy loss.[30] Women with systemic lupus erythematosus and aPL have increased risks for miscarriage compared to those with lupus and negative aPL.[31]

APS is treated with a combination of low dose heparin (5000–10,000 units subcutaneously every 12 hours) and low dose aspirin (81 mg PO daily) appears to be effective and may reduce pregnancy loss by 54% in women with APS.[32,33] Aspirin alone does not appear to reduce miscarriage rates.[34] Unfractionated heparin is preferred to low molecular weight heparin (LMWH) based on available data.[35]

However, two small series from Japan[36,37] have shown that abnormal antibodies do not guarantee normal chromosomes, and that approximately 30% of pregnancy losses in APS may be due to fetal aneuploidy. A placebo controlled trial is still required for patients with aPL and RPL in general, and for women losing euploid embryos in particular.

Immunotherapy

We do not currently offer immunotherapy for alloimmune disorders. Although some randomized double blinded studies have shown an increase with therapies, such as paternal leukocyte immunization, trophoblast immune infusion, intravenous intralipid therapy, and immunoglobulin infusion in successful pregnancy outcomes, others have not confirmed these results. A Cochrane review of 19 trials of various forms of immunotherapy did not show significant differences between treatment and control groups.[38] However, therapy may be beneficial in subgroups of patients. The relevant subgroups are described in the debates in Chapters 27, 28, 29, 30, and 31. Immunotherapy has not been assessed in patients losing euploid embryos.

Microbiologic Factors as a Cause of RPL

Certain infectious agents have been identified more frequently in cultures from women who have had spontaneous pregnancy losses.[39] These include *Ureaplasma urealyticum*, *Mycoplasma hominis,* and chlamydia. Other less frequent pathogens include toxoplasma gondi, rubella, HSV, measles, cytomegalovirus, coxsackievirus, and *Listeria monocytogenes*. It is important to be aware that none of these pathogens has been causally linked to RPL. Because of the association with sporadic pregnancy losses and the ease of diagnosis, some clinicians will test women with RPL and treat for the appropriate pathogen in both parents. The role of infective agents is fully described in Chapter 33.

Hereditary Thrombophilias

Thrombophilias are thought to be responsible for more than half of maternal venous thromboembolisms in pregnancy; however, ACOG recommends that only patients with a personal or family history of thromboembolic events should be tested.[40] The role of thrombophilias is described in Chapter 22, and the value of thromboprophylaxis debated in Chapters 23 and 24.

Genetic Factors as the Cause of RPL

There are a variety of genetic factors that may result in failure of a pregnancy to develop. These are described in Chapter 3. Broadly, genetic factors may be divided into embryonic x chromosomal aberrations derived from known parental chromosomal abnormalities and embryonic errors that arise de novo in apparently chromosomally normal parents.

Parental Chromosomal Disorders

If no fetal POC are available and the couple has a history of at least two consecutive or three nonconsecutive fetal losses, we recommend obtaining parental karyotypes. Parental chromosome anomalies occur in 3–5% of couples with RPL as opposed to 0.7% in the general population. This increased prevalence justifies investigating the parents. These chromosomal aberrations in the parents include translocations, inversions, and the relatively rare, ring chromosomes. Studies indicate that when the Robertsonian translocation is maternal, there is a greater risk that the fetus will exhibit an unbalanced phenotype.[41] Balanced reciprocal translocations are thought to directly contribute to both infertility and recurrent pregnancy loss (RPL).[42,43] However, Carp et al.[44] have karyotyped the abortus in patients with parental chromosomal aberrations and RPL. The subsequent live birth rate is as would be expected for women with RPL and no chromosomal aberrations. The aberrant chromosome was only found in 13% of subsequent miscarriages.[45]

Embryonic Aneuploidy and Recurrent Aneuploidy

The overall frequency of chromosome abnormalities in sporadic spontaneous abortions is at least 50%.[46–50] Of these abnormalities, most are numerical: 52% are trisomies, 29% are monosomy 45,X, 16% are triploidies, 6% are tetraploidies, and 4% are structural rearrangements.[51] The vast majority of embryonic aneuploidies are thought to result from maternal meiotic nondisjunction during oocyte development, although abnormalities arising from the sperm component are possible..

There is significant debate in the professional community as to how prevalent aneuploidy is among RPL embryos. Emerging data suggest that RPL patients may have lower rates of embryonic aneuploidy in first trimester miscarriages as compared to all women. For example, a study evaluating 4873 embryos via single nucleotide polymorphism (SNP) microarray showed the rate of aneuploidy found using trophectoderm biopsy at the blastocyst stage in RPL was significantly lower (32%) than the rate of aneuploidy found with cleavage stage biopsy (61%).[52] Additionally, the incidence of embryonic aneuploidy decreases with increasing numbers of misdcarriages.[37] However, other data from small studies suggest that the rate of aneuploidy in embryos in RPL is higher than 65%.[53,54] Therefore, the true rate of embryonic aneuploidy in couples with a diagnosis of RPL is currently a topic of great debate.

Evidence suggests that some couples are at risk for recurrent aneuploidy. Empirically, the birth of a trisomic infant places a woman at an approximately 1% increased risk for a subsequent trisomic conceptus.[55]. Germline mosaicism has been reported in recurrent cases of Down syndrome and may also be responsible for recurrent aneuploidy in some couples.[56] In RPL, repeat fetal aneuploidy has been shown in three of 30 patients in Sullivan et al.'s[57] series and eight of 43 patients in Carp et al.'s[58] series.

Preimplantation Genetic Testing

The role of PGS and PGD in RPL is hotly debated in Chapters 6 and 7. We feel that PGD for structural aberrations such as translocations and inversions is justified. In contrast, PGS is far more controversial. A 2007 publication in the *New England Journal of Medicine* by Mastenbroek et al. showed no benefit to PGS.[59] This was followed by major medical societies discouraging the routine use of PGS.[60] Since this time, newer technologies, such as microarrays, have been introduced that are capable of evaluating the ploidy status of all 23 pairs of chromosomes instead of the 9–14 pairs of chromosomes evaluated with older fluorescence *in situ* hybridization (FISH) technologies.[61] Additionally, performing embryo biopsy at the blastocyst, as opposed to the cleavage stage, seems to confer superior pregnancy rates.[62,63]

Recent data evaluating pregnancy rates in RPL patients using 23 chromosome microarrays are encouraging.[52,64] PGS as a treatment modality is currently widely utilized. Of 27,630 PGT IVF cycles reported over the past 10 years to the ESHRE PGD Consortium, collecting data from around the globe, 61% ($n = 16,806$) were performed for PGS.[61] Despite this high rate of utilization, there are no series reporting live birth rates or miscarriage rates in RPL specifically. Pregnancy rates are not a valid measurement in patients who conceive easily spontaneously. Large and well-conducted randomized controlled trials are necessary to firmly establish the efficacy of PGS and define which patient populations may benefit from these technologies. Furthermore, PGS is far from a full proof technology in determining the ploidy status of an embryo. Embryo mosaicism has been shown to be as high as 50% in cleavage stage embryos and as high as 10% in blastocysts.[65,66] Therefore, the cell taken at the time of embryo biopsy may not always be representative of the genetic composition of the embryo. Furthermore, technical limitations, such as failure to successfully amplify genomic DNA, genomic contamination, and the possibility for human error may be another source of diagnostic error. It is vital that providers explain to patients contemplating utilizing preimplantation genetic testing the risks, benefits, and alternatives of the technology in detail. PGS may be a viable option for couples with recurrent embryo aneuploidy and may reduce the incidence of future miscarriage.

Lifestyle Issues and Environmental Toxins

Couples experiencing recurrent pregnancy losses are often concerned those toxins within the environment may have contributed to their reproductive difficulty. It is important that health care providers, counseling patients about exposures to substances in the environment, have current and accurate information in order to respond to these concerns.

Cigarette Smoking

Cigarette smoking reduces fertility and increases the rate of spontaneous abortion. The data evaluating smoking and miscarriage are extensive and involve approximately 100,000 subjects. The studies suggest a clinically significant detrimental effect of cigarette smoking that is dose dependent, with a relative risk for miscarriage among moderate smokers (10–20 cigarettes a day) being 1.1–1.3.[67] Patients should be actively counseled to stop cigarette smoking prior to attempting pregnancy, and given adequate support to assist them in this task.

Alcohol Consumption

Alcohol consumption is associated with a risk of spontaneous abortion.[68] The minimum threshold dose for significantly increasing the risk of first trimester miscarriage appears to be two or more alcoholic drinks per week.[68,69] However, there is little evidence concerning recurrent miscarriage. When personal habits, cigarette smoking, and alcohol are utilized in the same individual, the risk of pregnancy loss may increase 4-fold. Couples should be counseled concerning these habits and strongly encouraged to discontinue these prior to attempting subsequent conception.[70]

Obesity

Obesity, defined as a body mass index over 30 has been shown to be an independent risk factor for first trimester miscarriage.[71] The association is strongest in women with BMI >40. The etiology of this phenomenon is unclear. However, many studies have linked obesity to a generalized increase in systemic inflammatory responses.[72] Patients should be actively encouraged to lose weight; however, the physician should be aware how difficult a task weight loss may be.

Caffeine Intake

Several studies have shown that caffeine in excess of 300 mg/day (three cups of coffee per day) is associated with a modest increase in spontaneous abortion, but it is not clear if this relationship is causal.[73]

Ionizing Radiation

The studies of atomic bomb survivors in Japan showed that *in utero* exposure to high-dose radiation increased the risk of spontaneous abortions, premature deliveries, and stillbirths.[74] Diagnostic x-rays in the first trimester delivering less than 5 rads are not teratogenic.[75] Large doses (360–500 rads) used in therapeutic radiation, however, induce abortion in offspring exposed *in utero* in the majority of cases. Adverse effects of chronic low-dose radiation on reproduction have not been identified in humans.[76]

Outcome

The treatment of RPL should be directed at the cause. Given the good outcome for most couples with unexplained recurrent miscarriage in the absence of treatment, it is difficult to recommend unproven therapies, especially if they are invasive and expensive. Explanation and appropriate emotional support are possibly the two most important aspects of therapy. However, this rule may not hold for patients with a poor prognosis or specific forms of pregnancy loss.

In approximately half of all cases of recurrent pregnancy loss, a complete evaluation will reveal a possible etiology. Abnormal findings during the evaluation should be corrected prior to attempting any subsequent pregnancy. If no cause can be found, the majority of couples will eventually have a successful pregnancy outcome with supportive therapy alone.[77] Once a pregnancy occurs, the patient should be monitored closely with evaluation of quantitative hCG levels at least twice and documentation of adequate progesterone levels. Early sonography should be scheduled and any encouraging results should be communicated to the couple. In women with a history of RPL, the presence of a normal embryonic heart rate between 6 and 8 gestational weeks that is confirmed with repeat sonography in one week is associated with a live birth rate of 82%.[78] Any subsequent failed pregnancies should have genetic testing on the POC. When aneuploidy is found, this can be reassuring to both the physician and patient that this loss was not due to a treatment failure or any patient activity.

A recent study evaluating 987 women with RPL found that the chances of achieving a live birth within 5 years of initial physician consultation was in excess of 80% for women under the age of 30 and approximately 60–70% for women ages 31–40.[7] However, the 20% of patients who do not conceive within 5 years and the 30–40% of women over the age of 31 also require our support and adequate treatment.

REFERENCES

1. The Practice Committee of the American Society for Reproductive Medicine. Evaluation and treatment of recurrent pregnancy loss: A committee opinion. *Fertil Steril* 2012;98:1103–11.
2. Stirrat GM. Recurrent miscarriage. *Lancet* 1990;336:673–5.
3. Jaslow CR, Carney JL, Kutteh WH. Diagnostic factors identified in 1020 women with two versus three or more recurrent pregnancy losses. *Fertil Steril* 2010;93:1234–43.
4. Practice Committee of the American Society for Reproductive Medicine. Aging and infertility in women. *Fertil Steril* 2006;86(5 Suppl 1):S248–52.
5. Stephenson M, Kutteh WH. Evaluation and management of recurrent early pregnancy loss. *Clin Obstet Gynecol* 2007;50:132–145.
6. Stephenson MD. Frequency of factors associated with habitual abortion in 197 couples. *Fertil Steril* 1996;66:24–9.
7. Lund M, Kamper-Jørgensen M, Nielsen HS et al. Prognosis for live birth in women with recurrent miscarriage: What is the best measure of success? *Obstet Gynecol* 2012;119:37–43.
8. Lathi RB, Gray Hazard FK, Heerema-McKenney A et al. First trimester miscarriage evaluation. *Semin Reprod Med* 2011;29:463–9.
9. Foyouzi N, Cedars MI, Huddleston HG. Cost-effectiveness of cytogenetic evaluation of products of conception in the patient with a second pregnancy loss. *Fertil Steril* 2012;98:151–5.
10. Bernardi LA, Plunkett BA, Stephenson MD. Is chromosome testing of the second miscarriage cost saving? A decision analysis of selective versus universal recurrent pregnancy loss evaluation. *Fertil Steril* 2012;98:156–61.
11. Sugiura-Ogasawara M, Ozaki Y, Katano K et al. Uterine anomaly and recurrent pregnancy loss. *Semin Reprod Med* 2011;29:514–21.
12. Jaslow CR, Kutteh WH. Effect of prior birth and miscarriage on the prevalence of acquired and congenital uterine anomalies in women with recurrent miscarriage: A cross-sectional study. *Fertil Steril* 2013;99:1916–22.
13. Stovall DW, Parrish SB, Van Voorhis BJ et al. Uterine leiomyomas reduce the efficacy of assisted reproduction cycles: Results of a matched follow-up study. *Hum Reprod* 1998;13:192–7.
14. Surrey ES, Lietz AK, Schoolcraft WB. Impact of intramural leiomyomate in patients with a normal endometrial cavity on *in vitro* fertilization-embryo transfer cycle outcome. *Fertil Steril* 2001;75:405–19.
15. Goldberg GM, Falcone T. Effect of diethylstilbestrol on reproductive function. *Fertil Steril* 1999;72:1–7.
16. American College of Obstetrics and Gynecologist. ACOG practice bulletin. Cervical insufficiency. *Int J Gynaecol Obstet* 2004;85:81–9.
17. Tuckerman E, Laird SM, Stewart R et al. Markers of endometrial function in women with unexplained recurrent pregnancy loss. *Hum Reprod* 2004;19:196–205.
18. Smith ML, Schust DJ. Endocrinology and recurrent early pregnancy loss. *Semin Reprod Med* 2011;29:482–90.
19. Shepard MK, Senturia YD. Comparison of serum progesterone and endometrial biopsy for confirmation of ovulation and evaluation of luteal function. *Fertil Steril* 1977;28:541–8.

20. Haas DM, Ramsey PS. Progestogen for preventing miscarriage. *Cochrane Database Syst Rev* 2008;CD003511.

21. Ghazeeri GS, Kutteh WH. Immunological testing and treatment in reproduction: Frequency assessment of practice patterns at assisted reproduction clinics in the USA and Australia. *Hum Reprod* 2001;16: 2130–5.

22. Kutteh WH, Yetman DL, Carr AC et al. Increased prevalence of antithyroid antibodies identified in women with recurrent pregnancy loss but not in women undergoing assisted reproduction. *Fertil Steril* 1999;71:843–8.

23. De Groot L, Abalovich M, Alexander EK et al. Management of thyroid dysfunction during pregnancy and postpartum: An endocrine society clinical practice guideline. *J Clin Endocrinol Metab* 2012;97:2543–65.

24. Mills JL, Simpson JL, Driscoll SG et al. Incidence of spontaneous abortion among normal women and insulin-dependent diabetic women whose pregnancies were identified within 21 days of conception. *N Engl J Med* 1988;319:1617–23.

25. Sills ES, Perloe M, Palermo GD. Correction of hyperinsulinemia in oligoovulatory women with clomiphene-resistant polycystic ovary syndrome: A review of therapeutic rationale and reproductive outcomes. *Eur J Obstet Gynecol Reprod Biol* 2000;91:135–41.

26. Dlugi AM. Hyperprolactinemic recurrent spontaneous pregnancy loss: A true clinical entity or a spurious finding? *Fertil Steril* 1998;70:253–5.

27. Hirahara F, Andoh N, Sawai K et al. Hyperprolactinemic recurrent miscarriage and results of randomized bromocriptine treatment trials. *Fertil Steril* 1998;70:246–52.

28. Hofmann GE, Khoury J, Thie J. Recurrent pregnancy loss and diminished ovarian reserve. *Fertil Steril* 2000;74:1192–5.

29. Kutteh WH. Immunology of multiple endocrinopathies associated with premature ovarian failure. *Endocrinologist* 1996;6:462–6.

30. Franklin RD, Kutteh WH. Antiphospholipid antibodies (APA) and recurrent pregnancy loss: Treating a unique APA positive population. *Hum Reprod* 2002;17:2981–5.

31. Kutteh WH, Lyda EC, Abraham SM et al. Association of anticardiolipin antibodies and pregnancy loss in women with systemic lupus erythematosus. *Fertil Steril* 1993;60:449–55.

32. Empson M, Lassere M, Craig JC et al. Recurrent pregnancy loss with antiphospholipid antibody: A systematic review of therapeutic trials. *Obstet Gynecol* 2002;99:135–44.

33. Kutteh WH. Antiphospholipid antibody-associated recurrent pregnancy loss: Treatment with heparin and low-dose aspirin is superior to low-dose aspirin alone. *Am J Obstet Gynecol* 1996;174:1584–9.

34. Pattison NS, Chamley LW, Birdsall M et al. Does aspirin have a role in improving pregnancy outcome for women with the antiphospholipid syndrome? A randomized controlled trial. *Am J Obstet Gynecol* 2000;183:1008–12.

35. Ziakas PD, Pavlou M, Voulgarelis M. Heparin treatment in antiphospholipid syndrome with recurrent pregnancy loss: A systematic review and meta-analysis. *Obstet Gynecol* 2010;115:1256–62.

36. Takakuwa K, Asano K, Arakawa M et al. Chromosome analysis of aborted conceptuses of recurrent aborters positive for anticardiolipin antibody. *Fertil Steril* 1997;68:54–8.

37. Ogasawara M, Aoki K, Okada S et al. Embryonic karyotype of abortuses in relation to the number of previous miscarriages. *Fertil Steril* 2000;73:300–4.

38. Scott JR. Immunotherapy for recurrent miscarriage [update of *Cochrane Database Syst Rev* 2000;CD000112]. *Cochrane Database Syst Rev* 2003;CD000112.

39. Penta M, Lukic A, Conte MP et al. Infectious agents in tissues from spontaneous abortions in the first trimester of pregnancy. *New Microbiol* 2003;26:329–37.

40. Lockwood C, Wendel G, Committee on Practice Bulletins—Obstetrics. Practice bulletin no. 124: Inherited thrombophilias in pregnancy. *Obstet Gynecol* 2011;118:730–40.

41. Boué A, Gallano P. A collaborative study of the segregation of inherited chromosome structural arrangements in 1356 prenatal diagnoses. *Prenat Diagn* 1984;4:45–67.

42. Chen CP, Wu PC, Lin CJ et al. Unbalanced reciprocal translocations at amniocentesis. *Taiwan J Obstet Gynecol* 2011;50:48–57.

43. Grati FR, Barlocco A, Grimi B et al. Chromosome abnormalities investigated by non-invasive prenatal testing account for approximately 50% of fetal unbalances associated with relevant clinical phenotypes. *Am J Med Genet A* 2010;152A:1434–42.

44. Carp HJA, Feldman B, Oelsner G et al. Parental karyotype and subsequent live births in recurrent miscarriage. *Fertil Steril* 2004;81:1296–301.
45. Carp HJA, Guetta E, Dorf H et al. Embryonic karyotype in recurrent miscarriage with parental karyotypic aberrations. *Fertil Steril* 2006;85:446–50.
46. Sugiura-Ogasawara M, Ozaki Y, Katano K et al. Abnormal embryonic karyotype is the most frequent cause of recurrent miscarriage. *Hum Reprod* 2012;27:2297–303.
47. Hassold T, Chen N, Funkhouser J et al. A cytogenetic study of 1000 spontaneous abortions. *Ann Hum Genet* 1980;44(Pt 2):151–78.
48. Werner M, Reh A, Grifo J et al. Characteristics of chromosomal abnormalities diagnosed after spontaneous abortions in an infertile population. *J Assist Reprod Genet* 2012;29:817–20.
49. Nayak S, Pavone ME, Milad M et al. Aneuploidy rates in failed pregnancies following assisted reproductive technology. *J Womens Health (Larchmt)* 2011;20:1239–43.
50. Coulam CB, Goodman C, Dorfmann A. Comparison of ultrasonographic findings in spontaneous abortions with normal and abnormal karyotypes. *Hum Reprod* 1997;12:823–6.
51. Boué A, Boué J, Gropp A. Cytogenetics of pregnancy wastage. *Annu Rev Genet* 1985;14:1–57.
52. Brezina PR, Tobler K, Benner AT et al. Evaluation of 571 *in vitro* Fertilization (IVF) Cycels and 4,873 Embryos Using 23-Chromosome Single Nucleotide Polymorphism (SNP) Microarray Preimplantation Genetic Screening (PGS). *Fertil Steril* 2012;97:S23–4.
53. Robberecht C, Pexsters A, Deprest J et al. Cytogenetic and morphological analysis of early products of conception following hystero-embryoscopy from couples with recurrent pregnancy loss. *Prenat Diagn* 2012;4:1–10.
54. Philipp T, Philipp K, Reiner A et al. Embryoscopic and cytogenetic analysis of 233 missed abortions: Factors involved in the pathogenesis of developmental defects of early failed pregnancies. *Hum Reprod* 2003;18:1724–32.
55. Stene J, Stene E, Mikkelsen M. Risk for chromosome abnormality at amniocentesis following a child with a non-inherited chromosome aberration. *Prenat Diagn* 1984;4:81–95.
56. Sachs ES, Jahoda MG, Los FJ et al. Trisomy 21 mosaicism in gonads with unexpectedly high recurrence risks. *Am J Med Genet Suppl* 1990;7:186–8.
57. Sullivan AE, Silver RM, LaCoursiere DY et al. Recurrent fetal aneuploidy and recurrent miscarriage. *Obstet Gynecol* 2004;104:784–8.
58. Carp HJA, Toder V, Orgad S et al. Karyotype of the abortus in recurrent miscarriage. *Fertil Steril* 2001;5:678–82.
59. Mastenbroek S, Twisk M, van Echten-Arends J et al. *In vitro* fertilization with preimplantation genetic screening. *N Engl J Med* 2007;357:9–17.
60. Practice Committee of Society for Assisted Reproductive Technology, Practice Committee of American Society for Reproductive Medicine. Preimplantation genetic testing: A Practice Committee opinion. *Fertil Steril* 2008;90:S136–43.
61. Harper JC, Wilton L, Traeger-Synodinos J et al. The ESHRE PGD Consortium: 10 years of data collection. *Hum Reprod Update* 2012;18:234–47.
62. Forman EJ, Tao X, Ferry KM et al. Single embryo transfer with comprehensive chromosome screening results in improved ongoing pregnancy rates and decreased miscarriage rates. *Hum Reprod* 2012;27:1217–22.
63. Schoolcraft WB, Fragouli E, Stevens J et al. Clinical application of comprehensive chromosomal screening at the blastocyst stage. *Fertil Steril* 2010;94:1700–6.
64. Wells D, Alfarawati S, Fragouli E. Use of comprehensive chromosomal screening for embryo assessment: Microarrays and CGH. *Mol Hum Reprod* 2008;14:703–10.
65. Munné S, Weier HU, Grifo J et al. Chromosome mosaicismin human embryos. *Biol Reprod* 1994;51:373–9.
66. Brezina P, Nguyen KHD, Benner AT et al. Aneuploid blastomeres may undergo a process of genetic normalization resulting in euploid blastocysts. *Hum Reprod* 2011;26(Suppl 1):i53–6.85.
67. Harlap S, Shiono PH. Alcohol, smoking, and incidence of spontaneous abortions in the first and second trimester. *Lancet* 1980;2:173–8.
68. Kline J, Shroat P, Stein ZA, Susser M, Warburton D. Drinking during pregnancy and spontaneous abortion. *Lancet* 1980;2:176–80.

69. Andersen AM, Andersen PK, Olsen J et al. Moderate alcohol intake during pregnancy and risk of fetal death. *Int J Epidemiol* 2012;41:405–13.

70. Ness RB, Grisso JA, Hrischinger N, Markovic N, Shaw LM, Day NL et al. Cocaine and tobacco use and the risk of spontaneous abortion. *N Engl J Med* 1999;340:333–9.

71. Smith ML, Schust DJ. Endocrinology and recurrent early pregnancy loss. *Semin Reprod Med* 2011;29:482–90.

72. Johnson AR, Justin Milner J, Makowski L. The inflammation highway: Metabolism accelerates inflammatory traffic in obesity. *Immunol Rev* 2012;249:218–38.

73. Dlugosz L, Bracken MB. Reproductive effects of caffeine: A review and theoretical analysis. *Epidemiol Rev* 1992;4:83–100.

74. Yamazaki JN, Schull WJ. Perinatal loss and neurological abnormalities among children of the atomic bomb. Nagasaki and Hiroshima revisited, 1949 to 1989. *JAMA* 1990;264:605–9.

75. Brent RL. The effects of embryonic and fetal exposure to x-ray, microwaves, and ultrasound. *Clin Perinatol* 1986;13:615.

76. Gardella JR, Hill JA 3rd. Environmental toxins associated with recurrent pregnancy loss. *Semin Reprod Med* 2000;18:407–24.

77. Brigham SA, Conlon C, Farquharson RG. A longitudinal study of pregnancy outcome following idiopathic recurrent miscarriage. *Hum Reprod* 1999;14:2868–71.

78. Hyer JS, Fong S, Kutteh WH. Predictive value of the presence of an embryonic heartbeat for live birth: Comparison of women with and without recurrent pregnancy loss. *Fertil Steril* 2004;82:1369–73.

42

Third Party Reproduction in Recurrent Pregnancy Loss

Gautam N. Allahbadia and Rubina Merchant

Introduction

A higher frequency of spontaneous miscarriage has been reported among infertile couples, as well as a higher prevalence of infertility among patients with recurrent spontaneous miscarriages, compared with the general population.[1,2] The risk of recurrent spontaneous miscarriage is much higher in patients with previous losses, being 17–25% after two consecutive losses and between 25% and 46% after three consecutive losses,[3] the risk of miscarriage increasing with age.[4]

Recently, assisted reproductive techniques (ART) have been used to prevent further miscarriages in women with recurrent miscarriage using either (i) screening or diagnosis of embryonic chromosomes prior to embryo replacement (preimplantation genetic screening [PGS]/preimplantation genetic diagnosis [PGD]) or (ii) surrogacy. While PGS/PGD assumes that the embryo is chromosomally abnormal, and that the mother should receive a chromosomally normal embryo, surrogacy assumes that the embryo is normal and that the maternal environment needs to be substituted.[5] In this chapter, we aim to highlight the role of third party reproduction as a treatment option for recurrent pregnancy loss (RPL).

Causes of RPL

Embryonic Causes

Aneuploidy in the embryo is the most common fetal cause of recurrent miscarriage, with the overall incidence being approximately 40%.[6] However, aging gametes is another cause. Aging gametes in the female genital tract before fertilization, maternal age, and the number of previous miscarriages are independent risk factors for a further miscarriage. A higher incidence of small amniotic sac syndrome and euploid miscarriages has been reported in infertility patients older than 35 years, the risk of miscarriage being highest among couples where the woman is ≥35 years of age and the man ≥40 years of age.[1] Patients >40 years, undergoing *in vitro* fertilization (IVF) have also presented a 29% spontaneous miscarriage following ultrasound evidence of a fetal heart beat.[7]

Parental Causes

The maternal causes of recurrent pregnancy loss are described in other chapters. In addition, the sperm from men with a history of idiopathic RPL have a higher percentage of DNA damage with a sperm DNA fragmentation index (DFI) of approximately 26% in male partners of couples experiencing idiopathic RPL. Men with a higher DFI are infertile, whereas men with lower DFI (26%) can enable conception but with resultant RPL.[8] Environmental factors, such as occupational and chemical exposure, stress, alcohol, and radiation have also been reported to be associated with an increased risk of recurrent miscarriages.[4]

Evaluation of defects in endometrial receptivity with native techniques based on endocrine parameters and new techniques based on microRNAs, proteomics, and epigenetics may help to unravel the maternal causes of RPL.[9] Pregnancies obtained after IVF and embryo transfer (IVF-ET) are at increased risk for an adverse outcome compared with natural pregnancies. Special investigations in ART include evaluation for inhibin-A, day 11 total beta-hCG, CA-125, PGS/PGD, and aneuploidy testing.[10] PGD for aneuploidy screening (PGD-AS) post-fertilization by ART techniques in selected groups of patients may help to detect and, possibly, eliminate the majority of chromosomally abnormal embryos, thereby increasing the chance of a healthy pregnancy.[11]

Standard semen parameters are poor predictors of fertility potential. Owing to the role of sperm factors in early embryonic development, and evidence of a high DFI in patients with a RPL, evaluation of sperm DNA integrity in idiopathic RPL is a useful diagnostic and prognostic marker with clinical implications.[8] However, even after exhaustive investigation using the most modern techniques, the cause of RPL often remains elusive.

Therapy

PGD-A Fool Proof Technique?

PGS or PGD may be indicated in women with repeated fetal aneuploidy or in the older patient.[5] By screening embryos for structural and numerical chromosomal abnormalities and selecting only normal embryos for transfer, PGS was envisioned and applied as a therapeutic tool for improving implantation and live birth rates from IVF and providing a means of attenuating pregnancy loss in recurrent pregnancy loss patients.[12] Chapters 6 and 7 debate the role of PGS in RPL. The inevitable threat of misuse of PGS for nondisease traits makes it is essential to select the application of PGS depending on the likelihood of an embryonic chromosome aberration. Preprocedure counseling is an integral part of the practice.[5]

Third Party Reproduction for RPL

Third party reproduction (TPR) involves the use of donor gametes (sperm or oocytes), embryos or surrogates by couples who may not be able to conceive with their own gametes or gestate a fetus, respectively.[13] Third party reproduction may be classified as

1. *Sperm donation.* The third party is a sperm donor, who provides sperm that can be used for insemination of the future mother or to fertilize an oocyte IVF with the transfer of the resulting embryo into the mother or a surrogate mother.

2. *Oocyte donation.* The third party is an oocyte donor, who donates oocytes for IVF with the transfer of the resulting embryo into the mother or a surrogate mother.

3. *Embryo donation.* The third party is an embryo donor, donating surplus embryos for use by a couple in need or a commissioned surrogate after the woman for whom they were originally created has successfully carried one or more pregnancies to term, or embryos specifically created for donation using donor eggs and donor sperm.

4. *Surrogacy.* The third party is a surrogate woman, used to carry a baby through pregnancy to term for a woman incapable of doing so.[13]

Sperm Donation for Recurrent Pregnancy Loss

Indications

Sperm donation may be indicated in severe male factor infertility due to: (i) a high risk of fertilization failure or two previous fertilization failures with conventional IVF. (ii) Semen parameters below the threshold for standard IVF treatment, for example, oligoasthenoteratozoospermia (OAT), severely oligozoospermic and teratozoospermic men (strict normal sperm morphology ≤5%) with a very high (>70%) frequency of defective sperm-ZP interaction and hence, a high risk of a low or zero fertilization rate in IVF. Severely impaired spermatogenesis (nonobstructive azoospermia), severe oligozoospermia and

OAT often have a genetic origin that necessitates sperm donation.[14] (iii) The absence of acrosomes or the presence of immotile spermatozoa. (iv) Genetic disorders such as Klinefelter's syndrome 47, XXY. (v) Sperm autoimmunity (high titers of antisperm antibodies/sperm-bound antibodies that interfere with gamete interaction).[14] (vi) When PGD is indicated in pregnancies that are at high risk of aneuploidy because of genetic factors associated with azoospermia, to avoid contamination by extraneous DNA in the case of PCR-based testing and to increase the number of embryos available for testing.[14]

Role of Sperm Donation

These factors usually present as infertility rather than RPL. However, if patients with RPL present with the above criteria, sperm donation may be indicated. Additionally, if DNA analyses from men with a history of RPL have a high percentage of DNA damage with a sperm DFI of 26% or above, sperm donation may be indicated. The question arises whether sperm donation is indicated in idiopathic RPL. In couples with a good prognosis, sperm donation is not indicated. The literature differs with regard to sperm aneuploidy. No increased incidence of aneuploidy or structural anomalies was found in the sperm of men whose partners had RPL above the level seen in normally fertile men.[15] Additionally, Carp et al.[16] have reported 99 parental chromosomal aberrations in RM, 55 maternal, 43 paternal, and one in both partners. However, Rubio et al.[17] analyzed 12 sperm samples from IVF couples with two or more miscarriages. Diploidy and disomy were assessed for chromosomes 13, 18, 21, X, and Y using fluorescence *in situ* hybridization. Sex chromosome disomy from RM significantly increased compared to controls (0.84% vs. 0.37%). Additionally, increases in disomy have been related to increased aneuploidy in the offspring.[18] The editor has described that in the Tel Hashomer registry, there were 62 cases of a change in the male partners of 1925 patients, 22 had three partners and one had five partners. In these cases, a change of the male partner had not alleviated the problem of RPL. Therefore, sperm donation should probably be limited to the indications above. Additionally, there is no series in literature on sperm donation in RPL.

Oocyte Donation

Indications

Oocyte donation may be indicated in: (i) carriers of genetic disorders, for example, 46, XY pure gonadal dysgenesis, Turner's syndrome (45, XO); (ii) repeated IVF failure with autologous oocytes; (iii) advanced maternal age; (iv) contraindications for spontaneous or induced ovulation, such as those with von Willebrand's disease.[19] Of these, advanced maternal age is the major indication in RPL.

Experience with Oocyte Donation for RPL

Simón et al.[20] reported that in 92 cycles of ovum donation, there were 64 implantations, 30 (32.6%) viable pregnancies, and 34 (37.0%) miscarriages. In Remohi et al.'s series, ovum donation was performed in eight RPL couples, in which the woman was a low responder to gonadotropins. Twelve cycles were performed. There was a 75% pregnancy rate and a delivery rate of 66.6%. The miscarriage rate was 11.1% per cycle. The authors suggested that the oocyte may be the origin of infertility in women with idiopathic recurrent miscarriages.[21] In their study, patients were down regulated with gonadotropin-releasing hormone analogs and supplemented with estradiol valerate for a minimum of 15 days until fertilized embryos from donor oocytes were transferred in IVF. Then, progesterone was added until day 100 of pregnancy. The results of oocyte donation compared favorably with low responders without a history of recurrent abortion undergoing this treatment during the study period. However, the live birth rates need to be compared to the spontaneous live birth rates for the patient's age and number of miscarriages.[21]

Issues with Oocyte Donation

Although oocyte donation is a successful option for achieving conception in these patients, the high risk of complications associated with pregnancies thus obtained, especially in women with genetic disorders and advanced maternal age, makes strict criteria for the selection of such patients and rigid protocols for the medical management of such pregnancies an absolute requirement.[19] For instance, although patients with Turner's syndrome may achieve high pregnancy rates, comparable to those observed in patients with other indications requiring oocyte donation, high miscarriage rates, potentially severe cardiovascular complications during pregnancy and early implantation failure often ensue. These complications may possibly be associated with a deficiency of X-linked genes regulating endometrial receptivity, and a subsequent high rate of cesarean section is commonly observed.[19]

Third party reproduction through oocyte donation is a long and labor intensive process with a significant amount of emotional, financial and physical involvement from all parties.[22] In order to ensure safety and success of the procedure, all the participants must be extensively screened medically and psychologically and a detailed understanding of the process by all parties involved should be achieved.[23] A written informed consent should be obtained from donors and recipients prior to commencing the program.

Embryo Donation

Indications

Embryo donation may be medically indicated in couples where both sperm and oocyte donation is mandatory to achieve a normal conception as in unexplained genetic disease and failure of ART due to poor fertilization or poor embryo quality. The embryos may be obtained from couples consenting to donate surplus embryos following self-use or specifically created by using a chosen sperm and oocyte donor.[13] Embryo donation may be offered as a viable treatment option in the event that all embryos are chromosomally abnormal following IVF-PGD/PGS. If pregnancies are miscarried despite the transfer of genetically normal embryos following IVF-PGD/PGS, there may be a role for embryo donation, but only if all the therapies for maternal causes of RPL have been exhausted.

Issues with Embryo Donation

Creation of embryos for therapy might fully be justified; however, wastage of surplus embryos, not intentionally created for future use, donation or research triggers ethical, legal, and moral issues that boil down to the moral status of the embryo. The main ethical issues concern the effect on offspring, consent and counseling of donors and recipients, avoidance of mixing embryos or gametes from different sources, and payment of donor expenses. The main legal issues concern whether embryo donation is viewed as gamete donation or adoption, the rearing rights and duties of donors and recipients in resulting offspring, liability, compensation issues, and the legality of monetary compensation for donors.[24]

Surrogacy

Surrogacy is a reproductive technology involving one woman (surrogate mother) carrying a child for another person(s) (commissioning person/couple), based on a mutual agreement requiring the child to be legally relinquished to the intended parent(s) or the commissioning couple/person following birth.[23] IVF allows the creation of embryos from the gametes of the commissioning couple and subsequent transfer of these embryos to the uterus of a surrogate host. Clinical pregnancy rates achieved in large series are up to 40% per transfer and series have reported live births in 60% of hosts.[25]

Indications

Apart from its indications in patients with congenital (Mayer–Rokitansky–Kuster–Hauser syndrome) or surgical absence of the uterus (hysterectomy) and various gynecological cancers, surrogacy may be offered as a treatment option in women with repeated IVF failure, high-order unexplained habitual abortions with a maternal cause, severe medical conditions, such as severe heart or renal disease, in which pregnancy is contraindicated or life-threatening, or following treatment for numerous oncological and nononcological conditions that result in uterine damage and poor reproductive outcomes.[23] Maternal causes of RPL that may benefit from surrogacy as a treatment option include autoimmune causes, anatomical uterine defects or Mullerian fusion defects following failed surgical correction and/or repeated miscarriage, advanced maternal age, and endocrine disorders that fail medical treatment. Oncological treatment for gynecologic cancers results in a reduction in the size of the uterus or possible damage of the uterine vasculature leading to decreased feto-placental blood flow. This may increase the risk for pregnancy-related complications, including spontaneous miscarriages, preterm labor and delivery, low birth weight infants, and placental abnormalities, and render these women unable to gestate, leaving surrogacy as the only option.[26] Surrogacy assumes that the embryo is normal and that the maternal environment needs to be substituted.[5]

Types of Surrogacy

Surrogacy may be of two types: (i) traditional surrogacy, where the surrogate or birth mother is also the oocyte donor, and hence, the genetic mother, and the intended father is the genetic father; pregnancy may be achieved by artificially inseminating the surrogate with the intended father's sperm; and (ii) gestational carrier surrogacy involving IVF, where the gametes from the intended parents or commissioning couple (the couple requesting surrogacy) are fertilized *in vitro* and the embryo transferred into the gestational carrier surrogate, who only "rents" the womb. In other words, the surrogate is not genetically linked to the child in any way. The child is legally adopted by the commissioning couple following delivery. While traditional surrogacy disables the genetic link between the intended mother and the child, gestational carrier surrogacy retains the genetic link with the offspring, retaining the surrogate as only the birth or gestational mother, unless the intended couple requires gamete donation or embryo donation.[13] Gestational carrier or IVF surrogacy, the most acceptable form of surrogacy practiced today, in contrast to traditional surrogacy, is largely complication-free without major ethical or legal complications with satisfactory treatment results and reassuring early results of the follow-up of children, commissioning couples and surrogates.[25]

In addition to the classification of surrogacy by parental roles, surrogacy can also be classified by financial compensation as (i) altruistic surrogacy that does not financially compensate the surrogate for her role apart from fees and costs associated with bringing an embryo to term and (ii) commercial surrogacy, which financially compensates a surrogate beyond expenses associated with the pregnancy, that is, the surrogate is paid for her gestational "services." Altruistic surrogacy is the most common among family members or close friends where the decision to be a surrogate stems from a willingness to help.[27]

Issues with Surrogacy

Surrogacy is, however, often beset with legal, social, ethical, and psychological complications. Some of the most significant problems that could result from improper surrogacy arrangements are: (i) failure to relinquish the baby immediately after birth; (ii) separation of a commissioning couple prior to treatment initiation; (iii) withdrawal of a patient from treatment following initial counseling of the implications of the treatment; (iv) poor response to follicular stimulation, particularly after Wertheim hysterectomy;[28] and (v) the possibility of the birth of a handicapped or genetically affected child and fear of rejection.[29] Hence, all the parties (commissioning couple, surrogate, and the gamete or embryo donor and recipients when employed) involved in a surrogacy arrangement should be bound by a surrogacy contract and thoroughly counselled on all the medical, legal, financial, ethical, and psychological aspects and risks and implications of the treatment. The implications of multiple pregnancy and the possibility that the surrogate host may spontaneously abort a pregnancy should be discussed with the commissioning couple prior to commencing the program. A written informed consent should be obtained from all third party participants.[23] Consents built upon effective lines of communication between clinical staff and legal counsel, assuring that parentage, relinquishment and recontact information in donor–recipient agreements are consistent with clinic consent documents, and desires of both parties are mandatory programs in all gamete donation. All decisions must be adequately documented and honored and long-term counseling needs should be addressed.[30] Prior to embarking on a surrogacy program, commissioning couples or alternatively, gamete donors, when employed, should be screened thoroughly to ensure that they do not transfer infection or a genetic disease to the offspring. Surrogates should likewise be screened and deemed physically, medically and psychologically fit to undertake the responsibility of carrying the pregnancy to term. The British Medical Association has adequately detailed issues for discussion with the commissioning couple and surrogate prior to signing a surrogacy contract.[22]

The guidelines for surrogacy, laid down by the "Guidelines for Accreditation, Supervision and Regulation of Art Clinics in India" include: (i) a child born through surrogacy must be adopted by the genetic (biological) parents unless they can establish through genetic (DNA) fingerprinting (of which the records will be maintained in the clinic) that the child is theirs; (ii) surrogacy by assisted conception should normally be considered only for patients for whom it would be physically or medically impossible/undesirable to carry a baby to term; (iii) payments to surrogate mothers should cover all genuine expenses associated with the pregnancy. Documentary evidence of the financial arrangement for surrogacy must be available. The ART center should not be involved in this monetary aspect; (iv) a surrogate mother should not be over 45 years of age. Before accepting a woman as a possible surrogate for a particular couple's child, the ART clinic must ensure (and put on record) that the woman satisfies all the testable criteria to go through a successful full-term pregnancy; (v) a relative, a known person, as well as a person unknown to the couple may act as a surrogate mother for the couple. In the case of a relative acting as a surrogate, the relative should belong to the same generation as the woman desiring the surrogate; (vi) a prospective surrogate mother must be tested for HIV and shown to be seronegative for this virus just before embryo transfer. She must also provide a written certificate that (a) she has not had a drug intravenously administered into her through a shared syringe; (b) she has not undergone blood transfusion; and (c) she and her husband (to the best of her/his knowledge) has had no extramarital relationship in the last 6 months. (This is to ensure that the person would not develop symptoms of HIV infection during the period of surrogacy.) The prospective surrogate mother must also declare that she will not use drugs intravenously, and not undergo blood transfusion excepting of blood obtained through a certified blood bank; and (vii) no woman may act as a surrogate more than thrice in her lifetime.[31]

Moreover, different interpretations of surrogacy in the various countries, based on their definition, application, social, religious and legal influences has complicated matters further, extending the practice across political borders and beyond judicial limits[23] necessitating a complete appraisal of the law of the land to protect all parties concerned and especially, the offspring to be.

Experience with Surrogacy for RPL

In 8 years' experience of an IVF surrogate gestational program, Raziel et al.[32] reported 33% and 12% pregnancy rates per patient and per transfer, respectively, in patients with IVF implantation failure, habitual abortions, and deteriorating maternal diseases, compared to 70% and 20%, respectively, in patients with Rokitansky syndrome and post-hysterectomy. The authors concluded that the existence or absence of the uterus in the commissioning mothers is irrelevant for their IVF performance and conception rates. In patients who conceived after more than three IVF cycles, an additional "oocyte factor" might be present.[32] Raziel et al.[33] reported a normal live birth in a patient with 24 prior pregnancy losses. The editor has advised surrogacy (unpublished) in a secondary aborter with 12 miscarriages, one primary aborter with six miscarriages and triplets of 25 weeks who died from prematurity, and a primary aborter with eight missed abortions including two euploid abortions, who continued miscarrying despite immunoglobulin therapy. In all three cases, the surrogate carrier delivered normal twins. The logic of surrogacy in patients with large numbers of miscarriages is due to the poor prognosis and low incidence of chromosomal aberrations.

Conclusion

Recurrent pregnancy loss is a frustrating and debilitating experience that leaves patients despairing and emotionally drained. Third party reproduction has a definite role to play in patents with a poor prognosis. Repeat aneuploidy following IVF-PGD/PGS may be an indication for third party reproduction with embryo donation if the maternal environment is supportive, or alternatively, surrogacy in patients with a maternal cause for recurrent miscarriage, such as a severe autoimmune disorder, which is resistant to treatment, and carrying a pregnancy is contraindicated. Oocyte donation may be offered as a treatment option in patients with exclusively maternal X-linked disorders without a related sperm chromosomal abnormality, advanced maternal age, and repeated failure with autologous oocytes, bearing in mind the future prognosis of the pregnancy, while sperm donation may an option in couples where the male partner has a sperm chromosomal abnormality. In balanced parental chromosome aberrations, it is uncertain which treatment mode is indicated.[5] However, ART with PGD/PGS or surrogacy may have a place only in those patients with a poor prognosis in whom ART will be shown to improve the subsequent live birth rate above the spontaneous rate.[5]

Individualizing the recurrence risk and building on an evidence-based approach in management and counselling should be the recommended clinical practice.[3] However, to date, there are no evidence-based trials. The patients who are selected for third party reproductive techniques are usually highly selected, and small in number. Hence, it has been impossible to devise a controlled trial of treatment.

REFERENCES

1. Jeve YB. Management of recurrent miscarriages. In: Arora S, Merchant R, Allahbadia GN, eds. *Reproductive Medicine: Challenges, Solutions and Breakthroughs*. New Delhi: Jaypee Brothers Medical Publishers Pvt Ltd; 2014. p. 443–52.
2. Coulam CB. Association between infertility and spontaneous abortion. *Am J Reprod Immunol* 1992;27:128–9.
3. Borrell A, Stergiotou I. Miscarriage in contemporary maternal-fetal medicine: Targeting clinical dilemmas. *Ultrasound Obstet Gynecol* 2013;42:491–7.
4. Leon S, Robert G, Nathan K. *Clinical Gynecologic Endocrinology and Infertility*. 6th edn. Baltimore: Lipincott Williams; 1999. p. 1044–52.
5. Carp HJA, Dirnfeld M, Dor J et al. ART in recurrent miscarriage: Preimplantation genetic diagnosis/screening or surrogacy? *Hum Reprod* 2004;19:1502–5.
6. Carp HJ. Recurrent miscarriage: Genetic factors and assessment of the embryo. *Isr Med Assoc J* 2008;10:229–31.
7. Deaton JL, Honore GM, Huffman CS et al. Early transvaginal ultrasonography following an accurately dated pregnancy: The importance of finding a yolk sac or fetal heart motion. *Hum Reprod* 1997;12:2820–3.
8. Kumar K, Deka D, Singh A et al. Predictive value of DNA integrity analysis in idiopathic recurrent pregnancy loss following spontaneous conception. *J Assist Reprod Genet* 2012;29:861–7.
9. Patel BG, Lessey BA. Clinical assessment and management of the endometrium in recurrent early pregnancy loss. *Semin Reprod Med* 2011;29:491–506.
10. Rai R, Tuddenham E, Backos M et al. Thromboelastography, whole-blood hemostasis and recurrent miscarriage. *Hum Reprod* 2003;18:2540–3.
11. Findikli N, Kahraman S, Saglam Y et al. Embryo aneuploidy screening for repeated implantation failure and unexplained recurrent miscarriage. *Reprod Biomed Online* 2006;13:38–46.
12. Go KJ, Patel JC, Cunningham DL. The role of assisted reproductive technology in the management of recurrent pregnancy loss. *Curr Opin Endocrinol Diabetes Obes* 2009;16:459–63.
13. Allahbadia G, Merchant R, Gandhi G. Third party reproduction: Current status and future. In: Dubey AK, ed. *Infertility: Diagnosis, Management and IVF*. New Delhi: Jaypee Brothers Medical Publishers Pvt Ltd; 2012. p. 370–91.
14. Merchant R, Gandhi G, Allahbadia GN. *In vitro* fertilization/intracytoplasmic sperm injection for male infertility. *Indian J Urol* 2011;27:121–32.
15. Rosenbusch B, Sterzik K. Sperm chromosomes and habitual abortion. *Fertil Steril* 1991;56:370–2.
16. Carp H, Feldman B, Oelsner G et al. Parental karyotype and subsequent live births in recurrent miscarriage. *Fertil Steril* 2004;81:1296–301.
17. Rubio C, Simón C, Blanco J et al. Implications of sperm chromosome abnormalities in recurrent miscarriage. *J Assist Reprod Genet* 1999;16:253–8.
18. Egozcue J, Blanco J, Vidal F. Chromosome studies in human sperm nuclei using fluorescence in-situ hybridization (FISH). *Hum Reprod Update* 1997;3:441–52.

19. Merchant R, Allahbadia GN. Can we define the indications for oocyte donation? In: Allahbadia GN, ed. *Donor Egg IVF*. New Delhi: Jaypee Brothers Medical Publishers Pvt Ltd; 2009. p. 11–9.
20. Simón C, Landeras J, Zuzuarregui JL et al. Early pregnancy losses in *in vitro* fertilization and oocyte donation. *Fertil Steril* 1999;72:1061–5.
21. Remohí J, Gallardo E, Levy M et al. Oocyte donation in women with recurrent pregnancy loss. *Hum Reprod* 1996;11:2048–51.
22. British Medical Association. *Changing Conceptions of Motherhood. The Practice of Surrogacy in Britain*. London: BMA Publications; 1996.
23. Merchant R, Allahbadia GN. Surrogacy: Ethical, psychological and legal implications. In: Allahbadia GN, ed. *Donor Egg IVF*. New Delhi: Jaypee Brothers Medical Publishers Pvt Ltd; 2009. p. 297–309.
24. Robertson JA. Ethical and legal issues in human embryo donation. *Fertil Steril* 1995;64:885–94.
25. Brinsden PR. Gestational surrogacy. *Hum Reprod Update* 2003;9:483–91.
26. Beski S, Gorgy A, Venkat G et al. Gestational surrogacy: A feasible option for patients with Rokitansky syndrome. *Hum Reprod* 2000;15:2326–8.
27. Meniru GI, Craft IL. Experience with gestational surrogacy as a treatment for sterility resulting from hysterectomy. *Hum Reprod* 1997;12:51–4.
28. Chang CL. Surrogate motherhood. *Formos J Med Humanit* 2004;5:48–62.
29. Balen AH, Hayden CA. British Fertility Society survey of all licensed clinics that perform surrogacy in the UK. *Hum Fertil* (Camb) 1998;1:6–9.
30. Lindheim SR, Porat N, Jaeger AS. Survey report of gamete donors' and recipients' preferences regarding disclosure of third party reproduction outcomes and genetic risk information. *J Obstet Gynaecol Res* 2011;37:292–9.
31. National Guidelines for Accreditation, Supervision and Regulation of ART Clinics in India. Indian Council of Medical Research, National Academy of Medical Sciences (India). 2005;68–69.
32. Raziel A, Schachter M, Strassburger D et al. Eight years' experience with an IVF surrogate gestational pregnancy programme. *Reprod Biomed Online* 2005;11:254–8.
33. Raziel A, Friedler S, Schachter M et al. Successful pregnancy after 24 consecutive fetal losses: Lessons learned from surrogacy. *Fertil Steril* 2000;74:104–6.

43

"Slippery Fetus": Recurrent Pregnancy Loss in Traditional Chinese Medicine

Aviv Messinger and Keren Sela

Introduction

Chinese medicine has a long history of gynecological references, dating back 2500 years. In the numerous canonical books, women's disorders have always received special attention in separate chapters dealing with specific diagnostic tools and treatment protocols using acupuncture and Chinese herbs to address common gynecological disorders. The clinical experience that evolved through the years and documented thoroughly in books, medical articles and passed on in clinics from Masters to disciples is the base upon which contemporary integrative Chinese medicine is now practiced. Throughout the decades and today, Chinese medicine in South East Asia is still the primary means of treatment for women's disorders.

In recent years, Chinese medicine has become popular in Western nations, leading to a novel approach, integrating the traditional knowledge and experience of the East with the research and technological advances of the West.

Chinese diagnosis is based on pattern discrimination formulated through clinical symptom and sign analysis. Diagnosis includes a thorough anamnesis encompassing the major complaint as well as a comprehensive and detailed inquiry of major systems such as digestive, urogenital, respiratory, cardio vascular, musculoskeletal, and more. Nutrition, stress management, sleep, physical exercise, and other health related factors are addressed as well. As cited in the article "Epidemiology of RPL" by Ole B Christiansen in the beginning of this book, factors such as obesity, overwork, stress, high consumption of alcohol or caffeine, frequent use of NSAIDS, infertility, and assistant reproductive techniques may be risk factors for recurrent pregnancy loss (RPL). Chinese medicine addresses these life habits.

In addition, a basic physical examination including pulse and tongue diagnosis and palpation are conducted. Together, all these lead the practitioner to formulate the basic patterns of disharmony and the treatment strategies.

The issue of recurrent pregnancy loss is described in all Chinese texts dealing with pregnancy disorders. Sun Si Miao—the famous Tang dynasty medical doctor—dedicated a chapter titled "Stirring Fetus and Repeated Miscarriages" in what is considered the first encyclopedic medical text dated to the seventh century AD.[1] In it, he describes six different herbal remedies given for habitual miscarriage, according to the specific symptoms and signs.

Fu Qing Zhu, a Qing dynasty practitioner, wrote the most important premodern gynecological text in which a chapter titled "small birth" describes five possible ethnologies for miscarriage and suggests appropriate treatment.[2]

Chinese medicine uses unique terminology to describe physiology and pathology. There is great emphasis on the interrelationship between different internal organs and functions. A healthy reproductive system relies on the optimal function of all other bodily systems. It is not uncommon to address gynecological disorders through treatment of digestive, cardiovascular, or mental emotional factors.

In this review, we will characterize the different Chinese syndromes and suggest possible herbal formularies as a mode of treatment. It is important to note that Chinese herbs need to be dispensed by a qualified Chinese herbalist within the framework of a complete treatment. The existing knowledge about the safety of these herbs during pregnancy is not complete and, as of date, we have no knowledge whether these herbs affect the embryo via the placental blood stream. Some qualified Chinese herbal practitioners choose to treat before pregnancy while others continue the use of herbs during the first trimester or in later stages of pregnancy. In either case, it is important to assure excellent quality of herbs from a known source that stand up to the highest safety regulations in each country. The availability of herbs may differ from country to country, depending on specific regulations.

Research into Chinese Medicine for RPL

The use of Chinese herbal medicines during pregnancy and postpartum is common in the Chinese community. A Taiwanese population-based cohort study[3] showed that 33.6% of pregnant women consumed herbal remedies. Women with a history of recurrent abortions were found to use more Chinese herbal medicines than others in the sample.

Despite the vast clinical experience, qualitative research regarding Chinese medicine treatment for RPL is limited and scanty. The few relevant studies described briefly below suggest possible mechanisms of action of Chinese herbs to prevent RPL.

There are, however, numerous studies regarding Chinese medicine and related topics to RPL, such as threatened miscarriage, implantation, polycystic ovarian syndrome (PCOS), endometriosis, and infertility, which show the efficacy of acupuncture and Chinese herbs in increasing implantation and ongoing pregnancy rates, and suggest possible mechanisms of action of Chinese medicine in regards to RPL.

Possible Mechanisms of Action of Chinese Herbal Remedies for RPL

Preliminary mice model studies of Chinese herbal remedies for RPL have shown different immunological influences as described below. These studies suggest possible biochemical mechanism of action of herbs. Lee et al. showed that the Korean herbal remedy, Cho Kyung Jong Ok Tang, induces type 2 shift in mice natural killer (NK) cells cytokine production that may explain the protective effect associated with its traditional use in unexplained RPL.[4] Lai et al. studied the frequently used Shou Tai Wan Pill for RPL and found that middle and high doses of the pills may shift Th1/Th2 cytokine towards Th2 bias, resulting in maternal–fetal immune tolerance.[5]

Nagamatsu et al.[6] researched the possible mechanism of action of a herbal remedy composed of two separate herbal formulas. They found that the Japanese herbal remedies Tokishakuyaku-San and Sairei-To enhanced the release of granulocyte–macrophage colony-stimulating factor, a cytokine working as an important mediator for intercellular communication in the embryonic development, in decidual stromal cells (DSCs). Fujii suggested that the clinical effect of these herbal medicines can be explained by enhancing Th1 cytokine release from peripheral blood mononuclear cells (PBMCs) and by suppressing the production of autoantibodies from B-cells.[7]

The same basic Japanese herbal remedy was studied by Kano et al. in a group of 61 women with antinuclear antibody (ANA) and anticardiolipin antibody (ACLA) positive recurrent spontaneous abortion.[8] The results showed a reduction of antibody titers and abortion rates following the use of the remedy.

These promising preliminary studies can be a foundation for identifying the complex pathways by which Chinese herbs may affect maternal–fetal immune tolerance.

Chinese Medicine for Threatened Miscarriage

The topic of threatened miscarriage can also shed light on RPL as similar Chinese herbal remedies are utilized in both cases. A Cochrane Review published in 2012 concluded that a combination of Chinese herbal and Western medicines was more effective than Western medicines alone for treating threatened miscarriage.[9] There is, however, insufficient evidence to assess the effectiveness of Chinese herbal medicines when used alone for treating threatened miscarriage.

Recently, a systematic review and meta-analysis was published by Li et al. in which they attempted to identify and describe adverse events of Chinese medicines when used for threatened miscarriage.[10] The meta-analysis demonstrated that loss of pregnancy was significantly lower in the combined Chinese medicines groups than in the Western medicines controls. No significant differences were found between these groups for adverse effects and toxicity or for adverse pregnancy and perinatal outcomes.

The quality, however, of the included studies in both reviews was poor and more high quality studies are necessary to further evaluate the effectiveness and toxicity of Chinese herbal medicines for threatened miscarriage.

Acupuncture for Threatened Miscarriage

Acupuncture is another major branch of Chinese medicine that is commonly used in cases of threatened miscarriage. As we will present later in this article, within fertility research, acupuncture demonstrates beneficial hormonal responses with decreased miscarriage rates, raising the possibility acupuncture may promote specific beneficial effects in early pregnancy. Due to lack of recommended medical treatment options for threatened miscarriage, acupuncture may have treatment benefits.[11]

Possible Mechanism of Action of Acupuncture

Traditionally, the field of gynecology in Chinese medicine was dominated by herbal medicine. Acupuncture protocols for women's disorders were later developed and assimilated into contemporary Chinese medicine.

The efficacy of acupuncture as an adjunctive treatment in infertility, endometriosis,[12] PCOS,[13] and *in vitro* fertilization (IVF),[14–16] as well as pregnancy related issues, such as nausea and vomiting,[17] pelvic girdle pain,[18] labor induction,[19] etc., have been investigated in numerous studies. The possible mechanisms of action of acupuncture derived from these studies may explain how acupuncture may prevent and assist in the treatment of RPL. Acupuncture may influence the secretion of gonadotropins via its effect on endogenous opioid peptides in the central nervous system, especially β-endorphin. Their action on GnRH and LH modulates the hypothalamus–pituitary–ovarian (HPO) axis.[20] In addition, acupuncture may modulate the hypothalamus–pituitary–adrenal axis, glucose and adipokine metabolism, and insulin secretion.[21,13]

Acupuncture affects uterine blood flow. It has been demonstrated that acupuncture can reduce uterine arterial blood flow impedance in infertile women,[22] which may explain the efficacy of acupuncture in increasing the implantation rate in IVF. Manheimer et al. published two reviews on the influence of acupuncture on IVF outcomes.[14,15] In 2008, a meta-analysis concluded that acupuncture increases clinical pregnancy and live birth rate. The updated Cochrane review from 2013 claimed that acupuncture had no effect. The difference between the two databases may be due to the inclusion of studies using several different sham acupuncture procedures in the 2013 database. As sham acupuncture has not been demonstrated to be inert, the ideal control group intervention in acupuncture studies has yet to be developed.

Chinese Clinical Experience and Differential Diagnosis of RPL

Modern integrative Chinese medicine indicates six fundamental syndromes corresponding to RPL.[23,24] The syndromes listed below summarize the essential clinical picture based on symptoms and signs, including tongue and pulse. Often these syndromes encompass specific medical diseases, as listed below.

1. Name of Syndrome: Qi and Blood Deficiency

Description and Etiology

Lack of nutrition and/or poor absorption leading to the weak uterine holding capacity of the fetus, which may result in RPL.

Clinical Symptoms and Signs

Repeated spontaneous abortions, scanty menstruation or amenorrhea, fatigue, general weakness, lassitude of spirit, dizziness, palpitations, insomnia, weak appetite, irregular bowel movements, and sallow complexion. Tongue is pale and pulse overall weak and deep.

Possible Western Diagnosis

Anemia, hypothyroid, malnutrition or eating disorders, anxiety.

Proposed Treatment: *Tai Shan Pan Shi San* (泰山盤石散)

Radix ginseng, Radix astragali, Radix angelica sinensis, Radix dipsaci, Radix scutellaria, Radix ligustici wallichii, Radix albus paeoniae lactiflorae, cooked Radix rhemannia, Rhizome atractylodis macrocephalae, Radix glycerrhizae, Fructus amomii, glutinous rice.

Remarks

Treatment must include lifestyle changes, such as nutritional recommendations, mild physical exercise, and adequate sleep.

2. Name of Syndrome: Liver and Kidney Yin Deficiency

Description and Etiology

Aging, enduring disease, long-term consumption of medication or drugs, long term stress or anxiety affect the quality of embryos leading to possible increased fragmentation and DNA mutations. Nourishment of the uterus is affected which may result in RPL.

Clinical Symptoms and Signs

Repeated spontaneous abortions, oligo-menorrhea, dry mouth and thirst, hot flushes, night sweat, insomnia, irritability, constipation, weak and sore low back and knees. Tongue is red, dry and has scanty fur and pulse is weak, rapid and thin.

Possible Western Diagnosis

Poor ovarian reserve, peri-menopause, hyperthyroid, autoimmune disorders, diabetes, stress.

Proposed Treatment: *Er Zhi Wan Jia Wei* (二至丸)

Fructus ligustri lucidi, Herba ecliptae, uncooked Radix rhemannia, Radix albus paeoniae lactiflorae, Radix scutellaria, Radix dioscoreae, Herba taxilli, Semen cuscutae, Radix dipsaci, Rhizome cimicifuga.

3. Name of Syndrome: Spleen and Kidney Qi and Yang Deficiency

Description and Etiology

Long term taxation and exhaustion, aging, enduring disease, long term consumption of medication or drugs result in exhaustion of the endocrine system affecting its ability to nourish and sustain a pregnancy. According to Chinese medicine physiology, the main component of this syndrome is the presence of internal or external cold that weakens and blocks the axis of endocrine communication.

Clinical Symptoms and Signs

Repeated spontaneous abortions, menstrual irregularities, edema, cold sensations, fatigue, lack of strength, loose stools, abdominal distension, pallor, weak and sore low back and knees, polyurea. Tongue is pale and swollen and pulse is weak, rapid and thin.

Possible Western Diagnosis

Adrenal and/or thyroid exhaustion, luteal phase insufficiency, chronic fatigue syndrome, severe anemia.

Proposed Treatment: Bu Shen Gu Chong Wan (補腎固衝丸)

Semen cuscutae, Radix dipsaci, Cortex eucommiae, cooked Radix rhemannia, Radix morindae officinalis, Cornu cervi degelatinatium, Radix angelica sinensis, Gelatinium corii asini, Fructus lycii, Radix codonopsitis pilosulae, Rhizome atractylodis macrocephalae, Fructus amomii, Fructus zizyphi jujubae.

Remarks

This syndrome requires warming techniques, such as moxibustion, warming nutrition, and avoiding exposure to cold.

4. Name of Syndrome: Stasis and Stagnation

Description and Etiology

Inhibited blood flow hinders the free and smooth transportation of nutrients and hormones to the target organs. Impaired blood flow may cause accumulation of toxins and oxidative factors leading to a higher tendency towards inflammation and pain and therefore a higher rate of RPL.

Clinical Symptoms and Signs

Repeated spontaneous abortions, severe dysmenorrhea, irregular menstrual cycle, dark menstrual blood with clots, mittleschmertz, chest, breast or rib side distention and pain, headaches, angry outbursts, type A personality. Tongue is dark purplish with distended under veins and pulse is strong, wiry, or tight.

Possible Western Diagnosis

Endometriosis, adenomyosis, clotting disorders, autoimmune diseases, hypertension, irritable bowel syndrome, trauma.

Proposed Treatment: Shao Fu Zhu Yu Tang (少腹逐郁汤)

Fructus foeniculi vulgaris, Rhizome zingiberis officinalis, Rhizome corydalis yanhusuo, Radix angelica sinensis, Radix ligustici wallichii, Myrrha, Cortex cinnamomi loureiroi, Radix rubrae paeoniae, Pollen typhae, Excrementum trogopteri seu pteromi.

Remarks

Physical activity to promote circulation is recommended. Use of antioxidants and avoidance of external toxins are beneficial.

The use of "blood invigorating" herbs is not recommended during pregnancy. This formula is to taken before pregnancy occurs and needs to be modified accordingly once the patient is pregnant.

5. Name of Syndrome: Accumulation of Fluids –"Damp and Phlegm"

Description and Etiology

Impaired metabolism of fluids can lead to accumulation of "phlegm" that thickens the mucous membranes in the body. Polycystic ovaries, fertility drugs and steroids can all aggravate the accumulation of fluids in the endometrium thus impairing implantation. PCOS is considered a risk factor for RPL as mentioned in Chapter 1 of this book. In ancient Chinese texts, this condition was referred to as "slippery fetus."

Clinical Symptoms and Signs

Repeated spontaneous abortions, overweight or obesity, possible profuse phlegm production and vaginal discharge, abdominal bloating, gastro intestinal disorders. Tongue is swollen and flabby with thick coating and pulse is slippery or full.

Possible Western Diagnosis

PCOS, diabetes, obesity, candidiasis.

Proposed Treatment: Chai Hu Ling Tang (柴胡苓汤)

Radix bupleuri, Rhizoma alismatis, Rhizoma pinelliae, Hoelen, Polyporus umbellatus, Rhizome atractylodes macrocephalae, Radix scutellariae, Radix panax ginseng, Radix glycyrrhizae, Ramulus cinnamomi cassiae, Zingiberis rhizoma, Jujubae fructus.

Remarks

A well-balanced sugar, gluten, and dairy free diet are a part of treatment.

6. Name of Syndrome: Bao Mai Disconnection

Description and Etiology

The Bao represents the emotional and mental connection between the chest area, house of the spirit and mind in Chinese thought, and the uterus. This reciprocal communication is essential for the proper function of all reproductive organs. According to Chinese medicine, mental and emotional well being is an important factor in proper endocrine function. As body and mind are connected and interdependent it is possible to affect the emotional factors via the physical body, and vice versa.

Clinical Symptoms and Signs

Anxiety, panic attacks, sleep disorders, chest pain and distention, palpitations, frequent vivid dreams, menstrual disorders, dyspareunia. Tongue and pulse differ according to additional symptoms.

Possible Western Diagnosis

Emotional and psychological trauma, sexual abuse, anxiety, phobias, memory of previous miscarriages.

Proposed Treatment: Tao Hong Si Wu Tang Jia Wei (桃紅四物湯)

Radix ligustici wallichii, Radix angelica sinensis, cooked Radix rhemannia, Radix albus paeoniae lactiflorae, Semen persica, Flos carthami tinctorii, Cortex albizziae julibrissin, Radix salvia miltiorrhizae, Radix polygalae tenuifoliae, Caulis polygoni multiflori, Fructus schizandrae chinensis.

Remarks

Integration of physiological counselling and body mind therapies, such as fertility yoga, Qi Gong, or Tai Qi are recommended.

Conclusion

The treatment of RPL in Chinese medicine has been developed over the centuries and is based on clinical practice. Evidence of efficacy of acupuncture and Chinese herbs has been gaining momentum in recent studies. Research on related topics that have been mentioned above imply that Chinese traditional therapies may influence RPL via the central nervous system, especially the HPO axis and uterine blood flow. Further high quality research is needed to establish the role of Chinese medicine and its mechanisms of action in the treatment of RPL.

Acupuncture is considered to be a safe modality of treatment and has little to no adverse side effects.[25,26] Specifically, acupuncture has been studied in various phases of pregnancy for the treatment of implantation of embryos, nausea and vomiting, pelvic girdle pain, labor induction, and pain relief during labor. In none of these studies were any maternal or obstetric negative side effects recorded.[27–31] In light of the potential efficacy and safety of Chinese medicine, acupuncture and herbal medicine should be considered as a useful adjunct to conventional treatment for RPL.

REFERENCES

1. Qian BJ, Fang JY. *Sun Si Miao*. Trans Wilms S. Chinese Medicine Database. 2008; Volume 2–4. p. 132–6.
2. Zhu FQ. *Gynaecology*. Trans Yang SZ, Liu DW. Boulder: Blue Poppy Press; 1996. p. 79–86.
3. Chuang CH, Chang PJ, Hsieh WS et al. Chinese herbal medicine use in Taiwan during pregnancy and the postpartum period: A population-based cohort study. *Int J Nurs Stud* 2009;46:787–95.
4. Lee HS, Cho KH, Kim TK et al. A traditional Korean herbal formula induces type 2 shift in murine natural killer cell cytokine production. *J Ethnopharmacol* 2011;134:281–7.
5. Lai M, You Z, Ma H et al. Effects of shoutai pills on expression of Th1/Th2 cytokine in maternal-fetal interface and pregnancy outcome. *Zhongguo Zhong Yao Za Zhi* 2010;35:3065–8.
6. Nagamatsu T, Fujii T, Matsumoto J et al. Theoretical basis for herbal medicines, Tokishakuyaku-San and Sairei-To, in the treatment of recurrent abortion: Enhancing the production of granulocyte-macrophage colony-stimulating factor in decidual stromal cells. *Am J Reprod Immunol* 2007;57:287–93.
7. Fujii T. Herbal factors in the treatment of autoimmunity-related habitual abortion. *Vitam Horm* 2002;65:333–44.
8. Kano T, Shimizu M, Kanda T. Differences in individual efficacy of two Sairei-to preparations (Sojyutu-Sairei-to and Byakujyutu-Sairei-to) on recurrent spontaneous abortions of autoimmune etiologies evaluated by antinuclear antibody and anticardiolipin antibody titers. *Am J Chin Med* 2010;38:27–36.
9. Li L, Dou L, Leung PC et al. Chinese herbal medicines for threatened miscarriage. *Cochrane Database Syst Rev* 2012;CD008510.
10. Li L, Dou LX, Neilson JP et al. Adverse outcomes of Chinese medicines used for threatened miscarriage: A systematic review and meta-analysis. *Hum Reprod Update* 2012;18:504–24.
11. Betts D, Smith CA, Hannah DG. Acupuncture as a therapeutic treatment option for threatened miscarriage. *BMC Complement Altern Med* 2012;12:20.
12. Rubi-Klein K, Kucera-Sliutz E, Nissel H et al. Is acupuncture in addition to conventional medicine effective as pain treatment for endometriosis? RCT cross-over trial. *Eur J Obstet Gynecol Reprod Biol* 2010;153:90–3.
13. Johansson J, Stener-Victorin E. Polycystic ovary syndrome: Effect and mechanisms of acupuncture for ovulation induction. *Evid Based Complement Alternat Med* 2013;2013:762615.
14. Manheimer E, Zhang G, Udoff L et al. Effects of acupuncture on IVF outcome: Systematic review and meta-analysis BMJ 2008;336:545–9.
15. Manheimer E, van der Windt D, Cheng K, Stafford K, Liu J, Tierney J et al. The effects of acupuncture on rates of clinical pregnancy among women undergoing *in vitro* fertilization: A systematic review and meta-analysis. *Hum Reprod Update* 2013;19:696–713.
16. Paulus WE, Zhang M, Strehler E et al. Influence of acupuncture on the pregnancy rate in patients who undergo ART. *Fertil Steril* 2002;77:721–4.
17. Smith C, Crowther C, Beilby J. Vomiting in early pregnancy: A randomized controlled trial. *Birth* 2002;29:1–9.
18. Elden H, Ladfors L, Olsen MF et al. Effect of acupuncture and stabilizing exercises as adjunct to standard treatment in pregnant women with pelvic girdle pain: Randomized single blind controlled trial. *BMJ* 2005;330:761.
19. Smith CA, Collins CT, Crowther CA et al. Acupuncture for induction of labor. *Cochrane Database Syst Rev* 2013;CD002962.
20. Chang R, Chung PH, Rosenwak Z. Role of acupuncture in the treatment of female infertility. *Fertil Steril* 2002;78:1149–53.
21. Magarelli PC, Cridennda DK, Cohen M. Changes in Serum cortisol and prolactin associated with acupuncture during controlled ovarian hyperstimulation in women undergoing *in vitro* fertilization embryo transfer treatment. *Fertil Steril* 2009;92:1870–9.

22. Stener-Victorin E, Waldenström U, Andersson SA et al. Reduction of blood flow impedance in the uterine arteries of infertile women with electro-acupuncture. *Hum Reprod* 1996;11:1314–7.

23. Flaws B. *Chinese Medical Obstetrics*. Boulder: Blue Poppy Press; 2005. p. 83–92.

24. Sela K, Saslove Y, Benjamin T et al. *The Clinical Guide of Chinese Gynaecology and Obstetrics* (in Hebrew). Tel Aviv: Sinteza Publications; 2011. p. 126–7.

25. Ernst E, White AR, Prospective studies of the safety of acupuncture: A systematic review. *Am J Med* 2001;110:481–5.

26. MacPherson H, Thomas K, Walters S et al. A prospective survey of adverse events and treatment reactions following 34,000 consultations with professional acupuncturists. *Acupunct Med* 2001;19:93–102.

27. Elden H, Ostgaard HC, Fagevik-Olsen M et al. Treatments of pelvic girdle pain in pregnant women: Adverse effects of standard treatment, acupuncture and stabilising exercises on the pregnancy, mother, delivery and the fetus/neonate. *BMC Complement Altern Med* 2008;8:34.

28. Wedenberg K, Moen B, Norling A. A prospective randomized study comparing acupuncture with physiotherapy for low-back and pelvic pain in pregnancy. *Acta Obstet Gynecol Scand* 2000;79:331–5.

29. Carlsson CP, Axemo P, Bodin A et al. Manual acupuncture reduces hyperemesis gravidarum: A placebo-controlled, randomized, single-blind, crossover study. *J Pain Symptom Manage* 2000;20:273–9.

30. Knight B, Mudge C, Openshaw S et al. Effect of acupuncture on nausea of pregnancy: A randomized, controlled trial. *Obstet Gynecol* 2001;97:184–8.

31. Kvorning N, Holmberg C, Grennert L et al. Acupuncture relieves pelvic and low-back pain in late pregnancy. *Acta Obstet Gynecol Scand* 2004;83:246–50.

44

A Patient's Perspective

Mindy Gross

I had six miscarriages in less than 3 years. In retrospect, this seems to be a physical impossibility. Although each miscarriage stands starkly alone in my mind, having six of them in such a short span of time produced a cumulative effect. Each presented me with peculiar challenges and carried its own unique message. On each occasion, I was in a different hospital either in America or in Israel, with different doctors and different walls to witness my misery. It was natural to begin getting that deja vu feeling, "haven't I been here before?" Yet, when I looked around, I was forced to admit that—"no, I had never been *here* before." Looking back, it seems as if each miscarriage demanded its own identity, its own space in my brain. Each refused to be lumped together with the others.

In retrospect, I had undergone six different and distinct losses. One might think that the loss becomes easier or at least less painful with each successive miscarriage. It does not. On the contrary, the physical pain is as fresh and as potent each time. The emotional suffering involved in the loss only increases. It has been said that humans can acclimate themselves to the most horrendous of circumstances; the "getting used to it" impulse seems to be very strong. This was not the case. I never got used to losing a nascent child.

Though each time I was more prepared on a practical level, I was never prepared on an emotional level. Each miscarriage came as a shock, though the physical symptoms often repeated themselves. The initial trouble always began suddenly, without warning a stain would appear. Foolishly, I would think, "could I just wish it away—make believe it didn't exist?" As the sharp pains in my back and cramping increased, I started to ramble, "could I have a nervous breakdown simultaneously with a miscarriage?" The hemorrhaging was merciless and as was now my custom, I grabbed some towels and headed to the car to take me to the hospital.

I had felt pregnant. I had experienced the morning sickness that seemed to last the whole day. Now I wish I had not. At least I would have been spared the pain of feeling the symptoms disappear. I was filled to the brim with disappointment. Miscarriage is a death, though perhaps not acknowledged as such by the world outside of the family who have suffered the loss. At the time of my miscarriages, I could not articulate this feeling, but it was very real. I was frightened by the fragility of life. I knew that I had experienced a touch of death, for something had died within me.

The trauma of miscarriage stems from lost hope that was so briefly, and so very vividly alive. For all of the frustration of infertility, it is one dimensional, monochromatic—negative, negative, negative, void and nothingness. Miscarriage by contrast is multichromatic. You have hope and a life inside you, and then it is lost, both the child and the hope. Surprisingly, I found that I never became jaded. No matter how many losses, each conception reawakened in me the belief that this time it was going to be different.

The assumption that children will arrive soon or easily, or at least whenever the couple desires them, is a normal assumption, but also a very dangerous one. My family and friends have children. They do not have miscarriages. So, although I may have known intellectually that miscarriages are not that uncommon, my unexpected complications were not part of my every day consciousness. Infertility and miscarriage are unfortunate things that happen to "other people." As it was too painful to imagine these difficulties in our own lives, when they did occur, I found that I was at a total loss. As the effects of one miscarriage seemed to spill over into the next miscarriage, one truth pervaded my thoughts, I was still barren.

Barren. What a horrible word. It conjures up images of the American southwest, of Arizona and Georgia O'Keeffe's paintings. One of O'Keeffe's favorite motifs is a dry horse's skull sitting on the desert's sand. No signs of life there. Some of the most wretched terrain on earth, incapable of creating and sustaining life. Barren. What a pitiful way to hear oneself described. The label "fruitless" was so contrary to the way I had perceived myself my whole life. I was always very fruitful, I was a producer. Now I was deficient. I did not have what it takes to "produce" in the most valuable of all endeavors, conceiving a child and sustaining a pregnancy.

Bitter. A word I never had an affinity for. Bittersweet chocolate is, to me, a very poor substitute for the real thing: gooey milk chocolate. Bitter implies something unappealing and most certainly not the ideal. Over the span of my years of infertility and often agonizing tests, I asked myself, "was I becoming bitter?" I resolved with all my heart that this was one sentiment that would have no place in my vocabulary. Bitterness was a particularly astringent emotion. One whose intensity I felt would be better put to use on other needs and emotions, particularly at such a sensitive time in my life. Bitterness twists one's core personality and corrodes a person's resources and strengths. I was concerned that becoming bitter would have held me back from full participation in and enjoyment of the births of my nieces and nephews as well as countless friends. It would have constricted my own flow of love and giving when that is, indeed, what I needed to do most.

All I wanted was to have a normal life. After having been married for 7 years and wanting children, "normal" by definition would mean a baby in my arms. Other women I know who have suffered pregnancy losses have also remarked that they too just wanted their lives to be "normal." I craved the ordinary, the mundane tasks of motherhood, but they continued to elude me. I also felt confused. I had not heard much about miscarriages before and even if they were relatively commonplace, they were not part of my lexicon. I read a book about women suffering from multiple miscarriages, which I could strongly relate to. Friedman and Gradstin in their book, "Surviving Pregnancy Loss" write: "when you lost your first pregnancy, everyone told you not to worry, it happens to a lot of people. Remember, you are young and healthy and have lots of time to have babies." But the authors continue, "other women have babies so easily; why not you? Lightening is not supposed to strike twice in the same place, and certainly not three or four times."

My earlier difficulties with conception often left me with a very frightening thought: "what if I never conceive?" With the miscarriages, I knew my situation was different. Somehow, I believed that in most cases when a woman conceives again and again, the likelihood is that sooner or later a pregnancy should sustain itself. I would periodically remind myself that there were women I knew who never even had the good fortune of having a hope to cling to. Yet, a nagging doubt was lodged in my consciousness and a subtle fear accompanied me wherever I went. My fear was based on the lesson that the miscarriages had taught me. Human existence is very fragile. There are no guarantees.

My body was out of control. First, it refused my command to become pregnant and then it refused to hold on to the pregnancy. As my infertility problems were unexpected, as until now I was a healthy female specimen, this bizarre turn of events caused me to lose my balance. I was young, athletic, never smoked, and only had an occasional glass of wine. Why was my body failing me? I felt that I was twirling in an almost dizzy fashion. Not only was my body out of control, but my life seemed to be spiraling in a direction I could not identify. Once the possibility of childlessness entered my mind, it never departed. It lurked in the shadows of my brain pushing to the fore at the most unexpected moments. Just when I was enjoying myself, actively engaged in the world around me, the sinking feeling would come rushing back: *I may never, ever give birth to a child. I may never, ever be a natural biological mother.* Paralysis seeped in. It was as if my body froze and my mind locked. Everything was now out of control. I would try to push the ugly thoughts out and concentrate on my life. I focused on my career, my family, my community and friends. But the thoughts were still there. The harsh fact of my being a "habitual aborter" lingered on and on. It aggressively invaded my consciousness and colored my perception of the world. In fact, the cumulative experiences of years of infertility and failed pregnancy had shaken me to my core. My world had suddenly become a whirlwind of intense and mighty emotions. Hope and despair would rage. I found that in the midst of my mundane activities, I was now insecure and frightened. Some of these emotions I felt quite powerfully for the first time in my life. I was distraught and disillusioned. The world had turned bleary.

On a particularly overcast and gloomy day in New York, I entered Brooks Brothers Department Store. Suddenly, I had an overwhelming need to buy a personal diary. The pocket diary I found was maroon and leather and was a present to myself, a consolation prize for bearing circumstances that would crumble many a strong individual. The gold leafed diary cost more than the budget would normally allow, even if it did bear the distinguished Brooks Brothers insignia. I distinctly remember the day that I bought it. I had been diagnosed with a "grapefruit size" ovarian cyst, the latest mishap in my uncontrollable reproductive system. I was nothing less than frenzied with my cyst surgery looming. With the diary in hand, I hurried to the corner of an enormous Hallmark card store in Manhattan and opened it to the back page. With a burning need, I wrote down the dates, locations, and treatments of the miscarriages. I also included the upcoming appointments, date of my cyst surgery, and all the various treatments I had undergone since the onset of my infertility problems. What if this information would be important some day? How would I remember all the details if I did not record it somewhere? My response to all my suffering at that time was the emotional equivalent of the diary's blank pages. I was silenced. No words could ever convey the emptiness I felt. But the precise week of each pregnancy loss, each doctor and each treatment would occupy the gold-leaf pages. Some empty lines would be filled in, in the not too distant future with the last and most crucial treatment that was yet to come. From time to time, I take out the diary to remember the tears that were shed in that Hallmark store. Amid the baubles and balloons, the shelves of colorful cards announcing every sort of happy occasion, I was occasionless. I wept and felt my precious lost souls wept with me. I stared in disbelief at the dates and the memories they evoked. I felt weighted down as I held the small maroon diary in my hand. The year 1986 was embossed in gold numbers on the front cover of the book. Could I have imagined what occasion would yet occur during that year?

A well-meaning friend had clipped an article from the local newspaper detailing an experimental treatment for multiple miscarriages. The treatment was initiated in the UK and was now being offered by a pioneering doctor in Israel. This was actually a rather frequent occurrence; concerned friends would drop by to relay information about some new and innovative medical technology they had learned of from the media. Of course, I very much appreciated their support, but as time passed and no experts had the answers I sought, and all the latest treatments had apparently failed, these suggestions only served as a constant reminder of my childlessness. I truly felt loved by all those who called and cared enough to keep me in their thoughts and prayers. No doubt, it was my pain and my insecurity about the future that made each suggestion so difficult. I was tired of being disappointed, sick of hanging my hope of becoming a mother on some new innovative medical treatment. Looking back, I think I was also tired of disappointing everyone around me. This particular newspaper article was especially ill timed; it arrived as the hemorrhaging of my sixth consecutive miscarriage worsened. As I lay on my bed, the only thing I could be sure of was that I did not want to look at, much less consider, any new "treatments." I certainly could not face another doctor. Each new doctor would need my medical history, and with each retelling, I found myself reliving. Six miscarriages, six different doctors, six different hospitals. Could I tell this sorrowful tale one more time? I crumpled the article and placed it in the wastepaper basket next to my bed amongst all of the tear-filled tissues. The cramping continued and I knew with certainty that I could not and would not ever have the energy to face another treatment protocol. In fact, the only thing I wanted was to survive this most recent hardship and sit very still, by myself, for a long, long time.

As the bleeding intensified, I could fool myself no longer. I needed a doctor. I turned to the wastepaper basket. The discarded ball of newspaper stared up at me. I felt it was actually challenging me— daring me to try once again. Suddenly, that rejected article became the focus of my anger, frustration and all my hope. My decision to take an experimental treatment was not an easy one. I was concerned with the unclear repercussions, but the confidence and sincere concern of my doctor helped me move forward. Treatments in general are not just the filling of prescriptions, scheduling doctors' appointments and undergoing procedures. The word treatment equals the word hope. It was therefore, very difficult for me to see any treatment as routine.

Infertility and pregnancy loss presented me with challenges and choices that were often painful and difficult to make. My personal suffering had been well hidden behind the guise of a "normal life." As a result, the life crisis that evolved with my pregnancy losses was often misunderstood.

Pregnancy loss creates isolation, an overwhelming feeling of sadness. I felt vulnerable and out of control. These are intense and powerful emotions that need to be recognized, identified, and dealt with. My own personal experience was that my spirit could be crushed or elated by the result of a blood test, because its results meant the difference between life and death in pregnancy, or between a healthy organ and a diseased one. Each doctor's visit became a focal point; a touchstone, a painful reality check as to how realistic it was to believe that motherhood was still within my grasp. Now nearly 20 years later from the birth of the first of my three children, writing this chapter still evokes such powerful emotions that it is as if it is in "real time." Tears flow freely. Painful, memories are now intertwined with joy that soars and knows no bounds. The years of infertility and multiple pregnancy loss will always be an integral part of my most essential self. That self came to motherhood with profound blessings from G-d and the pioneering and brave efforts of dedicated doctors and hospital staff, all to whom, I am forever grateful.

Epilogue

Howard J. A. Carp

In recurrent pregnancy loss (RPL), there are many questions unanswered. The physician and patient are often bewildered in the face of changing and conflicting information, as demonstrated by the various debates in this book. As Chapter 40 shows, there is not even agreement as to who should be investigated. The American Society of Reproductive Medicine[1] recommends investigation and treatment after two miscarriages, whereas the Royal College of Obstetricians and Gynaecologists[2] and the European Society of Human Reproduction and Embryology[3] recommend a minimum of three miscarriages.

Basically, there are two approaches. The first attempts to reach a more accurate diagnosis by separating maternal from embryonic causes, as shown in Chapter 41 (tailor made). The second approach is to take RPL as one homogeneous condition, examine treatment in a large cohort of patients, and rely on randomization to overcome the different causes of RPL. The second approach (evidence based) is often used to determine the value of treatment. For example, Laskin et al.[4] in an often quoted trial to show that steroids are ineffective included patients with two losses between 5 and 31 weeks. Ober et al.[5] in a paper often quoted to show that that paternal leucocyte immunization is ineffective included patients with nonconsecutive losses up to 29 weeks and may have rendered the immunizations ineffective by refrigeration.[6] The tailor made approach looks for subgroup analyses within the larger group of the meta-analysis, and uses further diagnostic tests to determine the right drug for the right person at the right time. An example is immunoglobulin therapy. If all patients are considered together, there is no effect.[7] However, if patients are selected according to time of administration (prior to pregnancy), there is a statistically significant benefit.[8] The next step would be a specific diagnostic test to determine which patient would respond to immunoglobulin and which would not. However, further specific diagnostic tests are not always available. In the light of current knowledge, if the tailor made approach is followed, patients losing aneuploid embryos should have preimplantation genetic screening (PGS), and those losing euploid embryos should have treatment shown to be effective in trials in which fetal aneuploidy has been excluded. To date, there are no such trials, either in PGS or treatment of maternal causes of RPL.

Hence, there are differences in treatment approach. One approach is that no treatment is to be prescribed until shown to be effective in high quality trials. It has even been claimed that it is the duty of the physician to protect patients from "unproven" treatment. However, the patient does not consult the physician for protection, but for help in order to deliver a child. In this age of patient autonomy, patients can demand cesarean section with no medical justification. Cosmetic surgery is provided with no medical indication. These operations have numerous side effects. Does the patient with RPL not have the same right to demand treatment, which many believe to be effective? Chapter 44 shows in a most eloquent manner the suffering that a patient goes through after six miscarriages. As Mindy Gross writes, she was treated by experimental treatment outside of any protocol. She now has three adult children. Should she have remained childless until we, the treating physicians, have proven to our satisfaction that treatment works? In the older patient, there may not be time to await the results of trials.

The patients demand for treatment has led to an anomalous situation. As paternal leucocyte immunization is not available in the U.S. due to the FDA not allowing treatment until efficacy is shown in a trial in the U.S., patients travel to Mexico to be immunized. The "pros and cons" of paternal leucocyte therapy are debated in this book, and efficacy has been shown in meta-analyses.

In many types of treatment, no evidence-based trials are possible. It is unlikely that a trial will ever be performed on surrogacy, as there will always be few patients requiring this form of treatment. Does that mean that surrogacy should not be allowed, or should patients be forced to travel, or act in clandestine ways?

The answers to these questions are difficult and not unique to RPL. Who has the last word on treatment, the physician or the patient?

REFERENCES

1. Practice Committee of the American Society for Reproductive Medicine. Evaluation and treatment of recurrent pregnancy loss: A committee opinion. *Fertil Steril* 2012;98:1103–11.
2. Royal College of Obstetricians and Gynaecologists. *The Investigation and Treatment of Recurrent Miscarriage. Guideline No 17*. London: RCOG Press; 2011.
3. Jauniaux E, Farquharson RG, Christiansen OB et al. Evidence-based guidelines for the investigation and medical treatment of recurrent miscarriage. *Hum Reprod* 2006;21:2216–22.
4. Laskin CA, Bombardier C, Hannah ME et al. Prednisone and aspirin in women with autoantibodies and unexplained recurrent fetal loss. *N Engl J Med* 1997;337:148–53.
5. Ober C, Karrison T, Odem RR et al. Mononuclear-cell immunisation in prevention of recurrent miscarriages: A randomised trial. *Lancet* 1999;354:365–9.
6. Clark DA, Banwatt D. Altered expression of cell surface CD200 tolerance-signaling molecule on human PBL stored at 4°C or 37°C correlates with reduced or increased efficacy in controlled trials of treatment of recurrent miscarriages. *Am J Reprod Immunol* 2006;55:392–3.
7. Porter TF, LaCoursiere Y, Scott JR. Immunotherapy for recurrent miscarriage. *Cochrane Database Syst Rev* 2006;CD000112.
8. Hutton B, Sharma R, Fergusson D et al. Use of intravenous immunoglobulin for treatment of recurrent miscarriage: A systematic review. *BJOG* 2007;114:134–42.

Index

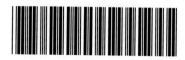

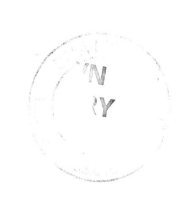